T0200523

INFECTIONS
in Cancer Patients

BASIC AND CLINICAL ONCOLOGY

Editor

Bruce D. Cheson, M.D.

National Cancer Institute
National Institutes of Health
Bethesda, Maryland

1. Chronic Lymphocytic Leukemia: Scientific Advances and Clinical Developments, *edited by Bruce D. Cheson*
2. Therapeutic Applications of Interleukin-2, *edited by Michael B. Atkins and James W. Mier*
3. Cancer of the Prostate, *edited by Sakti Das and E. David Crawford*
4. Retinoids in Oncology, *edited by Waun Ki Hong and Reuben Lotan*
5. Filgrastim (r-metHuG-CSF) in Clinical Practice, *edited by George Morstyn and T. Michael Dexter*
6. Cancer Prevention and Control, *edited by Peter Greenwald, Barnett S. Kramer, and Douglas L. Weed*
7. Handbook of Supportive Care in Cancer, *edited by Jean Klastersky, Stephen C. Schimpff, and Hans-Jörg Senn*
8. Paclitaxel in Cancer Treatment, *edited by William P. McGuire and Eric K. Rowinsky*
9. Principles of Antineoplastic Drug Development and Pharmacology, *edited by Richard L. Schilsky, Gérard A. Milano, and Mark J. Ratain*
10. Gene Therapy in Cancer, *edited by Malcolm K. Brenner and Robert C. Moen*
11. Expert Consultations in Gynecological Cancers, *edited by Maurie Markman and Jerome L. Belinson*
12. Nucleoside Analogs in Cancer Therapy, *edited by Bruce D. Cheson, Michael J. Keating, and William Plunkett*
13. Drug Resistance in Oncology, *edited by Samuel D. Bernal*
14. Medical Management of Hematological Malignant Diseases, *edited by Emil J Freireich and Hagop M. Kantarjian*
15. Monoclonal Antibody-Based Therapy of Cancer, *edited by Michael L. Grossbard*
16. Medical Management of Chronic Myelogenous Leukemia, *edited by Moshe Talpaz and Hagop M. Kantarjian*
17. Expert Consultations in Breast Cancer: Critical Pathways and Clinical Decision Making, *edited by William N. Hait, David A. August, and Bruce G. Haffty*
18. Cancer Screening: Theory and Practice, *edited by Barnett S. Kramer, John K. Gohagan, and Philip C. Prorok*

19. Supportive Care in Cancer: A Handbook for Oncologists: Second Edition, Revised and Expanded, *edited by Jean Klastersky, Stephen C. Schimpff, and Hans-Jörg Senn*

20. Integrated Cancer Management: Surgery, Medical Oncology, and Radiation Oncology, *edited by Michael H. Torosian*

21. AIDS-Related Cancers and Their Treatment, *edited by Ellen G. Feigal, Alexandra M. Levine, and Robert J. Biggar*

22. Allogeneic Immunotherapy for Malignant Diseases, *edited by John Barrett and Yin-Zheng Jiang*

23. Cancer in the Elderly, *edited by Carrie P. Hunter, Karen A. Johnson, and Hyman B. Muss*

24. Tumor Angiogenesis and Microcirculation, *edited by Emile E. Voest and Patricia A. D'Amore*

25. Controversies in Lung Cancer: A Multidisciplinary Approach, *edited by Benjamin Movsas, Corey J. Langer, and Melvyn Goldberg*

26. Chronic Lymphoid Leukemias: Second Edition, Revised and Expanded, *edited by Bruce D. Cheson*

27. The Myelodysplastic Syndromes: Pathobiology and Clinical Management, *edited by John M. Bennett*

28. Chemotherapy for Gynecological Neoplasms, *edited by Roberto Angioli, Pierluigi Benedetti Panici, John J. Kavanagh, Sergio Pecorelli, Manuel Penalver*

29. Infections in Cancer Patients, *edited by John N. Greene*

ADDITIONAL VOLUMES IN PREPARATION

19. Supportive Care in Cancer: A Handbook for Oncologists: Second Edition, Revised and Expanded, *edited by Jean Klastersky, Stephen C. Schimpff, and Hans-Jörg Senn*

20. Integrated Cancer Management: Surgery, Medical Oncology, and Radiation Oncology, *edited by Michael H. Torosian*

21. AIDS-Related Cancers and Their Treatment, *edited by Ellen G. Feigal, Alexandra M. Levine, and Robert J. Biggar*

22. Allogeneic Immunotherapy for Malignant Diseases, *edited by John Barrett and Yin-Zheng Jiang*

23. Cancer in the Elderly, *edited by Carrie P. Hunter, Karen A. Johnson, and Hyman B. Muss*

24. Tumor Angiogenesis and Microcirculation, *edited by Emile E. Voest and Patricia A. D'Amore*

25. Controversies in Lung Cancer: A Multidisciplinary Approach, *edited by Benjamin Movsas, Corey J. Langer, and Melvyn Goldberg*

26. Chronic Lymphoid Leukemias: Second Edition, Revised and Expanded, *edited by Bruce D. Cheson*

27. The Myelodysplastic Syndromes: Pathobiology and Clinical Management, *edited by John M. Bennett*

28. Chemotherapy for Gynecological Neoplasms, *edited by Roberto Angioli, Pierluigi Benedetti Panici, John J. Kavanagh, Sergio Pecorelli, Manuel Penalver*

29. Infections in Cancer Patients, *edited by John N. Greene*

ADDITIONAL VOLUMES IN PREPARATION

INFECTIONS
in Cancer Patients

edited by
John N. Greene
*University of South Florida College of Medicine
and Moffitt Cancer Center and Research Institute
Tampa, Florida, U.S.A.*

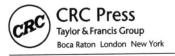

CRC Press
Taylor & Francis Group
Boca Raton London New York

CRC Press is an imprint of the
Taylor & Francis Group, an **informa** business

CRC Press
Taylor & Francis Group
6000 Broken Sound Parkway NW, Suite 300
Boca Raton, FL 33487-2742

First issued in paperback 2019

© 2004 by Taylor & Francis Group, LLC
CRC Press is an imprint of Taylor & Francis Group, an Informa business

No claim to original U.S. Government works

ISBN-13: 978-0-8247-5437-2 (hbk)
ISBN-13: 978-0-367-39429-5 (pbk)

This book contains information obtained from authentic and highly regarded sources. Reasonable efforts have been made to publish reliable data and information, but the author and publisher cannot assume responsibility for the validity of all materials or the consequences of their use. The authors and publishers have attempted to trace the copyright holders of all material reproduced in this publication and apologize to copyright holders if permission to publish in this form has not been obtained. If any copyright material has not been acknowledged please write and let us know so we may rectify in any future reprint.

Except as permitted under U.S. Copyright Law, no part of this book may be reprinted, reproduced, transmitted, or utilized in any form by any electronic, mechanical, or other means, now known or hereafter invented, including photocopying, microfilming, and recording, or in any information storage or retrieval system, without written permission from the publishers.

For permission to photocopy or use material electronically from this work, please access www. copyright.com (http://www.copyright.com/) or contact the Copyright Clearance Center, Inc. (CCC), 222 Rosewood Drive, Danvers, MA 01923, 978-750-8400. CCC is a not-for-profit organization that provides licenses and registration for a variety of users. For organizations that have been granted a photocopy license by the CCC, a separate system of payment has been arranged.

Trademark Notice: Product or corporate names may be trademarks or registered trademarks, and are used only for identification and explanation without intent to infringe.

Library of Congress Cataloging-in-Publication Data
A catalog record for this book is available from the Library of Congress.

Visit the Taylor & Francis Web site at
http://www.taylorandfrancis.com

and the CRC Press Web site at
http://www.crcpress.com

Preface

The field of infectious diseases in the cancer patient has undergone great metamorphosis and growth over the last decade. We have attempted to take an easy-to-read, well-organized approach to managing infections in oncological patients. With an emphasis on the underlying malignancy as the central theme, infections unique to that cancer and its therapy can be readily accessed and understood. Previous texts that emphasize organisms as the major theme are frequently hard to follow and less useful for management of the individual patient. By describing the major immune defects inherent to each malignancy and their therapy we allow for more accurate and timely diagnosis of the unique pathogens acquired. In addition, the malignancy and its therapy over time may alter the immune system and lead to anatomical changes that predispose to a changing spectrum of pathogens. For example, progressive growth of lung cancer can obstruct a major bronchus and result in postobstructive pneumonia, whereas radiation therapy to the lung may impair alveolar macrophage function and create lung paremchymal changes to form a cavity, both of which favor invasive aspergillus infection.

As patients are being treated with more aggressive chemotherapeutic regimens, profound immunosuppression for longer periods of time is occurring. This period of immunodeficiency is an open invitation to the invasion of a multitude of intrinsic and extrinsically acquired organisms. By understanding the period of vulnerability of the host throughout the periods of active malignancy growth, neutropenia, and cell-mediated immunodeficienies, the clinician can choose the appropriate antimicrobial agents to prevent or treat the most dangerous and most common infections.

Using a number of relevant and recent publications, the most important infections associated with each malignancy are presented. In addition, the susceptibility to different infections over the course of a chronic progressive malignancy is presented. For example, patients with newly diagnosed multiple myeloma are susceptible to pneumococcal infections of the respiratory tract. However, as the disease progresses and chemotherapy is used to control it, *Pseudomonas aeruginosa* infection of the respiratory tract becomes more prominent.

Neutropenia, the most common byproduct of cancer therapy can be broken down into periods of time when predominant pathogens change. Likewise, antimicrobial therapy must be altered to reflect this transition. For instance, gram-negative and gram-positive bacterial infections dominate the first week of neutropenia. During the second week, *candida sp* infections become important, followed by *aspergillus* infections into the third week. Therefore, changes in treatment are frequently necessary as neutropenia progresses.

In summary, the cancer patient's risk of infection can be tracked from diagnosis to cure or cancer-related death. By understanding the underlying immune status of each patient during cancer therapy, the best choices for infection management can be made. Using pictures to illustrate infectious disease presentations and easy-to-follow tables of pertinent groups of diseases, the clinician interested in cancer-related infections has a useful resource for patient evaluations and staff education.

We dedicate this book to all the patients who have valiantly battled cancer, endured the toxicity of its treatment, and overcome the ensuing microbial invasion during their most vulnerable moment.

John N. Greene

Contents

Preface   *iii*

Contributors   *ix*

Chapters

I. Introduction

1. Mechanisms of Host Defense   1
Dimitrios P. Agaliotis

2. Composition of the Normal Microbial Flora   15
John N. Greene

II. Infectious Complications of Hematologic Lymphoreticular Malignancies

3. Acute Lymphoblastic Leukemia   23
Jennifer Johnson and John Greene

4. Infection in Patients with Acute Myelogenous Leukemia   47
Indra Dé and Kenneth V.I. Rolston

5. Hairy Cell Leukemia   65
Nikolaos Almyroudis

6. Infections in Patients with Chronic Lymphocytic
   Leukemia   73
   Ana Maria Chiappori

7. Infections Associated with Chronic Myelogenous
   Leukemia   87
   James Riddell IV and Carol A. Kauffman

8. Infections in Patients with Myelodysplastic Syndromes   99
   Nadeem R. Khan

9. Infectious Complication in Multiple Myeloma   103
   Todd Groom and Joseph C. Chan

10. Non-Hodgkin's Lymphoma   127
    Teresa Field

11. Infections Unique to Hodgkin's Disease   145
    Karla Richards and John N. Greene

12. Infectious Complications in Stem Cell Transplant
    Recipients   151
    John N. Greene

III. **Infectious Complications of Solid Tumor Malignancies**

13. Infections in Patients with Brain Tumors   163
    Christoph Michael Stoll and Albert L. Vincent

14. Infections in Patients with Head and Neck Cancer   177
    Charurut Somboonwit and John N. Greene

15. Infections in Patients with Lung Cancer   187
    *Charurut Somboonwit, Charles Craig, and
    John N. Greene*

16. Infections Complicating Breast Cancer and Its
    Treatment   199
    Julia E. Richards and Larry M. Baddour

17. Infectious Complications of Gastrointestinal Cancer   219
    Albert L. Vincent and John N. Greene

18. Infections in Patients with Cancer of the Liver
    and Biliary Tract   227
    Carlos A. Castillo Albán and John N. Greene

Contents

19. Infections in Patients with Neuroendocrine Tumors   235
    John N. Greene

20. Infections in Patients with Bladder and Kidney Tumors   239
    Kadry R. Allaboun

21. Infections in Patients with Gynecological Malignancies   251
    Masoumeh Ghayouri, Cuc Mai, and Albert L. Vincent

22. Infections Related to the Management and Treatment
    of Sarcomas   263
    Wendy W. Carter and Douglas Letson

23. Infections Associated with Cutaneous Malignancy   271
    John S. Czachor

IV. **System Specific Infections in Cancer Patients**

24. Central Nervous System Infections in Cancer Patients   283
    Daniel Ginn and John N. Greene

25. Pulmonary Infections in Cancer Patients   289
    Charurut Somboonwit and John N. Greene

26. Cardiovascular Infections in Cancer Patients   307
    Bernhard Unsöld and John N. Greene

27. Gastrointestinal Infections in Cancer Patients   313
    Todd S. Wills

28. Genitourinary Infections in Cancer Patients   331
    Michael J. Tan and John N. Greene

29. Bone, Joint, and Soft Tissue Infections in Cancer
    Patients   337
    Lucinda M. Elko

30. Dermatological Infections in Cancer Patients   345
    Mary Evers and John N. Greene

V. **Infectious Complications of Cancer Treatment**

31. Infections Associated with Radiation Therapy   367
    Brent W. Laartz and John N. Greene

32. Complications of Surgery in Cancer Patients   373
    John N. Greene and Nick Nicoonahad

33. Catheter-Related Infections   379
     Ioannis Chatzinikolaou and Issam I. Raad

VI. **Unique Infections in Cancer Patients**

34. Fungal Infections in Cancer Patients   419
     Magnus Gottfredsson and John R. Perfect

35. Parasitic Diseases as Complications of Cancer   451
     Albert L. Vincent

36. HIV-Related Malignancies   471
     Kadry Allaboun and John N. Greene

IX. **Prevention of Infections in Cancer Patients**

37. Prevention of Infection in Cancer Patients   477
     Patrick Roth

38. Immunization Against Infectious Diseases in Cancer
     Patients   497
     Rama Ganguly and John N. Greene

39. Role of the Microbiology Laboratory   509
     Loveleen Kang and Ramon L. Sandin

     Index   *523*

Contributors

Dimitrios P. Agaliotis   Florida Hospital Cancer Institute, Orlando, Florida, U.S.A.

Carlos A. Castillo Albán   Universidad San Francisco de Quito, Quito, Ecuador

Kadry Allaboun   University of South Florida College of Medicine, Tampa, Florida, U.S.A.

Kadry R. Allaboun   Bradenton, Florida, U.S.A.

Nikolaos Almyroudis   Memorial Sloan Kettering Cancer Center, New York, New York, U.S.A.

Larry M. Baddour   Mayo Clinic, College of Medicine, Rochester, Minnesota, U.S.A.

Wendy W. Carter   Moffitt Cancer Center and Research Institute Tampa, Florida, U.S.A.

Joseph C. Chan   University of Miami School of Medicine, Miami, Florida, U.S.A.

Ioannis Chatzinikolaou   The University of Texas M. D. Anderson Cancer Center, Houston, Texas, U.S.A.

Ana Maria Chiappori   Cayatano Heredia University, Lima, Peru

Charles Craig   St. Joseph Mercy Health System, Ann Arbor, Michigan, U.S.A.

John S. Czachor   Wright State University School of Medicine and Miami Valley Hospital, Dayton, Ohio, U.S.A.

Indra Dé   The University of Texas M. D. Anderson Cancer Center, Houston, Texas, U.S.A.

Lucinda M. Elko   University of South Florida School of Medicine, Tampa, Florida, U.S.A.

Mary Evers   UHHS-Richmond Heights Hospital, Cleveland, Ohio, U.S.A.

Teresa Field   University of South Florida School of Medicine, Tampa, Florida, U.S.A.

Rama Ganguly   University of South Florida College of Medicine, Tampa, Florida, U.S.A.

Masoumeh Ghayouri   James A. Haley Veterans Hospital, Tampa, Florida, U.S.A.

Daniel Ginn   University of South Florida School of Medicine and Moffitt Cancer Center and Research Institute, Tampa, Florida, U.S.A.

John N. Greene   University of South Florida School of Medicine and Moffitt Cancer Center and Research Institute, Tampa, Florida, U.S.A.

Magnus Gottfredsson   Landspitali University Hospital, Reykjavik, Iceland

Todd Groom   University of Miami School of Medicine, Miami, Florida, U.S.A.

Daniel Ginn   University of South Florida School of Medicine and Moffitt Cancer Center and Research Institute, Tampa, Florida, U.S.A.

Jennifer Johnson   University of South Florida School of Medicine and Moffitt Cancer Center and Research Institute, Tampa, Florida, U.S.A.

Loveleen Kang   University of South Florida College of Medicine and Moffitt Cancer Center and Research Institute, Tampa, Florida, U.S.A.

Carol A. Kauffman   Veterans Affairs Ann Arbor Healthcare System, University of Michigan Medical School, Ann Arbor, Michigan, U.S.A.

Nadeem R. Khan   Infectious Diseases Private Practice, Tampa, Florida, U.S.A.

Douglas Letson   Moffitt Cancer Center and Research Institute, Tampa, Florida, U.S.A.

Cuc Mai   James A. Haley Veterans Hospital, Tampa, Florida, U.S.A.

Brent W. Laartz   University of South Florida School of Medicine and Moffitt Cancer Center and Research Institute, Tampa, Florida, U.S.A.

Nick Nicoonahad Shriner's Hospital, Tampa, Florida, U.S.A.

John R. Perfect Duke University Medical Center, Durham, North Carolina, U.S.A.

Issam I. Raad The University of Texas M. D. Anderson Cancer Center, Houston, Texas, U.S.A.

Julia E. Richards University of Tennessee Medical Center, Knoxville, Tennessee, U.S.A.

Karla Richards University of South Florida School of Medicine and Moffitt Cancer Center and Research Institute, Tampa, Florida, U.S.A.

James Riddell IV Veterans Affairs Ann Arbor Healthcare System, University of Michigan Medical School, Ann Arbor, Michigan, U.S.A.

Kenneth V. I. Rolston The University of Texas M. D. Anderson Cancer Center, Houston, Texas, U.S.A.

Patrick Roth Freiburg University, Freiburg, Germany

Ramon L. Sandin University of South Florida College of Medicine and Moffitt Cancer Center and Research Institute, Tampa, Florida, U.S.A.

Christoph Michael Stoll Städtisches Klinikum, Karlsruhe, Germany

Charurut Somboonwit University of South Florida School of Medicine and Moffitt Cancer Center and Research Institute, Tampa, Florida, U.S.A.

Michael J. Tan University of South Florida School of Medicine, Tampa, Florida, U.S.A.

Bernhard Unsöld Albert-Ludwigs University of Freiburg, Freiburg, Germany

Albert L. Vincent University of South Florida School of Medicine and Moffitt Cancer Center and Research Institute, Tampa, Florida, U.S.A.

Todd S. Wills University of South Florida School of Medicine, Tampa, Florida, U.S.A.

1

Mechanisms of Host Defense

Dimitrios P. Agaliotis
Florida Hospital Cancer Institute
Orlando, Florida, U.S.A.

INTRODUCTION

Evolution has resulted in the creation of a formidable panoply of host-nonspecific resistance to harmful foreign pathogens that can be the causes of infection and death. Multiple factors contribute to this resistance, and taken as a whole they seem to be the most powerful tools for the avoidance of invasion and systemic disease. Compared to the more complicated humoral and cellular immune system, the initial response of nonspecific defense mechanisms seems rather simple. However, considered as a whole, they are the strongest and most effective first-line defenses against further invasion and destruction by foreign intruders. These nonspecific host resistance factors include the normal indigenous microflora, genetic factors, natural secreted antibodies, mainly IgG and secretory IgA, the integrity of the skin and mucous membranes, normal excretory functions of mucous and other body fluids, cilia, complement, and lysozyme [1]. If the initial barrier is overcome, then the foreign invader will activate second-line mechanisms of defense, which are of varying specificity. These mechanisms include phagocytosis, natural killer cell activity, antigen-specific and antigen-nonspecific immune responses, natural anticoagulant mechanisms, humoral factors, nutrition, iron metabolism changes, and finally massive activation of cellular and humoral factors facilitated by acute-phase reactants, cytokines, and chemokines. First-line defense mechanisms serve also as temporizing factors prior to activation and preparation of a more specific and effective immune response against the foreign invader.

LOCAL OR MECHANICAL

Skin

Considering the risk factors for the development of infections in the immunocompromised host, such as the cancer patient, especially during treatment, the skin barrier integrity represents a major contributor of host defense [2]. When intact, this mechanical barrier is one of the first lines of defense against the invasion of microorganisms. Very few microorganisms have the ability to penetrate the skin on their own; they require other means to overcome this barrier. In the case of a cancer patient, these means may include an intravenous catheter, a surgical incision, a disruption of the skin by trauma, or also for the general population an arthropod vector sting. The skin has unfriendly conditions for pathogens, such as dryness and desiccating properties and mild acidic pH of 5 to 6. The normal skin flora also antagonize the proliferation of other pathogenic bacteria. The action of indigenous flora on skin secretions such as sebum creates a hostile acidic environment for bacteria. From a mechanical point of view, normal exfoliation of skin scales promotes the simultaneous shedding of microorganisms. Skin inflammation is associated with augmentation of water permeability and easier colonization by microorganisms. The number of skin-penetrating indwelling arterial and venous catheters has been described as a factor facilitating pathogen invasion in the immunocompromised host [2]. Hemorrhagic diathesis with resulting hematomas in association with mechanical skin disruption such as that due to needle sticks is also a factor that promotes increased skin permeability and pathogen invasion [2]. Thorough evaluation and careful examination of the skin is a very important part of the care of the cancer patient. Skin integrity disruption by rashes, petechiae, ecchymosis, hematomas, ecthyma, or catheter insertion sites can result in local and systemic infection. This clinical information is important in decision making regarding the choice of antibiotics, dosages, or the need to change treatment [3]. The importance of skin barrier integrity protection is well known to those caring for cancer patients with infections. On the other hand, the skin can also be a temporary carrier for pathogens. Currently, the mainstay in the prevention of patient cross contamination is thorough hand washing after examining patients and in between procedures [4]. Graft-versus-host disease (GVHD) in the allogeneic bone marrow, stem cell, or cord blood transplantation along with its immunocompromising effects changes the skin structure dramatically and may contribute to an increase risk of infection.

Varicella zoster virus infection develops in up to 50% of recipients of allogeneic or autologous hematopoietic stem cell transplantation (HSCT). Patients with GVHD are more susceptible to this infection primarily occurring more than five months after transplantation. The resultant skin injury may lead to bacterial or rarely fungal superinfection with or without dissemination. This further delineates the importance of skin integrity and health. Prophylactic use of intravenous *Varicella zoster* immunoglobulin within 48 to 96 hours of contact with a person with either chickenpox or shingles may protect from clinical development of this infection [5].

Mucous Membranes

A large number and a broad variety of microorganisms colonize the normal mucous membranes because of its innate moisture. On the other hand, normally sterile body fluids such as the cerebrospinal fluid have intense antimicrobial capabilities. Other body secretions such as tears, cervical mucous, and prostatic fluid are rather toxic to certain species of pathogens. Substances are found in these secretions that are effective against gram-positive bacteria and include lysozyme and *N*-acetyl muramyl-L-alanineamidase. Small cationic antimicrobial peptides or defensins also belong to the armamentarium of inhibitory agents in some body secretions [1]. The presence of IgG and more frequently secretory IgA on mucous membranes agglutinate the microorganisms or inhibit the attachment of microorganisms to host cell receptors. Secretory IgA is more resistant to proteolysis and is also known to bind intracellular pathogens.

Iron is a very important trace element in microorganism metabolism. Secretions that potentially come in contact with microorganisms have increased concentrations of ironbinding proteins that deprive pathogens of that important nutrient.

The intensity of chemotherapy regimens, especially in stem cell transplantation conditioning regimens, results in gastrointestinal injury and disruption of mucosal membrane integrity. This promotes invasion by colonizing microorganisms and translocation into the bloodstream [5]. Selection of resistant pathogens secondary to broad-spectrum antibiotic use and the immunocompromised state secondary to uncontrolled malignancy, chemotherapy, immune therapy, or graft-versus-host disease make the host vulnerable to bacterial and fungal invaders that cause significant morbidity and mortality.

In the hematologic transplantation setting, it is now common practice to keep not only the oral mucosa but most mucosal surfaces clean, free of trauma, and if possible with decreased numbers of colonizing pathogens. This is accomplished with rinses, frequent inspection, gentle cleaning, evaluation, and local treatment as needed for the oral mucosa, the vulvar, and perianal/perineum, and scrotal areas.

Severe stomatitis with oral mucositis may result from the reactivation of *Herpes simplex* virus (HSV), *candidiasis*, local anaerobic bacteria, or chemotherapy itself. Reactivation of oral herpes virus infection occurs in 70–80% of seropositive individuals following HSCT. Extension into the esophagus with the associated mucositis may result in increased risk for bacterial superinfection and bacteremia. Antiviral prophylaxis not only prevents reactivation but may also reduce herpes drug resistance [5]. This further demonstrates the importance of maintaining mucous membrane integrity for the prevention of infection.

Candida infections are common in neutropenic cancer patients, and they involve the mucosal surfaces of the oral cavity, causing thrush, of the esophagus (esophagitis), of the vagina, causing vaginitis, or the skin of the inguinal areas, causing intertrigo inguinalis. Invasion may result in bloodstream seeding and fungemia. The portal of entry is occasionally the interrupted mucosal lining of the gastrointestinal tract. *Candida* spp. proliferate on the mucosal surfaces as a result of the suppression of bacterial flora by the use of broad-spectrum antibiotics [5]. Candida infections will be discussed in more detail in another chapter.

The introduction of new chemotherapeutic agents such as the Taxanes in combination with other agents such as vinorelbine has resulted in new complications of mixed ischemic and infectious etiology in the gastrointestinal tract. In one study, 14 patients with metastatic breast cancer were treated with vinorelbine, docetaxel, and granlocyte-colony-stimulating factor in a phase I study. Three patients developed colitis/typhlitis symptoms, and two of them died, one from necrotic bowel and the other from neutropenic fever and colitis. In this study it is emphasized that damage of the GI mucosa in association with neutropenia may result in severe and occasionally lethal infectious complications [6]. Neutropenic enterocolitis (typhlitis) is a necrotizing colitis affecting the cecum. It is associated with granulocytopenia and fever. The disease seems to be more prevalent in children and is deemed to be responsible for 50% of surgical abdomens in children with leukemia. *Clostridia* species, *Enterobacteriaceae*, and *Pseudomonas* are the most common isolates [3]. A more detailed description of this entity is presented in another chapter. Perirectal cellulitis or abscess can readily occur in neutropenic patients who have hemorrhoids or rectal fissures. Prevention or treatment of typhlitis or perianal infections should include antibiotics with anaerobic and antipseudomonal activity.

Obstructed Sites (e.g., Prostatic Enlargement, Biliary Stones)

Urinary Tract

The most common pathophysiology of cystitis is via the ascending route. Host defenses against entry and proliferation of pathogens are the presence of normal perineal flora, the free flow of urine and adequate bladder emptying, and the intact mucosal epithelial lining, functional phagocytes, and eventually secretory IgG and IgA [7]. Urine is sterile in the healthy individual. Urine is toxic to certain bacteria owing to its pH, (possibly) urea, different solutes, or hypertonicity. A glycoprotein produced by the kidney serves as an anchor protein for many strains of bacteria that are attached to it and excreted along in the urine, so colonization is avoided. Lower urinary tract infections are avoided by urine flush four to eight times a day for bacteria that are not capable of attaching to the epithelial cells. There are exceptions to this rule, such as *Neisseria gonorrhoeae* and strains of *E. coli*. The anatomic structure of the urethra and mainly its length in the adult male of about 20 cm protects the male individual from bacterial contamination of the bladder. The introduction of bacteria into the male bladder through the urethra is possible by catheterization and instrumentation. The female urethra is only about 5 cm in the adult, and this cannot passively protect women from bladder infections, which are 14 times more common than in men. Prostatic enlargement due to benign hypertrophy or prostate cancer or other tumors originating within or outside the urinary tract obstructing urine flow constitute a barrier for complete emptying of this hollow organ, with stagnation and subsequent microorganism overgrowth. Paraneoplastic syndromes involving hypercalcemia or tumors or treatments of tumors that create a hyperuricemic state may be responsible for urinary stone formation and obstruction, with predisposition to urinary tract infections. Tumors involving the spinal cord or other conditions resulting in neurogenic bladder can also affect bladder emptying and urine stasis with infection. Urinary intestinal diversions also increase the bacterial urine load with a tendency to infection, especially when neutropenia coexists [7].

The mucinous urinary bladder layer is a formidable barrier against pathogen colonization of the bladder. Injury to the bladder mucosa by chemotherapy or instrumentation can predispose to infections. There is a strong correlation between rectal and periurethral isolates at the time of urinary catheterization and subsequent pathogen identification from an infected urinary tract following catheterization [9]. Dysuria or pyuria are not usually seen in neutropenic patients, and bacteremia may be the first finding in the neutropenic patient with urinary tract infection [7].

Urinary catheters occasionally need to be used in cancer patients undergoing HSCT as part of their conditioning regimen (i.e., when high-dose cyclophosphamide is given, hemorrhagic cystitis is avoided by continuous bladder irrigation). This type of instrumentation in males and females increases the risk of urinary tract infections (UTI). Urinary tract infections can result from cystoscopy when evaluating for bladder cancer. Asymptomatic candiduria is seen frequently in patients with urinary catheters. Although not usually requiring treatment, candiduria in patients with neutropenia should always be treated to avoid candidemia [8].

Vaginal secretions are usually under hormonal influence. Estrogens result in increased production of glycogen, which in turn is metabolized by acidogenic bacteria, especially lactobacilli, into lactic acid. The acidic environment of the vagina creates a hostile environment for other bacteria growth. Disturbed vaginal ecosystem by use of broad-spectrum antibiotics may result in increased pH and enteric pathogen overgrowth with resulting infection.

Biliary Tract

In the healthy individual, bile has antibacterial effects against certain pathogens. Obstruction of biliary flow may cause bacterial growth in the bile and subsequent ascending infection of the gall bladder or intrahepatic biliary system resulting in cholecystitis and/or cholangitis. It is important to detect cholelithiasis and or choledocholithiasis prior to instituting immunosuppressive therapy because of the high risk of cholangitis. Even without obstruction, protracted neutropenia may predispose to acalculus cholecystitis. As in the general population, cholecystitis or cholangitis may be a common cause of an acute abdomen in patients with neutropenia [7].

Foreign Devices (e.g., Endotracheal Tubes and Vascular Catheters)

Patients with cancer or following transplantation who require intensive care are at increased risk for serious infectious complications. Nosocomial pneumonia and ventilator-associated pneumonia are common in neutropenic patients in the intensive care unit (ICU). Pathogens causing nosocomial pneumonia following urgent endotracheal intubation seem to be identical to the isolates from the sputum at the time of intubation and at the time of diagnosis of pneumonia. It seems that emergency endotracheal intubation

contributes to the overall incidence of nosocomial pneumonia [10]. Previous antimicrobial therapy also has an impact on the type of pathogens isolated in patients with nosocomial pneumonia. *Pseudomonas aeruginosa* is more frequent in patients with previous antibiotic use, while the rate of ventilator-associated pneumonia caused by gram-positive cocci or *Hemophilus influenzae* is statistically lower [11].

Intubation and mechanical ventilation is well correlated with a poor prognosis in neutropenic ICU patients. This could be in part due to infections caused by the endotracheal tube and ventilator-associated nosocomial pneumonia. Many centers have tried to avoid endotracheal intubation in neutropenic cancer patients with acute respiratory failure by the use of noninvasive continuous positive airway pressure, with success in 25% of the cases [12].

The issue of the safety of tracheostomy in neutropenic patients has been studied. Stomal bleeding and infection, nosocomial pneumonias, and alveolar hemorrhage were reviewed. Neither stomal nor pulmonary infections attributable to the tracheostomy were noted. Although 73% of patients died in the ICU, there was no direct link between tracheostomy and death [13].

With regard to central venous catheters (CVC) and related temporary devices used to infuse cancer patients, the issue of infection has been studied and the literature seems to be at times contradictory. After the diagnosis of catheter-related infection is made, the most important question is if the catheter needs to be removed or not. Pathogen identification and host immune status are important in making this decision. Gram-negative bacteremia for example does not necessarily constitute a reason for catheter removal in a neutropenic patient. Catheter types, subcutaneous or nonsubcutaneous, have different risks of infections. The subcutaneous catheters are less prone to environmental or cutaneous contamination when not accessed and are less likely to be infected. Catheter location also plays a role in the risk of infection. Risk factors predisposing to CVC-related infection include prolonged catheterization, frequent manipulation of the catheter, improper aseptic insertion and maintenance techniques, prolonged high moisture in exit-site dressings, prolonged duration of needle left in subcutaneous ports, and multilumen CVCs. Impregnated and coated catheters have been used to prevent catheter-related infectious complications, but they are most effective in the short term after insertion.

In summary, CVCs are very important in the management of cancer patients for infusion of chemotherapeutic agents, blood products, antibiotics, and other medications and for nutritional support. Prevention and treatment of infections related to these catheters is extremely important; one must attempt to avoid removal, as these devices often are the lifeline for the critically ill cancer patient. Trained catheter care teams are critical in preventing CVC-related infections [14].

SYSTEMIC OR CELLULAR

Neutrophils

Polymorphonuclear leukocytes (PMNs) and mononuclear phagocytes as well as the complement system are important parts of the innate (natural) immune system of vertebrates. This mechanism encoded in germline genes enables the host to respond immediately to an invading agent regardless of previous exposure to that possible infectious challenge [15]. This early evolutionary part of the immune system has many similarities with immune systems in other organisms such as plants and insects. What makes vertebrates different from these multicellular organisms among others is the development of the acquired (adaptive) immunity. By this immunity, vertebrates can recognize and respond to a wide variety of "abnormal" antigens such as foreign infectious pathogens or cancer cells. The tools for this type of immunity are the B and T cells and antibodies. Time is of essence for the function of this adaptive immunity. Time is required for the processing of antigens and the production of specific antibodies. The innate natural immune system is much faster in response but has less specificity.

The pluripotent stem cell principally resides in the bone marrow. It carries on its surface the CD34 antigen and gives rise to all hematopoietic cell lines including neutrophil precursors. Two cellular functions of marrow cells that are inversely related are proliferation and differentiation. The more the cellular hematopoietic elements are differentiated, the less they proliferate, and vice versa. Neutrophils and their precursors obey the same rule. There is a proliferating pool and a maturing pool. The former mostly reside in the marrow and the latter in the peripheral blood, where they circulate or marginate and are mobilized. Granulocyte colony stimulating factor (G-CSF) not only stimulates proliferation and differentiation of the myeloid cells but also may enhance the functioning of neutrophils and prolong their survival. Proliferating precursor myeloid cells include the myeloblasts, promyelocytes, and myelocytes. The maturing pool consists of the metamyelocytes, myelocytes, bands, and neutrophils. Morphologically, the appearance of the characteristic primary and secondary neutrophil granules define the cell maturation. The mature functional neutrophil has surface Fc as well as complement receptors for phagocytosis, has oxygen-dependent antimicrobial activity, and demonstrates increased adhesiveness, cell motility, and chemotaxis [15].

Knowledge of neutrophil kinetics, along with changes in their functional status, is very important for the understanding of the natural immune deficiency in patients not only with cancer and hematologic malignancies but also with aplastic anemia or inherited neutropenic states. Daily production of mature PMNs in a healthy adult approximate 10^{11} cells. About 10 times that amount can be mobilized from the marrow reserves if need arises during infection or inflammation. Depletion of the above reserve may occur if there is a persistent stimulus, nutritional deficiency with deficient replacement of apoptotic cells, or alcohol intoxication. At times of need, the pool of stem cells will proliferate and differentiate when stimulated by colony stimulating growth factors (CSFs) produced by peripheral blood monocytes, stimulated lymphocytes, marrow stromal cells, and tissue macrophages. The neutrophils have an intravascular and extravascular half-life. The former is about 6–8 hours and the latter ranges from a few hours to several days. Five percent of the granulocytes (4×10^8 cells) are distributed in the circulating pool and the marginating pool. A kinetic balance exists between cell production, the marrow reserve, the circulating pool, and the marginating pool. Endotoxin or steroids acutely promote granulocyte release from the marrow reserve. Stress, epinephrine, ethanol, and hypoxia promote granulocytosis by demarginating the resting cells.

In most patients with cancer, immunodeficiency results from the reduction of the absolute number of available neutrophils called neutropenia. The number of circulating neutrophils correlates well with the total amount of neutrophils in their immune system. We define as normal a neutrophil count between 1,500 and 2,000 cells/mm^3. Probability of infection increases proportionately with the depth of neutropenia below 1,500 neutrophils/mm^3 and its duration. Over 80% of patients given intensive chemotherapy will develop fever (defined as $\geq 38.3°C$ at one recording or $38.0°C$ over at least one hour. Fever is documented as a result of infection in only 30% of patients, with bacteremia accounting for about half of the cases [2].

Drug therapy is frequently the reason for neutropenia. It occurs in a predictable fashion following chemotherapy or constitutes an idiosyncractic host reaction to a particular medication. Neutropenia can also develop from bone marrow failure, such as in aplastic anemia and myelodysplasia, or it can be hereditary, as in Kostmann's syndrome or cyclic neutropenia. Hypersplenism, which is associated with splenic sequestration of neutrophils and possibly immunologic destruction of these cells by antibodies, is another cause of neutropenia. Growth factors like G-CSF and GM-CSF have shortened the period of cytopenias after conventional doses of chemotherapy and in the more intensive bone marrow transplant setting. They are also used for the treatment of cytopenias of myelodysplasia and aplastic anemia with variable success. Major side effects include pain during the injection, occasional fevers, bone, muscle, or joint pains; they respond usually to acetaminophen, but the high costs of these agents limits their use in the impoverished patient [3]. Functional deficiency of neutrophils has been described in some myelodysplastic syndromes, so assessment of the neutrophil count alone in this patient population may not reflect their overall immune status when management of infectious complications is contemplated.

Granulocyte transfusions have been used in treatment of neutropenic febrile patients with life-threatening bacterial or fungal infections. Neutropenic patients with a documented bacterial infection who received daily granulocytic transfusions for the duration of their infection survived longer than nontransfused controls [16,17]. Complications of granulocyte transfusions include infection with cytomegalovirus, allosensitization to human leukocyte antigens, the cost of the procedure, and the increased incidence of pulmonary toxicity when transfusions are given along with amphotericin B infusions [18,19].

Humoral Immunity

The immune system has enabled us to survive by distinguishing between nonself and self and neutralizing or clearing harmful nonself elements from the host. Extracellular pathogens are attacked primarily by humoral immune responses. Humoral immunity constitutes part of the acquired or adaptive immunity characterizing only the vertebrates. Antibodies are produced by B lymphocytes, which are complex glycoproteins that exibit high specificity and bind to the biological molecules they are formed against. These molecules can be proteins or simple peptides, polysaccharides, or glycolipids, as are most bacterial toxins. Soluble antibodies are instrumental in the combat against extracellular pathogens with their exclusive antigen recognition and activation of the innate (general or nonspecific) host defense mechanisms, to which phagocytes and the complement system belong. Through somatic shuffling and rearrangements of gene components, millions of different gene combinations are efficiently created by each host to produce antibodies that can equally recognize millions of different antigens. Somatic mutation of genes coding for antibodies further expand antigen recognition and memory. A cell of the B-type lineage expresses only one antibody specificity. This results in the remarkable function of the immune system to regulate the responses against each antigen by promoting or restricting the proliferation and activation of cells reacting with the specific antigen. In immunization as an example, a select portion of lymphocytes persists as a pool of antigen-specific memory cells, which produce relatively quickly a more intense and longer immune response after a new challenge of the host with the same antigen [20].

Cell-Mediated Immunity

Foreign cellular elements, including host cells containing intracellular pathogens such as viruses, are recognized as "abnormal" and harmful and are eliminated primarily by the acquired (adaptive) immunity, which constitutes the cell-mediated immune system. Cellular immunity depends heavily on the TCR (T-cell receptor) for the specific recognition of cell surface foreign abnormal antigens and for activating the T-cell functions that result in killing of the foreign cells. Macrophages can also be recruited indirectly by the T cells to target and kill the foreign cells. This confirms the overlapping function of the more ancient nonspecific innate immune system with the more specific but slower reacting adaptive immune system. Recognition of foreign antigen and memory of a specific pathogen are both characteristics of the humoral and cell-mediated immunity [21]. The populations of T cells that directly destroy foreign cells are usually CD8+ and generally recognize a cell surface hybrid molecular structure consisting of MHC (major histocompatibility complex) class I molecules and nonself-origin peptides, derived primarily from intracellular proteins. The host's antigen presenting cells (APCs), which are mainly macrophages and dendritic cells, pick up foreign proteins and process them through a different cytoplasmic cascade for cell surface presentation as a new hybrid molecular structure consisting of a peptide coexpressed with MHC class II molecules. These peptides are eventually recognized by CD4+ T cells. These $\alpha\beta$ TCR$^+$ T cells expressing CD4+ are also referred to as Th cells. They produce cytokines that assist ("help") in antibody production, CD8+ or Tc cell activation and proliferation, and NK cell activation and expansion [21]. There are two subsets of Th cells called Th1 and Th2 cells. Th1 mainly secrete IL-2, IFN-γ and TNF α/β cytokines. Th1 cells are responsible for cytotoxicity and macrophage activation. They are beneficial in leishmaniasis, leprosy, viral infections, and allergy. They are detrimental in arthritis, autoimmunity, helminths, and organ transplantation. On the other hand, Th2 cells are secreting a whole other array of cytokines such as IL-4, IL-5, IL-6, IL-10, and IL-13. They help B cells and they activate eosinophils and mast cells. They are beneficial in arthritis, autoimmunity, helminths, pregnancy, and organ transplantation, and they are detrimental in allergy, viral infection, and leprosy [22]. The $\alpha\beta$ TCR T cells expressing CD8 are also called Tc cells and kill infected or neoplastic cells presenting a foreign peptide associated with MHC Class Ia molecules. This way cytotoxic T cells focus on the foreign cells rather than on normal host cells. As with the humoral immunity, T-cell immunity involves somatic gene component shuffling and rearrangement by which millions of different gene combinations are efficiently formed by the host to produce TCRs that can recognize equally millions of different antigens. Each T cell expresses in general only one antigen receptor specificity [20].

T-cell stimulation by a specific antigen activates two distinct mechanisms of signal transmission. The first selects the responding cell, triggering the specific TCR on the T-cell surface. The second signal has a costimulatory effect. This signal is generated by the APCs and is by itself insufficient, but it adds strength to the first signal and reduces the probability of unnecessary responses. Absence of a second signal usually results in anergy or cell death. Multiple regulatory cells as a complex network promote or harness the immune response by the secretion of cytokines and involvement of cell surface ligands. Removal or inactivation of self-reactive T cells and B cells result in avoidance of autoimmunity [20].

REFERENCES

1. Tramont CE, Hoover DL. Innate (general or non-specific) host defense mechanisms. Basic Principles in the Diagnosis and Management of Infectious diseases. Vol. 1. 5th ed. Philadelphia: Churchill-Livingstone, 2000:31.
2. Giamarellou H, Antoniadou A. Infectious complications of febrile leukopenia. Infections in the compromised host. Inf Dis Clin of N Am 2001; 15(2):457–482.
3. Finberg RW. Infection in cancer patients. Cancer Medicine and Hematology. Harvard Medical School Department of Continuing Education, October 26, 1999.
4. Serody JS, Shea TC. Prevention of infections in bone marrow transplant recipients. Nosocomial Infections. Inf Dis Clin of N Am 1997; 2(2):459–477.
5. Leather HL, Wingard JR. Infections following hematopoietic stem cell transplantation. Infections in the compromised host. Inf Dis Clin N Am 2001; 15(2): 483–520.
6. Ibrahim NK, Sahin AA, Dubrow RA, Lynch PM, Boehnke-Michaud L, Valero V, Buzdar AU, Hortobagyi GN. Colitis associated with docetaxel-based chemotherapy in patients with metastatic breast cancer. Lancet 2000; 355(9200):281–283.
7. Segal HB, Walsh TJ, Holland SM. Infections in the cancer patient. In: DeVita VT Jr, Hellman S, Rosenberg SA, eds. Cancer Principles and Practice of Oncology. 6th ed. Philadelphia: Lippincott Williams and Wilkins, 2001:2855–2858.
8. Ang BS, Telenti A, King B, Steckelberg JM, Wilson WR. Candidemia from a urinary tract source; microbiological aspects and clinical significance. Clin Infect Dis 1993; 17:662.
9. Koozeniowski OM. Urinary tract infections in the impaired host. Med Clin N Am 1991; 75:391.
10. Lowry FD, Carlisle PS, Adams A, Feiner C. The incidence of nosocomial pneumonia following urgent endotracheal intubations. Infect Control 1987; 8(6):245–248.
11. Rello J, Ausina V, Ricart M, Castella J, Prats G. Impact of previous antimicrobial therapy on the etiology and outcome of ventilator-associated pneumonia. Chest 1993; 104(4):1230–1235.
12. Hilbert G, Grimson D, Vargas F, Valentino R, Chene G, Boiron JM, Pigneux A, Reiffers J, Gbikpi-Benissan G, Cardinaud JP. Non-invasive continuous positive airway pressure in neutropenic patients with acute respiratory failure requiring intensive care unit admission. Crit Care Med 2000; 28(9):3185–3190.

13. Blot F, Nitenberg G, Guiguet M, Casetta M, Antoun S, Pico JL, Leclercq B, Escudier B. Safety of tracheostomy in neutropenic patients: a retrospective study of 26 consecutive cases. Intensive Care Med 1995; 21(8):687 690.
14. Greene JN. Catheter-related complications of cancer therapy. Infectious complications of cancer therapy. Inf Dis Clin N Am 1996; 10(2):255–295.
15. Nauseef WM, Clark RA. Granulocytic phagocytes. Basic Principles in the Diagnosis and Management of Infectious Diseases. 5th ed. Philadelphia: Churchill-Livingstone, 2000:89 112.
16. Herzig RH, Herzig GP, Graw RG, Bull MI, Ray KK. Successful granulocyte transfusion therapy for gram-negative septicima. N Engl J Med 1977; 296:701.
17. Alavi JB, Root RK, Djerassi I, Evans AE, Gluckman SJ, MacGregor RR, Guerry D, Schreiber AD, Shaw JM, Koch P, Cooper RA. A randomized clinical trial of granulocyte transfusions for infections in acute leukemia. N Engl J Med 1977; 296:706.
18. Young LS. Prophylactic granulocytes in the neutropenic host. Ann Intern Med 1982; 96:240.
19. Wright DG, Robichaud KJ, Pizzo PA, Deisseroth AB. Lethal pulmonary reactions associated with the combined use of amphotericin B and leukocyte transfusions. N Engl J Med 1981; 304:1185.
20. Restifo NP, Wunderlich JR. DeVita VT Jr, Hellman S, Rosenberg SA, eds. Essentials of Immunology. Cancer. Principles and Practice of Oncology. 6th ed. Lippincott Williams and Wilkins, 2001:43–77.
21. Johnson RM, Brown EJ. Cell-mediated immunity in host defense against infectious diseases. Basic Principles in the Diagnosis and Management of Infectious Diseases. Vol. 1. 5th ed. Philadelphia: Churchill-Livingstone, 2000:112–146.
22. Clayberger C, Krensky AM. T-cell immunity. Hematology. Basic Principles and Practice. 3d ed. Philadelphia: Churchill-Livingstone, 2000:98t.

2

Composition of the Normal Microbial Flora

John N. Greene
University of South Florida, School of Medicine
and Moffitt Cancer Center and Research Institute
Tampa, Florida, U.S.A.

Colonization of microbes in and on humans is normally a commensal relationship that is beneficial for both. However, cancer itself and its treatment disrupts the healthy balance between microbe and host. Because of damage to the skin, mucous membrane barriers and the immune system by the cancer itself, chemotherapy, radiation therapy, and intravenous catheters internal and external microbes can cause disease. Patients frequently develop nosocomial infections that are caused by normal endogenous flora at the time of admission, or by exogenous pathogens that are acquired and subsequently colonize the patient after admission to the hospital [1].

DIGESTIVE TRACT

The oropharynx is normally colonized with gram-positive bacteria, namely microaerophilic *Streptococci*. Oropharyngeal colonization with enteric gram-negative bacteria (GNB) seldom occurs in healthy individuals [2]. Even the introduction of a large inoculum of GNB into the mouths of healthy volunteers did not result in colonization [3]. However, with increasing age and illness including cancer, oropharyngeal colonization with GNB occurs more frequently [4]. One theory for this observation is that fibronectin normally found on the surface of epithelial cells allows for binding of gram-positive bacteria but not GNB [5]. With age and illness this protective barrier is damaged, allowing the surface of epithelial cells to be exposed. The exposed surface of these cells allows for the binding of GNB and their subsequent colonization [6]. Because of this phenomenon, pneumonia in the aged and the ill (including the patient with cancer) is more likely to be due to GNB than pneumonia in healthy people in the community.

Critically ill patients in the intensive care unit, with or without a ventilator, are especially at risk for GNB colonization of the oropharynx and GNB pneumonia. Ventilator-associated pneumonia is closely linked to preceding oropharyngeal colonization. In one study, 23% of colonized intensive care unit patients developed GNB pneumonia as compared to only 3% of noncolonized patients [2]. In another study, the percentage of pathogens colonizing the trachea and oropharynx prior to developing nosocomial pneumonia was 96% and 75%, respectively [6].

The most important endogenous source for GNB is the gastrointestinal (GI) tract. In healthy people, the colon contains more than 10^5 E. coli per gram of stool. Pseudomonas aeruginosa and Enterobacter can also be found in small numbers in the stool of some healthy people. In the setting of neutropenia, the only GNB colonizing the GI tract that preceded subsequent bacteremia in the majority of cases was P. aeruginosa. Because of its greater virulence and potential for translocation from GI tract to bloodstream, P. aeruginosa is the primary target of empiric antibiotics on the first day of neutropenia. Salads, especially lettuce and tomatoes, are a common source of P. aeruginosa [7]. Unless properly washed and prepared, these foods are restricted from patients with neutropenia.

The anaerobic flora of the GI tract far outnumber the aerobic flora, namely, E. coli, Streptococci, and Enterococci. The normal flora of the bowel contains more than 400 obligate anaerobic species in a total concentration of 10^{12} colony-forming units per gram of feces. The anaerobic flora protects against overgrowth of aerobic GNB. This phenomenon is known as "colonization resistance" [8]. A person with unimpaired microbial colonization resistance can resist colonization when an oral inoculum of 10^6 organisms is given [7]. Once resistance is reduced, such as with antibiotics, the inoculum required to induce colonization is only 10 to 100 organisms [7]. Normal flora provide protection against colonization by exogenous microorganisms and limit the concentration of indigenous pathogenic microbes [9]. Antibiotics that kill the anaerobic flora of the GI tract will increase the risk for subsequent GNB colonization, as well as infection. This has been most notably documented with P. aeruginosa and Salmonella species.

On the other hand, antimicrobials that lack antianaerobic activity can increase the risk of enterocolitis in the setting of neutropenia, primarily because of *Clostridium septicum*. Neutropenic enterocolitis (also known as typhlitis) develops primarily in the cecum and can mimic appendicitis. One of the reasons the cecum is particularly vulnerable is because it has the highest number of bacteria per gram of stool, primarily anaerobes. Although GNB play a role in the pathogenesis of typhlitis, *C. septicum* is the primary pathogen. This infection tends to occur in the first three weeks of neutropenia and arises from the patient's endogenous flora.

GENITOURINARY TRACT

Colonization of the vagina is usually made up of *Lactobacillus* and group *B Streptococci* in healthy women. Pregnant women are screened for vaginal colonization by group *B Streptococci* and treated, if they are present, to prevent neonatal bacteremia and meningitis. When lymphedema of the legs develops after surgical or radiation treatment for a gynecologic malignancy, recurrent cellulites of the legs can develop. The most common identified pathogen is group *B Streptococci* originating from chronic vaginal colonization.

Postmenopausal women, and those with underlying illnesses such as diabetes and cancer, may have a higher rate of vaginal and perineum colonization with GNB. Urinary tract infections from GNB can result from this contiguous site of colonization.

THE SKIN INTEGUMENT

Normally 10^3 to 10^4 microorganisms per cm^2 are found on the skin, while 10^6 organisms per cm^2 are found in the moist groin and axilla areas [10]. Washing decreases skin counts by 90%, but normal numbers are found again within 8 hours [10]. The normal flora of the skin includes coagulase-negative *Staphylococcus*, *Corynebacterium* species, *Propionobacterium* species, and a host of other bacteria, mostly gram positive.

Staphylococcus aureus can colonize the skin with the primary reservoir in the anterior nares. Twenty-five percent of the population at any given time is colonized with *S. aureus*. Colonization with *S. aureus* (including MRSA) can lead to subsequent surgical wound infection or catheter-related infections. Patients with underlying illness such as diabetes, HIV, and cancer have a higher incidence of *S. aureus* colonization and infection than those without those conditions. Since many patients with cancer require chemotherapy via a central venous catheter (CVC), skin flora mentioned above (especially coagulase-negative *Staphylococci* and *S. aureus*) can result in a CVC infection or bacteremia.

ANTIMICROBIAL EFFECTS

The suppression of endogenous GI flora in neutropenic patients to prevent nosocomial infections with antimicrobials has been explored over the last 30 years. Various antibiotics and antifungals, both absorbable and non-absorbable, have been used. Ultimately the practice has been abandoned in most cancer centers because of the concern for the emergence of multidrug-resistant pathogens and the failure to effect mortality rates [1]. Currently, oral flouroquinolones with antipseudomonal activity are being used for prophylaxis during the neutropenic period. Trials to establish efficacy and justify the expense of these prophylactic agents is ongoing. The exposure to antimicrobials in the weeks prior to the presentation of febrile neutropenia will determine the cause of breakthrough infection. When prophylactic flouroquinolones are administered, infections due to *viridans Streptococci*, coagulase-negative *Staphylococcus*, aerobic gram-positive bacilli, and multi-drug-resistant (MDR) GNB are expected. When a fungal infection develops while fluconazole is administered, nonalbicans *Candida* and molds are more likely.

NEUTROPENIA (DAY 0–7)

During the first week of neutropenia the primary source of infection is from the endogenous flora of the GI tract and skin. The usual documented infection is GNB bacteremia due to translocation from the GI tract. Several days later, under selective pressure from antipseudomonal antibiotics that lack gram-positive coverage, *viridans Streptococci*, coagulase-negative *Staphylococcus*, *Staphylococcus aureus* (including MRSA), Corynebacteria (non-JK and JK) cause bacteremia. All of the aforementioned bacteria primarily arise from the skin, except that *viridans Streptococci* and occasionally co-agulase-negative *Staphylococcus* tend to originate from the oropharynx and GI tract, especially when mucositis is present. Prior exposure to antibiotics that can alter the endogenous flora and exogenous flora can be acquired from hospital stays, especially in the intensive care unit. This history of exposure must be taken into consideration when choosing empiric antibiotics in the setting of febrile neutropenia.

NEUTROPENIA (DAY 7–14)

Infections occurring during the second week of neutropenia originate primarily from the GI tract. Under the selective pressure of antibiotics, which have broad activity against aerobic gram-positive bacteria and GNB, as well as anaerobes, yeasts emerge as significant causes of infection [11]. As the inoculum of *Candida albicans* and non-*albicans Candida* in the GI tract

increases, the risk of candidemia and dissemination increases accordingly [12]. In the 1960s a physician drank 10^{12} C. albicans during a monitored self-experiment [13]. Within two hours, he developed fevers, chills, and headache. Within three hours, his blood and urine were growing the same strain of C. albicans as ingested. Nystatin cured his self-induced infection. This serves as a vivid reminder that even with an intact GI tract and a normal immune system, translocation of Candida from GI tract to bloodstream can occur. Candida colonization of the GI tract is a common finding in patients with neutropenia, especially beyond two weeks, but does not predict subsequent candidemia except for C. tropicalis. There is a greater degree of candidemia in patients when C. tropicalis colonized the GI tract compared to other species of Candida [14].

In addition to Candida, other infections that can result from endogenous colonization during this period of neutropenia depend on the type and duration of antimicrobials given to the patient. By knowing the spectrum of activity of a given antibiotic and its duration of use, one can reliably predict the next infection and therefore empirically add or change antibiotics when necessary. However, awareness of noninfectious causes of fever is needed to prevent unnecessary antimicrobial additions and deletions. The same infections listed in the first week of neutropenia can occur during the second depending on the antimicrobials given.

NEUTROPENIA (DAY 14–BEYOND)

This is the most challenging period for clinicians trying to keep patients infection free until engraftment. The predominant pathogens causing infection will originate from the GI tract, skin, and respiratory tract. Exogenous sources of infection originating from contact with health care workers and the hospital environment become increasing important. The use of high-efficiency particulate air (HEPA) filtration can significantly reduce the risk of exogenous acquisition of fungi such as Aspergillus, Fusarium, and other molds. Molds acquired prior to neutropenia via inhalation, outside or inside the hospital, can cause sinopulmonary infection with a high mortality.

Reactivation of previously acquired pathogens can occur throughout this period of neutropenia. These include latent viruses such as Herpes simplex virus, Varicella zoster, Cytomegalovirus, Adenovirus, and BK virus.

Besides the latent pathogens that reactivate, endogenous and exogenous acquired bacteria and fungi that are resistant to the antimicrobials administered can cause serious infection. The bacterial pathogens of concern are multidrug-resistant (MDR) GNB (P. aeruginosa, Enterobacter, Klebsiella, E. coli, Citrobacter, Serratia, Stenotrophomonas, Acinetobacter and Alcaligines). MRSA, Bacillus species, Corynebacterium JK, Staphylococcus hemolyticum,

Vancomycin-resistant *Enterococci, Leuconostoc,* and *Pediococcus* are the primary gram-positive bacteria to cause infection. The latter three are resistant to Vancomycin. Anaerobic infections of the GI tract and oropharynx that may occur include *Clostridium* species, *Capnocytophaga ochracea,* and *Fusobacterium* species. Fungal infections during this period include nonalbicans *Candida* that are frequently resistant to fluconazole, as well as the molds.

STEM CELL TRANSPLANTATION (ALLOGENIC) (ENGRAFTMENT TO RESOLUTION OF GRAFT VERSUS HOST DISEASE (GVHD))

After engraftment, antimicrobials are discontinued and the normal endogenous flora in the GI tract and on the skin is allowed to return. The primary immunodeficiency is cell mediated, with loss of T lymphocyte, macrophage, and monocyte numbers and function from the treatment and prophylaxis for GVHD, namely, corticosteroids and cyclosporin A. Despite the resolution of neutropenia, there can be bacteremia, pneumonia, and central venous catheter-related infections due to GNB and gram-positive bacteria.

Reactivation of *Cytomegalovirus, Herpes simplex* virus, and *Varicella zoster* virus is prevented with prophylactic acyclovir in the latter two, and weekly antigen or PCR detection of CMV serum presence with the former. *BK* virus and *Adenovirus* can also reactivate and cause hemorrhagic cystitis.

The primary concern during this period is a sinopulmonary mold infection, usually acquired from the exogenous environment outside the hospital. *Aspergillus* species is most common, followed by *Fusarium, Scedosporium, Paecilomyces,* and *Zygomyces.*

Other rare causes of infection that can occur during this period from either endogenous reactivation or exogenous acquisition include *Pneumocystis carinii Mycobacterium tuberculosis,* nontuberculosus *Mycobacterium, Nocardia, Toxoplasma, Strongyloides, Cryptococcus,* and the endemic mycoses (*Histoplasma, Blastomyces, Coccioidomyces*). Respiratory virus infections from the community are dangerous when acquired during this period and include Respiratory *syncytial* virus, Influenza, *Parainfluenzae,* and *Adenovirus.* Finally, the risk of all these infections diminishes to the level of healthy noncancer patients, in most cases, with the resolution of neutropenia, GVHD, remission of the malignancy, and the cessation of all antimicrobials.

REFERENCES

1. Boyce JM. Treatment and control of colonization in the prevention of nosocomial infections. Infect Control Hosp Epidemiol 1996; 17:256–261.
2. Johanson WG, Pierce AK, Sanford JP. Changing pharyngeal bacterial flora of hospitalized patients. N Engl J Med 1969; 281:1137–1140.

3. Laforce FM, Hopkins J, Trow R. Human oral defenses against gram-negative rods. Am Rev Respir Dis 1976; 114:929.
4. Sveinbjornsdottir S, Gudmundsson S, Breim H. Oropharyngeal colonization in the elderly. Eur J Clin Microbiol Infect Dis 1991; 10:959–963.
5. Woods DE. Role of fibronectic in the pathogenesis of gram-negative bacillary pneumonia. Rev Infect Dis 1987; 9:386S–390S.
6. Bonten MJM, Weinstein RA. The role of colonization in the pathogenesis of nosocomial infections. Infect Control Hosp Epidemiol 1996; 17:193–200.
7. Remington JS, Schimpff SC. Occasional notes: please don't eat the salads. N Engl J Med 1981; 304(7):433–435.
8. Clasener HAL, Volaard EJ, van Saene HKF. Long-term prophylaxis of infection by selective decontamination in leukopenia and in mechanical ventilation. Rev Infect Dis 1987; 9:295–328.
9. Vollaard EJ, Clasener HAL. Mini review: colonization resistance. Antimicrob Agents Chemother 1994; 38(3):409–414.
10. Greene JN. The microbiology of colonizatiom, including techniques for assessing and measuring colonization. Infect Control Hosp Epidemiol 1996; 17:114–118.
11. Richet HM, Andremont A, Tancrede C, Pico JL, Jarris WR. Risk factors for candidemia in patients with acute lymphocytic leukemia. Rev Infect Dis 1991; 13:211–215.
12. Rahal JJ. Intestinal overgrowth by *Candida*: clinically important or not? Infect Dis Clin Pract 1993; 2:254–259.
13. Krause W, Matheis H, Wulf K. Fungemia and funguria after oral administration of Candida albicans. Lancet 1969; 1:598–599.
14. Wingard JR, Merz WG, Saral R. Candida tropicalis: a major pathogen in immunocompromised patients. Ann Intern Med 1979; 91:539–543.

3

Acute Lymphoblastic Leukemia

Jennifer Johnson and John Greene
University of South Florida School of Medicine
and Moffitt Cancer Center and Research Institute
Tampa, Florida, U.S.A.

INTRODUCTION

Acute lymphoblastic leukemia (ALL) accounts for 20% of acute leukemias diagnosed in patients over 20 years of age [1]. Although remarkable progress has been made in the treatment of childhood ALL, the prognosis for adults remains much less favorable [2]. Rates of complete remission currently range from 75 to 90% in adults with ALL, but disease-free survival is only 30 to 40% [3]. The inferior outcomes of ALL treatment in adults are due to the higher frequency of adverse genetic abnormalities seen in leukemic lymphoblasts as well as the greater severity of chemotherapy toxicity and higher incidence of comorbidities [4].

Although notable improvements have been made in the supportive care of patients with acute leukemia, infections remain the major cause of morbidity and mortality [6]. Half of patients presenting with ALL have fever and nearly a third have documented infection [3,5]. At the time of diagnosis, the predominant bacterial pathogens reflect those found in an outpatient setting, in particular β-hemolytic streptococci and *E. coli* [7]. Hospitalization causes a shift in the flora, with the appearance of colonization with gram-negative bacteria [8]. Chemotherapy-induced neutropenia places patients with ALL at risk for bacterial infections and herpetic reactivation early in their treatment course, with fungal infections generally occurring later. Although neutropenia occurring during induction therapy for ALL is not typically as prolonged as that occurring during AML induction, chemotherapy produces quantitative and qualitative suppression of the immune system over an extended period of time, often two to three years [9]. In addition, ALL in adults is punctuated by relapse in greater than 50% of cases, necessitating further courses of intensive chemotherapy and hospitalization [1].

EPIDEMIOLOGY

During induction therapy for ALL, the incidence of infection is 15–42%. Infectious mortality depends on the intensity of the induction regimen, the age of patients, and comorbidities, but ranges from 5 to 12% in most modern clinical trials [10–14]. Compared to AML, infectious complications during induction therapy for ALL are similar; however, they are somewhat lower during standard consolidation and maintenance therapy [15]. Most clinical trials report infection in approximately 25% of patients undergoing consolidation chemotherapy, with infectious mortality 2–5% during this phase [10–14].

The incidence and prevalence of infections in the patient with ALL has evolved over time owing to the intensification of therapy, changing epidemiological patterns, and the use of prophylactic antibiotics. While gram-negative organisms were the most frequently isolated pathogens prior to the 1980s, gram-positive organisms have since supplanted their role, now accounting for 55 to 60% of infectious episodes [16,17]. Enhanced access of skin flora via oral mucositis and intravascular devices may partially explain this phenomenon, along with selective pressure by prophylactic agents such as quinolones. Although *P. carinii* infections have decreased in ALL owing to the use of trimethoprim-sulfamethoxazole, fungal infections have increased in this group [18].

IMMUNITY AND INFECTION

Both quantitative and qualitative defects in immunity place the patient with ALL at increased risk for infection [19]. While neutropenia is not the sole factor predisposing to infection, it clearly remains an important one, particularly during induction chemotherapy. Patients with ALL typically experience neutropenia with median time to WBC recovery $>10^9$/L of 18 days

[20], although the duration of neutropenia is highly dependent on the intensity of the induction regimen [21]. The risk of infection correlates inversely with the number of circulating neutrophils [22] and increase with the duration of neutropenia. Also, infectious mortality is influenced by the trend in neutrophil count [23] as greater fatality occurs with declining counts during the infection.

Reduced bactericidal activity of neutrophils has been noted in patients with ALL undergoing induction chemotherapy, as well as in various stages of the disease [24]. In addition, defects in leukocyte function have been demonstrated in ALL patients. These abnormalities were noted prior to treatment, in remission, and during relape [25], indicating that functional impairment exists in the neutrophils of ALL patients even when their bone marrow exhibits normal morphology.

Disruption of other elements of the immune system result from displacement of immune cells from their original location by the leukemia in combination with the deleterious effects of chemotherapy. Profound alterations in humoral and cellular immunity can occur in ALL patients [19]. The hypogammaglobulinemia associated with intensive chemotherapy predisposes to both gram-positive and gram-negative bacterial infections, while abnormalities in T lymphocytes caused by corticosteroids and cytoreductive agents may predispose to infections with intracellular bacteria, fungi, viruses, and protozoa [26].

Treatment of ALL typically entails the administration of chemotherapy in various stages for 2 to 3 years, and many of these drugs have toxic effects on the immunocompetent blood cells. Anthracyclines, mitoxantrone, alkylating agents, and cytosine arabinoside exhibit a high degree of myelosuppressive activity, while methotrexate and epipodophyllotoxins cause a moderate amount of marrow suppression [27]. Inhibition of granulocyte phagocytosis and granulocyte bactericidal activity has been observed with daunorubicin, methotrexate, and vincristine [28]. In addition, adriamycin, cyclophosphamide, prednisone, procarbazine, and vincristine have been shown in vitro to decrease leukocyte-mediated antibody-dependent cellular cytotoxicity and natural killer cytotoxicity against cells infected by herpes simplex virus [29].

Corticosteroids are frequently used in the treatment of lymphoid malignancies for their lympholytic properties; however, immunomodulatory and anti-inflammatory effects may alter the incidence and detection of infection in patients with ALL. Administration of these compounds causes a redistribution of circulating lymphocytes, monocytes, eosinophils, and basophils to the lymphoid tissues, which compromises the ability of these cells to fight infection [30]. In addition, corticosteroids may dramatically reduce the inflammatory response and consequently fever and other usual clinical signs and symptoms of infection [12]. Absence of these features may delay prompt diagnosis and antimicrobial treatment.

The disruption of skin and mucosal barriers provides access for colonization and subsequent invasion of pathogens. Prolonged use of indwelling venous catheters increases the likelihood of infections with gram-positive organisms [15]. Ommaya reservoirs, often utilized for the intrathecal administration of chemotherapy for CNS prophylaxis, may serve as a portal of entry for pathogens. Anthracyclines and methotrexate are well known for causing mucositis of the oral cavity and digestive tract, which facilitates bacterial and fungal access to the bloodstream [19]. A corollary to the problem of mucositis is the observation that normal colonizing flora of the digestive tract can be displaced by more virulent organisms in the leukemia patient. One study in a hospital setting isolated enteric microorganisms from the oral flora of 62% of leukemia patients compared with 28% of control patients [8].

BACTERIAL INFECTIONS

Adults with ALL are most susceptible to bacterial infections during the initial intensive phase of treatment when neutropenia and mucositis are most severe. Although infections with gram-negative organisms continue to be associated with the highest mortality, gram-positives now account for the majority of bacterial infections, in large part because of the increase in catheter-related infections with *Streptococci* and coagulase negative Staphylococci in association with prophylactic quinolone therapy. Other bacterial pathogens frequently associated with indwelling catheters include *Corynebacterium* spp. and *Bacillus* spp. [31]. Cellulitis and subcutaneous tunnel infections as well as bacteremia may result from catheter-related infections.

The microbiologic spectrum of Ommaya reservoir infection also shows a predominance of gram-positive bacteria, particularly *Staphylococcus* and *Corynebacterium* species [32]. Bacterial meningitis is a potential complication and may occur in 7 to 50% of patients with the indwelling device [33]. Patients whose reservoir was punctured more than 20 times had a greater risk of acquiring infection than those accessed on fewer occasions [34]. Although most patients who develop Ommaya-related meningitis can be successfully treated via intravenous or intrathecal antibiotics, persistent infection may necessitate reservoir removal.

Bacteremia with viridans Streptococci, particularly *S. mitis*, has been reported in patients with ALL undergoing intensive chemotherapy. The clinical course is variable but may result in rapidly fatal sepsis owing to hypotension and acute respiratory distress syndrome (ARDS), with a mortality rate of 12% observed in two series [35,36]. Viridans streptococcal bacteremia appears to correlate highly with the presence of mucositis; neutropenia and high doses of cytosine arabinoside were other predisposing factors [35–37].

Vancomycin-resistant enterococci (VRE) represent another nosocomial gram-positive pathogen. Antianaerobic antibiotics as well as gastrointestinal colonization with VRE are associated with VRE bacteremia [38]. Compared to vancomycin-sensitive isolates, VRE bacteremia in patients with neutropenia is associated with a higher mortality and prompts central venous catheter removal.

While *C. difficile* colitis also has an association with the administration of antibiotics, pseudomembranous colitis has been observed following the administration of cytotoxic agents alone [39]. These results indicate that the symptom of diarrhea following chemotherapy with or without prior antibiotic exposure should prompt a search for toxin-producing *C. difficile* [40].

Listeria monocytogenes has a tropism for the nervous system and may cause meningitis, encephalitis, and brain abscess [41]. Suppression of cell-mediated immunity as a result of steroid administration as well as violation of the CNS during the administration of chemotherapy for CNS prophylaxis increase the risk of listerial infection in ALL. While meningitis is the most common manifestation of *L. monocytogenes* CNS infection, brain abscess has been reported in several patients with ALL [42].

Escherichia coli, Klebsiella, and *Pseudomonas aeruginosa* remain the most common gram-negative pathogens [43]. Although focal infections of the respiratory tract, skin, gastrointestinal tract, or genitourinary system may occur, sepsis caused by these endotoxin-producing organisms leads to hypotension, renal failure, and shock. Of additional concern is the isolation of quinolone-resistant *E. coli* from several cancer centers [44,45].

Pathogens that cause relatively mild infections in normal hosts may result in the development of life-threatening infection in the leukemia patient. A case of severe pneumonia caused by *Chlamydia pneumoniae* was reported in a woman with ALL undergoing induction chemotherapy [46]. Mechanical ventilation was required; however, she experienced full recovery after treatment with erythromycin.

Deeply invasive bacterial infection may be encountered in the setting of typhlitis, also known as neutropenic enterocolitis or ileocecal syndrome [47]. Most frequently observed after gastrointestinal mucosal injury due to chemotherapeutic agents, this syndrome consists of inflammation or necrosis of the ileum, cecum, or ascending colon. Abdominal distention, right-sided abdominal tenderness, diarrhea, and fever associated with neutropenia and thrombocytopenia are characteristic of the clinical presentation [48]. Perforation and sepsis may result, and *Clostridium septicum* is the most common blood culture isolate, although other pathogens including *C. difficile* may also play a causative role [49].

"New" gram-positive and gram-negative pathogens have emerged in the last decade as a cause of infection in neutropenic hosts. Adults with ALL who experience periods of profound neutropenia during intensive chemotherapy may be susceptible to infections with these microorganisms, many of which are normal nonpathogenic bacterial flora of the skin or environment. These organisms include *Stenotrophomonas maltophilia*, *Bacillus cereus*, *Stomatococcus mucilaginosus*, *Corynebacterium jeikeium*, *Rhodococcus* species, *Leuconstoc* species, *Burholderia cepacia*, and *Bartonella* species [16].

Stenotrophomonas (*Xanthomonas*) *maltophilia* may be associated with bacteremia or infections of the lungs, soft tissues, urinary tract, biliary tract, heart valves, and wounds [49]. Skin manifestations in the form of deep, tender infiltrates, presumably from septic emboli of *S. maltophilia*, have recently been described in two patients with ALL [50]. Because of its inherent resistance to imipenem and rapid development of resistance to other antibiotics, intensive combination therapy based on sensitivity testing is recommended.

Bacillus cereus may cause a fulminant sepsis in patients with ALL associated with neutropenia and high fever [51,52]. The organism has been noted to produce several hemolysins, which in some cases have been associated with massive intravascular hemolysis [51]. Localized infections such as pneumonia, endocarditis, osteomyelitis, meningitis, and soft tissue infections have also been described.

Stomatococcus mucilaginosus is part of the normal oral flora and has been recognized in recent years as an emerging pathogen in neutropenic patients [53]. Bacteremia may occur with complications such as septic shock, pneumonia, ARDS, and cutaneous manifestations. CNS infection, heralded by fever, headache, and lethargy, has also been described in several patients with ALL [54].

Corynebacterium jeikeium has been reported to cause sepsis in patients with ALL [55]. This organism is distinct from other frequently isolated diphtheroids and is usually resistant to many antibiotics. The risk factors for sepsis include the presence of a central venous catheter, exposure to multiple antibiotics, and profound or prolonged neutropenia [56]. Skin lesions and pulmonary lesions are reported in 48% and 36% of patients, respectively, and disease is ameliorated by recovery of the bone marrow.

VIRAL INFECTIONS

The predominant viral pathogens in patients with ALL are *herpes simplex*, *varicella zoster*, and *cytomegalovirus* [15]. Reactivation of latent herpes simplex virus (HSV) frequently occurs owing to defects in cell-mediated immunity mediated by cytotoxic chemotherapy [57]. Painful vesicular lesions are most commonly found in the oral cavity and perioral skin, although lesions may extend to the oropharynx and esophagus, resulting in odynophagia. However, vesicular lesions rapidly ulcerate with a white or black base and are easily misdiagnosed as thrush, chemotherapy-induced mucositis, or bacterial infection. Reactivation of herpes simplex virus may also occur less commonly in the genital and perianal areas. Although disseminated HSV infection is rare, lethal systemic HSV-1 infection with diffuse infiltration of the liver, colon, and esophagus has been reported [58]. Additionally, an association between mucocutaneous HSV infection and antibiotic resistant fever has been observed in neutropenic patients [59]. Empirical antiviral therapy may be indicated during neutropenic fever unresponsive to antibacterial agents when herpes infection is suspected.

Similar to HSV, infection with varicella zoster virus (VZV) is often the result of reactivation in adults, although young adults without a history of varicella infection may experience a fulminant or even life-threatening course [60]. Pain typically precedes vesicular lesions that appear in a dermatomal pattern with rare extension to other skin sites and internal organs. An abdominal-back pain syndrome has been reported in patients with ALL in which severe pain resembling pancreatitis or gut perforation preceded the appearance of a cutaneous papulovesicular rash and fever [61]. Prompt antiviral therapy should be initiated in the case of abdominal or back pain at the first appearance of vesicles, as visceral dissemination of VZV can be rapidly fatal.

Cytomegalovirus causes a diverse spectrum of clinical diseases including interstitial pneumonitis, esophageal and gastrointestinal ulcerations, pancreatitis, hepatitis, cholecystitis, and retinitis [62]. Patients at highest risk for these clinical entities are those undergoing bone marrow transplant; hence these infections will be described in greater detail in the corresponding chapter of this book.

Reactivation of human herpes virus-6 (HHV-6) has been reported in adults with ALL both during chemotherapy and following bone marrow transplant [63,64]. Although complications such as interstitial pneumonitis or marrow suppression have been observed in transplant recipients, reactivation of HHV-6 during chemotherapy may manifest as a skin exanthem without signs of systemic infection. Resolution of the exanthem often occurs with marrow recovery as well as treatment with ganciclovir.

Parvovirus B19 has been reported to cause intense cytopenia in ALL patients owing in part to the reduced compensatory capacity of the bone marrow induced by chemotherapy [65]. Although the erythroid lineage is usually most affected, concomitant thrombocytopenia and granulocytopenia have been reported during parvovirus B19 reactivation [66]. Giant pronormoblasts in bone marrow aspirates are considered diagnostic of infection with this virus. Complete hematologic recovery usually occurs; however, persistent parvovirus infection has been reported as a cause of severe chronic anemia in selected children with acute leukemia [67]. Intravenous immunoglobulin is indicated for the treatment of parvovirus B19–induced anemia in immuno-suppressed patients.

Community respiratory viruses such as respiratory syncytial virus (RSV), influenza virus, and parainfluenza virus may be a cause, of severe respiratory illness in hospitalized patients with ALL. One cancer center documented a 10% incidence of RSV infection in patients with acute leukemia during a period when RSV was prevalent in the community [68]. Patients with severe myelosuppression had the greatest risk of developing pneumonia, which had a mortality rate of 83%.

FUNGAL INFECTIONS

The rising incidence of fungal infections in patients with acute leukemia may be attributed in part to more frequent administration of prophylactic and empirical antibiotics, the use of indwelling venous catheters, and more intensive regimens with antineoplastic drugs resulting in longer periods of neutropenia [31]. Corticosteroids, a mainstay in the treatment of ALL, also predispose to fungal infections through suppression of cell-mediated immunity. Although fungal infections account for 2–20% of infections in this patient population, they may be the major cause of death in up to 45% of infectious fatalities [18,69]. The predominant pathogens are *Candida* and *Aspergillus*; however, infections due to *Mucor*, *Fusarium*, and *Trichophyton* spp. have been reported, particularly in patients undergoing intensive treatment or bone marrow transplantation.

Candida albicans is a component of the normal cutaneous and gastrointestinal flora. In one series, patients with the greatest risk for disseminated infection were those with high-level candidal colonization who were treated for microbiologically proven bacteremia [69]. Receipt of vancomycin and/or imipenem has also been identified as an independent risk factor for candidemia [70]. *Candida* spp. cause a spectrum of clinical syndromes, including oral thrush, esophagitis, catheter-related infections, urinary tract infections, bacteremia, and hepatosplenic candidiasis [15]. While *C. albicans* remains the most frequently encountered fungal pathogen, other species such as *C. tropicalis*, *C. parapsilosis*, *C. glabrata*, and *C. krusei* have emerged in recent years as important infectious agents [71].

Oral thrush is relatively common and usually easily managed. Disseminated candidiasis may be acute or chronic and is characterized by fever unresponsive to antibacterial agents [18]. The acute presentation involves fungemia, embolic skin lesions, visceral involvement, and sometimes shock [72]. Chronic disseminated candidiasis (CDC), also known as hepatosplenic candidiasis, must be suspected in patients who remain pyrexial after recovering from neutropenia. This entity is characterized by focal abscesses or granulomatous lesions in the liver and spleen, with infrequent involvement of the lungs, kidneys, and other tissues [73]. Other clinical manifestations include nonspecific gastrointestinal symptoms, leukocytosis, elevated C-reactive protein, and elevated serum alkaline phosphatase. In one analysis, independent factors related to the development of CDC in patients with acute leukemia were younger ages, duration of neutropenia ≥ 15 days, and the use of prophylactic quinolones [74]. High dose cytosine arabinoside has also been identified as a major risk factor [75]. Diagnosis is made most reliably by a demonstration of yeasts or pseudohyphae in biopsy specimens, but it may be suggested by characteristic target lesions on ultrasound or CT scan of the abdomen [76].

Because Aspergillus infection is usually acquired via inhalation of conidia, the respiratory tract is the most common site of disease; however, dissemination may occur to other body sites including the liver, spleen, brain, and heart [77]. Upper respiratory colonization frequently precedes invasive infection, and nasal culture yielding *A. flavus* or *A. fumigatus* has a positive predictive value of 91% for concurrent or subsequent invasive pulmonary infection [78]. While prolonged granulocytopenia is the primary predisposing factor [79], invasive aspergillosis occurring contemporaneously with bone marrow recovery has been reported in patients with ALL in complete remission [80]. An additional risk factor for patients with ALL is glucocorticoid therapy, as pharmacological doses of these agents have been shown directly to increase the growth rate of *A. fumigatus* and *A. flavus* independent of their immunomodulatory effects [81].

Initial findings of pulmonary aspergillosis on chest radiograph may be normal or nonspecific, but characteristic patterns include a patchy infiltrate or well-defined nodules, which progress to diffuse consolidation or cavitation [82]. Fever, pleuritic chest pain, and hemoptysis may be associated. Aspergillus rhinosinusitis should be suspected in patients who develop persistent fever, local nasal findings such as epistaxis or nasal discharge, symptoms of sinusitis, erythema or ulceration of the nose, sinuses, orbit, or hard palate, or unilateral tearing [83]. Biopsy is essential for diagnosis of both syndromes, and CT scan is desirable to elucidate the extent of disease and determine the best therapeutic approach.

The proportion of invasive yeast infections caused by non-*Candida* species in acute leukemia has increased [84]. Pathogens include *Malassezia furfur, Trichosporon* spp., *Blastoschizomyces capitatus, Rhodotorula rubra, Saccaromyces cerevisiae, Clavispora lusitaniae,* and *Cryptococcus* spp. Infections caused by these pathogens are associated with neutropenia and quinolone or fluconazole prophylaxis, and are more often fatal than infections caused by *Candida albicans*.

The molds Fusarium, Pseudoallescheria, Scedosporium, and Alternaria and the agents of zygomycosis (Mucor, Rhizopus, Absidia, Cunninghamella) are infrequent infectious pathogens that are most commonly isolated during periods of severe or prolonged neutropenia [31]. Although diagnosed more frequently in bone marrow transplant recipients, zygomycosis has been described in several patients with ALL undergoing induction chemotherapy [85,86]. Mucor infection may be cutaneous, rhinocerebral, pulmonary, or disseminated and is characterized by rapid progression, tissue necrosis, and vascular invasion. A gastrointestinal form of Mucor infection with involvement of the liver and small bowel has also been described [87,88]. Iron overload from blood transfusions and deferoxamine use increases the risk of zygomycotic infections because of its need for exogenous iron to grow.

Skin involvement occurs in more than 80% of cases of disseminated fusariosis, and typical lesions are erythematous macules, palpable and nonpalpable purpura, and flaccid pustules [89,90]. The spectrum of infection with *Scedosporium* species includes cutaneous, pulmonary, and disseminated disease, as well as meningoencephalitis [91,92]. In both instances of mold infection, pulmonary involvement may occur, and the disease is often fatal in the absence of bone marrow recovery [93,94]. As many of these molds are ubiquitous in the environment, epidemics have been traced to nearby construction activity and faulty ventilation systems as well as water-borne sources (i.e., shower heads) [95,96].

PROTOZOAL INFECTIONS

Cysts of *Pneumocystis carinii* are acquired in the respiratory tract early in life, and reactivation is provoked by defects in cell-mediated immunity [97]. Historically noted in children with ALL receiving corticosteroids and intensive chemotherapy [98], *P. carinii* pneumonia (PCP) is now relatively uncommon in this group owing to ubiquitous prophylaxis. The disease usually presents as acute hypoxia and dyspnea in association with bilateral interstitial pulmonary infiltrates. In adults with ALL, PCP generally occurs during consolidation or early maintenance therapy [26], although earlier presentations may occur with more intensive chemotherapy [99]. Because of the association of PCP with the tapering of steroids, many ALL protocols institute intermittent trimethoprim-sulfamethoxazole prophylaxis following induction [100].

PROPHYLAXIS OF INFECTION

Limiting infection begins with environmental measures designed to minimize microorganism transmission to the patient with leukemia. Hand washing is essential, and isolation measures may extend to total protective environments at some facilities [101]. Although chemotherapy-induced mucositis is difficult to avoid, ice chips have proven to be effective in reducing stomatitis due to fluorouracil [102].

Antibacterial prophylaxis has been mainly directed at gram-negative pathogens, given the high mortality of gram-negative sepsis. Oral trimetho-prim-sulfamethoxazole (TMP-SMX) is effective against most gram-negative enteric organisms (excluding *Pseudomonas aeruginosa*) as well as *P. carinii*. Although usually well tolerated, adverse effects may include myelosuppression, hypersensitivity, and predisposition to fungal infection [103]. The greatest benefits occur among patients experiencing neutropenia of greater than two weeks' duration [104], with no significant reduction in the incidence of fever or infection during shorter periods [105].

Recently, quinolones have been shown to be more effective than TMP-SMX and nonabsorbable antibiotics in preventing gram-negative sepsis [106,107]. The advantages of quinolones include their oral tolerability, broad antimicrobial spectrum, and sparing of intestinal anaerobic flora [108]. However, the emergence of quinolone-resistant organisms and inadequate coverage of the more prevalent gram-positive organisms are significant drawbacks. In addition, except in special cases of profound and prolonged neutropenia, the Infectious Diseases Society of America has recommended against routine antibacterial prophylaxis owing to the emergence of drug resistant bacteria and the fact that such prophylaxis has not been shown to reduce mortality [109].

Antiviral prophylaxis with acyclovir is effective in reducing reactivation of *herpes simplex* virus in seropositive patients. Because 25–66% of patients with the presence of the HSV antibody may experience reactivation during induction chemotherapy for acute leukemia, some authors have recommended acyclovir prophylaxis in these patients [57]. Other centers reserve antiviral prophylaxis for patients with a history of HSV reactivation. Notably, acyclovir prophylaxis has also been documented to reduce the incidence of bacteremias during induction therapy in adults with acute leukemia, presumably because of a decrease in mucosal injury [110].

A variety of agents including topical chorhexidine, oral polyenes, topical azoles, and systemic azoles have been shown to be effective in the prophylaxis of oropharyngeal candidiasis, but not disseminated disease [111]. A large multicenter randomized trial demonstrated the efficacy of fluconazole in preventing colonization and superficial infections by *Candida* species other than *C. krusei* in patients undergoing therapy for acute leukemia [112]. However, no significant difference could be detected in invasive fungal infections or mortality. Additionally, fluconazole lacks activity against *C. krusei*, some strains of *C. glabrata*, and molds. Some institutions have noted increased frequency of colonization with *C. krusei* and *C. glabrata* during fluconazole prophylaxis [113,114], although this observation has not been borne out at other institutions [115]. However, increased bacteremias have been observed in some centers instituting azole prophylaxis during neutropenia [116,117].

HEPA filtration is the only modality that has been shown to reduce the incidence of mold infection [118]. While itraconazole is effective against Aspergillus, no randomized trials have shown its effectiveness in prophylaxis of aspergillosis in acute leukemia patients. In addition, its erratic bioavalability in settings of neutropenia and mucositis limits the prophylactic use of oral itraconazole [119]. Intranasal amphotericin B reduced the frequency of invasive aspergillosis in neutropenic patients compared to historical controls in one study [120]. However, a subsequent randomized placebo controlled trial failed to replicate these findings, although Aspergillus colonization was markedly reduced by intranasal amphotericin B [121]. Trials investigating aerosol amphotericin B for prophylaxis of invasive aspergillosis have been similarly disappointing [122].

In summary, routine prophylaxis against bacterial and fungal infections is not recommended in most patients undergoing chemotherapy for ALL. However, in circumstances where the potential for infection is high in cases of profound or prolonged neutropenia, prophylaxis may be instituted if the potential for resistant organisms or mold infections is appreciated and outweighed [107].

HEMATOPOIETIC GROWTH FACTORS

The use of granulocyte colony stimulating factor (G-CSF) and granulocyte-macrophage colony stimulating factor (GM-CSF) has been investigated in the supportive care of patients with ALL. Growth factors have been used therapeutically during severe infection to accelerate neutrophil recovery [123]; additionally, trials are underway to evaluate which patients would most benefit from prophylactic administration. Data from published clinical trials have clearly demonstrated the safety of growth factors. Although receptors for G-CSF have been detected on leukemic blasts, there is no evidence to date indicating any increased risk of relapse in ALL patients treated with myeloid growth factors [124].

Growth factors have been employed at various stages in the treatment of ALL. When administered following induction or intensive consolidation chemotherapy, G-CSF has been shown significantly to accelerate granulocyte recovery and reduce febrile episodes and clinically documented infection [125]. Several clinical trials have also demonstrated the efficacy of G-CSF administered concomitantly with induction chemotherapy. Despite theoretical concerns that G-CSF might enhance myelosuppression due to stimulation of normal progenitor cells, two randomized controlled studies in ALL patients undergoing induction according to the German Multicenter Study Group for Adult ALL (GMALL) protocol demonstrated a significant reduction in the duration of neutropenia [126,127]. A trend toward reduction in episodes of febrile neutropenia and documented infections was also noted.

GM-CSF has been studied less rigorously in therapy for adults with ALL. Although more rapid recovery of the granulocyte count has been reported in ALL patients treated with GM-CSF following reinduction chemotherapy [128], no advantage has been observed in terms of incidence of febrile episodes or documented infection [128,129].

While more rapid marrow recovery has resulted in significantly fewer delays in completion of chemotherapy in most trials, this has not been shown to translate into improved leukemia-free survival. Similarly, despite the observed decrease in infections, the administration of G-CSF does not appear to have an appreciable effect on overall mortality. Further, the substantial cost of growth factors must be weighed against the observed decrease in infection rate, antibiotic use, and hospital time. Cost-benefit analyses of the use of G-CSF in children have shown either unchanged or slightly decreased hospital costs [130,131], but adult trials have yet to made. On the other hand, several authors feel that the administration of G-CSF may improve the quality of life [132].

The benefits of growth factors appear most evident in patients at highest risk for prolonged neutropenia [133], particularly those receiving chemotherapy regimens that involve high doses or multiple cycles of myelosuppressive drugs. Issues such as optimal scheduling and duration of therapy need to be addressed in clinical trials before prophylactic administration of G-CSF can be recommended for all patients with ALL.

GRANULOCYTE TRANSFUSIONS

The infusion of granulocytes in combination with antibiotic therapy has been studied in neutropic patients with infection. In the past, clinical responses were limited by the inability to obtain sufficient quantities of functional neutrophils, even when donors were pretreated with corticosteroids [134], and the practice was largely abandoned following the advent of hematopoietic growth factors. However, a recent clinical trial including patients with ALL evaluated G-CSF and utilized granulocyte transfusions in the treatment of neutropenia-related fungal infection [135]. Seventy-three percent of patients had favorable responses with a moderate incidence of adverse effects noted in both recipients and donors. Although this approach remains controversial, granulocyte infusions may have a role in selected cases, such as breakthrough septicemia or disseminated fungal infection in neutropenic patients [15].

However, the potential for the transmission of CMV as well as other infectious agents in donor leukocytes remains problematic, particularly in bone marrow transplant recipients.

CONCLUSION

ALL continues to be a therapeutic challenge, and the prevalence of high-dose chemotherapy regimens as well as bone marrow transplants has increased in pursuit of higher rates of leukemia-free survival. These more intensive regimens are closely connected with the greater incidence and severity of infections in this patient population. Because many treatment failures are due to infectious fatality, careful attention must be paid to recognizing the subtle signs and symptoms of infection that are so often suppressed by treatment-related modalities. Recent advances in techniques for the diagnosis of infection, antimicrobial agents, and prophylaxis including hematopoietic growth factors hold promise for mitigating infectious complicatons. Future research will further refine their role in improving outcomes for patients with ALL.

REFERENCES

1. Ong S, Larson R. Current management of acute lymphoblastic leukemia in adults. Oncology 1995; 9:433–442.
2. Hoelzer D. Treatment of acute lymphoblastic leukemia. Semin Hematol 1994; 31:1–15.
3. Pui C, Evans W. Acute lymphoblastic leukemia. N Engl J Med 1998; 339:605–615.
4. Hoelzer D. Acute lymphoblastic leukemia—progress in children, less in adults. N Engl J Med 1993; 329:1343–1344.
5. Extermann M. Acute leukemia in the elderly. Clinics in Geriatric Medicine 1997; 13:227–243.
6. Nedelkova M, Bacalova S, Georgieva B. Infectious complications and host immune defense in acute leukemia. Europ J Cancer 1981; 17:617–622.
7. Beam T, Allen J. Patterns of infections in untreated acute leukemia: impact of initial hospitalization. Southern Med J 1979; 72:282–286.
8. Galili D, Donitza A, Garfunkel A, Sela M. Gram negative enteric bacteria in the oral cavity of leukemia patients. Oral Surg Oral Med Oral Pathol 1992; 74:459–462.
9. Gokbuget N, Hoelzer D, Arnold R, Bohme A, Bartram C, Freund M, Ganser A, Kneba M, Langer W, Lipp T, Ludwig W, Maschmeyer G, Rieder H, Thiel E, Weiss A, Messerer D. Advances in the treatment of adult acute lymphocytic leukemia. Hematol Oncol Clin North Am 2000; 14:1307–1325.
10. Kantarjian H, Walters R, Keating M, Smith T, O'Brien S, Estey E, Huh Y, Spinolo J, Dicke K, Barlogie B, McCredie K, Freireich E. Results of the vin-

cristine, doxorubicin, and dexamethasone regimen in adults with standard- and high-risk acute lymphocytic leukemia. J Clin Oncol 1990; 8:994–1004.

11. Fiere D, Lepage E, Sebban C, Boucheix C, Gisselbrecht C, Vernant J, Varet B, Broustet A, Cahn J, Rigal-Huguet F, Witz F, Michaux J, Michallet M, Reiffers J. Adult acute lymphoblastic leukemia: a multicentric randomized trial testing bone marrow transplantation as postremission therapy. J Clin Oncol 1993; 11:1990–2001.

12. Hussein K, Dahlberg S, Head D, Waddell C, Dabich L, Weick J, Morrison F, Saiki J, Mertz E, Rivkin S, Grever M, Boldt D. Treatment of acute lymphoblastic leukemia in adults with intensive induction, consolidation, and maintenance chemotherapy. Blood 1989; 73:57–63.

13. Wiernik P, Dutcher J, Paietta E, Gucalp R, Markus S, Weinberg V, Azar C, Garl S, Benson L. Long-term follow-up of treatment and potential cure of adult acute lymphocytic leukemia with MOAD: a non-anthracycline containing regimen. Leukemia 1993; 7:1236–1241.

14. Hoelzer D, Thiel E, Loffler H, Buchner T, Ganser A, Heil G, Koch P, Freud M, Diedrich H, Ruhl H, Maschmeyer, G, Lipp T, Nowrousian M, Burket M, Gerecke D, Pralle H, Muller U, Lumscken C, Fulle H, Ho A, Kuchler R, Busch F, Schneider W, Gorg C, Emmerich B. Braumann D, Vaupel H, von Paleske A, Bartels H, Neiss A, Messerer D. Prognostic factors in a multicenter study for treatment of acute lymphoblastic leukemia in adults. Blood 1988; 71:123–131.

15. Bassan B. The management of infections in patients with leukemia. In: Henderson E, Lister T, Greaves M, eds. Leukemia. 6th ed. Philadelphia: W. B. Saunders, 1996:257–290.

16. Zinner S. Changing epidemiology of infections in patients with neutropenia and cancer: emphasis on gram-positive and resistant bacteria. Clin Infect Dis 1999; 29:490–494.

17. Gaytan-Martinez J, Mateos-Garcia E, Sanchez-Cortes E, Gonzalez-Llaven J, Casanova-Cardiel L, Fuentes-Allen J. Microbiologic findings in febrile neutropenia. Arch Med Res 2000; 31:388–392.

18. Anaissie E. Opportunistic mycoses in the immunocompromised host: experience at a cancer center and review. Clin Infect Dis 1992; 14(suppl 1):43–53.

19. Bodey G, Bolivar R, Fainstein V. Infectious complications in leukemia patients. Semin Hematol 1982; 19:193–226.

20. Garcia-Manero G, Kantarjian H. The hyper-CVAD regimen in adult acute lymphocytic leukemia. Hematol Oncol Clin North Am 2000; 14:1381 1398.

21. Pizzo P. Management of fever in patients with cancer and treatment-induced neutropenia. N Engl J Med 1993; 328:1323–1332.

22. Body G, Buckley M, Sathe Y, Freireich E. Quantitative relationship between circulating leukocytes and infection in patients with acute leukemia. Ann Intern Med 1966; 64:328–340.

23. Bodey G, Middleman E, Umsawadi T, Rodriguez V. Infection in cancer patients—results with gentamicin sulfate therapy. Cancer 1972; 23:1697–1701.

24. Gregory L, Williams R, Thompson E. Leukocyte function in Down's syndrome and acute leukemia. Lancet 1972; 1:1359 1361.

25. Pickering L, Anderson D, Choi S, Feigin R. Leukocyte function in children with malignancies. Cancer 1975; 35:1365–1371.

26. Chanock S. Evolving risk factors for infectious complications of cancer therapy. Hematol Oncol Clin North Am 1993; 7:771–793.

27. Chabner B, Longo D. Cancer chemotherapy and biotherapy. 2d ed. Philadelphia: Lippincott-Raven, 1996.

28. Giamarellou H, Antoniadou A. Infectious complications of febrile leukopenia. Infect Dis Clin North Am 2001; 15:457–482.

29. Bolivar R, Kohl S, Pickering L, Walters P. Effect of anti-neoplastic drugs on antibody dependent cellular cytotoxicity mediated by human leukocytes against *Herpes simplex* virus infected target cells. Cancer 1980; 46:1555–1561.

30. Schleimer R. An overview of glucocorticoid anti-inflammatory actions. Europ J Clin Pharmacol 1993; 45(suppl 1):3–7.

31. De Pauw B, Meunier F. Infections in patients with acute leukemia and lymphoma. In: Mandell G, Bennett J, Dolin R, eds. Principles and practice of infectious diseases. 5th ed. Philadelphia: Churchill Livingstone, 2000.

32. Ratcheson R, Ommaya A. Experience with the subcutaneous cerebrospinal-fluid reservoir. N Engl J Med 1968; 279:1025–1031.

33. Sutherland G, Palitang E, Marr J, Luedke S. Sterilization of ommaya reservoir by instillation of vancomycin. Am J Med 1981; 71:1068–1070.

34. Lishner M, Perrin R, Feld R, Messner H, Tuffnel P, Elhakin T, Matlow A, Curtis J. Complications associated with ommaya reservoirs in patients with cancer. Arch Intern Med 1990; 150:173–176.

35. Bochud P, Eggiman P, Calandra T, Van Melle G, Saghafi L, Francioli P. Bacteremia due to *Viridans streptococcus* in neutropenic patients with cancer: clinical spectrum and risk factors. Clin Infect Dis 1994; 18:25–31.

36. Burden A, Oppenheim B, Crowther D, Howell A, Morgenstern G, Scarffe J, Thatcher N. *Viridans streptococcal bacteremia* in patients with haematological and solid malignancies. Europ J Cancer 1991; 27:409–411.

37. Tasaka T, Nagai M, Sasaki K, Murata M, Taoka T, Ikeda K, Tanaka T, Takahara J, Irino S. *Streptococcus mitis septicemia* in leukemia patients; clinical features and outcome. Intern Med 1993; 32:221–224.

38. Edmond M, Ober J, Weinbaum D, Pfaller M, Hwang T, Sanford M, Wenzel R. Vancomycin-resistant *Enterococcus faecium bacteremia*: risk factors for infection. Clin Infect Dis 1995; 20:1126–1133.

39. Rampling A, Warren R, Bevan P, Hoggarth C, Swirsky D, Hayhoe F. Clostridium difficile in haematological malignancy. J Clin Pathol 1985; 38:445–451.

40. Cudmore M, Silva J, Fekety R, Liepman M, Kim K. Clostridium difficile colitis associated with cancer chemotherapy. Arch Intern Med 1982; 142:333–335.

41. Lorber B. Listeriosis. Clin Infect Dis 1997; 24:1–11.

42. Eckburg P, Montoya J, Vosti K. Brain abscess due to Listeria monocytogenes. Medicine 2001; 80:223–235.

43. Jagarlamudi R, Kumar L, Kochupillai V, Kapil A, Banerjee U, Thulkar S. Infections in acute leukemia: an analysis of 240 febrile episodes. Med Oncol 2000; 17:111 116.

44. Kern W, Andriof E, Oethinger M, Kern P, Hacker J, Marre R. Emergence of fluoroquinolone-resistant *Escherichia coli* at a cancer center. Antimicrob Agents Chemother 1994; 38:681–687.
45. Cometta A, Calandra T, Bille J, Glauser M. *Escherichia coli* resistance to fluoroquinolones in patients with cancer and neutropenia [letter]. N Engl J Med 1994; 330:1240–1241.
46. Heinemann M, Kern W, Bunjes D, Marre R, Essig A. Severe *Chlamydia pneumoniae* infection in patients with neutropenia: case reports and literature review. Clin Infect Dis 2000; 31:181–184.
47. Quigley M, Bethel K, Nowacki M, Millard F, Sharpe R. Neutropenic enterocolitis: a rare presenting complication of acute leukemia. Am J Hematol 2001; 66:213–219.
48. Nadiminti U, Greene J, Vincent A, Sandin R. Typhlitis in neutropenic patients: an analysis of thirty-nine patients in a cancer hospital. Infect Dis Clin Prac 2000; 9:153–156.
49. Marshall W, Keating M, Anhalt J, Steckelberg J. Xanthomonas maltophilia. An emerging clinical pathogen. Mayo Clin Proc 1989; 64:1097–1104.
50. Moser C, Jonsson V, Thomsen K, Albrectsen J, Hansen M, Prag J. Subcutaneous lesions and bacteraemia due to Stenotrophomonas maltophilia in three leukaemic patients with neutropenia. Br J Dermatol 1997; 136:949–952.
51. Arnaout M, Tamburro R, Bodner S, Sandlund J, Rivera G, Pui C, Ribeiro R. Bacillus cereus causing fulminant sepsis and hemolysis in two patients with acute leukemia. J Ped Hematol Oncol 1999; 21:431–435.
52. Musa M, Al Douri M, Khan S, Shafi T, Al Humaidi A, Al Rasheed A. Fulminant septicaemic syndrome of *Bacillus cereus*: three case reports. J Infect 1999; 39:154–156.
53. McWhinney P, Kibbler C, Gillespie S, Patel S, Morrison D, Hoffbrand A, Prentice H. *Stomatococcus mucilaginosus*: an emerging pathogen in neutropenic patients. Clin Infect Dis 1992; 14:641–646.
54. Goldman M, Chaudhary U, Greist A, Fausel C. Central nervous system infections due to *Stomatococcus* in immunocompromised hosts. Clin Infect Dis 1998; 27:1241–1246.
55. Fosi-Mbantenkhu J, Orett F. Predisposition to *Corynebacterium jeikeium* infection in acute lymphoblastic leukemia: a report of two cases in Trinidad. Med Ped Oncol 1994; 22:350–354.
56. Van der Lelie H, Leverstein-Van Hall M, Mertens M, Van Zaanen H, Van Oers R, Thomas B, Von dem Borne A, Kuijper E. *Corynebacterium* CDC group JK (*Corynebacterium jeikeium*) sepsis in haematological patients: a report of three cases and a systematic literature review. Scand J Infect Dis 1995; 27:581–584.
57. Bustamante C, Wade J. Herpes simplex virus infection in the immunocompromised cancer patient. J Clin Oncol 1991; 9:1015–1903.
58. Wirth K, Fetscher S, Neumann-Haefelin D, Herget G, Lubbert M. Fatal systemic herpes simplex virus type 1 infection during chemotherapy for acute lymphoblastic leukaemia. Br J Haematol 1999; 104:197–200.
59. Baglin T, Gray J, Marcus R, Wreghitt T. Antibiotic resistant fever associated

with herpes simplex infection in neutropenic patients with haematological malignancy. J Clin Pathol 1989; 42:1255–1258.

60. Ljungman P, Lonnqvist B, Gahrton G, Ringden O, Sundqvist V, Wahren B. Clinical and subclinical reactivations of *varicella-zoster* virus in immunocompromised patients. J Infect Dis 1986; 153:840–847.

61. Milone G, Di Raimondo F, Russo M, Cacciola E, Giustolisi R. Unusual onset of severe varicella in adult immunocompromised patients. Ann Hematol 1992; 64:155–156.

62. Wood M. Viral infections in neutropenia—current problems and chemotherapeutic control. J Antimicrob Chemo 1998; 41(suppl D):81–93.

63. Fujita H, Maruta A, Tomita N, Taguchi J, Sakai R, Shimizu A, Harada M, Ogawa K, Kodama F, Okubo T. Human herpesvirus-6–associated exanthema in a patient with acute lymphoblastic leukaemia. Br J Haematol 1996; 92:947–949.

64. Yoshikawa T, Suga S, Asano Y, Nakashima T, Yazaki T, Sobue R, Hirano M, Fukuda M, Kojima S, Matsuyama T. Human herpesvirus-6 infection in bone marrow transplantation. Blood 1991; 78:1381–1384.

65. Azzi A, Macchia P, Favra C, Nardi C, Zakrzewska K, Bartolomei C. Aplastic crisis caused by B19 virus in a child during induction therapy for acute lymphoblastic leukemia. Haematol 1989; 74:191–194.

66. De Renzo A, Azzi A, Zakrzewska K, Cicoira L, Notaro R, Rotoli B. Cytopenia caused by parvovirus in an adult ALL patient. Haematol 1994; 79:259–261.

67. Kurtzman G, Cohen B, Meyers P, Amunullah A, Young N. Persistent B19 parvovirus infection as a cause of severe chronic anemia in children with acute leukemia. Lancet 1988; 2:1159–1162.

68. Whimbey E, Couch R, Englund J, Andreeff M, Goodrich J, Raad I, Lewis V, Mirza N, Luna M, Baxter B, Tarrand J, Bodey G. Respiratory syncytial virus pneumonia in hospitalized adult patients with leukemia. Clin Infect Dis 1995; 21:376–379.

69. Guiot H, Fibbe W, van't Wout J. Risk factors for fungal infection in patients with malignant hematologic disorders: implications for empiric therapy and prophylaxis. Clin Infect Dis 1994; 18:525–532.

70. Richet M, Andremont A, Tancrede C, Pico J, Jarvis W. Risk factors for candidemia in patients with acute lymphocytic leukemia. Rev Infect Dis 1991; 13:211–215.

71. Wingard J. Importance of *Candida* species other than C, albicans as pathogens in oncology patients. Clin Infect Dis 1995; 20:115–125.

72. Maksymiuk A, Thongrasert S, Hopfer R, Luna M, Fainstein V, Bodey G. Systemic candidiasis in cancer patients. Am J Med 1984; 77:20–27.

73. Sanders S, Greene J, Sandin R. Disseminated candidiasis complicating treatment of acute leukemia. Infect Med 1999; 16:403–415.

74. Sallah S, Wan J, Nguyen N, Vos P, Sigounas G. Analysis of factors related to the occurrence of chronic disseminated candidiasis in patients with acute leukemia in a non–bone marrow transplant setting. Cancer 2001; 92:1349–1353.

75. Woolley I, Curtis D, Szer J, Fairley C, Vujovic O, Ugoni A, Spelman D. High

dose cytosine arabinoside is a major risk factor for the development of hepatosplenic candidiasis in patients with leukemia. Leuk Lymphoma 1997; 27:469–474.

76. Anttila V, Ruutu P, Bondestam S, Jansson S, Nordling S, Farkkila M, Sivonen A, Castren M, Ruutu T. Hepatosplenic yeast infection in patients with acute leukemia: a diagnostic problem. Clin Infect Dis 1994; 18:979–981.

77. Young R, Bennett J, Vogel C, Carbone P, DeVita V. Aspergillosis: the spectrum of the disease in 98 patients. Medicine 1970; 49:147–173.

78. Aisner J, Murillo J, Schimpff S, Steere A. Invasive aspergillosis in acute leukemia: correlation with nose cultures and antibiotic use. Ann Intern Med 1979; 90:4–9.

79. Gerson S, Talbot G, Hurwitz S, Strom B, Lusk E, Cassileth P. Prolonged granulocytopenia: the major risk factor for invasive pulmonary aspergillosis in patients with acute leukemia. Ann Intern Med 1984; 100:345–351.

80. Turner M, Russell L, Milne L, Parker A. Invasive aspergillosis in two patients with acute lymphoblastic leukaemia in complete remission. Postgrad Med J 1993; 69:408–410.

81. Ng T, Robson G, Denning D. Hydrocortisone-enhanced growth of Aspergillus species: implications for pathogenesis. Microbiol 1994; 140:2475–2479.

82. Gerson S, Talbot G, Lusk E, Hurwitz S, Strom B, Cassileth P. Invasive pulmonary aspergillosis in adult leukemia: clinical clues to its diagnosis. J Clin Oncol 1985; 3:1109–1116.

83. Talbot G, Huang A, Provencher M. Invasive aspergillus rhinosinusitis in patients with acute leukemia. Rev Infect Dis 1991; 13:219–232.

84. Kremery V, Krupova I, Denning D. Invasive yeast infections other than *Candida* spp. in acute leukemia. J Hosp Infect 1999; 41:181–194.

85. St-Germain G, Robert A, Ishak M, Tremblay C, Claveau S. Infection due to Rhizomucor pusillus: report of four cases in patients with leukemia and review. Clin Infect Dis 1993; 16:640–645.

86. Lerchenmuller C, Goner M, Buchner T, Berdel W. Rhinocerebral zygomycosis in a patient with acute lymphoblastic leukemia. Ann Oncol 2001; 12:415–419.

87. Suh I, Park C, Lee M, Lee J, Chang M, Woo J, Lee I, Ryu J. Hepatic and small bowel mucormycosis after chemotherapy in a patient with acute lymphoblastic leukemia. J Korean Med Sci 2000; 15:351–354.

88. Elnakadi I, Mehdi A, Franck S, Roger T, Larsimont D, Pector J. Cecal infarct: report of a case. Dis Colon Rectum 1998; 41:1585–1586.

89. Helm T, Longworth D, Hall G, Bolwell B, Fernandez B, Tomecki K. Case report and review of resolved fusariosis. J Am Ac Derm 1990; 23:393–398.

90. Boutati E, Anaissie E. Fusarium, a significant emerging pathogen in patients with hematologic malignancy: ten years' experience at a cancer center and implications for management. Blood 1997; 90:999–1008.

91. Berenguer J, Rodriguez-Tudela J, Richard C, Alvarez M, Sanz M, Gaztelurrutia L, Ayats J, Martinez-Suarez J. Deep infections caused by *Scedosporium prolificans*. Medicine 1997; 76:256–265.

92. Wood G, McCormack J, Muir D, Ellis D, Ridley M, Pritchard R, Harrison M.

Clinical features of human infection with *Scedosporium inflatum*. Clin Infect Dis 1992; 14:1027–1033.

93. Austen B, McCarthy H, Wilkins B, Smith A, Duncombe A. Fatal disseminated fusarium infection in acute lymphoblastic leukaemia in complete remission. J Clin Pathol 2001; 54:488–490.

94. Mardiak J, Danisovicova A, Trupl J, Sloboda J, Jesenska Z, Krcmery V. Three cases of fatal infection due to *Fusarium solani* in patients with cancer. Clin Infect Dis 1993; 17:930–932.

95. Loo V, Bertrand C, Dixon C, Vitye D, DeSalis B, McLean A, Brox A, Robson H. Control of construction-associated nosocomial aspergillosis in an antiquated hematology unit. Infect Control Hosp Epidemiol 1996; 17:360–364.

96. Levy V, Rio B, Bazarbach A, Hunault M, Delmer A, Zittoun R, Blanc V, Wolff M. Two cases of epidemic mucormycosis in patients with acute lymphoblastic leukemia. Am J Hematol 1996; 52:64–65.

97. Varthalitis I, Meunier F. Pneumocystis carinii pneumonia in cancer patients. Cancer Treat Rev 1993; 19:387–413.

98. Hughes W, Feldman S, Aur R, Verzosa M, Hustu O, Simone J. Intensity of immunosuppressive therapy and the incidence of *Pneumoncystis carinii* pneumonitis. Cancer 1975; 36:2004–2009.

99. Kritz A, Sepkowitz K, Weiss M, Telford P, Sogoloff H, Kempin S, Armstrong D, Gee T. Pneumocystis carinii pneumonia developing withn one month of intensive chemotherapy for treatment of acute lymphoblastic leukemia. N Engl J Med 1991; 325:661.

100. Hughes W, Rivera G, Schell M, Thornton D, Lott L. Successful intermittent chemoprophylaxis for Pneumocystis carinii pneumonitis. N Engl J Med 1987; 316:1627–1632.

101. Nagao T. Experience with protective isolation for infection prevention in the compromised host. Tokai J Exp Clin Med 1986; 11:23–28.

102. Mahood D, Dose A, Loprinzi C, Veeder M, Athmann L, Therneau T, Sorensen J, Gainey D, Mailliard J, Gusa N, Finck G, Johnson C, Goldberg R. Inhibition of fluorouracil-induced stomatitis by oral cryotherapy. J Clin Oncol 1991; 9: 449–452.

103. Dekker A, Rozenberg-Arska M, Verhoef J. Infection prophylaxis in acute leukemia: a comparison of ciprofloxacin with trimethoprim-sulfamethoxazole and colistin. Ann Intern Med 1987; 106:7–12.

104. Enno A, Darrel J, Hows J, Catovsky D, Goldman J, Galton D. Co-trimoxazole for prevention of infection in acute leukemia. Lancet 1978; 2:395–397.

105. Weiser B, Lange M, Fialk M, Singer C, Szatrowski T, Armstrong D. Prophylactic trimethoprim-sulfamethoxazole during consolidation chemotherapy for acute leukemia: a controlled trial. Ann Intern Med 1981; 95:436–438.

106. Bow E, Rayner E, Louie T. Comparison of norfloxacin with cotrimoxazole for infection prophylaxis in acute leukemia. Am J Med 1988; 84:847–854.

107. Winston D, Ho W, Nakao S, Gale R, Champlin R. Norfloxacin versus vancomycin/polymyxin for prevention of infections in granulocytopenic patients. Am J Med 1986; 80:884–890.

108. Del Favero A, Menichetti F. The new fluorinated quinolones for antimicrobial prophylaxis in neutropenic cancer patients. Eur J Cancer 1993; 29(suppl 1):2–6.

109. Hughes W, Armstrong D, Bodey G, Brown A, Edwards J, Feld R, Pizzo P, Rolston V, Shenep J, Young L. 1997 guidelines for the use of antimicrobial agents in neutropenic patients with unexplained fever. Clin Infect Dis 1997; 25:551 573.

110. Lonnqvist B, Palmblad J, Ljungman P, Grimfors G, Jarnmark M, Lerner R, Nystrom-Rosander C, Oberg G. Oral acyclovir as prophylaxis for bacterial infections during induction therapy for acute leukemia in adults. Support Care Cancer 1993; 1:129–144.

111. Uzun O, Anaissie E. Antifungal prophylaxis in patients with hematologic malignancies: a reappraisal. Blood 1995; 86:2063–2072.

112. Winston D, Chandrasekar P, Lazarus H, Goodman J, Silber J, Horowitz H, Shadduck R, Rosenfeld C, Ho W, Islam M, Buell D. Fluconazole prophylaxis of fungal infections in patients with acute leukemia. Ann Intern Med 1993; 118:495–503.

113. Wingard J, Mertz W, Rinaldi M, Johnson T, Karp J, Saral R. Increase in *Candida krusei* infection among patients with bone marrow transplantation and neutropenia treated prophylactically with fluconazole. N Engl J Med 1991; 325:1274–1277.

114. Hoppe J, Klingebiel T, Niethammer D. Selection of *Candida glabrata* in pediatric bone marrow transplant recipients receiving fluconazole. Pediatr Hematol Oncol 1994; 11:207–211.

115. Kunova A, Trupl J, Dluholcky S, Galova G, Krcmery V. Use of fluconazole is not associated with a higher incidence of *Candida krusei* and other non-*albicans Candida* species. Clin Infect Dis 1995; 21:226–227.

116. Viscoli C, Paesmans M, Sanz M, Castagnola E, Klastersky J, Martino P, Glauser M. Association between antifungal prophylaxis and rate of documented bacteremia in febrile neutropenic cancer patients. Clin Infect Dis 2001; 32:1532–1537.

117. Palmblad J, Lonnqvist B, Carlsson B, Grimfors G, Jarnmark M, Lerner R, Ljungman P, Nystrom-Rosander C, Petrini B, Oberg G. Oral ketoconazole prophylaxis for *Candida* infections during induction therapy for acute leukemia in adults: more bacteraemias. J Intern Med 1992; 231:363–370.

118. Rose H. Mechanical control of hospital ventilation and aspergillus infections. Am Rev Respir Dis 1972; 105:207–306.

119. Persat F, Marzullo C, Guyotat D, Rochet M, Piens M. Plasma itraconazole concentrations in neutropenic patients after repeated high-dose treatment. Eur J Cancer 1992; 28:838–841.

120. Jeffery G, Beard M, Ikram R, Chua J, Allen J, Heaton D, Hart D, Schousboe M. Intranasal amphotericin B reduces the frequency of invasive aspergillosis in neutropenic patients. Am J Med 1991; 90:685 692.

121. Cushing D, Bustamante C, Devlin A, Finley R, Wade J. Aspergillus infection prophylaxis: amphotericin B (AB) nose spray, a double blind trial. Proceedings of the 31st Interscience Conference on Antimicrobial Agents and Chemo-

therapy, Chicago, IL. Washington DC: American Society for Microbiology, September, 1991 (abstr 737).

122. Schwartz S, Behre G, Heinemann V, Wandt H, Schilling E, Arning M, Trittin A, Kern W, Boenisch O, Bosse D, Lenz K, Ludwig W, Hiddemann W, Siegert W, Beyer J. Aerosolized amphotericin B inhalations as prophylaxis of invasive aspergillus infections during prolonged neutropenia: results of a prospective randomized multicenter trial. Blood 1999; 93:3654–3661.

123. Lieschke G, Burgess A. Granulocyte colony-stimulating factor and granulo-cyte-macrophage colony-stimulating factor (second of two parts). N Engl J Med 1992; 327:99–106.

124. Hoelzer D. Acute lymphocytic leukemia in adults. In: Hoffman R, Benz E, Shattil S, Furie B, Cohen H, Silberstein L, McGlave P, eds. Hematology: Basic Principles and Practice. 3rd ed. Philadelphia: Churchill-Livingston, 2000:1089–1105.

125. Kantarjian H, Estey E, O'Brien S, Anaissie E, Beran M, Pierce S, Robertson L, Keating M. Granulocyte colony-stimulating factor supportive treatment following intensive chemotherapy in acute lymphocytic leukemia in first remission. Cancer 1993; 72:2950–2955.

126. Geissler K, Koller E, Hubmann E, Niederwieser D, Hinterberger H, Geissler D, Kyrle P, Knobl P, Pabinger I, Thalhammer R, Schwartzinger I, Mannhalter C, Jaeger U, Heinz R, Linkesch W, Lechner K. Granulocyte colony-stimulating factor as an adjunct to induction chemotherapy for adult acute lymphoblastic leukemia—a randomized phase-III study. Blood 1997; 90:590–596.

127. Ottmann O, Hoelzer D, Gracien E, Ganser A, Kelly K, Reutzel R, Lipp T, Busch F, Schwonzen M, Heil G, Wandt H, Koch P, Kolbe K, Heyll A, Bentz M, Peters S, Diedrich H, Dethling J, Meyer P, Nowrousian M, Loffler B, Weiss A, Kneba M, Foller A, Graf M, Hecht T. Concomitant granulocyte colony-stimulating factor and induction chemoradiotherapy in adult lymphoblastic leukemia: a randomized phase III trial. Blood 1995; 86:444–450.

128. Kantarjian H, Estey E, O'Brien S, Anaissie E, Beran M, Rios M, Keating M, Gutterman J. Intensive chemotherapy with mitoxantrone and high-dose cytosine arabinoside followed by granulocyte macrophage colony-stimulating factor in the treatment of patients with acute lymphoblastic leukemia. Blood 1992; 79:876–881.

129. Papamichael D, Andrews T, Owen D, Carter M, Amess J, Lister T, Rohatiner A. Intensive chemotherapy for adult acute lymphoblastic leukemia given with or without granulocyte-macrophage colony-stimulating factor. Ann Hematol 1996; 73:259–263.

130. Pui C, Boyett J, Hughes W, Rivera G, Hancock M, Sandlund J, Synold T, Relling M, Ribeiro R, Crist W, Evans W. Human granulocyte colony-stimulating factor after induction therapy in children with acute lymphoblastic leukemia. N Engl J Med 1997; 336:1781–1787.

131. Mitchell P, Morland B, Stevens M, Dick G, Easlea D, Meyer L, Pinkerton C. Granulocyte colony-stimulating factor in established febrile neutropenia: a randomized study of pediatric patients. J Clin Oncol 1997; 15:1163–1170.

132. Ottman O, Hoelzer D. Growth factors in the treatment of acute lymphoblastic leukemia. Leuk Res 1998; 22:1171–1178.
133. Welte K, Gabrilove J, Bronchud M, Platzer E, Morstyn G. Filgrastim (r-metHuG-CSF): the first 10 years. Blood 1996; 88:1907–1929.
134. Hubel K, Dale D, Liles W. Granulocyte transfusion therapy: update on potential clinical applications. Cur Opin Hematol 2001; 8:161–164.
135. Dignani M, Anaissie E, Hester J, O'Brien S, Vartivarian S, Rex J, Kantarjian H, Jendiroba D, Lichtiger B, Andersson B, Freireich E. Treatment of neutropenia-related fungal infections with granulocyte colony stimulating factor–elicited white blood cell transfusions: a pilot study. Leukemia 1997; 11:1621–1630.

4

Infection in Patients with Acute Myelogenous Leukemia

Indra Dé and Kenneth V. I. Rolston
The University of Texas M. D. Anderson Cancer Center
Houston, Texas, U.S.A.

INTRODUCTION

Infection is common among patients with acute leukemia [1]. The frequency and type of infections complicating acute myelogenous leukemia (AML) depends on the state of disease and the treatment status [2]. Two-thirds of patients with AML develop infection after remission induction chemotherapy, and one-third do so after consolidation therapy [3,4]. There is a marked reduction in the probability of infection once remission has been achieved and the bone marrow and peripheral blood have been repopulated with morphologically and functionally normal cells.

The most important factor that predisposes patients with AML to infection is neutropenia (Table 1). This may be the result of the underlying disease and is compounded by the use of intensive antineoplastic therapy. The risk of infection increases when the absolute neutrophil count (ANC) falls below $1000/mm^3$ [5]. The severity and duration of neutropenia are both important factors. It has been estimated that all patients with an ANC of $\leq 100/mm^3$ for 3 weeks will develop a serious infection. In addition to quantitative

TABLE 1 Predisposing Factors for Infection in Patients with Acute
Myelogenous Leukemia

Factor	Comment
Quantitative neutropenia (ANC $\leq$ 500/mm^3)	Chemotherapy-induced, underlying disease
Qualitative neutropenia (defects in neutrophil function)	Underlying disease IL-2 (?)
Disruption of anatomical barriers	
Mucosal surfaces	Chemotherapy, medical devices
Skin	Vascular access catheters and other medical devices, invasive procedures

neutropenia, patients with AML have defects in neutrophil function as well.
Studies in the early 1970s using morphologically mature neutrophils from
nonneutropenic patients with acute myelomonocytic leukemia showed that
these cells were able to phagocytize certain bacteria and fungi but failed to kill
them. This functional impairment was seen among patients not treated with
any chemotherapy and may be an intrinsic feature of the disease itself [6–8].
Mobilization of leukocytes in AML patients is also abnormal. In one study of
22 patients with AML, 17 had defect in leukocyte mobilization. Fourteen of
the 17 patients subsequently developed serious bacterial infections, 11 of them
being fatal. The leukocyte mobilization defect was present in treatment-naïve
as well as in treated patients with active leukemia, and it resulted more often in
infection and septic death and led to less frequent remissions [9,10]. Cell-
mediated immunity is usually not affected in therapy-naïve AML patients. In
general, humoral immunity is relatively unaffected in acute stages of therapy
for AML. As the disease progresses and/or as more intense chemotherapy is
administered, antibody-synthesizing capacity declines.

SPECIAL CONSIDERATIONS

Neutropenic patients including those with AML often fail to develop
symptoms and signs of infection because of their limited ability to mount
an inflammatory response. Only 8% of patients with severe neutropenia
(< 100/mL) who developed pneumonia produced purulent sputum, compared
to 84% who had adequate neutrophils (> 1000/mL) [11]. Neutropenic
patients with pneumonia may not show a pulmonary infiltrate on chest radiographs, and these patients may have meningitis without overt meningeal signs.

Fever may be the initial and in many cases the only sign of infection in neutropenic patients. Approximately 60% of febrile episodes in neutropenic patients are not associated with any signs or symptoms. Seventy percent respond to antibiotic therapy, suggesting that many of them are probably undetected infections [12]. Rarely, an infection may develop in the absence of fever, as with certain organisms like *Clostridium septicum*, or if the patient is receiving corticosteroids. Patients with AML frequently develop infection at unusual sites and/or with uncommon manifestations.

Typhilitis, an inflammatory process most commonly involving the caecum, occurs almost exclusively in patients with acute leukemia, especially children. Perirectal infections with extensive tissue necrosis extending to the rectum can occur in neutropenic patients, underscoring the importance of a perirectal examination in these patients. Meningitis is not common in neutropenic patients, and as noted above, when it occurs, it does not produce characteristic signs of infection. Organisms that are uncommon causes of meningitis in normal host, like *Escherichia coli, Pseudomonas aeruginosa, Enterococcus faecalis*, and *Clostridium perfringens*, can cause meningitis in this group of patients. Endocarditis is a rare infection in neutropenic patients. In a review of 420 patients with acute leukemia, none had endocarditis [13]. Fulminant endocarditis with unusual organisms like *Corynebacterium jeikeium* and *Bacillus* spp. with fatal outcome has been known to occur in acute leukemia patients with neutropenia. *Pseudomonas aeruginosa* can cause a variety of unusual infections including ecthyma of the lip, tonsil, and palate and multiple ecthyma gangrenosa lesions involving the skin, resembling septic emboli from endocarditis. Infection can disseminate rapidly in patients with severe neutropenia. Clinical and/or statistically derived prediction rules to identify such high-risk patients are unreliable, underscoring the importance of early, broad-spectrum antibiotic therapy in AML patients likely to have severe and prolonged neutropenia [14]. Finally, it is important to consider noninfectious causes of fever in these patients including the underlying leukemia, transfusion reactions, chemotherapy, (occasionally) antimicrobial therapy, colony-stimulating factors, or allergic/drug reactions.

ORGANISMS ASSOCIATED WITH INFECTION IN PATIENTS WITH AML

A large number of bacteria and fungi cause infections in patients with AML. The most common pathogens are listed in Table 2. Bacterial infections tend to occur more often during early phases of neutropenia, whereas fungal infections are recognized more often in patients with persistent neutropenia.

TABLE 2 Common Causes of Infection in Patients with
Acute Myelogenous Leukemia

BACTERIA
   Coagulase-negative staphylococci
   Staphylococcus aureus (including MRSA)
   Alpha-hemolytic (viridans) streptococci
   Enterococcus species (including VRE)
   Enterobacteriaceae (*E. coli, Klebsiella* spp., *Proteus* spp.,
      Serratia spp., *Citrobacter* spp., *Enterobacter* spp.)
   Pseudomonas aeruginosa
   Stenotrophomonas maltophilia
   Acinetobacter species
FUNGI
   Candida species
   Aspergillus species
VIRUSES
   Herpes viruses (HSV, VZV, CMV)
   Community respiratory viruses

BACTERIAL INFECTIONS

The spectrum of bacterial infection has undergone several periodic shifts in
the past four decades [15]. Enteric gram-negative bacilli (*Escherichia coli,
Klebsiella* spp., *Pseudomonas aeruginosa*), along with *Staphylococcus aureus*,
were the pathogens most frequently associated with bacteremia and serious
sepsis in the 1960s and 1970s. The spectrum then shifted to a predominance of
gram-positive organisms (coagulase-negative staphylococci, viridans streptococci, enterococci, etc.), and some centers reported gram-positive bacteremia rates of 60 to 70% [16,17]. The reasons for this shift are thought to be the
increased use of intravascular devices, prophylaxis with fluoroquinolones and
trimethoprim-sulfamethoxazole (TMP-SMX), which suppress gram-negative
but not gram-positive organisms, the prompt use of antimicrobial regimens
directed against gram-negative organisms when patients present with fever
and neutropenia, and chemotherapy-associated mucositis. In a recent report
of 42 patients with AML undergoing chemotherapy, gram-positive microorganisms accounted for 75.8% of blood isolates. Coagulase negative staph-
ylococcic and viridans streptococci accounted for more than half of the blood
isolates. Twelve percent of the bacteremic episodes were caused by gram-
negative organisms. The gram-negative bacteremia occurred in patients not
receiving fluoroquinolone prophylaxis, whereas all the patients with gram-
positive bacteremia were on fluoroquinolone prophylaxis at the time of the
bacteremic episode [18].

The pendulum may now be swinging back toward gram-negative bacillary infections. The most recent EORTC-IATG trial, conducted between 1997 and 2000, documented an increased incidence of single-agent gram-negative bacteremia from 6.5 to 12% in neutropenic patients. Also noticed was a decline in the prophylactic use of fluoroquinolones [19]. Similar trends are being seen at other institutions (R. Ramphal—personal communication; K. Rolston, unpublished data). Unfortunately, an alarming trend toward multidrug resistance has been observed among recent gram-negative isolates (*P. aeruginosa*, *Acinetobacter* spp., *Stenotrophomonas maltophilia*, etc.) [20].

Polymicrobial infections occur more often in patients with acute leukemia than other subsets of neutropenic patients. Currently, polymicrobial infections account for 25 to 30% of bacterial infections in neutropenic patients, and their frequency has almost doubled since the 1970s [16]. Approximately 80% of such infections have at least one gram-negative species isolated from microbiological cultures, and 33% are caused by multiple gram-negative species [21]. Most of these infections are tissue-based and manifest as pneumonias, perirectal infections or other necrotic soft-tissue infections, and neutropenic enterocolitis [22,23]. Approximately 8 to 12% of vascular catheter-related infections are also polymicrobial (gram-positives ± gram-negatives ± yeasts). In general, mortality rates are higher in polymicrobial infections than in single organism infections. Polymicrobial infections that include yeast, anaerobes, or *Pseudomonas aeruginosa* have mortality rates greater than 50% [21].

FUNGAL INFECTIONS

Fungal infections in patients with AML are caused most often by *Candida* spp. and *Aspergillus* spp. [24] (Table 2). Although *Candida albicans* is still the most commonly isolated species, there are several recent reports documenting the emergence of other *Candida* species as frequent and significant pathogens [25–27]. As with emerging bacterial organisms, these *Candida* species (*C. krusei, C. glabrata, C. lusitaniae*) are generally less susceptible to or resistant to currently available antifungal agents. Similarly, although *Aspergillus fumigatus* is the most common species, other species such as *A. terreus* are being isolated with increasing frequency and might be associated with greater resistance to antifungal agents. A large number of other yeasts and molds are capable of causing opportunistic infections in patients with AML (Table 3).

VIRAL INFECTIONS

Infections caused by herpes viruses such as herpes simplex virus (HSV-1 and HSV-2), varicella-zoster virus (VZV), cytomegalovirus (CMV), Epstein–Barr

TABLE 3   Uncommon and "Emerging" Pathogens in Patients with AML

GRAM-POSITIVE BACTERIA	FUNGI
Aerococcus species	Absidia species
Bacillus species	Acremonium species
Corynebacterium species	Alternaria species
Gemella species	Bipolaris species
Leuconostoc species	Blastoschizomyces capitatus
Micrococcus species	Curvularia species
Pediococcus species	Fusarium species
Rhodococcus species	Geotrichum species
Stomatococcus species	Malassezia furfur
	Pseudoallescheria species
	Rhizopus species
	Rhodotorula species
	Scedosporium species
	Trichosporon species
GRAM-NEGATIVE BACTERIA	
Alcaligenes xylosoxidans	
Burkholderia cepacia	
Chyseobacterium meningosepticum	
Flavimonas oxyzihabitans	
Methylobacterium species	
Pseudomonas spp. (P. putida, P. fluorescens)	

virus (EBV), and Human herpes virus-6 (HHV-6) are not uncommon in AML patients. Although most of these infections are localized, they are frequently recurrent, and when they disseminate, they can be associated with substantial morbidity and mortality. The role of other viruses (influenza, parainfluenza, respiratory syncitial virus, adenovirus, etc.) as significant causes of infection in patients with AML is less clear, but recent data indicate that these viruses are infrequent but important pathogens [28,29]. Increased awareness and newer diagnostic techniques are likely to shed further light on the role that these viruses play in such patients. Several epidemiological studies at large cancer treatment centers are evaluating these and other viral pathogens in high-risk patients.

INFECTIONS CAUSED BY SPECIFIC PATHOGENS

Gram-Positive Organisms

Coagulase-negative staphylococci are the most frequently isolated organisms from neutropenic cancer patients including those with AML [15,30]. The predominant species is *Staphylococcus epidermidis*, although *Staphylococcus hominis* and *Staphylococcus haemolyticus* are often isolated. The frequent occurrence of infections by these normal skin flora may be attributed to the increased use of intravascular devices, surgery, and trauma. The GI tract is also a major source of coagulase-negative staphylococci in febrile neutropenic patients gaining access to the bloodstream through chemotherapy-damaged mucosa. Bacteremia, often catheter-related, is the most common manifestation of staphylococcal infection. Skin and soft tissue infections including surgical wound infections and cellulitis are also common. Although thought to be low-virulence organisms, these organisms can occasionally cause serious, sometimes fatal infections, like septic thrombophlebitis and visceral abscesses in neutropenic patients. Therefore positive blood cultures, if obtained properly, should not be discounted as a contaminant in these patients.

Some institutions have documented a decline in infections caused by *Staphylococcus aureus* [31]. Mortality is higher with methicillin-resistant strains of *S. aureus* (MRSA) than with methicillin-susceptible strains [32]. Infections caused by methicillin-resistant strains are more likely in patients receiving antibacterial prophylaxis or prolonged treatment with broad-spectrum antibacterial agents [33]. The recent emergence of *Staphylococcus* spp. with reduced susceptibility or resistance to vancomycin is of great concern.

The treatment of Staphylococcal infection should be guided by antimicrobial susceptibility. *Staphylococcus aureus* isolates are susceptible to methicillin more often (60–80%) than coagulase-negative staphylococci (5–15%). Methicillin-susceptible strains can be treated with a semisynthetic penicillin (naficillin, oxacillin). Most broad-spectrum agents used for empiric therapy in febrile neutropenic patients (cefepime, imipenem, meropenem, piperacillin-tazobactam) are also active against these isolates [34]. Vancomycin is a suitable alternative in patients with serious beta-lactam allergy and for methicillin-resistant strains. Older agents (tetracyclines, TMP/SMX, rifampin) and newer agents (linezolid, quinopristin-dalforpristin) are also useful for the treatment of staphylococcal infections.

Once considered commensals, viridans (alpha-hemolytic) streptococci are common causes of infection in patients with AML. Common predisposing factors include profound neutropenia, oral mucositis often as a result of cytosine arabinoside therapy, antimicrobial prophylaxis (TMP/SMX, quinolones), and histamine type 2 antagonists [35]. The predominant species are *Streptococcus mitis*, *Streptococcus sanguis*, *Streptococcus salivarius*, and *Streptococcus milleri*. Bacteremia is the most common infection, and it usually responds favorably to therapy. A more serious form of infection can also occur. In 1990, Arning et al. [36] published a report of eight cases of *Streptococcus mitis* bacteremia in acute leukemia patients, most of whom subsequently developed acute respiratory distress syndrome. Engel et al. [37] showed increased levels of proinflammatory cytokines, such as IL1, IL-6, and TNF-α, in patients with neutropenia and alpha-hemolytic streptococcal toxic shock syndrome with death rates up to 30%, despite appropriate antibiotics and clearance of bacteremia.

There is increasing concern that antibiotic resistance in viridans streptococci is increasing, with 13% of the isolates resistant to penicillin, 17% to ceftriaxone, and more than 33% to macrolides [38]. Resistance to vancomycin and aminoglycosides has also been reported [39,40]. Empiric antibiotic therapy should be based on local susceptibility patterns of clinical isolates.

Infections caused by beta-hemolytic streptococci (*S. pyogenes*, *Streptococcus* groups B, C, G, F) are uncommon in patients with AML, as are infections with *Streptococcus pneumoniae*. Most beta-hemolytic streptococci remain penicillin-susceptible (although penicillin and vancomycin tolerance has been reported). Up to 60% of pneumococcal isolates can have low-level penicillin resistance, and 15 to 25% demonstrate high-level penicillin resistance. Most broad-spectrum agents (cefepime, imipenem, meropenem) used for empiric therapy in patients with AML are active against these organisms [34].

Enterococcus species now rank as the third most common gram-positive organisms after coagulase-negative staphylococci and *Streptococcus* spp. [16]. This increased frequency is associated with increased use of extended spectrum cephalosporins to which the organisms are naturally resistant, increased use of fluoroquinolone prophylaxis, increases in empiric glycopeptide therapy, and prolonged hospital stay. The infections most commonly caused by these organisms are bacteremias, urinary tract, wounds, and intra-abdominal infections. *Enterococcus faecalis* is the predominant species, being isolated in 60 to 75% of enterococcal infections. Most isolates are susceptible to penicillin, ampicillin, and vancomycin. Aminoglyocosides provide synergistic activity when used in combination with these antibiotics and are recommended for serious enterococcal infections. Infections with *E. faecium* are rising, and they are more common in neutropenic patients. These organisms are often resistant to the penicillins, aminoglycosides, and glycopeptides and represent a treatment dilemma when all three resistance patterns are seen in the same strain. Several reports have documented that vancomcyin-resistant enterococci (VRE) are encountered more frequently in neutropenic cancer patients, including those with AML [41]. Infection with VRE occurs almost exclusively in patients with fecal colonization. A recent study from the University of Texas M. D. Anderson Cancer Center documented VRE fecal colonization rates of 59/1000 in patients with acute leukemia, with approximately 34% of these patients developing bacteremia following subsequent chemotherapy [42]. Until recently, the treatment of multidrug resistant VRE posed a significant problem, showing very few therapeutic options. Two new agents have now been approved for the treatment of infections caused by VRE. These include quinopristin-dalfopristin, and the oxazolidinone linezolid. Neither of these agents is bactericidal against VRE, and the response rate (55 to 65%) is substantially lower than those achieved for standard enterococcal infections using bactericidal combinations [43]. Agents under evaluation for resistant gram-positive organisms including MRSA and VRE include daptomycin and oritavancin.

There is a growing list of "new" gram-positive pathogens that cause a variety of infections in AML patients (Table 3). These include *Corynebacterium jeikeium*, *Stomatococcus mucilaginosus*, *Bacillus* spp., *Rhodococcus equi*, *Aerococcus* spp., and *Gemella* spp. Organisms with intrinsic vancomycin resistance including *Leuconostoc* spp., *Pediococcus* spp., and *Lactobacillus* spp. are uncommon but appear to be increasing in frequency. Knowledge of local epidemiology and susceptibility/resistance patterns is vital for the appropriate management of these infections.

Gram-Negative Bacilli

The overall frequency of infections caused by enteric, gram-negative bacilli has declined substantially in recent years, particularly in patients with AML, who often receive fluoroquinolone prophylaxis [15–17]. Currently, approximately 15 to 20% of documented single-organism bacterial infections are caused by gram-negative bacilli [16]. As indicated earlier, approximately 80% of polymicrobial infections have a gram-negative component, increasing the overall frequency of gram-negative infections to 35 to 45 percent [16,21]. Although gram-negative infections are being documented less often, the proportion of infections caused by various gram-negative species has not changed much [20]. *Escherichia coli*, *Pseudomonas aeruginosa*, and *Klebseilla* spp. are the three most common organisms isolated, accounting for 60% of all gram-negative infections. Other, so-called secondary gram-negative pathogens include *Enterobacter* spp., *Serratia* spp., *Citrobacter* spp., *Acinetobacter* spp., and *Stenotrophomonas maltophilia*. Many other gram-negative organisms are capable of causing opportunistic infections in neutropenic patients with AML. The clinical characteristics of these infections are not unique, and fever is the most consistent, and often the only, manifestation. Overall, gram-negative infections are associated with substantially greater morbidity and mortality than gram-positive infection [44].

Particular attention needs to be focused on *P. aeruginosa*. In addition to an overall decline in documented gram-negative infections, some institutions have also reported a disproportionate decline in infections caused by *P. aeruginosa* [45]. However, data from several European and American centers indicate that this is still a common pathogen in neutropenic patients [20,46–49]. Consequently, empiric therapy in neutropenic AML patients should include potent pseudomonal coverage. Two large reviews of *P. aeruginosa* bacteremias in cancer patients conducted at The University of Texas M. D. Anderson Cancer Center have revealed several important facts including the following:

> These infections are most common in patients with acute leukemia, especially AML.
>
> A substantial proportion of these infections (50%) are community acquired.
>
> Response to appropriate antimicrobial therapy is in the range of 75 to 80%.
>
> Factors associated with poor response rates include the presence of septic shock, persistent neutropenia, deep tissue involvement (pneumonia, enterocolitis, perirectal infection, soft tissue infection with ≥5 cm necrosis), and inappropriate initial therapy [50,51].

Infections caused by nonaeruginosa *Pseudomonas* spp. (*P. fluorescens*, *P. putida*, *P. stutzeri*) and *S. maltophilia* are being documented with greater frequency in patients with acute leukemia. This may be partly due to the fact that most quinolones used for antimicrobial prophylaxis in such patients have variable or poor activity against these organisms [52]. *Stenotrophomonas maltophilia* and *Alcaligenes* spp. are among the most resistant gram-negative organisms encountered in clinical practice today, and therapy is often a challenge.

Anaerobic Infections

Anaerobes are seldom isolated from neutropenic patients including those with AML. The reasons for this are poorly understood. It is customary to consider anaerobes as potential pathogens among patients with central nervous system infections, mucositis, pneumonia (particularly following aspiration), typhlitis/enterocolitis, intra-abdominal/pelvic abscesses, and perirectal infections. *Clostridium* spp. have been associated with necrotizing fascitis, enterocolitis, disseminated infections, and severe sepsis. Toxin-mediated pseudomembranous colitis secondary to *Clostridium difficile* is the most common gastrointestinal infection among patients with leukemia. Both antineoplastic chemotherapy and repeated courses of antimicrobial therapy predispose patients to this infection.

Fungal Infections

The most common yeast infection in neutropenic patients including those with AML is candidiasis [24–26]. The incidence of this infection has decreased substantially ever since the practice of using azoles (fluconazole, itraconazole) for antifungal prophylaxis in such patients became widespread [26]. The clinical spectrum of candidiasis consists of local and systemic infections. Local manifestations include thrush, esophagitis, vaginitis, and urinary tract infection (UTI). Epiglottitis is a rare form of locally invasive *Candida* infection seen predominantly in leukemic patients. Systemic infections include candidemia (often vascular catheter related), acute (hematogenous) dissemination, and chronic (hepatosplenic) systemic candididasis. Patients with hematogenous dissemination may develop various end organ infections including endophthalmitis, osteomyelitis, cutaneous lesions, septic arthritis, hepatic, splenic, or renal abscesses, and endocarditis [53]. As indicated earlier, many studies have documented the changing epidemiology of *Candida* infections with decreasing isolation rate of *C. albicans* and increasing isolation rates of other *Candida* species.

Aspergillosis is the most common mold infection in patients with AML. Infection rates appear to be increasing, since azole prophylaxis, particularly with fluconazole, is ineffective for the prevention of this infection. Aspergillosis can also have localized or invasive manifestations. Localized infection include primary cutaneous infection, sinusitis, tracheobronchitis, and aspergilloma. Invasive infections include pulmonary aspergillosis, sino-orbital infection, and disseminated infection, including cerebral aspergillosis. The epidemiology of *Aspergillus* infections may also be changing, with increasing isolation rates of *A. terreus* and other nonfumigatus species [53].

A large number of yeasts and molds have been responsible for occasional infection in patients with AML. These include *Trichosporon beigellii, Malassezia furfur, Fusarium* spp., the *Zygomycetes, Bipolaris*, and other dematiaceous fungi. A detailed description of infections caused by these uncommon organisms is presented in another chapter.

TREATMENT OF INFECTIONS IN PATIENTS WITH AML

Empiric Therapy

The administration of empiric, broad-spectrum antimicrobial therapy when AML patients develop a febrile neutropenic episode is considered standard [14]. Several therapeutic choices exist (Table 4). Individual institutions need to tailor the use of specific antimicrobial agents based on local epidemiology and susceptibility/resistance patterns. Many experts still favor combination regimens that are potentially bactericidal over single-agent therapy (monotherapy), especially in high-risk patients, such as those with AML undergoing remission induction chemotherapy. However, most clinical trials have not demonstrated the superiority of combination regimens over currently available, broad-spectrum agents used for monotherapy [14]. Combination reg-

TABLE 4 Choices for Empirical Therapy in AML Patients with Fever and Neutropenia

---

COMBINATION REGIMENS (WITHOUT VANCOMYCIN)
  Aminoglycoside + antipseudomonal penicillin, extended-spectrum cephalosporin, carbapenem or quinolone
COMBINATION REGIMENS (WITH VANCOMYCIN)[a]
  Vancomycin + extended spectrum cephalosporin, carbapenem, monobactam, antipseudomonal penicillin, or quinolone (± aminoglycoside)
SINGLE-AGENT REGIMENS (MONOTHERAPY)
  Extended-spectrum cephalosporin
  Carbapenem

---

[a] No data yet on combinations replacing vancomycin with newer agents—linezolid or quinopristin/dalfopristin.

imens may reduce the overall emergence of resistant organisms, but they may be associated with increased toxicity and costs.

Combinations that do not include initial use of a glycopeptide generally consist of an aminoglycoside (amikacin, tobramycin, gentamicin) along with an extended spectrum cephalosporin (cefepime, ceftazidime), a carbapenem (imipenem, meropenem), an antipseudomonal penicillin ± a beta-lactamase inhibitor (piperacillin/tazobactam) or a quinolone (ciprofloxacin). When more potent gram-positive coverage is needed, combining vancomycin with beta-lactams or a quinolone might be indicated. Based on current susceptibility patterns and the epidemiology of infections among patients with AML, cefepime, imipenem, and meropenem are the most appropriate agents for monotherapy [34,54]. Combination therapy might be preferable in certain situations such as polymicrobial infections, complicated tissue-based infections (pneumonia, enterocolitis, perirectal infections), or infections caused by *P. aeruginosa*.

Approximately 55 to 85% of patients will respond to the initial regimen [14]. It is customary to treat for approximately 72 to 96 hours before making modifications, in order to allow enough time for the initial regimen to produce a response. Modifications depend upon the clinical setting (e.g., suspected catheter-related infection, abdominal focus, etc.) and microbiological data. The most common modifications include the addition of a glycopeptide if not used initially, or the addition of an antifungal agent. The choice of antifungal agent will depend upon the use of antifungal prophylaxis and the nature of the suspected fungal infection (yeast vs. mold). In general, amphotericin B or one of its lipid preparations is used in this setting. Newer agents (voriconazole, caspofungin, etc.) are also being evaluated for empirical antifungal use in persistently febrile neutropenic patients [55].

The length of therapy depends upon the type of infection (UTI, bacteremia, pneumonia, etc.) and the persistence of, or recovery from, neutropenia. Most experts continue therapy until all signs and symptoms have resolved, the patient has been afebrile for 4 or 5 days, and cultures (if initially positive) have been rendered negative. Some experts recommend continuing therapy until resolution of neutropenia (ANC $\geq 500/mm^3$ for 2 days).

Specific Therapy

Among patients with microbiologically documented infections (bacteria, fungal, viral), therapy can be tailored to the specific pathogen isolated based on local susceptibility patterns. The agents used most often, and newer options, are listed in Table 5. The isolation of a specific pathogen, particularly if it is a gram-positive organism, does not necessarily permit the use of narrow-spectrum agents, in severely neutropenic patients, since these patients often have occult gram-negative or polymicrobial infections. Our antifungal armamentarium is expanding, and several newer triazoles and echinocandins have either recently become available or are nearing approval. The need to

TABLE 5 Therapeutic Agents for the Treatment of Systemic Infections in AML Patients

---

ANTIBACTERIAL AGENTS
  Narrow-spectrum (gram-positive)
    Penicillin, nafcillin or oxacillin
    Vancomycin
    Linezolid, quinopristin/dalfopristin
  Narrow-spectrum (gram-negative)
    Aminoglycosides
    Aztreonam
  Narrow-spectrum (anaerobic)
    Metronidazole, clindamycin
  Broad-spectrum
    Meropenem, imipenem
    Cefepime, ceftazidime
    Piperacillin/tazobactam
ANTIFUNGAL AGENTS
  Polyenes
    Amphotericin B (including lipid preparations)
  Azoles
    Fluconazole, itraconazole, voriconazole
  Echinocandins
    Caspofungin

develop newer antiviral agents has reached its peak, since our ability to treat most viral infections is rather limited.

ANTIMICROBIAL PROPHYLAXIS

Antibacterial prophylaxis has been shown to reduce the frequency and severity of gram-negative infections, but to have no impact on or occasionally to lead to an increase in gram-positive infection [56]. It is only recommended among patients anticipated to have severe neutropenia for >14 days. The quinolones (ofloxacin, ciprofloxacin) and TMP/SMX have been used most often for prophylaxis. The newer quinolones (gatifloxacin, moxifloxacin) need to be evaluated, since they have much more potent and expanded gram-positive activity [57–59]. The emergence of resistant organisms is a significant drawback of prophylaxis strategies [60].

Antifungal prophylaxis (fluconazole) has been shown to reduce the frequency of infections caused by *Candida* spp. [61]. Mold infections have proven to be much more difficult to prevent. Some of the newer antifungal agents with activity against filamentous fungi are being evaluated for the prevention of fungal infections.

SUMMARY

Patients with AML are at increased risk for developing infections, particularly during periods of severe and prolonged neutropenia. The spectrum of infections in these patients undergoes periodic changes, and it is important to detect epidemiological shifts early on. The prompt administration of empirical, broad-spectrum, antimicrobial therapy is associated with response rates ranging from 65 to 85 percent. Most patients not responding to the initial regimen will respond to therapeutic modifications, and the infection-related mortality is approximately 3 percent. Newer strategies for infection prevention need to be developed, particularly for fungal and some viral infections. These issues will continue to challenge clinicians who care for these patients.

REFERENCES

1. Hersh EM, Bodey GP, Nies BA, Freireich EJ. Causes of death in acute leukemia. A ten-year study of 414 patients from 1954–1963. JAMA 1965; 193:105–109.
2. Burke PJ, Braine GH, Rathbun HK, Owen AH Jr. The clinical significance and management of fever in acute myelocytic leukemia. Johns Hopkins Med J 1976; 139:1–12.
3. Bishop JF, Matthews JP, Young GP, Szer J, Gillett A, Joshua D, Bradstock K, Enno A, Wolf MM, Fox R, Cobcroft R, Herrman R, Van Der Weyden M,

Lowenthal RM, Page F, Garson OM, Juneja S. A randomized study of high-dose cytarabine in induction in acute myeloid leukemia. Blood 1996; 87:1710–1717.

4. Mayer RJ, Davis RB, Schiffer CA, Berg DT, Powell BL, Schulman P, Omura GA, Moore JO, McIntyre OR, Frei E III. Intensive post remission chemotherapy in adults with acute myeloid leukemia. N Engl J Med 1994; 331:896–903.

5. Bodey GP, Buckley M, Sathe YS, Freireich EJ. Quantitative relationships between circulating leukocytes and infection in patients with acute leukemia. Ann Intern Med 1966; 64:328 340.

6. Cline MJ. Defective mononuclear phagocyte function in myelomonocytic leukemia and in some patients with lymphoma. J Clin Invest 1973; 52:2815–2819.

7. Cline MJ. A test of individual phagocyte function in a mixed population of leukocytes. Identifications of a neutrophil abnormality in acute myelocytic leukemia. J Lab Clin Med 1973; 81:311 315.

8. Lehrer RI, Cline MJ. Leukocyte candidacidal activity and resistance to systemic candidiasis in patients with cancer. Cancer 1972; 72:1211–1217.

9. Holland JF, Senn HJ, Banerjee T. Quantitative studies of localized leukocyte mobilization in acute leukemia. Blood 1971; 37:499–511.

10. Senn HJ, Holland JF. Leukocyte mobilization in health and acute leukemia. Blood 1967; 30:888.

11. Sickles EA, Green WH, Wiernik PH. Clinical presentations of infection in granulocytopenic patients. Arch Intern Med 1875; 135:715–719.

12. Bodey GP. Unusual presentations of infection in neutropenic patients. Int J Antimicrob Agents 2000; 168:93–95.

13. Roberts WC, Bodey GP, Wertlake PT. The heart in acute leukemia. A study of 420 autopsy cases. Am J Cardiol 1968; 21:388–412.

14. Hughes WT, Armstrong D, Bodey GP, Bow EJ, Brown AE, Calandra T, Feld R, Pizzo PA, Rolston KVI, Shenep JL, Young LS. 2002 Guidelines for the use of antimicrobial agents in neutropenic patients with cancer. Clin Infect Dis 2002; 34:730–751.

15. Koll BS, Brown AE. The changing epidemiology of infections at cancer hospitals. Clin Infect Dis 1993; 17(suppl 2):S322–S328.

16. Rolston KVI, Bodey GP. Infections in patients with cancer. In: Holland JF, Frei E, eds. Cancer Medicine e5. Hamilton, Ontario: BC Decker, 2000:2407–2432.

17. Zinner SH. Changing epidemiology of infections in patients with neutropenia and cancer: emphasis on gram-positive and resistant bacteria. Clin Infect Dis 1999; 29:490–494.

18. Madani TA, Al-Abdullah NA, Al-Sanousi AA, Ghabrah TM, Afandi SZ, Bajunid HA. Methicillin-resistant *Staphylococcus aureus* in two tertiary-care centers in Jeddah, Saudi Arabia. Infect Control Hosp Epidemiol 2001; 22:211 216.

19. DeBock R, Cometta A, Kern N, Aoun M, Caballero D, Engelhard D, Schaffner A, Galazzo M, Paesmans M, Vandenbergh M, Viscoli C Incidence of single agent gram-negative bacteremias (SAGNB) in neutropenic cancer patients (NCP) in EORTC-IATG trials of empirical therapy for febrile neutropenia. 41st ICAAC st, Chicago 2001, Session 079, Poster 773, 445.

20. Rolston KVI, Tarrand JJ. *Pseudomonas aeruginosa*—still a frequent pathogen

in patients with cancer: 11-year experience from a comprehensive cancer center. Clin Infect Dis 1999; 29:463–464.

21. Elting LS, Bodey GP, Fainstein V. Polymicrobial septicemia in the cancer patient. Medicine 1986; 65:218–225.

22. Rolston KVI, Bodey GP. Diagnosis and management of perianal and perirectal infection in the granulocytopenic patient. In: Remington J, Swartz MN, eds. Current Clinical Topics in Infectious Diseases. Boston: Blackwell Scientific, 1993:164–171.

23. Gomez L, Martino R, Rolston KV. Neutropenic enterocolitis: spectrum of the disease and comparison of definite and possible cases. Clin Infect Dis 1998; 27:695–699.

24. Dismukes WE. Established and emerging invasive mycoses. Infect Dis Clin Pract 1998; 7(suppl 1):S35–S41.

25. Perfect JR, Schell WA. The new fungal opportunists are coming. Clin Infect Dis 1996; 22(suppl 2):S112–S118.

26. Abi-Said D, Anaissie E, Uzon O, Raad I, Pinzcowski H, Vartivarian S. The epidemiology of hematogenous candidiasis caused by different *Candida* species. Clin Infect Dis 1997; 24:1122–1128.

27. Nguyen MH, Peacock JE Jr, Morris AJ, Tanner DC, Nguyen ML, Snydman DR, Wagener MM, Rinaldi MG, Yu VL. The changing face of candidemia: emergence of non–*Candida albicans* species and antifungal resistance. Am J Med 1996; 100:617–623.

28. Couch RB, Englund JA, Whimbey E. Respiratory viral infections in immunocompetent and immunocompromised persons. Am J Med 1997; 102:2–9.

29. Whimbey E, Englund JA, Couch RB. Community respiratory virus infections in immunocompromised patients with cancer. Am J Med 1997; 102:10–18.

30. Rolston KC, Raad I, Whimbey E, Bodey GP. The changing spectrum of bacterial infections in febrile neutropenic patients. In: Klastersky JA, ed. Febrile Neutropenia. Berlin: Springer-Verlag, 1998:53–56.

31. Whimbey E, Kiehn TE, Brannon P, Blevins A, Armstrong D. Bacteremia and fungemia in patients with neoplastic disease. Am J Med 1987; 82:723–730.

32. Horvathova Z, Spanik S, Sufliarsky J, Mardiak J, Pichna P, Pichnova E, Krajcik S, Mraz M, Chmelik B, Dacok J, Beresova J, Krupova I, Hrachova A, Trupl J, Kunova A, Krcmery V Jr. Bacteremia due to methicillin-resistant staphylococci occurs more frequently in neutropenic patients who received antimicrobial prophylaxis and is associated with higher mortality in comparison to methicillin-sensitive bacteremia. Internl J Antimicrob Agents 1998; 10:55–58.

33. Boyce JM. Methicillin-resistant *Staphylococcus aureus*. Detection, epidemiology, and control measures. Inf Dis Clin North Am 1989; 3:901–913.

34. Diekema DJ, Coffman SL, Marshall SA, Beach ML, Rolston KVI, Jones RN. Comparison of activities of broad spectrum beta-lactam compounds against 1,128 gram-positive cocci recently isolated in cancer treatment centers. Antimicrob Agents Chemother 1999; 43:940–943.

35. Elting LS, Bodey GP, Keefe BH. Septicemia and toxic shock syndrome due to viridans streptococci: a case-control study of predisposing factors. Clin Infect Dis 1992; 14:1201–1207.

36. Arning M, Gehrt A, Aul C, Runde V, Hadding U, Schneider W. Septicemia due to *Streptococcus mitis* in neutropenic patients with acute leukemia. Blut 1990; 61:364–368.
37. Engel A, Kern P, Kern WV. Levels of cytokines and cytokine inhibitors in the neutropenic patient with alpha-hemolytic streptococcus shock syndrome. Clin Infec Dis 1996; 23:785 789.
38. Doern GV, Ferraro MJ, Brueggemann A, Ruoff KL. Emergence of high rates of antimicrobial resistance among viridans group streptococci in the United States. Antimicrob Agents Chemother 1996; 40:891–894.
39. Kaufhold A, Potgieter E. Chromosomally mediated high-level gentamicin resistance in *Streptococcus mitis*. Antimicrob Agents Chemother 1993; 37:2740–2742.
40. Shlaes DM, Marino J, Jacobs MR. Infection caused by vancomycin-resistant *Streptococcus sanguis* II. Antimicrob Agents Chemother 1984; 25:527–528.
41. Edmond MB. Ober JF, Weinbaun DL, Pfaller MA, Hwang T, Sanford MD, Denzel RP. Vancomycin-resistant *Enterococcus faecium* bacteremia: risk factors for infections. Clin Infect Dis 1995; 20:1126–1133.
42. Matar MJ, Tarrand J, Raad II, Rolston KV. Vancomycin-resistant-enterococci (VRE) in cancer patients: rates of colonization, infection sites, species differentiation and antibiotic susceptibilities. Abstract #59. 39th Annual Meeting Infectious Diseases Society of America. San Francisco, CA, Oct. 25–29, 2001.
43. Raad I, Hachem R, Hanna H, Girgawy E, Rolston K, Whimbey E, Husni R, Bodey G. Treatment of vancomycin-resistant enterococcal infections in the immunocompromised host: quinupristin-dalfopristin in combination with minocycline. Antimicrob Agents Chemother 2001; 45:3202–3204.
44. Elting LS, Rubenstein EB, Rolston KVI, Bodey GP. Outcomes of bacteremia in patients with cancer and neutropenia: observations from two decades of epidemiological and clinical trials. Clin Infect Dis 1997; 25:247–259.
45. Pizzo PA. Drug therapy: management of fever in patients with cancer and treatment-induced neutropenia. N Engl J Med 1993; 328:1323–1332.
46. Coullioud D, Van der Auwera P, Viot M, Lasset C. Prospective multicentric study of the etiology of 1051 bacteremic episodes in 782 cancer patients. Support Care Cancer 1993; 1:34–46.
47. Escande MC, Herbrecht R, French Study Group. Prospective study of bacteremia in cancer patients: results of a French multicentre study. Support Care Cancer 1998; 6:273–280.
48. Berhgmans T, Crokaert F, Markiewicz E, Sculier JP. Epidemiology of infections in the adult medical intensive care unit of a cancer hospital. Support Care Cancer 1997; 5:234–240.
49. Al-Bahar S, Pandita R, Dhabhar B, Al-Bahar E. Febrile neutropenia in cancer patients in Kuwait: microbial spectrum and outcome. Support Care Cancer 1994; 2:400–402.
50. Chatzinikolaou I, Abi-Said D, Bodey GP, Rolston KVI, Tarrand JJ, Samonis G. Recent experience with Pseduomonas aeruginosa bacteremia in patients with cancer. Arch Intern Med 2000; 160:501–509.
51. Bodey GP, Jadeja L, Elting L. Pseudomonas bacteremia: retrospective analysis of 410 episodes. Arch Intern Med 1985; 145:1621 1629.

52. Khadori N, Elting L, Wong E, Schable B, Bodey GP. Nosocomial infections due to *Xanthomonas maltophilia* (*Pseudomonas maltophilia*) in patients with cancer. Rev Infect Dis 1990; 12:997–1003.

53. Rolston K. Overview of systemic fungal infections. Oncology 2001; 15(suppl): 11–14.

54. Jacobson K, Rolston K, Elting L, LeBlanc B, Whimbey E, Ho DH. Susceptibility surveillance among gram-negative bacilli at a cancer center. Chemother 1999; 45:325–334.

55. Walsh TJ, Pappas P, Winston DJ, Lazarus HM, Petersen F, Raffalli J, Yanovich S, Stiff P, Greenberg R, Donowitz G, Schuster M, Reboli A, Wingard J, Arndt C, Reinhardt J, Hadley S, Finberg R, Laverdiere M, Perfect J, Garber G, Fioritoni G, Anaissie E, Lee J. The National Institute of Allergy and Infectious Diseases Mycoses Study Group. Voriconazole compared with liposomal amphotericin B for empirical antifungal therapy in patients with neutropenia and persistent fever. N Engl J Med 2002; 346:225–234.

56. Cruciani M, Rampazzo R, Malena M, Lazzarini L, Todeschini G, Messori A, Concia E. Prophylaxis with fluoroquinolones for bacterial infections in neutropenic patients: a meta-analysis. Clin Infect Dis 1996; 23:795–805.

57. Rolston KVI, LeBlanc B, Ho DH. In vitro activity of gatifloxacin against gram-positive isolates from cancer patients. Abstract #360. 39th Annual Interscience Conference on Antimicrobial Agents and Chemotherapy. San Francisco, CA, September 26–29, 1999.

58. Rolston KVI, LeBlanc B, Ho DH. In vitro activity of gatifloxacin against gram-negative isolates from cancer patients. Abstract #359. 39th Annual Interscience Conference on Antimicrobial Agents and Chemotherapy. San Francisco, CA, September 26–29, 1999.

59. Rolston KVI, LeBlanc BM, Balakrishnan M, Ho DH. In-vitro activity of moxifloxacin against gram-negative isolates from cancer patients. Abstract #2324. 40th Interscience Conference on Antimicrobial Agents and Chemotherapy. Toronto, Ontario, Canada, September 17–20, 2000.

60. Kern WV, Andriof E, Oethinger M, Kern P, Hacker J, Marre R. Emergence of fluoroquinolone-resistant *Escherichia coli* at a cancer center. Antimicrob Agents Chemother 1994; 38:681–687.

61. Winston DJ, Chandrasekar PH, Lazarus HM, Goodman JL, Silber JL, Horowitz H, Shadduck RK, Rosenfeld CS, Ho WG, Islan MF. Fluconazole prophylaxis of fungal infections in patients with acute leukemia. Results of a randomized placebo-controlled, double-blind, multicenter trial. Ann Intern Med 1993; 118:495–503.

5

Hairy Cell Leukemia

Nikolaos Almyroudis
Memorial Sloan Kettering Cancer Center
New York, New York, U.S.A.

Hairy cell leukemia (HCL) is a chronic lymphoproliferative disorder in which the malignant cells originate from the B-cell lymphocytic line. HCL typically manifests with varying degrees of cytopenias and splenomegaly. Occasionally, peripheral, abdominal, and less commonly mediastinal lymphadenopathy may be present. The distinctive feature of this type of leukemia is the presence of abnormal mononuclear cells with characteristic cytoplasmic projections (hairy cells) circulating in the peripheral blood or infiltrating the bone marrow [1,2].

Infections are a major complication of HCL. They are the presenting manifestation in 28% of patients, while up to 70% of patients will develop infections during the course of the disease [2,3]. Infections were the leading cause of death in 62.5–67% of patients, even though in more recent reports mortality due to infections seems to decline [1,4,5].

The immune defect in patients with HCL is multifactorial and not completely elucidated yet. Granulocytopenia plays a major role in the development of an infection and is usually caused by translocation of enteric flora. The low white blood cell count is due to HCL, in the presence or absence of infiltration of bone marrow by leukemic cells, splenomegaly, or cytotoxic chemotherapy. Granulocytopenia in HCL is moderate (at the level of 500–1500 cells/μL) in 40.9% of patients and profound (<500 cells/μL) in 39.0% of patients [5]. Disrupted first-line barriers due to mucositis or the presence of foreign bodies such as central venous catheters serve as portals of entry for the pathogenic organisms. Functional defects of granulocytes in patients with HCL have been demonstrated as well. The ability of neutrophils to kill *Candida guilliermondi* and *Staphylococcus aureus* in vitro is defective [6]. Monocytopenia is another prominent feature of HCL that has been considered even more important in the pathogenesis of infections, particularly by opportunistic pathogens [7]. Monocytes are undetectable in 55.5% of patients and at the level of 1–500 cells/μL in 42.3% [5,8]. Monocytes are important components of the immune response against intracellular pathogens [9]. Besides the defect in the production of monocytes, functional abnormalities are also present. In vivo, subnormal migration of monocytes at experimental "skin windows" (Rebuck skin windows) was found in patients with HCL [8,10,11], and the absence of monocyte chemotaxis and oxidative burst activity were demonstrated in vitro [12]. In a small study including four patients, impaired granuloma formation was observed in response to an infectious challenge. Lesions appeared as focal necrosis or focal microabscesses and consisted of polymorphonuclear infiltration around an area of central necrosis containing few macrophages [13]. Additionally, the absolute number of natural killer cells is decreased and their activity severely impaired [14]. More recently, a significant decrease in the peripheral blood dendritic cells was demonstrated [15]. The above data indicates a critical impairment in the innate immune response.

To what degree T-cell dysfunction contributes to the immune defect in HCL is not completely understood. There is a marked T-cell imbalance with an increased number of suppressor cells with a low helper-to-suppressor ratio [16]. T-cell lymphocytes are abnormally activated [17] and nonresponsive, possibly owing to inadequate antigen presentation due to the absence of circulating monocytes [18]. Delayed hypersensitivity to recall antigens is impaired, and there is no antibody-dependent cellular cytotoxicity [19]. In contrast, the serum immunoglobulin levels are normal in most patients [7,20].

The majority of infections in patients with HCL are due to pyogenic bacteria and are accompanied by higher mortality among all infectious episodes [1,3,4,7]. According to different studies, the incidence of pyogenic infections in patients with HCL varies between 52 and 64% among the total number of culture-positive infectious episodes [4,21]. *P. aeruginosa* and the other enteric gram-negative bacilli are the most frequent gram-negative bacteria isolated, with *Staphylococcus* species representing the majority of the gram-positives [3,7,22].

The relative frequency of nonpyogenic infections in patients with HCL is 36–41% [3,21]. The higher incidence of infections due to mycobacterial, fungal, and viral pathogens is only comparable to that in patients with Hodgkin's disease and is higher than that in patients with chronic lymphocytic leukemia and acute leukemias [21].

Nontuberculous mycobacterial infections are documented in almost all studies. *M. kansasii* is the most prevalent species, and *M. avium-intracellulare*, *M. gordonae*, *M. scrofulaceum*, *M. chelonae*, *M. fortuitum*, and *M. malmoense* complicate the course of HCL less frequently [3,7,13,23,24].

Nontuberculous mycobacteriosis in HCL is typically disseminated and is accompanied by a high mortality rate [7,23,26]. The lungs are involved in the vast majority of the disseminated cases in addition to supraclavicular, mediastinal, and abdominal lymph nodes, and the liver, spleen, bone marrow [7,23] and occasionally the skin [27]. High-yield culture specimens are the lymph nodes. Bone marrow, liver, spleen, and lungs are also useful sites. Frequently the diagnosis requires invasive procedures such as thoracotomy and laparotomy [23]. Remarkably enough, the PPD skin testing may be useful in the diagnosis of Mycobacterial infections since it was positive in several, though not all, reported cases [4,7,28].

M. tuberculosis has also been reported as complicating HCL [1,3, 24,25,29]. The discrepancy on its incidence among different studies most likely reflects the different levels of tuberculosis in a given population. Finally, *M. bovis* axillary lymphadenitis has been described following bacillus Calmette–Guerin vaccination [7].

Besides the usual fungal pathogens that are commonly seen in patients with leukemia, such as *Candida* species and *Aspergillus* species [3,29], unique pathogens found in patients with HCL include *Histoplasma capsulatum* [1,3,22,28,29], *Coccidioides immitis* [13,24], *Cryptococcus neoformans* [1,3,22,29], *Blastomyces dermatitidis* [13], *Sporothrix schenkii* [30], and *Pseudallescheria boydii* [7]. Like mycobacterial infections, fungal infections are usually disseminated. *Pneumocystis carinii* has been described as well, although less commonly [1,3,22,29].

Viral infections occur with low frequency in patients with HCL. The herpes simplex virus, herpes zoster, and cytomegalovirus are the major viral pathogens; the latter causes primarily pneumonia [3,4,7,24]. Other nonpyogenic infections that have been described in patients with HCL are due to *Legionella* [29,31–33], *Mycoplasma pneumoniae* [29], *Listeria monocytogenes* [33], *Rhodococcus aurantiacus* [34], *Toxoplasma gondii* [7,29,35], and *Strongyloides stercoralis* [4].

Pneumonia and septicemia are the most common infections observed in patients with pyogenic infections, followed by skin and soft tissue infections, urinary tract infections, and rectal or other abscesses [1,3,7,22,29].

Several diagnostic problems may arise in the management of HCL as a result of the unique clinical features of this type of leukemia. Clinicians should keep in mind that fever very rarely complicates HCL as a constitutional complaint [1,2]. Any febrile illness should trigger an extensive workup for an infectious source before it is attributed to leukemia per se. In addition to bacterial cultures and a chest x-ray, investigation of a febrile episode should include a tuberculin skin test (PPD), fungal culture, and appropriate serologies for the previously mentioned pathogens as well as a specific stain for pneumocystis carinii of the sputum. If the diagnosis remains elusive, bronchoscopy or invasive procedures for tissue diagnosis from the involved sites should be done without delay [2,29]. Diagnosis of such febrile episodes may still be difficult [28], and a significant percentage of cases eventually meet the criteria for fever of unknown origin [7,22]. The institution of empirical antituberculosis drug therapy in such cases, especially when there is a more insidious presentation with persistent fever, weight loss, and malaise, has been considered a reasonable approach by some authors [2]. In one study of 13 patients of whom seven had tuberculosis, four others responded to empirical antituberculous therapy [25].

Besides the common causes of noninfectious fever, other clinical syndromes should be included when diagnosing persistent fever in patients with HCL. These are the various autoimmune syndromes that develop during the course of HCL that can be accompanied by fever, such as vasculitis, polyarteritis, arthritis, or erythema nodosum. Two discrete syndromes have been described. The first one is mild and includes arthritis or arthralgias, nodular skin lesions, and low-grade fever, while the other one is more severe and can be progressive. It is characterized by weight loss, malaise, and fever that can take the form of a fever of unknown origin with frequent involvement of lungs, liver, intestine, or kidney and may resemble polyarteritis nodosa [2,29]. Both syndromes should be included in the differential diagnosis of HCL patients with fever.

Granulomatous disease of the liver, spleen, and lungs is not uncommon in patients with HCL [13,36]. This is due to the greater incidence of nontuberculous mycobacteriosis, tuberculosis, and fungal infections. In a number of reports, though, the workup failed to reveal the cause of these granulomas. Even though there is no evidence, it has been suggested that such cases are probably infectious in etiology [36].

Cutaneous lesions develop in 56% of patients during the course of HCL. Including skin and soft tissue infections, 58% of these lesions are infectious in origin, predominantly from bacterial pathogens [37]. Rashes can be due to nontuberculous mycobacteria and disseminated deep mycoses. Sweet's syndrome and hairy cell leukemia cutis have also been reported but are extremely rare [37,38]. Various forms of rashes due to vasculitis or other autoimmune syndromes have been described but are infrequent. Finally, pleural effusions, ascites, and meningeal or central nervous system involvement rarely occur in HCL as a result of infiltration by neoplastic cells [39]. The most frequent cause of neurologic complications in patients with HCL is by far infection [40].

The treatment of HCL has radically changed during the last few decades. Interestingly enough, splenectomy, a widely used treatment modality in the past that now has been abandoned, was associated with a decrease in the rate of infections in HCL. This was presumably due to an increase in the granulocyte count as a result of this procedure [22,28]. The purine analogs 2-deoxycoformycin (2-dCF) and 2-chlorodeoxyadenosine (2-CdA) are newer compounds that are currently the drugs of choice for HCL. Myelosuppression involving transient neutropenia is a frequent toxicity of these compounds [41,42]. In addition, both induce a decrease in the total lymphocyte count, primarily affecting the T-cells. In one study, the CD4+ and CD8+ T-lymphocyte counts were decreased to less than 200 cells/μL for at least 6 months after treatment with 2-dCF was completed. Full recovery of CD4+ occurred at a median time of 54 months [43]. Similar was the effect of 2-CdA on the CD4+ cells, a median time to recovery being 40 months [44]. Surprisingly, opportunistic infections associated with these low counts were uncommon among patients treated with these compounds.

In conclusion, patients with HCL have an increased susceptibility to infections. Treatment should start promptly whenever infection is suspected, and if the fever persists and cultures remain negative a thorough workup should be done for mycobacterial, fungal, viral, or other opportunistic pathogens.

REFERENCES

1. Bouroncle BA. Leukemic reticuloendotheliosis (hairy cell leukemia). Blood 1979; 53(3):412–436.
2. Lembersky BC, Golomb HM. Hairy cell leukemia: clinical features and therapeutic advances. Cancer Metastasis Rev 1987; 6(3):283–300.
3. Golomb HM, Hadad LJ. Infectious complications in 127 patients with hairy cell leukemia. Am J Hematol 1984; 16(4):393–401.
4. Mackowiak PA, Demian SE, Sutker WL, Murphy FK, Smith JW, Tompsett R, Sheehan WW, Luby JP. Infections in hairy cell leukemia. Clinical evidence of a pronounced defect in cell-mediated immunity. Am J Med 1980; 68(5):718–724.
5. Frassoldati A, Lamparelli T, Federico M, Annino L, Capnist G, Pagnucco G, Dini E, Resegotti L, Damasio EE, Silingardi V. Hairy cell leukemia: a clinical review based on 725 cases of the Italian Cooperative Group (ICGHCL).

Italian Cooperative Group for Hairy Cell Leukemia. Leuk Lymphoma 1994; 13(3-4):307-316.

6. Child JA, Cawley JC, Martin S, Ghoneim AT. Microbicidal function of the neutrophils in hairy-cell leukaemia. Acta Haematol 1979; 62(4):191-198.

7. Stewart DJ, Bodey GP. Infections in hairy cell leukemia (leukemic reticuloendotheliosis). Cancer 1981; 47(4):801-805.

8. Janckila AJ, Wallace JH, Yam LT. Generalized monocyte deficiency in leukaemic reticuloendotheliosis. Scand J Haematol 1982; 29(2):153-160.

9. Cline MJ, Lehrer RI, Territo MC, Golde DW. UCLA Conference. Monocytes and macrophages: functions and diseases. Ann Intern Med 1978; 88(1):78-88.

10. Yam LT, Chaudhry AA, Janckila AJ. Impaired marrow granulocyte reserve and leukocyte mobilization in leukemic reticuloendotheliosis. Ann Intern Med 1977; 87(4):444-446.

11. Seshadri RS, Brown EJ, Zipursky A. Leukemic reticuloendotheliosis. A failure of monocyte production. N Engl J Med 1976; 295(4):181-184.

12. Nielsen H, Bangsborg J, Rechnitzer C, Jacobsen N, Busk HE. Defective monocyte function in Legionnaires' disease complicating hairy cell leukaemia. Acta Med Scand 1986; 220(4):381-383.

13. Rice L, Shenkenberg T, Lynch EC, Wheeler TM. Granulomatous infections complicating hairy cell leukemia. Cancer 1982; 49(9):1924-1928.

14. Trentin L, Zambello R, Agostini C, Ambrosetti A, Chisesi T, Raimondi R, Bulian P, Pizzolo G, Semenzato G. Mechanisms accounting for the defective natural killer activity in patients with hairy cell leukemia. Blood 1990; 75(7):1525-1530.

15. Bourguin-Plonquet A, Rouard H, Roudot-Thoraval F, Bellanger C, Marquet J, Delfau-Larue MH, Divine M, Farcet JP. Severe decrease in peripheral blood dendritic cells in hairy cell leukaemia. Br J Haematol 2002; 116(3):595-597.

16. Lauria F, Foa R, Matera L, Raspadori D, Tura S. Membrane phenotype and functional behaviour of T lymphocytes in hairy cell leukemia (HCL). Semin Oncol 1984; 11(4):409-412.

17. Kluin-Nelemans JC, Kester MG, Oving I, Cluitmans FH, Willemze R, Falkenburg JH. Abnormally activated T lymphocytes in the spleen of patients with hairy-cell leukaemia. Leukemia 1994; 8(12):2095-2101.

18. Van De Corput L, Falkenburg JH, Kluin-Nelemans JC. T-cell dysfunction in hairy cell leukemia: an updated review. Leuk Lymphoma 1998; 30(1-2):31-39.

19. Hersh EM, Quesada J, Keating MJ, Rasmussen S, Murphy SG, Gschwind C, Morgan J. Host defence factors and prognosis in hairy cell leukemia. Leuk Res 1982; 6(5):625-637.

20. Hansen DA, Robbins BA, Bylund DJ, Piro LD, Saven A, Ellison DJ. Identification of monoclonal immunoglobulins and quantitative immunoglobulin abnormalities in hairy cell leukemia and chronic lymphocytic leukemia. Am J Clin Pathol 1994; 102(5):580-585. .

21. Golomb HM, Hanauer SB. Infectious complications associated with hairy cell leukemia. J Infect Dis 1981; 143(5):639-643.

22. Bouza E, Burgaleta C, Golde DW. Infections in hairy-cell leukemia. Blood 1978; 51(5):851–859.

23. Bennett C, Vardiman J, Golomb H. Disseminated atypical mycobacterial infection in patients with hairy cell leukemia. Am J Med 1986; 80(5):891–896.

24. Libshitz HI, Shuman LS, Gresik MV, Heaston DK. Pneumonia in hairy-cell leukemia. Radiology 1981; 139(1):19–24.

25. Marie JP, Degos L, Flandrin G. Hairy-cell leukemia and tuberculosis. N Engl J Med 1977; 297(24):1354.

26. Gallo JH, Young GA, Forrest PR, Vincent PC, Jennis F. Disseminated atypical mycobacterial infection in hairy cell leukemia. Pathology 1983; 15(3):241–245.

27. Castor B, Juhlin I, Henriques B. Septic cutaneous lesions caused by Mycobacterium malmoense in a patient with hairy cell leukemia. Eur J Clin Microbiol Infect Dis 1994; 13(2):145–148.

28. Rex JH, Harris RL, Wheeler T, White M, Bradshaw W, Williams TW Jr. Granulomatous disease complicating hairy cell leukemia. Tex Med 1985; 81(7):31–33.

29. Westbrook CA, Golde DW. Clinical problems in hairy cell leukemia: diagnosis and management. Semin Oncol 1984; 11(4 suppl 2):514–522.

30. Kumar S, Kumar D, Gourley WK, Alperin JB. Sporotrichosis as a presenting manifestation of hairy cell leukemia. Am J Hematol 1994; 46(2):134–137.

31. Cordonnier C, Farcet JP, Desforges L, Brun-Buisson C, Vernant JP, Kuentz M, Dournon E. Legionnaires' disease and hairy-cell leukemia. An unfortuitous association? Arch Intern Med 1984; 144(12):2373–2375.

32. Berlin G, Fryden A, Maller R, Malm C, Vikrot O. Legionnaires' disease in leukaemic reticuloendotheliosis. Scand J Haematol 1980; 25(2):171–174.

33. Fang GD, Stout JE, Yu VL, Goetz A, Rihs JD, Vickers RM. Community-acquired pneumonia caused by Legionella dumoffii in a patient with hairy cell leukemia. Infection 1990; 18(6):383–385.

33a. Salata RA, King RE, Gose F, Pearson RD. Listeria monocytogenes cerebritis, bacteremia, and cutaneous lesions complicating hairy cell leukemia. Am J Med 1986; 81(6):1068–1072.

34. Prinz G, Ban E, Fekete S, Szabo Z. Meningitis caused by Gordona aurantiaca (Rhodococcus aurantiacus). J Clin Microbiol 1985; 22(3):472–474.

35. Knecht H, Rhyner K, Streuli RA. Toxoplasmosis in hairy-cell leukaemia. Br J Haematol 1986; 62(1):65–73.

36. Bendix-Hansen K, Bayer Kristensen I. Granulomas of spleen and liver in hairy cell leukaemia. Acta Pathol Microbiol Immunol Scand [A] 1984; 92(3):157–160.

37. Carsuzaa F, Pierre C, Jaubert D, Viala JJ. Cutaneous findings in hairy cell leukemia. Review of 84 cases. Nouv Rev Fr Hematol 1994; 35(6):541–543.

38. Finan MC, Su WP, Li CY. Cutaneous findings in hairy cell leukemia. J Am Acad Dermatol 1984; 11(5 pt 1):788–797.

39. Bouroncle BA. Unusual presentations and complications of hairy cell leukemia. Leukemia 1987; 1(4):288–293.

40. Kimmel DW, Hermann RC Jr, O'Neill BP. Neurologic complications of hairy cell leukemia. Arch Neurol 1984; 41(2):202–203.

41. Catovsky D, Matutes E, Talavera JG, O'Connor NT, Johnson SA, Emmett E, Corbett L, Swansbury J. Long term results with 2′deoxycoformycin in hairy cell leukemia. Leuk Lymphoma 1994; 14(suppl 1):109–113.
42. Hoffman MA, Janson D, Rose E, Rai KR. Treatment of hairy-cell leukemia with cladribine: response, toxicity, and long-term follow-up. J Clin Oncol 1997; 15(3):1138–1142.
43. Seymour JF, Talpaz M, Kurzrock R. Response duration and recovery of CD4+ lymphocytes following deoxycoformycin in interferon-alpha-resistant hairy cell leukemia: 7-year follow-up. Leukemia 1997; 11(1):42–47.
44. Seymour JF, Kurzrock R, Freireich EJ, Estey EH. 2-chlorodeoxyadenosine induces durable remissions and prolonged suppression of CD4+ lymphocyte counts in patients with hairy cell leukemia. Blood 1994; 83(10):2906–2911.

6

Infections in Patients with Chronic Lymphocytic Leukemia

Ana Maria Chiappori
Cayatano Heredia University
Lima, Peru

INTRODUCTION

CLL is the most frequent hematological malignancy in the Western Hemisphere, accounting for 30% of all leukemias [1–3] and for an annual incidence of 1.8 to 3.0 per 100,000 in the U.S. [4,5]. The main characteristic of CLL is a monoclonal proliferation with progressive accumulation of functionally incompetent, long-lived small lymphocytes of B cell (95%) or T cell (5%) lineage [6–8]. It initially develops in the bone marrow and peripheral blood; in later stages it accumulates in the lymphatic organs [6]. The clinical course is variable, with patient survival ranging from only a few years to 15 years [7,8].

Because of this immunological incompetence, infections in CLL patients have long been recognized as a common cause of morbidity and mortality. Up to 80% of patients will suffer infectious complications, accounting for approximately 60% of death in these patients [2,9]. The predisposition to infections in CLL patients has many components, including both immunodeficiency related to the leukemia itself (humoral and cellular immune dysfunction) and the results of cumulative immunosuppresion related to

CLL treatment [3]. The goal of this chapter is to describe the pathogenesis of the immunodeficiency associated with B-CLL and the infectious complications of the disease per se and its forms of treatment.

FACTORS INCREASING INFECTIONS SUSCEPTIBILITY

B-CLL has been described as lying at the crossroads of hematology, immunology, and oncology for at least three major reasons: it is the prototype of human malignancies that primarily involve defects in the induction of apoptosis; CLL patients develop a severe immunodeficiency with progressive hypogammaglobulinemia; and they have a high prevalence of autoimmune phenomena [10].

HYPOGAMMAGLOBULINEMIA

Hypogammaglobulinemia is a well-known feature in patients presenting with CLL. Since the association was first described in 1955 [11,12], many authors have reported the impaired ability of CLL patients to produce normal amounts of immunoglobulins. The frequency of hypogammaglobulinemia depends on the duration and stage of the disease, and it has been reported in 19 to 75% of the patients [11–22]. The pathogenesis of hypogammaglobulinemia in B-CLL is poorly understood, and data concerning helper and suppressor lymphocytes, natural killer and ADCC (antibody-dependent cellular cytotoxicity) activity are contradictory [23,24]. Although the defect is probably multifactorial, hypogammaglobulinemia may be considered to be the result of a dysfunction of nonclonal CD5- B cells (decrease due to progressive dilution or inhibition) [1,25–27]. This is a rare phenomenon in other B cell malignancies including acute lymphoblastic leukemia, nodular and diffuse lymphomas, hairy cell leukemia, and prolymphocytic leukemia, although reciprocal depression of the nonclonal Ig subsets is common in multiple myeloma [26]. This decrease or inhibition of normal CD5-negative B cells could also explain the classical inability of B cell CLL to respond to new antigenic challenges [28]. Patients with early forms of the disease tend to have defective specific antibody responses to infection or immunization [29].

Hypogammaglobulinemia is the most important immune defect in CLL and carries a poor prognosis. Susceptibility to bacterial infections, especially *Streptococcus pneumoniae*, *Staphylococcus aureus*, and *Escherichia coli* [30] is greatly increased in CLL as in primary immunoglobulin deficiency [13]. The risk of infection may increase with longer duration of the disease [9] and may be due to the natural history of the disease and the therapeutic measures taken until then. Indeed, these factors may worsen the level of hypogammaglobulinemia [24].

IMPAIRMENTS IN CELL-MEDIATED IMMUNITY

B-CLL is a malignancy of a mantle zone-based subpopulation of anergic, self-reactive, activated CD 5+ B cells [31], and it is characterized by the accumulation of circulating clonal B cells. This accumulation occurs not as a consequence of their continued, augmented proliferation but of their enhanced viability and life span [32]. B-CLL is the prototype of human malignancy that primarily involves defects in the induction of apoptosis or programmed cell death [10,31].

The lack of expression of important glycoproteins on the surface of the B-CLL malignant cells directly correlates with clinical immune dysfunction. Decreases in major histocompatibility complex (MHC) molecules or activation ligands (as CD 80) directly impair their ability to function as antigen-presenting cells (APCs) [32]. As weak APCs, the malignant cells do not stimulate potent T cell helper activity, which leads to deficient humoral and cellular immune responses [32]. Because the tumor cells act as the major accessory cells, and are inefficient antigen presenting cells, the accumulating malignant B cell population per se is a hurdle to the production of normal antibodies and leads to a progressive and severe hypogammaglobulinemia [10,31].

Cell-mediated immune function is altered in CLL patients; however, it is not always clear which defects are primary to the disease itself and which are chemotherapy induced [1,5]. Recent evidence offers insight into the profound alterations in the T cells of CLL patients and the role of clonal T cell populations in the pathogenesis of this disease [3]. Cellular immunity defects lead to impaired immune responses to intracellular bacteria or viral infection, autoimmune disorders, and secondary neoplasms associated with B-CLL [30,32].

GRANULOCYTOPENIA AND PHAGOCYTIC CELL DEFECTS

Relative neutropenia is present in untreated CLL patients, but in general the granulocyte count and function in patients with CLL is normal or slightly decreased. Lymphoid infiltration of the bone marrow, suppression of granulocyte progenitors by cellular or humoral mediators, and myelotoxicity from chemotherapy are factors contributing to the pathogenesis of granulocytopenia. Chemotherapy-induced neutropenia may predispose these patients to infections with gram-positive and gram-negative organisms [3,5, 23,27].

There have been reports of severe impairments of most granulocyte functions in CLL patients with a history of infections. Defective granulocyte chemotaxis has been reported as a predicting factor of infections in this group of patients. Additionally, significant beta-glucuronidase, lysozyme, and myeloperoxidase enzyme deficiencies have been reported in monocytes of untreated CLL patients. These deficiencies may resolve with hematological remission. With the widespread use of combination cytotoxic chemotherapy for advanced disease, it is expected that neutropenia and qualitative phago-cytic cell defects will contribute more to the risk of infection in this group of patients [3,5,23,27].

COMPLEMENT ACTIVITY

Complement activity in CLL patients is abnormal and associated with shortened survival, severe infections, and increased incidence of autoimmune disorders. The type of infection depends on which component is the defective one [3,5,23,27]. For instance, deficiencies in C1, C4-C2 are associated with pneumococcal infections. Deficiencies of C3, C5, C6, C7, or C8 are related to neisserial infections [33]. Complement plays a crucial role in the control of bacterial infections caused by *S. pneumoniae*, *H. influenza*, and *E. coli* as opsonization with complement is necessary for interaction with neutrophils. Decreased levels of complement proteins have been reported in 100% of patients with advanced CLL and in 40% of patients in earlier stages of the disease [27,34]. Specifically, decreased levels of C3b have been reported in patients who have received corticosteroids [15,27].

MUCOSAL IMMUNITY

There is little information about the integrity of the mucosal immune system and the relationship between systemic immune dysfunction and mucosal immune defects. Mucosal antibodies are the primary line of defense against sinopulmonary infections. Defects in mucosal defenses have been associated with a high incidence of sinopulmonary infection, especially with encapsu-lated organisms [5].

SPLENECTOMY

Splenectomy is infrequently performed in CLL patients except those with autoimmune hemolytic anemia, immune thrombocytopenia, splenomegaly, and cytopenia secondary to hypersplenism [1,27]. Splenectomy may be responsible for severe infections with encapsulated bacteria, such as pneu-mococci [23]. Because autoimmune phenomena associated with CLL follow-ing splenectomy result in improved hematological parameters and survival benefit, its role may be upgraded in the future [35].

Infections Associated with Conventional or Standard Chemotherapy

Prior to the development of purine analogs such as fludarabine, conventional or standard therapy for CLL consisted of an alkylating agent with or without the addition of corticosteroids. The most frequent alkylating agent used alone is chlorambucil, while cyclophosphamide is the one most frequently used in multiagent chemotherapy combinations [27]. Two of the most frequent toxicities of alkylating agents are myelosuppression and immunosuppression. Neutropenia has been described along with selective suppression and depression of B lymphocytes as well as suppression of lymphocyte function mediated by T cells. Additionally, corticosteroids are also well known for their immunosuppressive effects including decreased antibody formation and direct lymphotoxicity and lymphopenia [27].

Therefore it is not surprising that in patients with CLL and their inherent immunocompromised status, treatment with myelosuppressive and immunosuppressive drugs such as alkylating agents and corticosteroids results in an increased risk of infection. Infections are more common in pretreated than in untreated patients and remain the major cause of morbidity and mortality in patients with chronic lymphocytic leukemia [5].

Clinical studies dealing with their incidence have yielded inconclusive results [36]. In 1973 Twomey estimated that 84% of patients with CLL will sustain infectious complications ranging in severity from moderate to life threatening at some time in their disease course and that infections account for 63% of deaths in this patient population [2]. More recently, Itala et al. estimated that the incidence of infection was 0.47 per patient-year [17]. Molica et al. described that among 125 patients followed over 10 years, the crude rate of severe infections was 0.1 per patient-year. The 5 year risk of developing a severe infection in that study was 26%, with 29.5% of patient deaths attributed to infections [36]. More importantly, the same study [36] found that the risk of infection increased with low IgG levels (57.1%) and even more with both low IgG levels and advanced (stage C) disease (68%). Most of these studies used different diagnostic criteria for infection and cause of death and examined selected populations from tertiary care centers. Despite these limitations, they allow us to establish the stage of the underlying leukemia, neutrophil count, immunoglobulin level, and prior treatment using cytotoxic agents as important factors for the type and severity of infections in CLL [3].

The majority of infections complicating the course of CLL patients treated with conventional chemotherapy are of bacterial origin and mucosal-lined structures. The respiratory tract is the most frequent site or portal of entry for such infections [5,23]. For this reason, pneumonia is the commonest and most severe infection in patients with CLL. Sinusitis is also common. Bacteremia/septicemia is typically seen in patients with profound neutropenia. Other sites of infection reported include kidney, skin, soft tissues, bowel, peritoneal cavity, and meninges [3,5,23].

Bacterial infections caused by encapsulated organisms such as *S. pneumoniae* are common. *S. aureus* infections are prominent in some series, while increased numbers of gram-negative infections are more frequent in others. Frequent fatal bacteremias or pneumonias caused by *P. aeruginosa* have been described in the setting of advanced disease and profound and prolonged myelosuppression, similar to that seen in acute leukemias [3,5, 23,37]. Other frequently reported pathogens include *H. influenzae*, *Legionella* spp., and *Salmonella* spp. Mycobacterial infections, or those caused by *Listeria monocytogenes*, *Nocardia* spp., or *P. carinii*, are rare in CLL patients treated with conventional chemotherapy [3,5,23]. Viral and fungal infections are far less common than bacterial infections. However, infections due to fungi (*Candida* and *Aspergillus*) and those due to viruses (herpesvirus, especially herpes simplex and varicella zoster) are also associated with advanced-stage disease and severe and prolonged neutropenia [3,5,23,37].

Infections in CLL Patients Treated with Fludarabine

The activity of fludarabine both in previously untreated and in previously treated patients with CLL is excellent, and response rates range between 75 and 80% for the former and 50 to 60% for the latter [38–41]. After intravenous injection, fludarabine is dephosphorylated to F-ara-A and enters the cell, were it is rephosphorylated by deoxycytidine kinase (dCk) to the triphosphate (F-ara-ATP) that inhibits DNA synthesis, ribonucleotide reductase, and a variety of enzymes required for DNA synthesis and repair, as well as RNA synthesis. Recent data also suggests that it acts primarily by activating apoptosis [39,42]. In most patients, fludarabine causes quantitative and qualitative (functional) T cell abnormalities [5], the most frequent being the rapid development of lymphocytopenia, with CD4 cells primarily affected [41]. After as early as two cycles of therapy, profound and prolonged suppression of the CD4 counts can occur [5,39] and may persist 1 to 2 years after discontinuation of therapy. Lesser effects are seen on CD8 and NK cells. The CD4/CD8 ratio remains either unchanged or somewhat decreased [5,42].

Fludarabine has been used not only as a single agent but also in combinations with corticosteroids and alkylating agents with various results. Although mostly well tolerated, fludarabine use in all these different settings has been associated with the development of serious infections [5,38,39,41,43,44]. A retrospective review of over 400 untreated and previously treated patients (chlorambucil with or without prednisone) at the M. D. Anderson Cancer Center who went on to receive fludarabine (with or without prednisone) has been published [45]. Infections occurred more often in previously treated patients (58% vs. 34%) and fludarabine in this group of previously treated patients may be associated with infections involving T cell dysfunction. These infectious include listeriosis, pneumocystosis, mycobacterial infections, and opportunistic fungal and viral infections (cutaneous zoster more often in patients with CD4 counts less than 50 cells/mL). Rather than the previously recognized pattern of infections predominantly caused by encapsulated pathogens [11], this study revealed the emergence of a new spectrum of pathogens (*Listeria monocytogenes*, *Pneumocystis carinii*, cytomegalovirus, herpes simplex virus, varicella zoster virus, and mycobacteria). Typically associated with T cell dysfunction, these organisms were most frequently observed in fludarabine-treated patients [45]. Similar patterns of opportunistic infections have been reported by several other investigators [5,38,39,43–45]. In these previously treated patients, immunosuppression (mainly lymphopenia and lymphocyte dysfunction) may persist for more than 1 year after the end of antineoplastic therapy [28]. Additionally, a multivariate analysis identified advanced stage (Rai III or IV), previous chemotherapy, creatinine greater than 1.4 mg/dL and absolute granulocyte count less than 1000 cells/µL as independent risk factors associated with major infection.

Until recently, only a French CLL prospective randomized study comparing fludarabine to CHOP and CAP analyzed but did not confirm a significantly higher risk of infection among fludarabine treated patients [39,43]. CALGB 9011, a recently published intergroup study that prospectively randomized previously untreated CLL patients to fludarabine, chlorambucil, or the combination, was specifically designed to determine whether the incidence and type of infections in fludarabine-treated patients are different from infections in CLL patients treated with traditional alkylator-based therapy [43]. Of a total of 1107 infections (241 major infections), more than 70% occurred in those receiving fludarabine. Patients receiving the combination drug regimen had more infections (including major infections) than those receiving either drug alone. Among the single drug arms, there were more infections on the fludarabine arm, particularly more major infections and herpesvirus infections [43] than in the chlorambucil arm. Among the parameters identified as risk factors for infections in the previous retrospective review [45], the intergroup study found that neutropenia was more common with major infections but did not differ among the treatment arms, and that there was no association between the incidence of infection and the Rai stage of CLL. Only patients treated with fludarabine and chlorambucil who experienced a decline in creatinine clearance were at greater risk of having at least one major infection and also had more major infections [43]. Although patients with low IgG levels (<500 mg/dL) had more infections, correlation with treatment arms were nonsignificant.

In summary, infections in fludarabine-treated patients include bacterial infections common to CLL patients in addition to a variety of opportunistic pathogens, such as *Listeria*, *Nocardia*, and *Mycobacterium* species. Fungal infections, often disseminated, are most often caused by Candida or Aspergillus species. Reports of *Pneumocystis carinii* infections are common. Lastly, herpesvirus infections, especially VZV, are frequent in fludarabine-treated patients [5,38–40,43–45], and as many as 30 to 50% of them occur after completion of initial therapy [43].

Bone Marrow Therapy

The use of bone marrow transplant for patients with CLL is a relatively new approach when compared with the use of this therapy for other hematological malignancies. There have been several factors that deterred the use of this procedure in patients with CLL, including the long natural history of the disease, the significant procedure-related mortality of BMT, and the median age at diagnosis of 55 years, which make patients ineligible for transplant [46,47]. Over the past ten years, there have been major improvements in the transplantation procedures and supportive care, allowing the use of either autologous or allogeneic BMT in patients with CLL [48–51]. Although there are reports showing complete remissions with BMT, it is still premature to evaluate long-term disease-free and overall survival in patients with CLL before BMT gains widespread acceptance as a new therapy for this disease [46].

Prophylaxis

The risk of infection and prophylactic strategy in CLL patients depends on the different stages of the disease and the type of treatment [23,52]. Patients with early-stage disease usually do not require intensive chemotherapy, so antimicrobial prophylaxis is not recommended. Patients with advanced disease receiving cytotoxic chemotherapy are at high risk for infection, and antibacterial, antifungal, and antiviral prophylaxis should be considered.

Antibacterial Prophylaxis

Anaissie et al. [45] have developed a prophylactic strategy for patients with CLL treated with fludarabine. They advised patients to avoid unpasteurized milk, soft cheeses, raw vegetables, and undercooked poultry or meat, known to contain *L. monocytogenes*, preventing life-threatening listeriosis in patients at risk. They recommend the use of amoxicillin and clavulanate for early signs of infection, to cover encapsulated organisms. Acyclovir is used for mucocutaneous herpes infections, especially if CD4 counts are less than 50 cells/mL, to shorten the course of herpetic infection and decrease the severity of postherpetic neuralgia. True antimicrobial prophylaxis should be used only for patients at highest risk for infections, such as patients with advanced Rai stage renal dysfunction, an absolute granulocyte count less than 1000 cells/μL, and previous cytotoxic therapy. Antifungal prophylaxis is indicated when persistent (more than 10 to 14 days) and profound neutropenia (less than 100 neutrophils) is present. Voriconazole is recommended because of the risk of Aspergillosis. Antibacterial prophylaxis with trimethoprim-sulfmethoxazole is used against *P. carinii* pneumonia and listeriosis. In addition, Sudhoff et al. [53] recommended adding oral ciprofloxacin for the duration of therapy-induced neutropenia (less than 500 cells/μL) to avoid gram-negative septicemia. The duration of antimicrobial prophylaxis has not been well established [45,53], but it is important to consider continuing with prophylaxis as long as the risk for major infections persists, including in patients with low CD4 counts or concomitant steroid therapy.

Immunoglobulin Replacement

The benefit of using intravenous immunoglobulin (IVIG) as a supportive measure in CLL patients is still controversial. A large randomized double-blind prospective trial comparing placebo with IVIG in patients with an increased risk of infection due to hypogammaglobulinemia, a history of infection, or both by the Cooperative Group for the Study of Immunoglobulin in CLL was completed. The study found significantly fewer moderately severe bacterial infections in patients who received immunoglobulin (400 mg/kg every 3 weeks) than in the placebo group. But minor and severe bacterial infections remained unchanged. Also, no reduction in mortality was noted [3,17,54,55].

Vaccination

Several studies have reported a suboptimal response of CLL patients to immunization related to impaired antibody production and defects in antigen presentation [5,32,56]. More than 30 years ago Shaw et al. demonstrated poor serological response in patients who received diphteria, typhoid, influenza, and mumps vaccines. None of these patients received steroids or cytotoxic agents before vaccination [57]. The Gribabis group reported antibody response of influenza vaccine in 43 CLL patients. An antibody response to the vaccine occurred in 81% of patients. Hypogammaglobulinemic patients responded less frequently than their counterparts with normal immunoglobulin levels. Because of a decrease in antibody levels, reimmunization with influenza vaccine at 1 month is recommended [58]. Jacobson et al. [59] found a significantly lower serological response to pneumococcal vaccine in CLL patients than in multiple myeloma patients and in normal controls. Therefore select patients with early-stage disease and normal immunoglobulin levels show better serological response to vaccine and may benefit most from vaccines. Immunization may be ineffective in refractory CLL and advanced-stage disease, because the lack of an adequate antibody response correlates with an advanced stage of disease and hypogammaglobulinemia [3,56–59].

Growth Factors

Neutropenia is expected in more than 50% of patients treated with fludarabine [53,60]. It has been found in 74% of the initial fludarabine treatment cycles in pretreated patients with Rai III and IV, along with an increase in the incidence of infectious complications during the first three courses of treatment [61]. Neutropenia usually improves with the continuation of chemotherapy so the use of G-CSF as an attempt to stimulate myelopoiesis to reduce the risk of infectious complications can be justified in patients with known risk factors for major infections [23,62,63].

CONCLUSIONS

The neoplastic component of CLL is of great interest. Patients with this disease are still dying, mostly from infectious complications. The continuing changes in therapeutic schemes have resulted in a change in the spectrum of infections. More effective prophylaxis and therapy has reduced infectious complications in patients with CLL. Goals for the future include a prolonged control of the disease and improving the immunological status of patients with CLL.

REFERENCES

1. Foon KA, Raik R, Gale RP. CLL: new insights into biology and therapy. Ann Int Med 1990; 113:525–539.
2. Twomey JJ. Infections complicating multiple myeloma and CLL. Arch Intern Med 1973; 132:562–565.
3. Tsiodras S, Samonis G, Keating MJ, Kontoyiannis DP. Infection and Immunity in CLL. Mayo Clin Proc 2000; 75:1039–1054.
4. Surveillance Epidemiology Results, Incidence and Mortality Data: 1973–1977. NCI Monograph 57. Bethesda, MD: NCI, 1981:10.

5. Morrison Vicki A. The infectious complications of chronic lymphocytic leukemia. Semin Oncol 1998; 25:98–106.
6. De Lima M, O'Brien S, Lerner S, Keating M. Chronic lymphocytic leukemia in the young patient. Seminars in Oncology 1998; (1):80–97.
7. Galton DAG. The pathogenesis of CLL. Can Med Assoc 1996; J 94:1005.
8. Dameshek W. CLL, an accummulative disease of immunologically incompetent lymphocytes. Blood 1967; 29:566.
9. Fairley GH, Scott RB. Hypogammaglobulinemia in chronic lymphocytic leukemia. Br Med J 1961; 2:920–924.
10. Caligaris-Cappio F. Biology of chronic lymphocytic leukemia. Rev Clin Exp Hematol 2000; 4(1):5 21.
11. Lenders JWM, DePauw BE, Bogman MJ, Haanen C. Blut 1984; 48:171–175.
12. Brem TH, Morton ME. Defective gamma globulin formation. Ann Int Med 1955; 43:465 479.
13. Cone L, Uhr JW. Immunological deficiency disorders associated with chronic lymphocytic leukemia and multiple myeloma. J Clin Invest 1964; 43:2241–2248.
14. Hudson RP, Wilson SJ. Hypogammaglobulinemia and chronic lymphocytic leukemia. Cancer 1960; 13:200–204.
15. Ultmann JE, Fish W, Osserman E, Gellhorn A. The clinical implications of hypogammaglobulinemia in patients with chronic lymphocytic leukemia and lymphocytic lymphosarcoma. Ann Int Med 1959; 51:501–516.
16. Videbaek A. Some clinical aspects of leukemia. Acta Haematol 1960; 24:54–58.
17. Itala M, Helenius H, Nikoskelaien J, Remes K. Infections and serum IgG levels in patients with chronic lymphocytic leukemia. Eur J Haematol 1992; 48:266–270.
18. Rozman C, Monserrat E, Vinolas N. Serum immunoglobulins in B-CLL. Natural history and prognostic significance. Cancer 1988; 61:279–283.
19. Foa R, Catovsky D, Brozovic M, Marsh G, Ooyirilangkumaran T, Cherchi M, Galton DA. Clinical staging and immunological findings in chronic lymphocytic leukemia. Cancer 1979; 44:54 58.
20. Ben-Bassat I, Many A, Modan M, Peretz C, Ramot B. Serum immunoglobulins in chronic lymphocytic leukemia. Am J Med Sci 1979; 278:4–9.
21. Whelan CA, Willoughby R, McCann SR. Relationship between immunoglobulin levels, lymphocyte subpopulations and Rai staging in patients with BCLL. Acta Haematol 1983; 69:217 223.
22. Rai KR, Montserrat E. Prognostic factors in chronic lymphocytic leukemia. Semin Hematol 1987; 24:252–256.
23. Morra E, Nosari A, Montillo M. Infectious complications in chronic lymphocytic leukaemia. Hematol Cell Ther 1991; 41:145 151.
24. Foa R. Pathogenesis of the immunodeficiency in chronic lymphocytic leukemia 1993. In: Cheson BD, ed. Chronic Lymphocytic Leukemia: Scientific Advances and Clinical Developments. New York: Marcel Dekker, 1993:147–166.
25. Apostopoulos A, Simeonidis A, Zoumbos N. Prognostic significance of immune function parameter in patients with chronic lymphocytic leukemia. Eur J Haematol 1990; 44:39 44.

26. Dighiero G. An attempt to explain disordered immunity and hypogammaglobulinemia in CLL. Nouv Rev Fr Hematol 1988; 30:283–288.
27. Molica S. Infections in chronic lymphocytic leukemia: risk factors, and impact on survival and treatment. Leukemia and Lymphoma 1994; 13:203–214.
28. Hardy RR, Hayakawa K. Development and physiology of Ly-1 B and its human homolog Leu-1 B. Immunol Rev 1986; 93:53–80.
29. Chapel MH. Hypogammaglobulinemia and chronic lymphocytic leukemia. In: Pritsch O, Maloum K, Dighiero G, eds. Basic biology of autoimmune phenomena in chronic lymphocytic leukemia. Sem in Oncol 1998; (1):34–41
30. Rozman C, Monserrat E. Chronic lymphocytic leukemia. N Engl J Med 1995; 333:1052–1057.
31. Caligaris-Cappio F, Hamblin TJ. B-cell chronic lymphocytic leukemia: a bird of a different feather. Clin Oncol 1999; 17(1):399–408.
32. Bartik MM, Welker D, Kay NE. Impairments in immune cell function in B-cell chronic lymphocytic leukemia. Semin Oncol 1998; 25:27–33.
33. Ross SC, Densen P. Complement deficiency states and infection: epidemiology, pathogenesis and consequences of neisserial and other infections in immune deficiency. Medicine (Baltimore) 1984; 63:243–273.
34. Jaksic B, Rundek T, Planinc-Peraica A, Brugiatelli M. Changes in serum immunoglobulin concentration in B-chronic lymphocytic leukemia (B-CLL). XXII Congress of the International Society of Hematology, Milan, August 28–September 2, 1988:323.
35. Cusack JC Jr, Seymour JF, Lerner S, Keating MJ, Pollock RE. Role of splenectomy in chronic lymphocytic leukemia. J Am Coll Surg 1997; 185:237–243.
36. Molica S, Levato D, Levato L. Infections in chronic lymphocytic leukemia. Analysis of incidence as a function of length of follow-up. Haematologica 1993; 78(6):374–377.
37. Batlle M, Ribera JM, Oriol A, Rodriguez L, Cirauqui B, Xicoy B, Grau J, Feliu J, Flores A, Milla F. Pneumonia in patients with chronic lymphocytic leukemia. Med Clin (Barc) 2001; 116(19):738–740.
38. Keating MJ, O'Brien S, Koller LC, Lerner S, Beran M, Robertson LE, Freireich EJ, Estey E, Kantarjian H. Long-term follow-up of patients with chronic lymphocytic leukemia (CLL) receiving fludarabine regimens as initial therapy. Blood 1998; 92(4):1165–1171.
39. Fenchel K, Bergmann L, Wijermans P, Engert A, Pralle H, Milrou PS, Dichl V, Hoelzer D. Clinical experience with fludarabine and its immunosuppressive effects in pretreated chronic lymphocytic leukemias and low-grade lymphomas. Leukemia and lymphoma, 1995; (18):485–492.
40. Bergmann L, Fenchel K, John B, Milrou PS, Hoelzer D. Immunosuppressive effects and clinical response of fludarabine in refractory chronic lymphocytic leukemia. Annals of Oncology 1993; 4:371–375.
41. Keating MJ. Chronic lymphocytic leukemia. Sem in Oncol 1999; 26(5 suppl 14): 107–114.
42. Ross SR, McTavish D, Faulds D. Fludarabine. A review of its pharmacological properties and therapeutic potential in malignancy. Drugs 1993; 45:737–759.

43. Morrison V, Rai KR, Peterson BL, Kolitz JE, Elias L, Appelbaum FR, Hines JD, Shepherd I, Martell RE, Larson RA, Schiffer CA. Impact of therapy with chlorambucil, fludarabine, or fludarabine plus chlorambucil on infections in patients with chronic lymphocytic leukemia: intergroup study cancer and leukemia group B 9011. Journal of Clinical Oncology 2001; 19(16):3611–3621.
44. O'Brien SM, et al. Results of the fludarabine and cyclophosphamide combination regime in chronic lymphocytic leukemia. Journal of Clinical Oncology 2001; 19(5):1414–1420.
45. Anaissie EJ, Kontoyiannis D, O'Brien S, et al. Infections in patients with chronic lymphocytic leukemia treated with fludarabine. Ann Intern Med 1998; 129:559 566.
46. Byrd JC, et al. Old and new therapies in chronic lymphocytic leukemia: now is the time for a reassessment of therapeutic goals. Sem in Oncol 1998; 25(1):65–74.
47. Rai KR, Sawitsky A, Cronkite EP, et al. Clinical staging of chronic lymphocytic leukemia. Blood 1975; 46:219–234.
48. Binet JL, Auguier A, Dighiero G, et al. A new prognostic classification of CLL derived from a multivariate survival analysis. Cancer 1981; 48:198–216.
49. Lee JS, Dixon DO, Kantarjian HM, et al. Prognosis of CLL: a multivariate regression analysis of 325 untreated patients. Blood 1987; 69:929–936.
50. Montserrat E, Rozman C. Chronic lymphocytic leukemia: prognostic factors and natural history. Baillieres Clin Haematol 1993; 6:849 866.
51. Montserrat E, Gomis F, Vallespi T, et al. Presenting features and prognois of CLL in younger adults. Blood 1991; 78:1545–1551.
52. O'Brien S, Kantarjian H, Beran M, et al. Results of fludarabine and prednisone therapy in 264 patients with chronic lymphocytic leukemia with multivariate analysis–derived prognostic model for response to treatment. Blood 1993; 82: 1700–1965.
53. Sudhoff T, Arning M, Schneider W. Prophylactic strategies to meet infectious complications in fludarabine-treated CLL. Leukemia 11 Apr 1997; 2(suppl):S38–41. Review.
54. The Cooperative Group for the Study of Immunoglobulin in Chronic Lymphocytic Leukemia. Intravenous immunoglobulin for prevention of infection in CLL A randomized control trial. New Engl J Med 1988; 319:902–907.
55. Chapel H, Dicato M, Gamm H, et al. Immunoglobulin replacement in patients with chronic lymphocytic leukemia: a comparison of two dose regimens. Br J Haematol 1994; 88:209–212.
56. Cone L, Uhr JW. Immunological deficiency disorders associated with chronic lymphocytic leukemia and multiple myeloma. J Clin Invest 1964; 43:2241–2248.
57. Shaw RK, Szwed C, Boggs DR, et al. Infection and autoimmnunity in chronic lymphocytic leukemia. Arch Intern Med 1960; 106:467–478.
58. Gribabis DA, Panayiotidis P, Boussiotis VA, et al. Influenza virus vaccine in B-cell chronic lymphocytic leukemia patients. Acta Haematol 1994; 91:115–118.
59. Jacobson DR, Ballard HS, Silber R, et al. Antibody response in pneumococcal immunization in patients with chronic lymphocytic leukemia. Blood 1998; 72(suppl 1):205a.

60. O'Brien MER, Matutes E, Cunningham D, et al. Fludarabine in lymphopro-
    liferative disorders: the Royal Marsden hospital experience. Leuk Lymphoma
    1994; 14(suppl 2):17–24.
61. Keating MJ, Kantarjian H, Talpaz M, et al. Fludarabine: a new agent with major
    activity against CLL. Blood 1989; 74:19–25.
62. O'Brien S, Kantarjian H, Beran M, et al. Fludarabine and granulocyte colony-
    stimulating factor (G-CSF) in patients with chronic lymphocytic leukemia. Leu-
    kemia 1997; 11:1631–1635.
63. Vadhan-Raj S, Velasquez WS, Butler JJ, et al. Stimulation of myelopoiesis in
    chronic lymphocytic leukemia and in other lymphoproliferative disorders by
    recombinant human granulocyte-macrophage colony-stimulating factor. Am J
    Haematol 1990; 33:189–197.

7

Infections Associated with Chronic Myelogenous Leukemia

James Riddell IV and Carol A. Kauffman
Veterans Affairs Ann Arbor Healthcare System
University of Michigan Medical School
Ann Arbor, Michigan, U.S.A.

INTRODUCTION

Chronic myelogenous leukemia (CML) is a disease in which hematopoietic stem cells are transformed into malignant clones as a result of a chromosomal translocation. As a result of this translocation, the cells constitutively produce a fusion protein, which leads to a dysregulated expansion of circulating cells from the bone marrow. Functional abnormalities of the immune system occur as this abnormal population of cells expands and puts the patient at risk for infectious complications. The risk varies from minimal to major depending on the phase of the disease that the patient is experiencing. Thus a patient in the early asymptomatic chronic phase will likely have no more infections than any other person without leukemia. In contrast, patients in blast crisis and those who have received a hematopoietic stem cell transplant (HSCT) are at as much risk as any other patient in these respective groups. The following is a synthesis of what is known regarding the immune defects observed in the several phases of CML and a review of specific infectious processes that have been reported either as case reports or as small series.

CHARACTERISTICS OF CML

The advent of sophisticated molecular investigative techniques has allowed clinicians to understand the genetics and pathophysiology of CML in substantial detail [2]. As early as 1960, it was known that there was a shortening of chromosome 22, the so-called Philadelphia chromosome, associated with the disease. In 1973, this was further defined as a translocation of the long arms of chromosomes 9 and 22. As a result of this translocation, the fusion protein BCR-ABL, a tyrosine kinase that is constitutively active in the cytoplasm of hematopoietic progenitors, is produced; its unregulated activity leads to malignant transformation of the hematopoietic progenitor cells [1–4].

CML is a triphasic illness consisting of a chronic phase that lasts for 3 to 5 years on average, followed by an accelerated phase that culminates in blast crisis similar to that seen with acute leukemias. During the chronic phase, when the diagnosis is established in the majority of patients, a variety of abnormalities are observed on the peripheral blood smear [4]. These include leukocytosis (white blood cells >25,000/μL and often >100,000/μL), anemia, and thrombocytosis. The differential reveals cells in all stages of the granulocytic series and often an increased number of basophils. Most patients are asymptomatic during this phase of the disease and are often diagnosed when a complete blood count is obtained for an unrelated reason. In others, the diagnosis is made after they see a physician for fatigue, anorexia, and weight loss. Hepatosplenomegaly is commonly noted at the time of diagnosis.

The accelerated phase is a transition between the chronic and blast phases. It can be defined by a need for increasing cytotoxic therapy to control the white blood cell and platelet counts, increasing splenomegaly, and worsening fatigue, anorexia, fever, and night sweats [3]. It is a harbinger of blast crisis, which is rapidly fatal if not treated. Patients in blast crisis are similar to other patients with acute myeloid or acute lymphoid leukemias; they have fever, night sweats, weight loss, and bone pain, and they develop marked anemia, thrombocytopenia, and leukemic infiltrates in many viscera and the skin. Most patients develop a myeloid blast crisis, but in as many as 25% of CML patients, a lymphoid blast crisis develops, and in some patients, the cell lineage is not clear [4]. The median survival once the blast phase supervenes is only 3 to 6 months.

TREATMENT OF CML

Treatment in the past utilized cytoreductive therapy with hydroxyurea or busulfan to decrease the white blood cell count during the chronic and accelerated phases. Remission in this circumstance translated into reducing the white blood cell count to near normal levels but was not associated with any changes in the genetic aberrations [1,3]. Once the patient entered blast crisis, aggressive chemotherapeutic regimens had to be undertaken, but the outcome was dismal. Infections are a major complication in this group of patients.

A major step forward was taken when it was shown that HLA-matched allogeneic bone marrow transplantation could cure CML [1,2,5,6]. Success rates are higher with HLA-matched sibling donor transplants than with HLA-matched unrelated donors [1], and older patients generally do less well than those younger than 50 years of age [3,4]. To succeed, transplantation has to be accomplished as early as possible and certainly before the patient enters the accelerated and blast crisis phases of the disease [3,5,6]. Whereas previously infections were not a major complication of CML until blast crisis occurred, they assume great importance once transplantation is performed.

For patients for whom no donor is available or who, for some other reason, are not candidates for HSCT, therapy with interferon alpha (IFN-α) has proved very useful. Both clinical and cytogenetic remissions are induced with IFN-α therapy, and a small proportion of patients are cured [7]. Older adults respond well but do have more side effects [8]. Early treatment during the chronic phase of CML is associated with better outcomes. Treatment with IFN-α is not associated with an increase in complications due to infection and indeed might help protect against some viral infections.

Recently, a specific inhibitor of the BCR-ABL tyrosine kinase has been developed. Imatinib mesylate (Gleevec, Novartis, Basel, Switzerland) has been shown to induce both cytogenetic and clinical responses in a large proportion of patients who had previously failed IFN-α therapy [9]. Even later stages of the disease appear to respond. Overall, it appears that this agent will dramatically change the course of CML for many patients, but data on long-term survival have not yet been evaluated. If the effect of imatinib mesylate is long-lasting, it seems likely that even fewer patients will suffer infectious complications related to CML.

CML-ASSOCIATED IMMUNE DEFECTS

Humoral Immunity

Humoral immunity appears to be intact in patients with CML [10]. Immunoglobulin levels are usually in the normal range and remain normal, even after cytoreduction therapy [11,12]. Primary and secondary antibody responses also have been shown to be normal in patients with CML. Heavy chain gene rearrangements have been found in late chronic phase CML and seem to predict impending blast crisis [13]; however, there are no data to suggest that these rearrangements lead to dysfunction of the immunoglobulin molecule.

Cell-Mediated Immunity and Cytokine Production

Abnormalities of cell-mediated immunity have been described by some, but not all, investigators in patients in chronic phase CML [11,12,14,15]. Delayed-type hypersensitivity has been noted to be normal in most patients with CML [11,12]. However, in vitro lymphocyte stimulation with phytohemagglutinin and pokeweed antigen has been shown to be decreased in a small number of patients [11,15]. The proportion of T cells with the CD4 marker are low and those with the CD8 marker are high at the time of diagnosis, but both return to normal values during remission induced by IFN-α or hydroxyurea treatment [16]. A decreased proportion of interferon-gamma (IFN-γ) positive CD4 cells, interleukin-4 (IL-4) positive CD4 cells, and IFN-γ/IL-4 double positive CD4 cells has been noted in CML patients who have not received any treatment [14]. Values return toward normal after treatment with hydroxyurea. A specific defect in T cell responsiveness to mycobacterial antigens has been well described in one patient who had both CML and tuberculosis [15]. Production of the cytokines TNF-α and IFN-γ is low in chronic phase CML patients who have not received any therapy, but it increases to normal levels when a sustained remission has been produced [16,17].

Neutrophil Function

It has been known for almost half a century that neutrophils from some patients in the chronic phase of CML have decreased phagocytic capability and that the abnormalities return to normal with remission [18–22]. Metabolic activities of neutrophils are normal in some treatment-naive individuals but markedly deficient in others [23–25]. The ability of neutrophils to respond to chemoattractants has also been noted to be abnormal in some patients with CML [24–25]. Specifically, this appears to be a defect in the ability to degranulate in response to fLMP-type chemoattractants and is associated with decreased fLMP receptors on the neutrophil surface.

Natural Killer Cell Function

Natural killer cell populations diminish as CML progresses [26] and may be involved in malignant transformation in advanced CML [27]. The NK cells from CML patients appear to be functionally defective in vitro in cytotoxicity and target cell binding assays; these defects can be restored in vitro with the addition of IL-2 [17,28].

Relationship of Immune Defects to Risk of Infection

Although the above defects in cell-mediated immunity, cytokine production, and neutrophil and natural killer cell function have been well described, most patients in the chronic phase of CML do not appear to be at great risk for infection when compared with patients who have chronic lymphocytic or acute leukemia. In regard to the defects in neutrophil function, the large number of circulating cells may compensate for defects that may be present in some but not all of the cells. The in vitro cell-mediated immune defects have not been consistently noted by all investigators, and the ultimate test for cell-mediated immunity in vivo, the delayed hypersensitivity skin test reaction, appears not to be diminished. Finally, some of the immune deficiencies that have been described may lead to an inability to handle a certain type of pathogen but not cause overwhelming risk for infection with normal flora of the gastrointestinal tract, for example, as occurs in acute leukemia.

Clearly, patients in the blast phase of CML are at great risk for infection because of neutropenia and the effects of aggressive chemotherapeutic regimens on the gastrointestinal tract and the marrow. Immune defects in this phase are the same as those noted in other patients with acute leukemias. Likewise, those who undergo HSCT have the same defects in immune response as other transplant recipients. In addition, there is some suggestion that T cell function may not return as promptly in those who undergo HSCT for CML as in those who have undergone transplantation for acute lymphocytic or myeloid leukemias [29].

INFECTIONS IN CML

Infections in Chronic Phase CML

There appears to be no overwhelming predisposition to infection in most patients with chronic phase CML. Infection is rarely a presenting manifestation of CML. Large reviews of infectious complications of leukemia and reviews of infections due to specific organisms show no cases or only a few cases of CML or do not separate out CML from other chronic leukemias [30–36]. It is likely that the paucity of reports highlighting infectious complications of CML reflects the fact that CML is not associated with profound immune suppression. It is also likely that only a few cases of CML are included in large reviews because of the relative rarity of this form of leukemia compared with other types and because most patients in chronic phase CML are not in hospital and not receiving aggressive chemotherapy.

There may be an increased risk for infection with mycobacteria in patients in chronic phase CML. An early report noted a higher rate of disseminated tuberculosis among patients with CML when compared with patients with other types of leukemias [37]. This high rate has not been affirmed since that report, and that report may be unique because the patients studied had developed leukemia following the Hiroshima atomic bomb blast. An incidence of systemic atypical mycobacterial infections of 3.9% among patients with CML was reported, also from Japan [38]. Although this was an inordinately high rate, it represented only three cases. The author reviewed three other cases previously reported [39–41]. Four of the six patients had been treated with corticosteroids prior to the development of infection with *Mycobacterium kansasii* and *Mycobacterium avium* complex, and two had busulfan lung injury and pulmonary alveolar proteinosis [40,41].

It appears that patients with CML may have an increased risk for CMV pneumonia, but it is not as high as that noted with some other leukemias [42]. In a large series from the M. D. Anderson Cancer Center, the incidence of CMV pneumonia was 2.3% among patients with CML, compared with 8.8% in those with chronic lymphocytic leukemia. The mortality rate was the highest among CML patients (78%). Although it is not clear from the data presented, it appears that most of these patients had been treated with high-dose cytotoxic therapy, and many were in blast crisis. Isolated case reports note the occurrence of various fungal and bacterial infections in patients in chronic phase CML [43,44]. Although in chronic phase CML, these patients had received cytotoxic therapy prior to development of the infection.

Infections in Blast Crisis

The real concern for infection arises when the patient enters the blast phase of the disease. At this point, the patient is hospitalized, aggressive chemotherapy is given, and neutropenia and mucositis ensue. Bacterial infections are the primary concern and arise most often from the gastrointestinal tract or intravenous catheters. Even in this circumstance, various series of infections in neutropenic patients and patients with acute leukemias tend to have small numbers of patients with CML in blast phase in comparison with patients with acute myelogenous leukemia, likely reflecting the more common occurrence of the latter type of leukemia [45–47]. As noted above, it is likely that most of the patients with CML who were reported with CMV pneumonia were actually in blast crisis [42].

The approach to the diagnosis of infection in CML patients in blast crisis does not differ from that for any other neutropenic patient. Similarly, approaches to prophylaxis, empiric treatment, and therapy for established infections are not unlike those for other acute leukemias. These topics are covered in depth in the chapters devoted to infections in acute leukemias.

Infections Posttransplantation

Not surprisingly, given the importance of allogeneic bone marrow transplantation for treatment of CML, there are more data available on infections in patients with CML who have undergone HSCT [48–63]. Many of the large series dealing with a variety of infectious complications of HSCT include a large number of CML patients; however, the relative proportion of patients with CML in each series often reflects the numbers of patients with CML who are transplanted at each transplant center. Several points emerge when evaluating the epidemiology and risks for many of the infections seen in CML posttransplantation. Infections tend to occur late after engraftment, usually at day + 100, and a major risk factor that emerges is the presence of chronic GVHD in almost all of the patients.

Several types of infections in HSCT recipients for whom CML is the underlying malignancy appear to be reported more often than expected. CMV pneumonia seems to occur disproportionately more often in patients with CML than in those with other leukemias. Data from the M. D. Anderson Medical Center reveal that 11% of patients with CML, but only 6% of those with acute leukemias, developed CMV pneumonia [53]. Most patients developed CMV infection late after transplant (after day + 100), and many had extensive GVHD and were on high doses of immunosuppressive agents. A similarly disproportionately high number of cases of toxoplasmosis has been reported among CML patients who have undergone HSCT [54]. In one series from Germany, six of eight cases of toxoplasmosis were in CML patients, all but one of whom had GVHD and all but one of whom had received a matched unrelated donor transplant. Onset in most patients was after day + 100.

A major problem among all HSCT recipients is the development of fungal infections. The almost universal use of fluconazole prophylaxis posttransplant has led to a marked reduction in systemic *Candida* infections [50,60,62], but unfortunately the incidence of infections with *Aspergillus* and other filamentous molds has increased markedly [50,62]. This increase has occurred mostly late in the posttransplant period and is strongly associated with the development of GVHD and the need for increased immunosuppression [58,59,61,63]. In several recent series on filamentous fungal infections in HSCT patients, CML is the most common underlying malignancy [58,59]. It is unlikely that there are specific factors related to the underlying CML that predispose to the relatively large number of filamentous fungal infections seen in this group of transplant recipients. It is much more likely that the increase in filamentous fungal infections reflects the frequent occurrence of GVHD in CML patients. When aspergillosis or other filamentous fungal infections do occur in CML patients posttransplant, the outcomes are poor [58,59,63].

The approach to the diagnosis of specific infections and recommendations for treatment of these infections in CML patients are the same as those for other HSCT recipients. Likewise, prophylaxis and empirical treatment guidelines for CML patients who have undergone HSCT do not differ from those for patients with other leukemias. These topics are covered in depth in the chapters dealing with transplantation.

CONCLUSIONS

Among the leukemias, CML is unique in that there are no major specific defects in host immune defenses against infecting microorganisms, and consequently infections are not an important complication until the disease progresses to blast crisis. When this occurs, infections become a major cause of morbidity and mortality. Those patients who undergo HSCT are at major risk for all of the bacterial, viral, parasitic, and fungal infections found in other transplant recipients. Perhaps there is a higher risk of late CMV pneumonia and toxoplasmosis in those transplant recipients whose underlying disease was CML; however, these increases may reflect only the greater propensity for graft versus host disease, especially in those receiving unrelated donor cells, among the CML population. Infections may assume an even less important role as more CML patients are treated with imatinib mesylate, especially if long-term survival rates verify the remarkable success noted in early studies of this new approach.

REFERENCES

1. Sawyers CL. Chronic myeloid leukemia. N Engl J Med 1999; 340:1330–1340.
2. Faderl S, Talpaz M, Estrov Z, O'Brien S, Kurzrock R, Kantarjian HM. The biology of chronic myeloid leukemia. N Engl J Med 1999; 341:164–172.
3. Faderl S, Talpaz M, Estrov Z, Kantarjian HM. Chronic myelogenous leukemia: biology and therapy. Ann Intern Med 1999; 131:207–219.
4. Cortes JE, Talpaz M, Kantarjian H. Chronic myelogenous leukemia: a review. Am J Med 1996; 100:555–570.
5. Thomas ED, Clift RA, Fefer A, Appelbaum FR, Beatty P, Bensinger WI, Buckner CD, Cheever MA, Deeg HJ, Doney K, Flournoy N, Greenberg P, Hansen JA, Martin P, McGuffin R, Ramberg R, Sanders JE, Singer J, Stewart P, Storb R, Sullivan K, Weiden PL, Witherspoon R. Marrow transplantation for the treatment of chronic myelogenous leukemia. Ann Intern Med 1986; 104:155–163.
6. Goldman JM, Apperley JF, Jones L, Marcus R, Goolden AWG, Batchelor R, Hale G, Waldmann H, Reid CD, Hows J, Gordon-Smith E, Catovsky D, Galton DAG. Bone marrow transplantation for patients with chronic myeloid leukemia. N Engl J Med 1986; 314:202–207.

7. Wetzler M, Kantarjian H, Kurzrock R, Talpaz M. Interferon-α therapy for chronic myelogenous leukemia. Am J Med 1995; 99:402–411.
8. Cortes J, Kantarjian H, O'Brien S, Robertson LE, Pierce S, Talpaz M. Results of interferon-alpha therapy in patients with chronic myelogenous leukemia 60 years of age and older. Am J Med 1996; 100:452–455.
9. Kantarjian H, Sawyers C, Hochhaus A, Guilhot F, Schiffer C, Gambacorti-Passerini C, Niederwieser D, Resta D, Capdeville R, Zoellner U, Talpaz M, Druker Bfor the International ST1571 CML Study Group. Hematologic and cytogenetic responses to imatinib mesylate in chronic myelogenous leukemia. N Engl J Med 2002; 346:645 –652.
10. Hersh EM, Gutterman JU, Mavligit GM. Effect of haematological malignancies and their treatment on host defence factors. Clin Haematol 1976; 5:425–448.
11. Ghalaut VS, Ghalaut PS, Kharb S. Immunological assessment in patients of leukaemia. Indian J Pathol Microbiol 1999; 42:471–474.
12. DiBella NJ, Brown GL. Immunologic dysfunction in the myeloproliferative disorders. Cancer 1978; 42:149–158.
13. Spencer A, Szydlo SA, Grand FH, Goldman JM, Melo JV. Abnormal patterns of immunoglobulin heavy chain gene DNA fingerprinting during chronic phase chronic myeloid leukemia. Leuk Lymphoma 1999; 32:299–307.
14. Tsuda H, Yamasaki H. Type I and Type II T cell profiles in chronic myelogenous leukemia. Acta Haematol 2000; 103:96–101.
15. Vila LM, Rios-Olivares E, Rios Z, Melendez M, Garcia M, Pichardo B. Abnormal immunological response to *Mycobacterium tuberculosis* antigens in a patient with chronic myelocytic leukemia and active tuberculosis. PRHSJ 1998; 17:345–352.
16. Guarini A, Breccia M, Montefusco E, Petti MC, Zepparoni A, Vitale A, Foa R. Phenotypic and functional characterization of the host immune compartment of chronic myeloid leukaemia patients in complete haematological remission. Br J Haematol 2001; 113:136–142.
17. Chang W-C, Hsiao MH, Pattengale PK. Natural killer cell immunodeficiency in patients with chronic myelogenous leukemia. Nat Immun Cell Growth Regul 1991; 10:57–70.
18. Braude AI, Feltes J, Brooks M. Differences between the activities of mature granulocytes in leukemic and normal blood. J Clin Invest 1954; 33:1036–1046.
19. Brandt L. Adhesiveness to glass and phagocytic activity of neutrophiic leukocytes in myeloproliferative disorders. Scand J Haemat 1965; 2:126–136.
20. Penny R, Galton DAG. Studies on neutrophil function. Pathological aspects. Brit J Haemat 1966; 12:633 645.
21. Sbarra AJ, Shirley W, Selvaraj RJ, McRipley MJ, Rosenbaum E. The role of the phagocyte in host-parasite interactions. III The phagocytic capabilities of leukocytes from myeloproliferative and other neoplastic disorders. Cancer Res 1965; 25:1199–1206.
22. Rosner F, Valmont I, Kozinn PJ, Caroline L. Leukocyte function in patients with leukemia. Cancer 1970; 25:835–842.

23. Cramer E, Auclair C, Hakim J, Feliu E, Boucherot J, Troube H, Bernard J-F, Bergogne E, Boivin P. Metabolic activity of phagocytosing granulocytes in chronic granulocytic leukemia: ultrastructural observation of a degranulation defect. Blood 1977; 50:93–106.

24–25. Radhika V, Thennarasu S, Naik NR, Kumar A, Advani SH, Bhisey AN. Granulocytes from chronic myeloid leukemia (CML) patients show differential response to different chemoattractants. Am J Hematol 1996; 52:155–164.

26. Pierson BA, Miller JS. CD56$^{+bright}$ and CD56^{+dim} natural killer cells in patients with chronic myelogenous leukemia progressively decrease in number, respond less to stimuli that recruit clonogenic natural killer cells, and exhibit decreased proliferation on a per cell basis. Blood 1996; 88:2279–2287.

27. Nakajima H, Zhao R, Lund TC, Ward J, Dolan M, Hirsch B, Miller JS. The BCR/ABL transgene causes abnormal NK cell differentiation and can be found in circulating NK cells of advanced phase chronic myelogenous leukemia patients. J Immunol 2002; 168:643–650.

28. Fujimiya Y, Chang W-C, Bakke A, Horwitz D, Pattengale PK. Natural killer (NK) cell immunodeficiency in patients with chronic myelogenous leukemia. II Successful cloning and amplification of natural killer cells. Cancer Immunol Immunother 1987; 24:213–220.

29. Diamond HR, Souza MHFO, Bouzas LFS, Tabak DG, Campos MM, Camara FP, Rumjanek VM. Deficit of T-cell recovery after allogeneic bone marrow transplantation in chronic myeloid leukemia patients. Anticancer Res 1995; 15:1553–1560.

30. Miller SP, Shanbrom E. Infectious syndromes of leukemias and lymphomas. Am J Med Sci 1963; 246:420–428.

31. Levine AS, Shimpff SC, Graw RG, Young RC. Hematologic malignancies and other marrow failure states: progress in the management of complicating infections. Sem Hematol 1974; 11:141–202.

32. Singer C, Kaplan MH, Armstrong D. Bacteremia and fungemia complicating neoplastic disease. A study of 364 cases. Am J Med 1977; 62:731–742.

33. Chatzinikolaou I, Abi-Said D, Bodey GP, Rolston KVI, Tarrand JJ, Samonis G. Recent experience with *Pseudomonas aeruginosa* bacteremia in patients with cancer. Retrospective analysis of 245 episodes. Arch Intern Med 2000; 160:501–509.

34. Shah MK, Sebti A, Kiehn TE, Massarella SA, Sepkowitz KA. *Mycobacterium haemophilum* in immunocompromised patients. Clin Infect Dis 2001; 33:330–337.

35. Boutati EI, Anaissie EJ. *Fusarium*, a significant emerging pathogen in patients with hematologic malignancy: ten years' experience at a cancer center and implications for management. Blood 1997; 90:999–1008.

36. Sebti A, Kiehn TE, Perlin D, Chaturvedi V, Wong M, Doney A, Park S, Sepkowitz KA. *Candida dubliniensis* at a cancer center. Clin Infect Dis 2001; 32:1034–1048.

37. Morrow LB, Anderson RE. Active tuberculosis in leukemia. Malignant lymphoma and myelofibrosis. Arch Pathol 1965; 79:484–493.
38. Akiyama H, Maruyama T, Uetake T, Kawaguchi K, Sakamaki H, Onozawa Y. Systemic infection due to atypical mycobacteria in patients with chronic myelogenous leukemia. Rev Infect Dis 1991; 13:815–818.
39. Grillo-Lopez AJ, Rivera E, Castillo-Staab M, Maldonado N. Disseminated M kansasii infection in a patient with chronic granulocytic leukemia. Cancer 1971; 28:476–481.
40. Green D, Dighe P, Ali NO, Katele GV. Pulmonary alveolar proteinosis complicating chronic myelogenous leukemia. Cancer 1980; 46:1763–1766.
41. Watanabe K, Sueishi K, Tanaka K, Nagata N, Hirose N, Shigematsu N, Miake S, Yoshida M. Pulmonary alveolar proteinosis and disseminated a typical mycobacteriosis in a patient with busulfan lung. Acta Pathol Jpn 1990; 40:63–66.
42. Nguyen Q, Estey E, Raad I, Rolston K, Kantarjian H, Jacobson K, Konoplev S, Ghosh S, Luna M, Tarrand J, Whimbey E. Cytomegalovirus pneumonia in adults with leukemia: an emerging problem. Clin Infect Dis 2001; 32:539–545.
43. Mochizuki T, Sugiura H, Watanabe S, Takada M, Hodohara K, Kushima R. A case of disseminated trichosporonosis: a case report and immunohisto-chemical identification of fungal elements. J Med Vet Mycol 1988; 26:343–349.
44. Nenoff P, Kellermann S, Borte G, Horn L-C, Ponisch W, Winkler J, Haustein U-F. Pulmonary nocardiosis with cutaneous involvement mimicking a metastasizing lung carcinoma in a patient with chronic myelogenous leukaemia. Eur J Dermatol 2000; 10:47–51.
45. Anaissie E, bodey GP, Kantarjian H, Ro J, Vartivarian SE, Hopfer R, Hoy J, Rolston K. New spectrum of fungal infections in patients with cancer. Rev Infect Dis 1989; 11:369–378.
46. Bodey GP, Rodriquez V, Chang H-Y, Narboni G. Fever and infection in leukemic patients. A study of 494 consecutive patients. Cancer 1978; 41:1610–1622.
47. Bodey GP, Elting L, Kassamali H, Lim BP. Escherichia coli bacteremia in cancer patients. Am J Med 1986; 81(suppl 1A):85–95.
48. Marron A, Carratala J, Gonzalez-Barca E, Fernandez-Sevilla A, Alcaide F, Gudiol F. Serious complications of bacteremia caused by viridans strepto-cocci in neutropenic patients with cancer. Clin Infect Dis 2000; 31:1126–1130.
49. Schwella N, Schwerdtfeger R, Schmidt-Wolf I, Schmid H, Siegert W. Pneumococcal arthritis after allogeneic bone marrow transplantation. Bone Marrow Transplantation 1993; 12:165–166.
50. Ninin E, Milpied N, Moreau P, Andre-Richet B, Morineau N, Mahe B, Vigier M, Imbert B-M, Morin O, Harousseau J-L, Richet H. Longitudinal study of bacterial, viral, and fungal infections in adult recipients of bone marrow transplants. Clin Infect Dis 2001; 33:41–47.
51. Cone RW, Huang M-LW, Corey L, Zeh J, Ashley R, Bowden R. Human

herpesvirus 6 infections after bone marrow transplantation: clinical and virologic manifestations. J Infect Dis 1999; 179:311–318.

52. Yoshikawa T, Asano Y, Ihira M, Suzuki K, Ohashi M, Suga S, Kudo K, Horibe K, Kojima S, Kato K, Matsuyama T, Nishiyama Y. Human herpesvirus 6 viremia in bone marrow transplant recipients: clinical features and risk factors. J Infect Dis 2002; 185:847–853.

53. Nguyen Q, Champlin R, Giralt S, Rolston K, Raad I, Jacobson K, Ippoliti C, Hecht D, Tarrand J, Luna M, Whimbey E. Late *cytomegalovirus* pneumonia in adult allogeneic blood and marrow transplant recipients. Clin Infect Dis 1999; 28:618–623.

54. Roemer E, Blau IW, Basara N, Kiehl MG, Bischoff M, Gunzelmann S, Kirsten D, Sanchez H, Wocker EL, Fauser AA. Toxoplasmosis, a severe complication in allogeneic hematopoietic stem cell transplantation: successful treatment strategies during a 5-year single-center experience. Clin Infect Dis 2001; 32:e1–e8.

55. Darrisaw L, Hanson G, Vesole DH, Kehl SC. *Cunninghamella* infection post bone marrow transplant: case report and review of the literature. Bone Marrow Transplantation 2000; 25:1213–1216.

56. Leleu X, Sendid B, Fruit J, Sarre H, Wattel E, Rose C, Bauters F, Facon T, Jouet J. Combined anti-fungal therapy and surgical resection as treatment of pulmonary zygomycosis in allogeneic bone marrow transplantation. Bone Marrow Transplantation 1999; 24:417–420.

57. Cairoli R, Marenco P, Perego R, de Cataldo F. *Saccharomyces cerevisiae* fungemia with granulomas in the bone marrow in a patient undergoing BMT. Bone Marrow Transplantation 1995; 15:785–786.

58. Baddley JW, Stroud TP, Salzman D, Pappas PG. Invasive mold infections in allogeneic bone marrow transplant recipients. Clin Infect Dis 2001; 32:1319–1324.

59. Ribaud P, Chastang C, Latge J-P, Baffroy-Lafitte L, Parquet N, Devergie A, Esperou H, Selimi F, Rocha V, Derouin F, Socie G, Gluckman E. Survival and prognostic factors of invasive aspergillosis after allogeneic bone marrow transplantation. Clin Infect Dis 1999; 28:322–330.

60. Marr KA, Seidel K, White TC, Bowden RA. Candidemia in allogeneic blood and marrow transplant recipients: evolution of risk factors after the adoption of prophylactic fluconazole. J Infect Dis 2000; 181:309–316.

61. Wald A, Leisenring W, van Burik J-A, Bowden RA. Epidemiology of *Aspergillus* infections in a large cohort of patients undergoing bone marrow transplantation. J Infect Dis 1997; 175:1459–1466.

62. van Burik J-A, Leisenring W, Myerson D, Hackman RC, Shulman HM, Sale GE, Bowden RA, McDonald GB. The effect of prophylactic fluconazole on the clinical spectrum of fungal diseases in bone marrow transplant recipients with special attention to hepatic candidasis. An autopsy study of 355 patients. Medicine 1998; 77:246–254.

63. Marr KA, Carter RA, Crippa F, Wald A, Corey L. Epidemiology and outcome of mould infections in hematopoietic stem cell transplant recipients. Clin Infect Dis 2002; 34:909–917.

8

Infections in Patients with Myelodysplastic Syndromes

Nadeem R. Khan
Infectious Diseases Private Practice
Tampa, Florida, U.S.A.

OVERVIEW OF MYELODYSPLASTIC SYNDROMES

Hematopoiesis in myelodysplastic syndromes (MDS) is ineffective, resulting in pancytopenia in spite of having a cellular marrow. This group of acquired blood disorders often progress to acute leukemia and are characterized by pancytopenias and low reticulocyte counts. The bone marrow is normocellular to hypercellular with cells showing morphological or dysplastic changes. Myeloid cells in MDS have not lost the ability to proliferate and differentiate but do undergo an abortive maturation resulting in inadequate production of mature red blood cells. According to the French–American–British classification, MDS can be divided into five types based on morphological characteristics: RA (refractory anemia), RARS (refractory anemia with ringed sideroblasts), RAEB (refractory anemia with excess blasts), RAEB-t (refractory anemia with excess blasts in transformation), and CMML (chronic myelomonocytic leukemia). RAEB-t has the highest rate of leukemic transformation (50%), as compared to the other subtypes [1]. Currently, the classification of RAEB-t has been deleted and AML exists when the bone marrow blast exceeds 20% of cells (instead of 30% of cells).

PATHOPHYSIOLOGY AND IMMUNOLOGICAL ABNORMALITIES IN MDS

Because MDS is a clonal disorder that most often, but not always [2], affects lymphohematopoietic progenitor cells at various stages of differentiation [3,4], lymphoid cells may be derived from the malignant clone [5–7]. Most frequently, the B cells are clonal, but cases with involvement of T cells have been reported [5]. Alterations of the immune system are frequently observed [8], including a peripheral blood lymphocytopenia with reduced numbers of CD4 T cells [9]. T cells may show reduced response to mitogens [10], B cells may have deficient receptors for C3d [11], and the serum levels of soluble IL-2 (interleukin-2) receptors can be increased [12]. Activity of natural killer cells may be reduced with failure to respond to IF (interferon) and deficient IF production [13]. Lymphoid and plasma cell neoplasias not infrequently coexist in MDS patients [14]. A third of the patients can have a polyclonal rise in serum immunoglobulin levels, and in 12% of MDS patients a coexisting monoclonal gammopathy has been found [15]. In 19% of cases, the serum immunoglobulin levels were reduced [15]. Autoantibodies were most frequently found in patients with CMML [15,16]. The significance of the immunological abnormalities is still not clear, whether they are age-related changes also found in elderly patients without MDS, whether they are due to repeated infections frequently occurring in MDS patients, whether they occur secondary to abnormal macrophage function, or lastly whether they are due to the clonal origin of the lymphoid cells [17].

Most patients are neutropenic at some stage of their disease, and those who are not are likely to have disordered granulocyte function [18]. Regardless of the proposed mechanisms, MDS patients with impaired immunity have three characteristic findings: an increased susceptibility to infection, autoimmunity, and an increased incidence of malignant neoplasms [17]. The risk of infection in MDS patients cannot be attributed to neutropenia alone. Infection rates for patients with comparable neutrophil counts were strongly associated with a MDS subgroup. Pomeroy et al. concluded that neutrophils may be more dysfunctional in RAEB and RAEB-t than in RA or RS [19]. It has been previously shown that patients with MDS may have poorly granulated neutrophils or neutrophils that have decreased myeloperoxidase activity despite a normal number of granules [18,20].

SPECIFIC INFECTIONS IN PATIENTS WITH MDS

The infections common in MDS are those commonly seen in neutropenics, with gram-negative bacteremia and bacterial bronchopneumonias being most frequent. Fungal and mycobacterial infections may be seen, but they are rare except as a consequence of treatment [21,22]. Bacterial infections may be seen in the absence of neutropenia, especially in CMML, where a neutrophilic leukocytosis is the rule. A characteristic of infection in patients with MDS is the ability to form a collection of large quantities of pus within various tissues, with very little systemic reaction [23]. Poor bacterial killing by dysplastic neutrophils associated with normal neutrophil chemotaxis is probably responsible for both the accumulation of pus and its limited systemic effect [23].

Pomeroy et al. found 188 infections in 66 (77%) of 86 MDS patients [19]. Forty-one percent of these infections were skin and lung infections. Urinary tract infections and bacteremias were also common, with 13 of the 22 bacteremias showing a recognized distant focus. Infection rates were found to be higher in patients with less than or equal to 1,000 neutrophils/μL blood. This is one of the very few studies done to evaluate the incidence of infections in the MDS patient. Pomeroy et al. also showed that the patients with RAEB and RAEB-t were more likely to die from infections than other subtypes of MDS. Lung, skin, urinary tract, and bloodstream were the most common sites of infection. Fungal and viral infections were infrequently diagnosed and occurred primarily in patients receiving immunosuppressive therapy. In this study, death from infection was common, accounting for 64% of deaths in patients with MDS that had not progressed to acute leukemia and was much more common than transformation to acute leukemia [19]. The infections related to treatment of MDS that transform to acute leukemia will be dealt with in another chapter.

CONCLUSIONS

Infection is a major cause of morbidity and death in MDS. Patients with RAEB and RAEB-t are at particularly high risk, as are patients who are neutropenic or receiving immunosuppressive therapy. Clinicians should aggressively evaluate patients with MDS and fever for infection with organisms associated with deficient neutrophil defenses.

REFERENCES

1. Castro-Malaspina H, O'Reily RJ. Harrison's Principles of Internal Medicine. 14th ed. New York: McGraw-Hill, 1998:672 678.
2. Kere J, Ruutu T, De la Chapelle A. Monosmy 7 in granulocytes and monocytes in myelodysplastic syndrome. NEJM 1987; 316:499.
3. Jacobs A. Genetic lesions in preleukemia. Leukemia 1991; 5:277.
4. Sato Y, Suda T, Suda J, Saito M, Miura Y. Erythroid- and myeloid-lineage involvement in chronic myelomonocytic leukemia. Exp Hematol 1987; 15:316.
5. Janssen JWG, Buschle M, Layton M, Drexler HG, Lyons J, van den Berghe H, Heimpel H, Kubanek B, Kleihauer F, Mufti GJ, et al. Clonal analysis of

myelodysplastic syndromes: evidence of multipotent stem cell origin. Blood 1989; 73:248.

6. Raskind WH, Tirumali N, Jacobson R, Singer J, Fialkow PJ. Evidence for multistep pathogenesis of a myelodysplastic syndrome. Blood 1984; 63:1318.
7. Stark AN, Scott CS, Bhatt B, Roberts BE. Myelodysplatic syndrome coexisting with acute lymphoblastic leukemia. J Clin Pathol 1986; 39:729.
8. Colombat PH, Renoux M, Lamagnere JP, Renoux G. Immunologic indices in myelodysplastic syndromes. Cancer 1988; 61:1075.
9. Byone AG, Scott CS, Ford P, Roberts BE. Decreased T-helper cells in the myelodysplastic syndromes. Br J Hematol 1983; 54:97.
10. Baumann MA, Milson TJ, Patrick CW, Libnoch JA, Keller RH. Immunoregulatory abnormalities in myelodysplastic disorders. Am J Hematol 1986; 22:17.
11. Anderson RW, Volsky DJ, Greenburg B, Knox SJ, Bechtold T, Kuszynski C, Harada S, Purtilo DT. Lymphocyte abnormalities in preleukemia-1. Decreased NK activity, anomalous immunoregulatory cell subsets and deficient EBV receptors. Leuk Res 1983; 7:389.
12. Zwierzina H, Herold M, Schollenberger S, Geissler D, Schmalzl F. Detection of soluble IL-2 receptor in the serum of patients with myelodysplastic syndromes: induction under therapy with GM-CSF. Br J Hematol 1991; 79:438.
13. Tagaki S, Kitawaga S, Takeda A, Minato N, Takaku F, Miuro Y. Natural killer-interferon system in patients with proleukaemic states. Br J Haematol 1984 Sep; 58 (1): 71–81.
14. Copplestone JA, Mufti GJ, Hamblin TJ, Oscler DG. Immunological abnormalities in myelodysplastic syndromes. II. Coexistent lymphoid or plasma cell neoplasia: a report of 20 cases unrelated to chemotherapy. Br J Hematol 1986; 63:149.
15. Mufti GJ, Figes A, Hamblin TJ, Oscler DG, Copplestone JA. Immunological abnormalities in myelodysplastic syndromes. I. Serum immunoglobulins and autoantibodies. Br J Hematol 1986; 63:143.
16. Solal-Celigny P, Desaint B, Herrera A, Chastang C, Amar M, Vroclans M, Brousse N, Mancilla F, Renoux M, Bernard JF, et al. Chronic myelomonocytic leukemia according to FAB classification: analysis of 35 cases. Blood 1984; 63:634.
17. Koeffler HP. Myelodysplastic syndromes. Hematology/Oncology Clinics of North America. Saunders 1992; 6:3, 609.
18. Ruutu T. Granulocyte function in the myelodysplastic syndromes. Scand J Hematol 1986; 36(suppl 45):66–70.
19. Pomeroy C, Oken MM, Rydell RE, Filice GA. Infection in the myelodysplastic syndromes. Am J Med 1991; 90:338–344.
20. Martin S, Baldock S, Ghoneim A, Child JA. Defective neutrophil function and microbicidal mechanisms in the myelodysplastic disorders. J Clin Pathol 1983; 36:1120–1128.
21. Hunt BJ, Andrews V, Pettingale KW. The significance of pancytopenia in military tuberculosis. Postgrad Med J 1987; 63:801–804.
22. Reboli AC, Reilly RF, Jacobson RJ. Aspergillus myositis in a patient with myelodysplastic syndrome. Mycopathologia 1987; 97:117–119.
23. Williamson PJ, Oscier DG, Mufti GJ, Hamblin TJ. Pyogenic abcesses in the myelodysplastic syndrome. Br Med J 1989; 299:375–376.

9

Infectious Complications in Multiple Myeloma

Todd Groom and Joseph C. Chan
University of Miami School of Medicine
Miami, Florida, U.S.A.

INTRODUCTION

Multiple myeloma (MM) is a neoplastic disease of B cell lineage resulting in the overproliferation of malignant plasma cells. These plasma cells produce a homogenous monoclonal immunoglobulin (Ig) or an excessive amount of monoclonal free light chain or both. These proteins are known as monoclonal proteins, or M proteins. Production of M protein is the hallmark in the laboratory diagnosis of MM. M protein can be detected in blood or in urine. MM accounts for 8–10% of all hematologic malignancies. It is estimated that 14,000 new cases of MM will be diagnosed each year, and more than 11,200 of those patients will eventually die of the disease. Unfortunately, almost all patients with MM who initially respond to chemotherapy eventually relapse. The median survival of MM with standard therapy is approximately 4 years [1].

There are at least two different sets of established criteria to confirm the diagnosis of MM: (1) Durie and Salmon, (2) Kyle and Greipp [2,3]. These systems of diagnosis disagree mostly among the earlier stages of the disease spectrum. Minimal criteria for the diagnosis of MM consist of more than 10% plasma cells in the bone marrow or a plasmacytoma and one of the following: (1) more than 30 g/L of M protein in the serum, (2) M protein in the urine, or (3) lytic bone lesions. These findings must not be related to metastatic carcinoma, lymphoma, connective tissue disorders, or chronic infection.

The clinically apparent stages of MM may be preceded by an asymptomatic period of variable duration. Patients with a serum M protein less than 30 g/L, bone marrow plasma cells less than 10%, and no evidence of anemia, hypercalcemia, renal failure, or bone lesions are considered to have monoclonal gammopathy of undetermined significance (MGUS). Up to 25% of patients with MGUS will eventually progress to overt myeloma at a rate of 1% per year. Other patients may be classified as having smoldering multiple myeloma (SMM) if their serum M protein is 30 g/L or higher, their plasma cells in the bone marrow 10% or more, but they do not have significant anemia, bone lesions, hypercalcemia, or renal insufficiency. Patients with SMM are more likely to transform into MM than patients with MGUS [2]. Few patients may have solitary plasmacytoma of bone alone, but some have only extramedullary plasmacytoma. Patients with localized plasmacytomas, either solitary bone or extramedullary, tend to survive longer than those with classical MM. The median survivals are 10 years and 16 years, respectively. If they have a residual MGUS after radiation therapy, these patients will eventually develop overt MM. The complete opposite clinical spectrum from solitary plasmacytomas is plasma cell leukemia. This condition is characterized by rapid proliferation of the malignant clone of the plasma cells and represents the occasional manifestation of the terminal phase of the disease.

VIRUSES AND PATHOGENESIS

A viral etiology of certain malignancies has been well established, but the link between a viral infection and the development of MM has been more difficult to prove [4]. Three different viruses have been implicated: hepatitis C, human immunodeficiency virus (HIV), and human herpesvirus type 8 (HHV-8). A causative role for the hepatitis C virus in the development of certain lymphoproliferative disorders has been proposed. This controversial theory relied on observational data demonstrating a high rate of B cell non-Hodgkin's lymphoma in hepatitis C–infected patients. However, the incidence of MM among hepatitis C–infected patients is very small and remains statistically insignificant, leading most investigators to doubt any potential causative role for this virus [5,6].

Malignancies are quite common at the later stages of HIV infection, but an association with MM has not yet been well defined. Approximately 50 cases of MM have been reported among HIV-infected patients [7,8]. The development of MM is significantly more common in HIV-infected patients, with an incidence 4 to 12 times that of the normal population. Since clinical manifestations are quite similar in both diseases, such as anemia, recurrent bacterial pneumonia, hyperglobulinemia, and renal insufficiency, the diagnosis of MM may be missed because these signs and symptoms are often attributed to HIV [9,10]. The diagnosis of MM can only be established in an HIV-infected patient by performing specific laboratory tests to identify a monoclonal protein in blood or urine. Thus the true incidence of MM may be higher than the reported figures.

HHV-8 has recently attracted much attention as a possible or important contributor in the pathogenesis of MM [11–13]. This virus has been implicated as a causative factor for Kaposi's sarcoma, body cavity lymphoma, and multicentric Castleman's disease [14]. An increasing body of evidence suggests that it may also play an important role in MM [15,16]. Cultures of bone marrow aspirates from patients with MM have demonstrated the presence of HHV-8. It has also been found in marrow-derived dendritic cells in patients with either MM or MGUS [17]. The use of nested-PCR has confirmed the presence of HHV-8 DNA and the presence of circulating antibodies to nuclear HHV-8 antigens in myeloma patients [18]. Furthermore, this virus secretes an interleukin 6 (IL-6) homolog. This homolog has been demonstrated to stimulate and support the growth of myeloma cells in vitro. It is now widely accepted that IL-6 is the predominant growth factor essential for the growth and survival of myeloma cells [19]. It is believed that this multipurpose cytokine acts as a paracrine growth factor that is produced in large quantities by marrow stromal cells in the presence of myeloma cells. It also supports the expansion of the myeloma cell population by preventing apoptosis even in the presence of dexamethasone. The ultimate effect of IL-6 is an enhanced growth of malignant cells with a resulting increase in tumor burden. High serum levels of IL-6 may differentiate patients with MM from those with MGUS [20]. Further research is necessary to evaluate the role of HHV-8 in the pathogenesis of MM.

CLINICAL PRESENTATION AND NATURAL HISTORY

Clinical presentation of patients affected by MM can be quite variable (Table 1). They usually seek medical attention because of (1) bone pain due to lytic bone lesion(s), (2) weakness and fatigue due to anemia or azotemia, (3) mental confusion due to hypercalcemia, (4) neurologic symptoms from hyperviscosity or peripheral neuropathy, or (5) recurrent bacterial infections due to impairment of host defense mechanisms [1,21–24]. A few patients may present with cryoglobulinemia or hemorrhagic manifestations because of the unusual physicochemical properties of their paraproteins. Up to 20% of

TABLE 1 Clinical Presentations of Multiple Myeloma

Bone pain	Plasmacytomas
Bone marrow failure	Amyloidosis
Recurrent infections	Hyperviscosity syndrome
Renal failure	Hemorrhagic diathesis
Hypercalemia	Peripheral neuropathy

patients have no symptoms at the time of the diagnosis, and their condition is often discovered serendipitously [25].

Multiple myeloma has a progressive course with a median survival of 6 months without treatment. To assess for infectious complications, the clinical course of MM treated with traditional chemotherapy can be divided into four phases: the pretreatment and the initial induction phase (which include all newly diagnosed cases), the plateau or stable phase with or without maintenance therapy, the refractory phase requiring more intense chemotherapy, and the late accelerated or terminal phase [25]. If the patient's clinical parameters warrant chemotherapy, the initial treatment with melphalan (an alkylating agent) and prednisone is usually continued in 6-week cycles for at least a year or until the patient reaches the plateau phase. The plateau phase is defined as a period when serum and urine M protein levels are stable and there is no clinical progression of the disease. The patient may not be in remission from the chemotherapeutic intervention. More intense chemotherapy is often administered when the disease becomes progressive again, and this can contribute to a higher infection risk. The refractory phase may be stabilized by some of the newer treatment modalities such as thalidomide and arsenic trioxide. Eventually, those patients who survive the many complications from their MM up to this point may still deteriorate into an aggressive terminal phase that is characterized by rapid tumor growth, pancytopenia, worsening of renal failure and hypercalcemia. Patients in this terminal phase are usually refractory to treatment and their survival rarely exceeds 6 months.

CHEMOTHERAPY

Throughout the last three decades, various combinations of chemotherapeutic agents more aggressive than melphalan/prednisone (MP) have been used to treat patients with MM. The overall response rate with MP remains at about 50%, but the 5-year survival rate in patients treated with MP is only 24%. In the hopes of achieving higher response rates, various combinations of chemotherapeutic agents have been studied. For example, the combination of vincristine, carmustine (BCNU), melphalan, cyclophosphamide, and prednisone (VBMCP) has produced a better objective response in up to 72% of treated patients. However, there was no survival benefit [26]. In a meta-analysis of 18 published trials, no difference in survival was shown between MP and the other more aggressive combinations [27].

Perhaps the greatest advance in the treatment of MM has been the use of very-high-dose chemotherapy followed by autologous hematopoietic stem-cell transplantation (auto-HSCT). Although it is still not a cure, the 5-year survival has improved to over 50%. In a randomized trial by the French Myeloma Group, the use of high-dose chemotherapy and auto-HSCT was superior to conventional chemotherapy with regards to response rate (81% vs. 57%), complete response (22% vs. 5%), 5-year event-free survival (28% vs. 10%) and overall survival rate (52% vs. 12%) [28].

The use of peripheral stem cells has replaced bone marrow in most hematopoietic transplants. Various purging techniques are used to reduce any residual myeloma cells in the stem cell harvest. Selecting hematopoietic progenitor cells that express the CD34 cell surface marker can significantly reduce the burden of myeloma cells in the autograft. Unfortunately, residual tumor cells are still detectable even after 5-log depletion of myeloma cells. Therefore it would appear that no patients are cured [29]. Despite this drawback, auto-HSCT is still considered standard therapy for patients younger than 65 with good performance status. Some cancer centers actually harvest enough stem cells initially for two transplantations in tandem. The use of tandem auto-HSCT appears to offer a better result because more intense chemotherapy can be given than with a single transplant.

Allogeneic HSCT (allo-HSCT) may lead to prolonged disease-free survival in a relatively small percentage of patients; however, the high early-transplantation-related mortality has limited the role of this procedure. The advantage of allo-HSCT is a disease-free graft; the disadvantage is graft-vs. -host disease (GVHD). The use of a T cell–depleted allograft may reduce the severity of GVHD but has not shown any improvement in survival benefit [30]. Recently, allo-HSCT was demonstrated to have another advantage over auto-HSCT. The graft itself has been shown to possess antitumor activity. This so-called graft-vs.-myeloma (GVM) effect was further enhanced by the infusion of donor lymphocytes to recipient after transplantation [31]. At the present time, it is not clear whether GVM and GVHD represent two interdependent processes or two separate pathological processes involving distinct T cell clones. Ideally, one should minimize GVHD while at the same time maximizing the GVM effect. Studies are currently under way to clarify the interaction between these two T cell–related phenomena.

The infectious complications for those myeloma patients randomized early to receive either auto-HSCT or allo-HSCT are quite similar to those of other patients who are treated with stem cell transplantations for other hematological malignancies. On the other hand, the risk of bacterial infections, especially those caused by encapsulated organisms, remains higher among the HSCT recipients with MM unless the underlying Ig and B cell defects are corrected by HSCT. These issues are covered in more detail in another chapter.

NEWER TREATMENT MODALITIES

Newer modalities of treatment such as thalidomide and arsenic trioxide are being used to prepare patients for HSCT or treatment for patients with relapse. The exact mechanism of action of thalidomide in MM is unclear, although it has known antiangiogenic and immunomodulatory properties [32]. In vitro studies have demonstrated that thalidomide can induce apoptosis and maturation arrest in myeloma cells. Clinically it has been used primarily in refractory or relapsing patients, in which the combination of thalidomide and dexamethasone has produced significant response rates of up to 70% [33,34]. Studies are ongoing to further define the role of this agent as part of a chemotherapeutic regimen (salvage vs. first-line treatment).

The use of arsenicals in lymphoproliferative disorders is still being investigated, although preclinical data suggests a possible role for arsenic trioxide (As_2O_3) as adjunctive treatment for MM. The mechanism of action is unknown, although experimental studies suggest a direct cytotoxic action as well as a possible inducer of apoptosis [35].

The use of interferon (IFN) in multiple myeloma has been studied for approximately twenty years, and its role in the treatment of MM remains controversial. Through its broad-range effects on cell growth and immune regulation, IFN-α has been shown to have a potent antitumor effect in animal models of MM [36]. The wide array of mechanisms attributed to this cytokine include inhibition of cell-cycle proliferation, decreased IL-6 receptor expression, and stimulation of tumor mRNA degradation. Clinically IFN-α has been used in induction treatment as both a single agent and with combination chemotherapy, but its use appears to be more promising as an agent to maintain the plateau phase following conventional chemotherapy or hematopoietic transplantation. There is a prolongation of the plateau phase along with a modest increase in overall survival with the use of IFN-α as part of this treatment [37,38]. Significant rates of toxicity (flulike symptoms, fatigue, cardiotoxicity, nausea, etc.) have resulted in the frequent reduction of dosage or the premature discontinuation of treatment. Thus the potential benefits of this agent as part of the standard therapy may be underestimated.

Even more exciting is the use of molecular biological techniques to produce more effective treatments while minimizing toxicities associated with standard chemotherapeutic agents. DNA vaccines were developed to target specific idiotype tumor proteins/antigens to kill autologous tumor cells in a MHC-restricted fashion. The hope is to develop vaccines using genetic carriers specifically tailored to each patient's specific idiotype M protein produced by the myeloma cells [39]. The possibility of using whole myeloma cells as the antigenic source for immunotherapy is also currently being investigated.

IMMUNE DEFECTS IN MULTIPLE MYELOMA

Infections arise in patients with MM either because of the underlying host defects induced by the disease itself or the damages directly or indirectly related to therapeutic interventions. Both the humoral and the cell-mediated immune (CMI) defenses are compromised in MM. This is manifested as a quantitative deficiency of circulating B cells, low levels of polyclonal immunoglobulin (Ig) and specific antibodies, as well as an inadequate response to immunization [40]. It has been hypothesized that immunological responses of the host play an important role in controlling proliferation of the malignant clone. Overt myeloma and more aggressive stages of the disease develop when the immunoregulatory system is overwhelmed or somehow fails its mission. This hypothesis explains why the measurable immune defects of a myeloma patient often parallel the underlying myeloma progression or remission [41].

B CELL CHANGES

Most patients with MM have polyclonal Ig levels less than 20% of normal individuals. A variety of mechanisms including decreased numbers of B cells, the presence of suppressor B cells, the direct effect of macrophages, disturbed T cell control, and a number of inhibitory soluble factors have all been implicated in the development of isotopic immunoglobulin suppression [41]. Paraproteins produced in this disease have been implicated to block the production of specific antibodies of the same class. This immunoregulatory role of the paraproteins and the low levels of circulating B cells appear to be related to the stage of the disease, being more pronounced with greater tumor burden. The ability to mount a primary immune response is severely depressed as evidenced by a prolonged induction time for IgM production and decreased peak antibody titers. Myeloma cells are thought to release an unidentified soluble RNA-containing factor that alters the expression of normal Ig receptors on the surface of normal B cells, thus impairing recognition of foreign antigen and subsequent antibody formation. Therefore myeloma patients respond poorly to primary immunization such as pneumococcal polysaccharide vaccines. Specific antibody titers to recalled antigens such as tetanus-diphtheria toxins, and antibodies against some common gram-positive and gram-negative bacteria, may also be reduced. It has been demonstrated that there is a correlation between increased infection risk to *Streptococcus pneumoniae* (Sp) and *Escherichia coli* (*E. coli*) and reduced titers of antipneumococcal and anti–*E. coli* lipopolysaccharide antibodies in patients with MM [42].

CELL-MEDIATED IMMUNITY

Abnormalities in CMI have been demonstrated in MM patients. CD4+ helper T cells are decreased, but the CD8+ subset of lymphocytes, including suppressor or cytotoxic T cells, are increased in numbers, leading to a reverse helper-to-suppressor ratio similar to those in patients infected by the human immunodeficiency virus (HIV) [41]. There is also a loss of antigen-experienced T and B cells and defective differentiation of "pre-B" and "pre-T" cells to more mature forms [43]. Myeloma patients also have suppressed delayed hypersensitivity responses. The significance of these CMI abnormalities and their relationship to the pathogenesis or complications of this disease are unclear. Clinically, these defects are subtle and do not usually predispose untreated myeloma patients to infection with opportunistic fungi, protozoa, or viruses, with the possible exception of varicella zoster. Even the increased incidence of shingles in myeloma patients may be just age-related and not necessarily a disease-related phenomenon.

OTHER IMMUNE DEFECTS

Natural killer (NK) cells are capable of a direct cytotoxic response to tumor cells without the requirement of major histocompatibility complex restriction. Studies have shown that both NK cell numbers and NK cell activity are increased in myeloma patients. These changes are directly related to disease stage, suggesting that these cells may play an important regulatory function against the malignant clone.

Macrophages from myeloma patients inhibit polyclonal Ig production upon antigen presentation in vitro. Interestingly, this inhibitory effect was not abolished upon removal of these cells, suggesting that macrophages from myeloma patients release a soluble factor that inhibits B cell expansion and antibody production. It has been demonstrated that there exists an inverse relationship between the level of serum paraprotein and monocyte function in patients with MM [44].

Granulocyte dysfunction and low levels of certain components of circulating complement have been occasionally observed in myeloma patients [45]. Phenotypically these granulocytes demonstrate impaired chemotaxis and have decreased numbers of receptors for IgG and C3b. Interestingly, these observed abnormalities do not seem to correlate with a higher incidence of infection. Neutropenia before chemotherapeutic treatment is quite rare and it does not seem to be a significant contributing factor for serious infections.

TIMING OF INFECTIONS

There is an association of pretreatment risk factors and early mortality during the induction phase of chemotherapy. These risk factors include renal insufficiency with >2 mg/dL of creatinine, poor performance status, and advanced age. Uremia has been associated with an increased susceptibility to infections due to substantial impairment of phagocytic functions of neutrophils and reduced T and B lymphocyte functions. Other contributing factors such as metabolic acidosis, malnutrition, and iron overload are often present among patients with chronic renal insufficiency [46]. Poor renal function is often a reflection of the severity of the underlying myeloma. The incidence of MM increases with increasing age. Less than 2% of the patients were under 40 years of age when it was first diagnosed at the Mayo Clinic before 1971. 69% of the male patients in that study were older than 60. A French study demonstrated a much shorter median survival among myeloma patients over the age of 85 (9 months) compared to those between the ages of 75 and 84 (30 months). Infection at diagnosis is associated with a higher death rate [20].

Infectious complications of MM are often life threatening. Nearly 70% of patients with myeloma die as a result of an infection [47–49]. Because of the preexisting defects in host defense and the coexisting medical complications such as renal insufficiency, the first 2 months of chemotherapy are a particularly high–risk period for infection. During this time, almost half of the patients experience at least one significant infection, and the overall infection incidence is 4.68 infections per patient-year (Table 2). These early infections are often severe, fatality approaching one third of the infected patients. Even those who survive have to either delay further treatment or require dose re-

TABLE 2 Incidence of Infection in Relation to Treatment and Response Status in Multiple Myeloma

Period of observation	No. of infections per patient year
Pretreatment	1.50
First 2 months of chemotherapy	4.68
During objective response	0.44
Nonresponse or relapse	1.31
Overall	1.46

Source: Adapted from Ref. 50.

TABLE 3 Relative Risk of Various Infections During Different Phases of Multiple Myeloma[a]

Disease stage	Induction stage	Plateau phase	Auto-HSCT,[b] first 100 days	Auto-HSCT, >100 days (remission)	Allo-HSCT, first 100 days	Allo-HSCT, >100 days (remission)
Pathogen						
BACTERIA						
S. pneumoniae	+++	+	++	+	++	+
S. aureus	++	+	++	+	++	+
Coag. Neg. Staph.	+	+	++	+	+++	+
E. coli	++	+	++	+	+++	+
Klebsiella pneumoniae	++	+	++	+	+++	+
Enterococcus spp.	+	0	++	+	++	+
Listeria monocytogenes	+	0	+	0	+	+
"SPACE" organisms[c]	+	0	++	+	+++	+
MYCOBACTERIUM						
M. tuberculosis	0	+	0	+	+	+
M. fortuitum-chelonii	0	0	+	0	++	+
VIRUSES						
Cytomegalovirus	0	0	+	++	+	+++
Varicella zoster	+	+	+	++	++	+++
FUNGI						
Candida species	+	+	++	+	+++	++
Aspergillus species	0	0	++	+	+++	+
Other molds	0	0	+	+	++	+
Pneumocystis carinii	0	0	0	+	+	++

[a] 0, no increase in risk compared to age-matched non-myeloma patients. +, slight increase in risk. ++, moderate increase in risk. +++, significant increase in risk.
[b] Auto-HSCT, autologous hematopoietic stem-cell transplantation. Allo-HSCT, allogeneic hematopoietic stem-cell transplantation.
[c] SPACE, Serratia, Pseudomonas, Acinetobacter, Citrobacter, and Enterobacter species.

duction in chemotherapy, leading to added morbidity or a shortened event-free period. In the study from the Minneapolis Veterans Administration Medical Center reported in 1981, infection was infrequent during the plateau phase, even though most patients continued to receive maintenance chemotherapy [50]. Neither the rate of infectious complications nor the nature of the infection in MM is uniform throughout the course. Therefore they cannot be assessed as a single entity: the risks for various infections differ significantly depending on the phase of the disease and the modality of treatment of the underlying malignancy (Table 3). For example, the risk for opportunistic infections due to cytomegalovirus (CMV) or aspergillus species is much higher within the first 100 days after allo-HSCT than with auto-HSCT [51–54], which in turn is higher than the traditional MP treatment. On the other hand, a patient who is in remission after a successful auto-HSCT is likely to be less susceptible to encapsulated bacterial infections than a patient who is in the induction phase of MP treatment, because of the normalization of the level of polyclonal Ig and B cell function [55].

RESPIRATORY INFECTIONS

About 27% of myeloma patients present with a bacterial infection. As with other patients with hypogammaglobulinemia, infections involving the respiratory tract, the urinary tract, and soft tissue are the most common. The majority of the pneumonias are due to either *Streptococcus pneumoniae* (Sp) or *Haemophilus influenzae* (Hi). Infections due to these two encapsulated organisms are expected in patients who are deficient in opsonizing antibodies against these organisms. Most of these infections are highly invasive. The mortality of bacteremic pneumococcal pneumonia has been consistently reported at ≥20% even among penicillin-susceptible strains. It is likely that the actual mortality may be higher among patients infected by the multiply antimicrobial-resistant strains of *Streptococcus pneumoniae* [56].

The incidence of invasive disease due to *Haemophilus influenzae* type b (Hib) has declined by 98% since the introduction of the Hib conjugate vaccines in 1989. Among adults in the United States, between the ages 40–59 and 60–79, the annual incidence of Hib invasive diseases were 0.03 and 0.07 per 100,000 population in 1994–1995. In the same year, the incidence of invasive disease due to non-b typable Hi was slightly higher at 0.33 and 1.01 per 100,000 population, respectively [57]. The important role that was once played by typable strains of *Haemophilus influenzae* in causing infections in MM patients will certainly be less significant in this country.

The evaluation and management of community-acquired pneumonia (CAP) in a myeloma patient is usually not much different from those in any other patient. The subject of CAP management has been written about extensively. Comprehensive management guidelines are available on the Internet from various government and professional organizations [58]. Guidelines for the diagnosis and management of CAP such as those published by the Infectious Diseases Society of America (IDSA) have incorporated practically all clinical considerations including but not limited to underlying risk factors of the hosts, seasonal and geographic variations, and antimicrobial resistance. According to the latest IDSA guidelines, most myeloma patients with CAP should qualify for inpatient care because their risk scores are usually more than 90 according to the Pneumonia Patient Outcome Research Team (PORT) prediction rule [59]. PORT scores of 90 or higher put them into the highest two risk categories, classes IV and V. Every attempt should be made to establish an etiological diagnosis in a myeloma patient. The rationales and the test procedures required are well summarized and they will not be reiterated here. Even though the IDSA document was designed for immunocompetent patients, the recommended empirical antibiotic therapy, using a combination of β-lactam and a macrolide, applies very well to the myeloma patient. A third-generation (3rd G) cephalosporin such as cefotaxime or ceftriaxone should be the β-lactam of choice unless the local penicillin resistance rate among Sp isolates is very low. Monotherapy with a fluoroquinolone with enhanced Sp activity, such as levofloxacin, gatifloxacin, or moxifloxacin, should be used with caution because there is very little published data on the efficacy among MM patients. Furthermore, a seriously ill elderly patient with renal insufficiency may have a higher incidence of cardiac and metabolic toxicities from these fluoroquinolones, such as prolonged QT intervals, torsades de pointe, and hypo- or hyperglycemia [60].

When relevant information on the infectious agent and the corresponding drug-susceptibility profile becomes available, pathogen-directed antimicrobial therapy should replace the empirical therapy. Treatment for pneumococcal pneumonia should be continued with either parenteral cefotaxime or ceftriaxone unless the Sp isolate has a minimal inhibitory concentration (MIC) of ≤1.0 μg/mL for penicillin. For those relatively susceptible isolates, high doses of penicillin or ampicillin have been used successfully in patients without any extrapulmonary involvement other than blood. With patients with meningitis due to Sp, penicillin or ampicillin can only be used if the penicillin MIC is ≤0.06 μg/mL [61]. There have not been any controlled trials that have addressed the optimal duration of treatment in this situation. The expected response to treatment among myeloma patients may be slower because of their reduced immunological capacity and the severity of the infection. Common clinical judgment dictates that myeloma patients with serious pneumococcal pneumonia should be continued on a parenteral antibiotic at least until 2 or 3 days after near normalization of objective findings including respiratory symptoms, fever, partial pressure of oxygen, and peripheral leukocyte counts. Early substitution with oral antibiotic should probably be avoided, because most early switch trials did not include patients with hematological malignancies.

The increased incidence of respiratory infections for a myeloma patient continues unabated after hospitalization. However, the infecting pathogens usually shift from the encapsulated organisms to mostly gram-negative bacilli such as *Klebsiella pneumoniae* and *Pseudomonas aeruginosa*. Even though gram-negative bacteremia is rarely detected as a consequence of nosocomial pneumonia in most hospital surveys, sepsis has been reported quite frequently among myeloma patients with the same infection [48]. A poorer outcome may be associated with *Staphylococcus aureus* pneumonia because of its high virulence and drug resistance profile.

URINARY TRACT INFECTIONS

Bacteriuria is very common in elderly patients because of age-related physiological changes. Asymptomatic bacteriuria in elderly patients is not a simple bacterial colonization even though treatment is not indicated. Most patients with asymptomatic bacteriuria develop both a granulocytic response in the form of pyuria and an immunological response with measurable antibody production against the specific bacterial isolate in their urine culture [62]. It is not surprising that urinary tract infection is the second most common infection in myeloma patients, given their relatively advanced age and their poor mucosal defense. Furthermore, many myeloma patients have other urological complications such as neurogenic bladder from cord compression or renal calculi from hypercalcemia. It has been observed that the incidence of urinary tract infection could increase fourfold when indwelling urinary catheters were introduced to these patients [47]. Urinary tract infections tend to be more severe in myeloma patients than in other age-matched patients with similar comorbid conditions such as renal insufficiency. Bacteremia accompanying the infection should be suspected, and the outcome is often worse. A large proportion of induction phase gram-negative sepsis in myeloma patients is probably a consequence of a urinary tract infection. The duration of antibiotic treatment should follow the guidelines for complicated cystitis or pyelonephritis. Obviously, patients with gram-negative sepsis should be treated with at least 2 weeks of effective antimicrobial therapy. Eradication of urinary pathogens is dependent on the concentration of the administered antibiotic in the urine. Myeloma patients with renal insufficiency may have lower urinary antibiotic concentrations and thus a slower eradication rate. Therefore the duration of treatment may have to be prolonged. Unfortunately, there is no well-controlled clinical trial to address this issue.

Escherichia coli is still the most common urinary pathogen in patients with MM, followed by other enterobacteriaceae such as *Proteus mirabilis* and *Klebsiella pneumoniae*. Antibiotic susceptibility of these community uropath-

ogens has decreased significantly [63]. The prevalence of resistance to ampicillin, trimethroprim/sulfamethoxazole, (TMP/SMX), or 6-fluoroquino-
lone (6FQ) can be as high as 30, 15, and 3%, respectively [64]. These figures
are probably much worse among myeloma patients who are receiving one of
those antibiotics as prophylaxis. The choice of antibiotics empirically for
suspected urosepsis in myeloma patients is dependent on the history of drug
allergy, recent antibiotic use or prophylaxis, and the local susceptibility pattern of the common uropathogens listed above. In general, a 3rd G cephalosporin such as cefotaxime, ceftriaxone, or ceftazidime with or without an
added aminoglycoside should be chosen. In institutions where extended spectrum β-lactamases (ESBL) are commonly found among Escherichia coli and
Klebsiella species, cefepime or a carbapenem such as imipenem or meropenem
should replace the 3rd G cephalosporins listed above. The antibiotic combinations containing a β-lactam and a β-lactamase inhibitor (βL/βLI) such as
piperacillin/tazobactam or ticarcillin/clavulanate may not be as effective
against these ESBL-producing enterobacteriaceae. On the other hand, piper-
acillin/tazobactam may be more effective than any cephalosporin if an enterococcal infection is suspected. Aminoglycosides can be given once daily at
dosages of 5–7 mg/kg and should be adjusted to the patient's renal function.
There is a slightly higher rate of nephrotoxicity with the 7 mg/kg dosage, so it
should be reserved for suspected Pseudomonas aeruginosa infection [65]. After
the initial 48 to 72 hours of antibiotic treatment, when the drug-susceptibility
information of the gram-negative isolates is available, aminoglycosides can
usually be discontinued to avoid nephrotoxicity. Many recent trials have demonstrated the successful treatment of febrile neutropenic patients with a single agent such as cefepime or a carbapenem [66]. The necessity to enhance the
bactericidal activities of the highly potent cephalosporins or carabapenems
may be limited to highly resistant organisms or highly unstable neutropenic
patients.

SOFT TISSUE INFECTION

Most soft tissue infections in myeloma patients are either cutaneous abscesses
or simple cellulitis. Unless there is another epidemiological factor involved,
such as concurrent diabetes mellitus, animal bite, or traumatic exposure to
brackish inland waters, the majority of these infections are caused by Staphylococcus aureus or Streptococcus pyogenes. These organisms should be susceptible to treatment with oxacillin, nafcillin, or cefazolin. However, reports
of community-acquired oxacillin-resistant Staphylococcus aureus (ORSA)
infections are accumulating rapidly, and vancomycin or linezolid may be necessary for the patients who have not responded to oxacillin or cefazolin treatment after 48 to 72 hours [67]. Clinical specimens are often not available for
culture in soft tissue infections; objective response to treatment may be the

only reliable means of assesing the appropriateness of the chosen antibiotic. Occasionally, the pathogenic organism can be identified from blister fluids, blood cultures, or aspirates of an abscess [68]. In that case, antibiotic treatment should be directed against the isolated organism(s).

MULTIPHASIC PATTERN OF INFECTIONS

The spectrum of bacterial infection varies with the phase of the illness and treatment (Table 3). Encapsulated organisms are the commonest bacterial infections during the induction phase, and *Streptococcus pneumoniae* continues to be an important pathogen throughout the illness, gram-negative bacteria usually take over the lead 2 to 6 months into chemotherapy [47,69]. Pathogens other than *E. coli* and *Klebsiella* spp., such as *Serratia marcescens*, *Pseudomonas aeruginosa*, *Acinetobacter* spp., *Citrobacter* spp., and *Enterobacter* spp. (SPACE), may predominate once the myeloma patient is hospitalized. These organisms have been associated with primary sepsis, nosocomial pneumonia, nosocomial urinary infections, and wound infections. The SPACE organisms carry the chromosome-mediated type I β-lactamase, and they can be highly resistant to all the 3rd G cephalosporins [70]. A carbapenem should be used empirically to treat infections caused by these organisms until susceptibility is available. After prolonged or repetitive hospitalizations, less common bacterial isolates may predominate as the infecting pathogens. These include but are not limited to *Stenotrophomonas maltophilia*, *Alcaligenes xylosoxidans*, *Bacillus* spp., *Bacteroides* spp., and *Corynebacterium* spp. Many of these organisms are not susceptible to the standard recommended empirical antibiotics, and early treatment failures are not uncommon.

Gram-positive organisms such as *Staphylococcus aureus*, coagulative-negative staphylococci, and enterococcus spp. will share an equally important role with these less common nosocomial gram-negative organisms. The increasing presence of indwelling catheters and other implantable infusion devices has served as a nidus for gram-positive infections. More than half of the *Staphylococcus aureus* isolates and more than 75% of coagulative-negative staphylococci in large hospitals are resistant to oxacillin (ORSA), so vancomycin or linezolid are the more reliable first-line gram-positive agents. *Enterococcus faecium* can be resistant to both ampicillin and vancomycin (VRE), and the treatment may be limited to either linezolid or quinupristin-dalfopristin combination, unless the isolate remains susceptible to tetracycline [71]. When selecting an empirical antibiotic for an infected myeloma patient, the following must be considered: the leukocyte count, the most likely site of infection, any recent or current antibiotic usage, and the antibiotic susceptibility patterns of the hospital.

Infections during neutropenia are expected in myeloma patients, given their immunological deficiencies combined with myeloablative conditioning therapy. Neutropenic fever should be treated empirically with broad-spectrum antibiotics at the onset of fever [66]. During the pre-engraftment phase of HSCT, patients typically develop neutropenic fever. Prolonged neutropenia is associated with an increased risk of fungal infections. The most common fungal infections during this phase are caused by *Candida* spp. and *Aspergillus* spp. Recent post-mortem data found invasive aspergillosis as the leading cause of death in patients with multiple myeloma receiving high-dose chemotherapy [72]. A European study found that 31 patients with Durie-Salmon stage 2 (6%) or 3 (94%) multiple myeloma developed invasive aspergillosis with a mortality rate of 45% [54]. The median time between multiple myeloma and invasive aspergillosis diagnosis was eight months. Sixteen patients (51%) had a neutrophil count $\leq 500/mL$ for a median duration of 19 days. Fourteen patients (45%) had recently received corticosteroid therapy, and 11 (36%) high doses of melphalan. The lung was involved in 28 cases and the sinus in three. The major risk factors for invasive aspergillosis was prolonged neutropenia (longer than 2 weeks) and high doses of steroids in this nonallograft population. Empirical antifungal therapy is recommended if the neutropenic patients do not respond to broad-spectrum antibiotics after 72 hours.

Reactivation of latent herpes viruses such as CMV, varicella zoster virus (VZV), and herpes simplex virus (HSV) is common during the pre-engraftment and the early postengraftment (first 100 days) phases of HSCT [51,52,73]. The risk for VZV infection is highest during the late engraftment period (>100 days after HSCT) because the recurrence rate increases with GVH disease. In recipients of HSCT, VZV infection can present with visceral involvement without any cutaneous manifestations [74]. Strategies to prevent and to treat these opportunistic fungal and viral infections are presented in another chapter.

PROPHYLAXIS AND PREVENTION

Recent clinical trials have shown that intensive chemotherapeutic regimens combined with HSCT can be administered to patients aged up to 76 years and to those with renal failure [75,76]. These findings greatly increase the number of patients eligible for this form of therapy, thereby placing most myeloma patients early on at similar risks of infections as seen in other recipients of HSCT. Therefore recent guidelines to limit mortality and morbidity by preventing opportunistic infections among HSCT recipients apply to most myeloma patients practically at the time when the diagnosis is confirmed [77,78]. These guidelines are comprehensive and well referenced, and their recommendations will not be reproduced here. Readers should consult these guidelines routinely for prophylactic and preventive measures for a myeloma patient. They are available readily on the Internet free of charge.

The best example of antimicrobial prophylaxis is the use of trimetho-prim/sulfamethoxazole (TMP/SMX) in both organ transplantation and advanced HIV infection. A small trial enrolling only 57 patients has demonstrated a reduction in infection-associated mortality in myeloma patients who received TMP/SMX 160/800 mg twice daily during the first two months of induction chemotherapy [79]. However, 25% of the recipients of TMP/SMX had to discontinue prophylaxis because of skin rashes, nausea, and vomiting. There are no data on the role of antimicrobial prophylaxis in the prevention of infection in either the plateau phase of the disease or among individuals who require more intensive treatment because of disease relapse.

Immunologloglobulin (Ig) replacement therapy was considered logical for patients with suppression of nonparaprotein Ig class in MM even as early as 1963 [80]. However, results were poor owing both to the low dose that can be given by the intramuscular route and to the lack of compliance with these painful weekly injections. This raised the possibility of intravenous Ig (IVIG) replacement therapy in patients with secondary antibody deficiency disorders. A randomized double-blind, placebo-controlled trial of IVIG was undertaken in a group of 82 selected patients with stable myeloma. Half the patients received 400 mg/kg IVIG or an equivalent volume of placebo (0.4% albumin) every 4 weeks for up to 1 year. Although most of the patients suffered an infection by the end of the study, IVIG delayed the time to the first infection, and there was a significant reduction of serious infections (19 in 449 patient-months vs. 38 in 470 patient-months). At the same time, infusion-related adverse reactions occurred in 12% of IVIG recipients compared to 5% of placebo. Most of these reactions were chills, fever, sleepiness, flushing, and anxiety. Three patients developed hypotension and responded to reduction in the rate of the infusion and the administration of hydrocortisone [81]. They were not observed in this particular trial, but other investigators were concerned with the probability of increases in plasma and whole blood viscosity, increases in thromboembolic events, and deterioration in renal function associated with the administration of high-dose of IVIG to patients with MM. Few oncologists question the clinical efficacy of IVIG replacement therapy in well-selected myeloma patients, but most hesisate to administer such costly prophylaxis routinely. The issue of the cost-effectiveness of prophylactic IVIG in patients with B cell lymphoproliferative diseases has not been settled [82,83].

FUTURE DIRECTIONS

Infectious complications affect the outcome of multiple myeloma in every stage and practically every modality of treatment for this disease. Although the long-term results of treating this plasma-cell malignancy are still disappointing, restoration of the humoral immune dysfunction was accomplished in the few patients that achieved complete remission. Ultimately, reduction in infectious complications will rely on improved therapy of the disease itself. We hope that in the near future more studies will be carried out to improve our understanding of the following questions: First, can polyclonal Ig suppression in MM be corrected in any way other than reducing tumor burden? Second, what is the exact risk of invasive pneumococcal infection in a myeloma population where most individuals have been previously immunized before the onset of the malignancy? Will antipneumococcal antibodies behave like secondary recalled antigens such as tetanus among individuals who received the polysaccharide or the conjugated vaccines before the illness? Third, will the application of highly specific assays, such as real-time PCR, to detect various pathogens such as herpesviruses and molds, direct preemptive antimicrobial therapy more appropriately [84,85]? Fourth, will the development of potent antiviral agents against HHV8 be helpful to halt the progression of the disease and hence the infectious complications as well?

REFERENCES

1. Bataille R, Harousseau J-L. Multiple myeloma. N Eng J Med 1997; 336:1657–1664.
2. Durie BGM. Staging and kinetics of multiple myeloma. Semin Oncol 1986; 13:300–309.
3. Greipp PR. Advances in the diagnosis and management of myeloma. Semin Hematol 1992; 29:24–45.
4. Pagano JS. Viruses and lymphomas. N Engl J Med 2002; 347:78–79.
5. Hausfater P, Cacoub P, Rosenthal E, Bernard N, Loustaud-Ratti V, Le Lostec Z, Laurichesse H, Turpin F, Ouzan D, Grasset D, Perrone C, Cabrol MP, Piette JC. Hepatitis C virus infection and lymphoproliferative diseases in France: a national study. Am J Hematol 2000; 64:107–111.
6. Hausfater P, Cacoub P, Sterkers Y, Thibault V, Amoura Z, Nguyen L, Ghillani P, Leblond V, Piette JC. Hepatitis C virus infection and lymphoproliferative diseases: prospective study on 1,576 patients in France. Am J Hematol 2001; 67:168–171.
7. Pouli A, Lemessiou H, Rontogianni D, Papanastassiou C, Tsakanikas S, Gerassimou A, Stamatelou M. Multiple myeloma as the first manifestation of acquired immunodeficiency syndrome: a case report and review of the literature. Ann Hematol 2001; 80:557–560.
8. Jin DK, Nowakowski M, Kramer M, Essex DW. Hyperviscosity syndrome secondary to a myeloma-associated IgG1k paraprotein strongly reactive against the HIV p24 antigen. Am J Hematol 2000; 64:210–213.
9. Pulik M, Genet P, Jary L, Lionnet F, Jondeau K. Acute myeloid leukemias,

multiple myelomas, and chronic leukemias in the setting of HIV infection. AIDS Pat Care STDs 1998; 12:913 919.

10. Yee TT, Murphy K, Johnson M, Abdalla SH, Patton GS, Lee CA, Mehta AB. Multiple myeloma and human immunodeficiency virus-1 (HIV-1) infection. Am J Hematol 2001; 66:123 125.

11. Parravicini C, Lauri E, Baldini L, Neri A, Poli F, Sirchia G, Moroni M, Galli M, Corbellino M. Kaposi's sarcoma-associated herpesvirus infection and multiple myeloma. Science 1997; 278:1969–1970.

12. Masood R, Zheng T, Tulpule A, Arora N, Chatlynne L, Handy M, Whitman J Jr, Kaplan M, Dosik M, Ablashi DV, Gill PS. Kaposi's sarcoma-associated herpesvirus infection and multiple myeloma. Science 1997; 278:1970–1971.

13. Brousset P, Meggetto F, Attal M, Delsol G. Kaposi's sarcoma-associated herpesvirus infection and multiple myeloma. Science 1997; 278:1972.

14. Belec L, Mohamed AS, Authier F-J, Hallouin M-C, Soe AM, Cotigny S, Gaulard P, Gherardi RK. Human herpesvirus 8 infection in patients with POEMS syndrome-associated multicentric Castleman's disease. Blood 1999; 93:3643–3653.

15. Fukuzawa M, Oguchi S, Saida T. Kaposi's varicelliform eruption of an elderly patient with multiple myeloma. J Am Acad Dermatol 2000; 42:921–922.

16. Sjak-Shie NN, Vescio RA, Berenson JR. The role of human herpesvirus-8 in the pathogenesis of multiple myeloma. Hematol-Oncol Clin North Am 1999; 13:1159–1167.

17. Rettig MB, Ma HJ, Vescio RA, Pold M, Schiller G, Belson D, Savage A, Nishikubo C, Wu C, Fraser J, Said JW, Berenson JR. Kaposi's sarcoma-associated herpesvirus infection of bone marrow dendritic cells from multiple myeloma patients. Science 1997; 276:1851 1854.

18. Gao S-J, Alsina M, Deng J-H, Harrison CR, Montalvo EA, Leach CT, Roodman GD, Jenson HB. Antibodies to Kaposi's sarcoma-associated herpesvirus (Human herpesvirus 8) in patients with multiple myeloma. J Infect Dis 1998; 178:846–849.

19. Anderson KC, Lust JA. Role of cytokines in multiple myeloma. Semin Hematol 1999; 36(1 suppl 3):14–20.

20. Murakami H, Takada S, Hatsumi N, Yokohama A, Saitoh T, Uchiumi H, Maehara T, Matsushima T, Tsukamoto N, Morita K, Tamura J, Sawamura M, Karasawa M. Multiple myeloma presenting high fever and high serum levels of lactic dehydrogenase, CRP, and interleukin-6. Am J Hematol 2000; 64:76–77.

21. Rodon P, Linassier C, Gauvain J-B, Benboubker L, Goupille P, Maigre M, Luthier F, Dugay J, Lucas V, Colombat P. Multiple myeloma in elderly patients: presenting features and outcome. Eur J Haematol 2001; 66:11–17.

22. Blade J, Kyle RA, Greipp PR. Presenting features and prognosis in 72 patients with multiple myeloma who were younger than 40 years. Br J Haematol 1996; 93:345–351.

23. Kapadia SB. Multiple myeloma: a clinicopathologic study of 62 consecutively autopsied cases. Medicine 1980; 59:380–392.

24. Oshima K, Kanda Y, Nannya Y, Kaneko M, Hamaki T, Suguro M, Yamamoto

R, Chizuka A, Matsuyama T, Takezako N, Miwa A, Togawa A, Niino H, Nasu M, Saito K, Morita T. Clinical and pathologic findings in 52 consecutively autopsied cases with multiple myeloma. Am J Hematol 2001; 67:1–5.

25. Oken MM. Multiple myeloma. Med Clinic N America 1984; 68:757–787.

26. Oken MM, Harrington DP, Abramson N, Kyle RA, Knospe W, Glick JH. Comparison of melphalan and prednisone with vincristine, carmustine, melphalan, cyclophosphamide, and prednisone in the treatment of multiple myeloma. Results of Eastern Cooperative Oncology Study E2479. Cancer 1997; 79: 1561–1567.

27. Gregory WM, Richards MA, Malpas JS. Combination chemotherapy versus melphalan and prednisolone in the treatment of multiple myeloma. An overview of published trials. J Clin Oncol 1992; 10:334–342.

28. Attal M, Harousseau JL, Stoppa AM, Sotto JJ, Fuzibet JG, Rossi JF, Casassus P, Maisonneuve H, Facon T, Ifrah N, Payen C, Bataille R. Autologous bone marrow transplantation versus conventional chemotherapy in multiple myeloma. A prospective, randomized trial. N Eng J Med 1996; 335:91–97.

29. Lemoli RM, Fortuna A, Motta MR, Rizzi S, Giudice V, Nannetti A, Martinelli G, Cavo M, Amabile M, Mangianti S, Fogli M, Conte R, Tura S. Concomitant mobilization of plasma cells and hematopoietic progenitors into peripheral blood of multiple myeloma patients: positive selection and transplantation of enriched CD34+ cells to remove circulating tumor cells. Blood 1996; 87:1625.

30. Bensinger WI, Buckner D, Gahrton G. Allogeneic stem cell transplantation for multiple myeloma. Hematol-Oncol Clin North Am 1997; 11(1):147–157.

31. Bensinger WI. Allogeneic hematopoietic cell transplantation for multiple myeloma. Biomed Pharmacother 2002; 56:133–138.

32. Hideshima T, Chauhan D, Shima Y, Raje N, Davies FE, Tai YT, Treon SP, Lin B, Schlossman RL, Richardson P, Muller G, Stirling DI, Anderson KC. Thalidomide and its analogs overcome drug resistance of human multiple myeloma cells to conventional therapy. Blood 2000; 96:2943–2950.

33. Kyle RA, Rajkmur SV. Therapeutic application of thalidomide in multiple myeloma. Semin Oncol 2001; 28:583–587.

34. Meierhofer C, Dunzendorfer S, Wiedermann CJ. Theoretical basis for the activity of thalidomide. Biodrugs 2001; 15:681–703.

35. Dai J, Weinberg RS, Waxman S, Jing Y. Malignant cells can be sensitized to undergo growth inhibition and apoptosis by arsenic trioxide through modulation of the glutathione redox system. Blood 1999; 93:268–277.

36. Cooper MR, Welander CE. Interferons in the treatment of multiple myeloma. Cancer 1987; 59:594–600.

37. Hjorth M, Westin J, Dahl IMS, Gimsing P, Hippe E, Holmberg E, Lamvik J, Nielsen JL, Lofvenberg E, Palva IP, Rodjer S, Talstad I, Turesson I, Wisloff F, Zador G. Interferon-alpha 2b added to melphalan-prednisone for initial and maintenance therapy in multiple myeloma. A randomized, controlled trial. Ann Intern Med 1996; 124:212–222.

38. Salmon SE, Crowley JJ, Grogan TM, Finley P, Pugh RP, Barlogie B. Combination chemotherapy, glucocorticoids, and interferon alfa in the treatment of

multiple myeloma: a Southwest Oncology Group study. J Clin Oncol 1994; 12:2405 2414.

39. Ruffini PA, Biragyn A, Kwak LW. Recent advances in multiple myeloma immunotherapy. Biomed Pharmacother 2002; 56:129–132.

40. Jacobsen DR, Zolla-Pazner S. Immunosuppression andinfection in multiple myeloma. Semin Oncol 1986; 13:282–290.

41. Munshi NC. Immunoregulatory mechanisms in multiple myeloma. Hematol-Oncol Clin North Am 1997; 11:51–69.

42. Lawson HA, Stuart CA, Paull AM. Observations on the antibody content of the blood in patients with multiple myeloma. N Engl J Med 1955; 252:13–18.

43. Pileri A, Ferrero D, Massaia M, Dianzani U, Boccadoro M. Advances in biology of multiple myeloma: cell kinetics, molecular biology and immunology. Eur J Hematol 1989; 43(suppl 51):30–34.

44. Mainwaring CJ, Williams MA, Singer CRJ, Lush RJ, Smith JG, Haynes CL, Kelsey SM. Monocyte dysfunction in patients with multiple myeloma and lymphoplasmacytic disorders is related to serum paraprotein levels. Br J Haematol 1999; 105:948–954.

45. Hopen G, Glette J, Halstensen A, Kalager T, Schreiner A, Solberg CO. Granulocyte function in malignant monoclonal gammopathy. Scand J haematol 1983; 31:133 143.

46. Pesanti EL. Immunologic defects and vaccination in patients with chronic renal failure. Infect Dis Clin North Am 2001; 15:813–832.

47. Doughney KB, Williams DM, Penn RL. Multiple myeloma: infectious complications. South Med J 1998; 81:855–858.

48. Meyers BR, Hirschman SZ, Axelrod JA. Current patterns of infection in multiple myeloma. Am J Med 1972; 52:87 92.

49. Salonen J, Nikoskelainen J. Lethal infections in patients with hematological malignancies. Eur J Haematol 1993; 51:102–108.

50. Perri RT, Hebbel RP, Oken MM. Influence of treatment and response status on infection risk in multiple myeloma. Am J Med 1981; 71:935–940.

51. Holmberg LA, Boeckh M, Hooper H, Leisenring W, Rowley S, Heimfeld S, Press O, Maloney DG, McSweeney P, Corey L, Maziarz RT, Appelbaum FR, Bensinger W. Increased incidence of cytomegalovirus disease after autologous CD34-selected peripheral blood stem cell transplantation. Blood 1999; 94:4029–4035.

52. Fassas AB-T, Bolanos-Meade J, Buddharaju LN, Rapoport A, Cottler-Fox M, Chen T, Lovchik JC, Cross A, Tricot G. Cytomegalovirus infection and non-neutropenic fever after autologous stem cell transplantation: high rates of reactivation in patients with multiple myeloma and lymphoma. Br J Haematol 2001; 112:237–241.

53. Ketterer N, Espinouse D, Chomarat M, Dumontet C, Moullet I, Rieux C, Neidhardt-Berard E-M, Boufia F, Coiffier B, Salles G. Infections following peripheral blood progenitor cell transplantation for lymphoproliferative malignancies: etiology and potential risk factors. Am J Med 1999; 106:191–197.

54. Lortholary O, Ascioglu S, Moreau P, Herbrecht R, Marinus A, Casassus P, De

Pauw B, Denning DW. Invasive aspergillosis as an opportunistic infection in nonallografted patients with multiple myeloma: a European organization for research and treatment of cancer. Clin Infect Dis 2000; 30:41–46.

55. Steingrimsdottir H, Gruber A, Bjorkholm M, Svensson A. Immune reconstitution after autologous hematopoietic stem cell transplantation in relation to underlying disease, type of high-dose therapy and infectious complications. Haematologica 2000; 85:832–838.

56. Feikin DR, Schuchat A, Kolczak M, Barrett Nl, Harrison LH, Lefkowitz L, McGeer A, Farley MM, Vorgia DJ, Lexau C, Stefonek KR, Patterson JE, Jorgenson JH. Mortality from invasive pneumococcal pneumonia in an era of antibiotic resistance, 1995–1997. Am J Public health 2000; 90:223–229.

57. Bisgard KM, Kao A, Leake J, Strebel PM, Perkins BA, Wharton M. *Haemophilus influenzae* invasive disease in the United States, 1994–1995: near disappearance of a vaccine-preventable childhood disease. Emerg Infect Dis 1998; 4:229–237.

58. Bartlett JG, Dowell SF, Mandell LA, File TM Jr, Musher DM, Fine MJ. Practice guidelines for the management of community-acquired pneumonia in adults. Clin Infect Diseases 2000; 31:347–382. www.idsociety.org.

59. Fine MJ, Auble TE, Yealy DM, Hanusa BH, Weissfeld IA, Singer DE, Coley CM, Marrie TJ, Kapoor WN. A predication rule to identify low-risk patient with community-acquired pneumonia. N Engl J Med 1997; 336:243–250.

60. Rubinstein E, Camm J. Cardiotoxicity of fluoroquinolones. J Antimicrob Chemotherapy 2002; 49:593–596.

61. Kaplan SL, Mason EO Jr. Management of infections due to antibiotic-resistant *Streptococcus pneumoniae*. Clin Microbiol Rev 1998; 11:628–644.

62. Nicolle LE. Urinary tract infection in long-term-care facility residents. Clin Infect Dis 2000; 31:757–761.

63. Carratala J, Fernandez-Seilla A, Tubau F, Dominguez MA, Gudiol F. Emergence of fluoroquinolone-resistant Escherichia coli in fecal flora of cancer patients receiving norfloxacin prophylaxis. Antimicrob Agents Chemother 1996; 40:503–505.

64. Kahlmeter G. The ECO•SENS Project: a prospective, multinational, multicentre epidemiological survey of the prevalence and antimicrobial susceptibility of urinary tract pathogens—interim report. J Antimicrob Chemother 2000; 46(suppl 1): 15–22.

65. Fishman DN, Kaye KM. Once-daily dosing of aminoglycoside antibiotics. Infect Dis Clin North Am 2000; 14:475–487.

66. Hughes WT, Armstrong D, Bodey GP, Bow EJ, Brown AE, Calandra T, Feld R, Pizzo PA, Rolston KVI, Shenep JL, Young LS. 2002 guidelines for the use of antimicrobial agents in neutropenic patients with cancer. Clin Infect Dis 2002; 4:730–751. www.idsociety.org.

67. Chambers HF. The changing epidemiology of *Staphylococcus aureus*? Emerg Infect Dis 2001; 7:178–182.

68. Bishara J, Gabay B, Samra Z, Hodak E, Pitlik S. Cellulitis caused by *Citrobacter diversus* in a patient with multiple myeloma. Cutis 1998; 61:158–159.

69. Savage DG, Lindenbaum J, Garrett TJ. Biphasic pattern of bacterial infection in multiple myeloma. Ann Intern Med 1982; 96:47–50.
70. Bush K. New beta-lactamases in gram-negative bacteria: diversity and impact on the selection of antimicrobial therapy. Clin Infect Dis 2001; 32:1085–1089.
71. Weinstein RA. Controlling antimicrobial resistance in hospitals: infection control and use of antibiotics. Emerg Infect Dis 2001; 7:188–192.
72. Paradisi F, Corti G, Cinelli R. Infections in multiple myeloma in IDCNA. Cunha BA June 2001; 15:373–384.
73. Meyers KD, Flournoy N, Thomas ED. Infection with herpes simplex virus and cell-mediated immunity after marrow transplant. J Infect Dis 1980; 142:338–346.
74. Yagi T, Karasuno T, Hasegawa T, Yasumi M, Kawamoto S, Murakami M, Uosima N, Nakamura H, Hiraoka A, Masaoka T. Acute abdomen without cutaneous signs of varicella zoster infection as a late complication of allogeneic bone marrow transplantation: importance of empiric therapy with acyclovir. Bone Marrow Transplant 2000; 25:1003–1005.
75. Siegel DS, Desikan KR, Mehta J, Singhal S, Fassas A, Munshi N, Anaissie E, Naucke S, Ayers D, Spoon D, Vesole D, Tricot G, Barlogie B. Age is not a prognostic variable with autotransplants for multiple myeloma. Blood 1999; 93:51–54.
76. Barlogie B, Jagannath S, Desikan KR, Mattox S, Vesole D, Siegel DS, Tricot G, Munshi N, Fassas A, Singhal S, Mehta J, Anaissie E, Dhodapkar D, Naucke S, Cromer J, Sawyer J, Epstien J, Spoon D, Ayers D, Cheson B, Crowley J. Total therapy with tandem transplants for newly diagnosed multiple myeloma. Blood 1999; 93:55–65.
77. Dykewicz CA. Summary of the guidelines for preventing opportunistic infections among hematopoietic stem cell transplant recipients. Clin Infect Diseases 2001; 33:139–144.
78. Centers for Disease Control and Prevention. Guidelines for preventing opportunistic infections among hematopoietic stem cell transplant recipients: recommendations of CDC, the Infectious Disease Society of America, and the American Society of Blood and Marrow Transplantation. MMWR Morb Mortal Wkly Rep 2000; 49(RR-10):1 128. www.cdc.gov/mmwr/preview/mmwrhtml/rr4910al.htm.
79. Oken MM, Pomeroy C, Weisdorf D, Bennett JM. Prophylactic antibiotics for the prevention of early infection in multiple myeloma. Am J Med 1996; 100:624–628.
80. Fahey J, Scoggin R, Uts J, Swed C. Infection antibody response and gamma-globulin components in multiple myeloma and macroglobulinemia. Arch J Med 1963; 35:698–707.
81. Chapel JM, Lee M, Hargreaves R, Pamphilon DH, Prentice AG. Randomized trial of intravenous immunoglobulin as prophylaxis against infection in plateau-phase multiple myeloma. Lancet 1994; 343:1059–1063.
82. Weeks JC, Tierney MR, Weinstein MC. Cost effectiveness of prophylactic administration of intravenous immune globulin in chronic lymphocytic leukaemia. N Engl J Med 1991; 324:81–86.

83. Gill TM, Feinstein AR. A critical appraisal of the quality of quality-of-life measurements. JAMA 1994; 272:619–626.
84. Mackay JM, Arden KE, Nitsche A. Real-time PCR in virology. Nucleic Acids Res 2002; 30:1292–1305.
85. Kami M, Fukui T, Ogawa S, Kazuyama Y, Machida U, Tanaka Y, Kanda Y, Kashima T, Yamazaki Y, Hamaki T, Mori S, Akiyama H, Mutou Y, Sakamaki H, Osumi K, Kimura S, Hirai H. Use of real-time PCR on blood samples for diagnosis of invasive aspergillus. Clin Infect Dis 2001; 33:1504–1512.

10

Non-Hodgkin's Lymphoma

Teresa Field
University of South Florida School of Medicine
Tampa, Florida, U.S.A.

INTRODUCTION

Non-Hodgkin's lymphomas (NHL) are a diverse group of diseases. They are the fifth most common cancers in the U.S. with 55,000 new cases diagnosed each year. The incidence has increased since the 1970s by approximately 3% each year [1,2].

There have been several classification schemes that group NHL by their clinical, morphological, and genetic features [3,4]. These range from indolent lymphomas, which comprise 40% of the group, to the more rapidly growing high-grade or aggressive types. The most common forms are follicular cell, an indolent form accounting for 22% of the cases, and diffuse large B cell lymphoma, comprising 31% of the NHL.

Infectious complications in NHL result from a multitude of factors. Non-Hodgkins lymphoma consists of a spectrum of diseases, each having different treatment regiments, which in turn give different incidences of infections. Treatments include single agent chemotherapy, combination chemotherapy, monoclonal antibodies, radioimmunoantibodies, high-dose chemotherapy with autologous stem cell rescue, and allogeneic stem cell transplantation. Each of these approaches has a different risk profile for developing infectious complications. Chemotherapy is usually administered monthly and the risk of infection increases with each successive cycle.

NHL occurs in patients of all ages and with a variety of comorbid conditions. All of these factors affect the host defenses, including neutrophil function and neutropenia, cellular (T cell/monocyte-macrophage defects) and humoral (B lymphocytes, hypogammaglobulinemia) immune defects, mucosal damage (mucositis and enteritis), skin barrier breakdown, and changes in the endogenous flora [5–8].

Additionally, exogenous factors such as use of central venous catheters, growth factors, H_2-antagonists, parenteral nutrition, and prophylactic antimicrobials contribute to the risk of infectious complications during NHL treatment.

NEUTROPHILS AND NEUTROPENIA

Neutropenia is common in the treatment of NHL. The classic paper by Bodey [9,10] demonstrated that the risk of infection due to neutropenia depends on the extent of the neutropenia as well as the duration of the neutropenic period. If the neutrophils are less than $100/\mu L$, 47% of the patients who develop sepsis will die, whereas 14% of patients with neutrophils greater than $1000/\mu L$ succumb to sepsis. Similarly, the majority of patients with a duration of neutropenia greater than 1 week developed fever, versus 30% of the patients if the duration was less than 1 week.

The duration of the neutropenia impacts the risk of developing specific infections. Early infections generally are bacterial. As time progresses the risk of developing fungal infections increases.

In addition to the increased risk of developing infectious complications, neutropenic patients have difficulty mounting an inflammatory response such that most patients will have fever as their only sign of infection. In many series of febrile neutropenia, only 30% of the episodes identified a microbiologically documented infection. Along the same lines, early in the course of pneumonia, 50% of the neutropenic patients have a normal chest radiograph [11]. Common sites of infection include blood (bacteremia), the oral phanynx, the lower respiratory tract, skin, sinus, and GI tract [10,12].

Most agents used for NHL suppress neutrophil counts, although to different degrees, for varying lengths of time, and can affect the neutrophils directly by impairing their function. Etoposide, cytoxan, vincristine, and steroids are commonly used, and they exert a direct myelotoxic effect [13,14]. These drugs are used singly and in combination on a cyclic basis. The risk of neutropenia increases with each successive cycle of chemotherapy.

Cyclophosphamide, doxorubicin, vincristine, and prednisone (CHOP) is a standard treatment regimen for intermediate grade NHL, and 28–51% of the patients develop neutropenia of less than $500/\mu L$ within 5 to 7 days [7,8]. In one retrospective study, 126 of 577 patients developed febrile neutropenia, 56% during the first cycle [15]. Age of the patients was a clear risk factor with 65% of the febrile neutropenic episodes occurring in patients greater than 65 years old.

Cyclophosphamide, vincristine, and prednisone (CVP), used for follicular NHL, has a smaller chance of neutropenia on the order of 12–20% [7,16].

INDOLENT NHL

Indolent NHL accounts for 25 to 40% of the cases of NHL with an expected median survival of 7 to 10 years. Approximately 24 to 31% will transform into a high-grade NHL that decreases survival times considerably [17]. Initial treatment strategies include watchful waiting, oral alkylating agent monotherapy (cholorambucil or cyclophosphamide), and combination chemotherapy (CVP–cyclophosphamide, etoposide also known as (VP-16) and prednisone). Eighty percent of patients treated achieve a complete or partial remission. Upon recurrence, a significant number of patients can achieve a response to salvage therapies, although the duration is shorter on each successive remission. In one retrospective series, only 10% of the deaths were due to causes not related to the lymphoma [19]. Brice et al. [18] studied patients with follicular NHL and low tumor burden randomized to watchful waiting, an alkylating agent, or interferon alfa-2b treatment. There was a similar overall survival, time to progression, response to salvage chemotherapy, and rates of histologic transformation to a more aggressive lymphoma in all three cohorts. There were 38 deaths in the 199 patients enrolled; 31 were due to progression of the lymphoma, which is consistent with most other studies' findings.

More recently developed treatments include the use of purine nucleoside analogs such as fludarabine singly and in combination, Rituximab, a chimeric anti-CD20 antibody, radioimmunotherapy, high-dose chemotherapy with autologous stem cell rescue, and allogeneic stem cell transplant using high-dose or nonmyeloablative induction regimes [20,21].

FLUDARABINE

Fludarabine, an inhibitor of DNA repair, is used singly and in combination in the treatment of low-grade NHL. It is most effective in treating follicular NHL. Chemotherapy regimes for NHL utilizing fludarabine demonstrate an increase in the number of opportunistic infections, although to a lesser extent

TABLE 1 Common Toxicity Grades

			Toxicity Grade		
	0	1	2	3	4
Blood					
Neutrophils (×10⁹/L)	Normal	1.5–2.0	1.0–1.5	0.5–1.0	<0.5
Infection					
Infection, febrile neutropenia	None	Mild	Moderate	Severe	Life threatening
Infection without neutropenia	None	Mild, no active treatment	Moderate, localized requiring local or oral treatment	Severe, systemic requiring IV antibiotics or hospitalization	Life threatening

than reported in patients treated for chronic lymphocytic leukemia (CLL) [22]. Fludarabine use causes a marked decrease in the CD4+ lymphocytic subsets. Lazzarino et al. [23], utilizing the single agent fludarabine, reported a median decrease in CD4+ counts from 484/μL to 198/μL in 24 patients. Eleven patients had infectious complications, but none were hospitalized. These included two lobar pneumonias, one herpes zoster infection, six febrile episodes, three upper respiratory tract infections, one urinary tract infection, two herpes simplex infections, and one cellulitis. Flinn et al. [24] reported comparable results, with CD4+ lymphocytes decreasing from 799/μL to 134/μL in 45 low-grade NHL patients using a combination of fludarabine and cyclophosphamide. Grade III neutropenia (neutrophils < 1000/μL) developed in 12 patients and Grade IV neutropenia in five patients. Early in the study, one patient developed *Pneumocystis carinis* (PCP) pneumonia, resulting in the utilization of prophylactic trimethoprim-sulfamethoxazole (TMP-SMX). Infections included cryptococcal pneumonia, dermatomal herpes zoster, cellulitis, and sinusitis.

Clinical trials treating low-grade NHL with single-agent fludarabine reported 10–55% incidences of Grade III/IV neutropenia (Table 1) [25–30]. Infectious complications varied. Solal-Celigny et al. [30] studied 54 patients with follicular NHL and noted 41% with Grade III neutropenia, none with Grade IV (neutrophils < 500/μL) neutropenia, eight (15%) Grade I infections, and five Grade II infections (four pneumonias, one CMV).

Fludarabine has been used in combinations with DNA damaging agents, such as cyclophosphamide, mitoxantron, or ifosphamide, which enhances its activity in vitro. These combinations also increased the incidence of neutropenia, which ranged from 18 to 80% [31–34]. McLaughlin and Hagemeister [35] studied the combination of fludarabine, mitoxantrone, and dexamethasone in 51 patients. They noted 12% infections, with significant instance of opportunistic infections: six herpes zoster, PCP pneumonia confirmed in two and suspected in four, and one atypical mycobacterium. As a result, they recommend PCP prophylaxis in subsequent trials.

RITUXIMAB

Rituximab is a chimeric anti-CD20 monoclonal antibody targeted to a surface antigen on B cells. Phase I trials demonstrated activity against indolent NHL, and a large efficacy trial confirmed these results. As it has mild side effects, is easily tolerated, and is given on an outpatient basis, it is an attractive choice for treatment. The Food and Drug Administration approved its use in 1997.

McLaughlin et al. [36] studied 166 patients with low-grade NHL receiving single-agent Rituximab for four once-weekly infusions. The overall response was 48%, with 12% complete remissions. B cell counts were monitored and became undetectable in all but 16 patients after the first dose, returning to normal in 9 to 12 months. They reported 13 Grade I/II neutropenias and seven Grade I/II leukopenias. The majority of the infectious complications consisted of bacterial infections (37/68). Most were minor infections, Grade I/II (61/68). Viral infections included 10 herpes simplex and five herpes zoster. Locations of infections were 19 in the respiratory tract, three in the urinary tract, three in the gastrointestinal and bacteremias.

Davis and Grillo-López [37] studied 60 patients in a phase II trial retreated with a second 4 week course of rituximab. Again, the infectious complications were moderate with only two patients requiring hospitalization for infectious reasons. There was one patient with Grade III neutropenia during the treatment course and one patient with Grade III neutropenia 1 month after concluding treatment.

Sweetenham et al. [38] performed a retrospective review and cost analysis of the treatment of indolent NHL with combination chemotherapy (CHOP) vs. fludarabine vs. rituximab. The overall response was similar in each modality, and comparable to published reports, ranging from 44 to 62%. Neutropenia, of all grades, was 41% with CHOP, 62% with fludarabine, and none with rituximab. In their analysis, only CHOP had hospital stays attributable to neutropenia (24 days/48 patients). The incidence of fever and infections was 27% with CHOP, 18% with fludarabine, and 25% with rituximab. Hospital stays attributable to infectious causes were 48 days/50 patients for CHOP, 39 days/48 patients for fludarabine, and 6 days/64 patients with rituximab. Not surprisingly, the cost of fever and infection contributed a significant component to the total cost of the treatment of all adverse events. This was 34% with CHOP and 57% with fludarabine. In rituximab it was 29% of the cost of adverse events.

RADIOIMMUNOCONJUGATES

In order to improve response rates and their duration, therapies with radioisotope conjugated antibodies have been investigated. The cytotoxic effect to the indolent NHL via the unconjugated anti-CD 20 antibody is coupled to that of the radioisotope emissions. Two radioimmunoconjugates ^{131}I-tositumomab (Bexxar) and ^{90}Y ibritumomab (Zevalin) have been investigated in phase III, prospective multicenter trials.

In the pivotal trial of ^{131}I-tositumomab, Kaminski et al. [39] studied 60 heavily pretreated patients with indolent or transformed NHL and achieved an overall response rate of 65%. It was well tolerated and the majority of the toxicity was hematological. The median neutrophil nadir was 800/µL at 43 days after infusion. The median time to recovery was 74 days. Grade IV neutropenia was seen in 20% (12/60). Infections were seen in 15 patients for a total of 31 infections; 12 of the 15 received antimicrobials. Only one patient was hospitalized with febrile neutropenia.

A phase III prospective randomized trial compared ^{90}Y ibritumomab to the unconjugated rituximab [40]. Patients with indolent or transformed NHL were randomized and the overall response rate in the ^{90}Y ibritumomab group was 80% versus 56% in the rituximab group. Infectious toxicities consisted of five patients (7%) hospitalized in the ^{90}Y ibritumomab group—one with febrile neutropenia, two with urinary tract infections, one with gastroenteritis, and one with sepsis. Only one (1%) patient from the rituximab group was hospitalized. CD19+ lymphocyte counts were assessed and fell by the fourth week after treatment and recovered by 6 months in the ^{90}Y ibritumomab group and 9 months in the rituximab group.

INTERMEDIATE/AGGRESSIVE NHL

Intermediate grade NHL is common, and diffuse large B cell NHL accounts for 31 to 40% of the total number of NHL cases. This disease is progressive, and, unlike the indolent NHL, it is treated on diagnosis.

In addition to the classification systems noted above, the intermediate/high grade NHLs are categorized by the International Prognostic Index (IPI), which divides patients into risk groups based on age, performance status, stage, extra-nodal involvement, and lactate dehydrogenase level on presentation. Survivals based on these factors range from 73% at 5 years for low IPI index to 26% at 5 years for the high IPI group [41]. Recent studies and retrospective analysis of previously reported studies can stratify patients according to their IPI index, thus assessing for subgroups that would benefit from more aggressive therapies.

High-grade non-Hodgkin's lymphomas are treated with combination chemotherapy, and long-term complete remissions occur in approximately 30 to 35% of the patients. These are administered cyclically every 3 to 4 weeks for a total of 6 to 8 cycles [42]. Chemotherapy-induced neutropenia and infectious complications are the majority of the major toxicities, resulting in dose reductions and thus decreased efficacy. Multiple combinations of agents have been investigated as initial chemotherapy, but none were found to be superior to CHOP when compared in a phase III prospective randomized trial of 899 patients [43]. Overall survival and disease-free survival were similar in all four regimes studied and were 50–54% and 41–52%, respectively. There were differences in toxicities that favored CHOP. Most of the toxicities were due to neutropenia and subsequent infectious complications. The fatal toxicity varied between 1 and 5%, and Grade 4 toxicity was 31 to 54%.

Coiffier [44] reported on several of the French studies that included over 3000 patients with greater than 9 year followup treated with variants of CHOP including a higher dosage of cyclophosphamide. Severe neutropenia Grade IV occurred in the majority of the patients, and over 80% had at least one episode of febrile neutropenia. Most of the toxic deaths were complications of febrile neutropenia.

Chrischilles et al. [15] analyzed retrospectively 577 cases of NHL treated with CHOP at 12 different community practices. They found 126 patients hospitalized with febrile neutropenia, and 56% of these occurred in the first cycle and 73% took place within the first two cycles. The average length of stay was 8.3 days in the 88 patients with one hospital stay and 15.9 days for the patients with multiple hospitalizations. The two variables that were significantly associated with hospitalization and length of stay were age greater than 65 and utilization of hemopoietic growth factors. There were 17 deaths, none of which were attributed to infection.

Coiffier et al. [45] studied the addition of rituximab to CHOP in a multicenter randomized trial of 398 patients over age 60 with diffuse large cell NHL. CHOP and rituximab (CHOP + R) had a CR of 76% compared with 63% using CHOP alone. At 2 years of followup, the addition of rituximab increased disease-free survival, although the two curves began to converge. The incidence of adverse events was comparable in both groups. The decrease in neutrophils was similar and was Grade IV with a median of $400/\mu L$. There were 20 deaths related to infection. Fever of any grade occurred in 69% receiving CHOP + R and 59% receiving CHOP. Grade III/IV fever occurred in 2% getting CHOP + R and 5% getting CHOP. Total infections were 65% in both groups. Grade III/IV infection was 12% in the CHOP + R group and 20% in the CHOP group. There was more herpes zoster in the CHOP + R group, nine vs. two recieving CHOP.

Although most patients can achieve a remission on induction chemotherapy and one third can be cured, relapse of NHL occurs, 70% of the relapses taking place within the first 2 years [46]. The 5 year disease free survival for salvage chemotherapy is 10–20% if the relapse occurs within the first year and is greater if relapse develops later.

The second-line chemotherapy regimes all have similar response rates, and the remissions are shorter in duration, usually less than 1 year [42]. Patients with chemosensitive disease proceed to high-dose chemotherapy with autologous stem cell rescue if they are eligible.

Infectious toxicity profiles of these salvage regimens are similar. Gutierrez et al. [47] studied 131 patients with relapsed NHL utilizing EPOCH (etoposide, vincristine and doxorubicin, cyclophosphamide, and prednisone). Grade IV neutropenia (ANC $< 500/\mu L$) occurred in 30% of patients and was brief, usually less than 4 days. Febrile neutropenia requiring hospitalization occurred in 18% of the cycles. In this study, 65% of infections were bacterial and 21% due to herpes simplex or herpes zoster, and there were 14% fungal infections including five cases of candidemia and two cases of pulmonary aspergillosis. The fungal infections accounted for two of the three infection-related deaths.

HEMOPOIETIC GROWTH FACTORS

A major source of morbidity and mortality in the treatment of aggressive NHL is myelotoxicity, Methods that would ameliorate this could allow delivery of the full treatment course with fewer infectious complications. Hemopoietic growth factors, granulocyte colony-stimulating factor (G-CSF), and granulocyte-macrophage colony stimulating factor (GM-CSF) decrease the duration of the neutropenia seen following administration of chemotherapy and thus decrease the time of greatest risk of infectious complications. In addition, their use decreases the delays in proceeding to the next treatment cycle and permits more intense chemotherapy regimens to be delivered. There have been multiple studies in solid tumors to determine whether their use decreases the infectious risk associated with neutropenia. It is recommended that they be used if the chemotherapy is associated with a 40% incidence of Grade IV neutropenia and after febrile neutropenia is documented in a previous cycle [48–50]. Several randomized studies in NHL demonstrate decreased duration of neutropenia and less febrile neutropenia in patients receiving hematopoietic growth factor support [51,52].

G-CSF

Zinzani et al. [51] reported a clinical trial of 158 untreated patients with aggressive NHL who were more than 60 years old and randomized them to combination chemotherapy VNCOP-B (cyclophosphamide, mitoxantrone, vincristine, etoposide, bleomycin, and prednisone) with or without G-CSF. The two groups had a similar response rate. The extent of neutropenia differed, 23% (18/77) of the G-CSF group vs. 55.5% (40/72) in the controls. Infectious complications differed also. There were 5% (4/77) infections in the G-CSF group; all were minor and utilized oral antibiotics. In the control group, there were 21% (15/72) infections; 10 were minor and five were major, requiring hospitalization and intravenous antibiotics. Documented infections included one enterococcal infection, three staphylococcal infections, and one *Pneumocystis carinii* (PCP) pneumonia.

Pettengel et al. [52] studied 80 patients randomized to receive G-CSF vs. placebo during VAPEC-B (vincristine, adriamycin, prednisolone, etoposide, cyclophosphamide, bleomycin) chemotherapy. The prednisolone is given at

50 mg for 5 weeks, 25 mg for 5 weeks, and titrated off during 2 weeks. Pro-phylactic cotrimoxazole and ketoconazole were given. The extent of neutro-penia and the incidences of fever differed between the two groups. Grade III neutropenia was 37% (15/41) in the G-CSF patients and 85% (33/39) in the controls. Grade IV neutropenia was 22% in the G-CSF and 72% in the controls. Fever was also greater in the controls 44% (17/39) than with G-CSF 22% (9/41). However, there were no significant differences in documented infections (seven in G-CSF group, five in control group), days of hospitali-zation (20 in each group), or need for more than 3 days of intravenous antibiotics (nine in G-CSF group, 12 in the control group). Delivery of the chemotherapy was delayed due to neutropenia in 19 of the control group and only two of the G-CSF group. The authors felt there was an advantage to hemopoietic growth factor utilization, as it allowed timely delivery of the full course of treatment. They attributed the similar infectious profile to the use of prophylactic antibiotics, which would decrease the observed infectious rate, particularly infections associated with prolong steroid use.

GM-CSF

Gerhartz et al. [53] investigated 125 patients with aggressive NHL random-ized to receive GM-CSF after induction chemotherapy with COP-BLAM (cyclophosphamide, doxorubicin, bleomcin, vincristine, procarbazind, and prednisolone). The prednisolone was given days 1 through 5, and patients did not receive prophylactic antibiotics. This study did demonstrate a reduction in the duration of neutropenia, days with fever (2.1 vs. 4.0), and days of hospitalization for infection (3.5 vs. 8.0). The group receiving GM-CSF had 28 infections in 16/59 patients compared with 69 infections in 30/66 patients in the control group. The numbers of bacteremia and pulmonary infections were similar to those found in other studies, 10 in the GM-CSF group and 22 in the control. Each group had the same number of positive cultures, 18% in the GM-CSF group and 19% in the control. The lack of prophylactic antibiotics in this clinical trial unmasked the fever and infectious complications as compared to the study by Pettengell [52], thus this study demonstrated a reduction in infection with growth factor use, in addition to allowing timely delivery of chemotherapy. There were no differences in survival between the two groups.

Bergmann et al. [54] also studied the effect of GM-CSF after chemo-therapy in patients with aggressive NHL. This was a smaller, randomized pilot study using VACPE (vincristine, doxorubicin, cyclophosphamide, prednisone—given days 1 through 7—and etoposide). In the first two cycles of chemotherapy, there were significant differences in Grade IV neutropenia 20/37 (54%) in the GM-CSF group versus 28/30 (93%) in the control group.

The duration of Grade IV neutropenia was shorter, 2 days in the GM-CSF group and 4.5 days in the control. There were no differences in the incidence of febrile neutropenia, utilization of systemic antibiotics, or survival.

PROGNOSTIC MODELS

There have been several studies to formulate models that could predict both the risk of developing neutropenia following chemotherapy and the severity of the infectious complications [6,55,56]. These studies included 40% of the patients with hematological malignancies. The goal was to identify low-risk cohorts that would be eligible for alternative treatment regimens such as outpatient treatment and oral vs. intravenous antibiotics. Of note, approximately 21 to 30% of the febrile incidents in these studies had a microbiologically identified source, which is consistent with most published reports.

Several groups have developed prognostic models specifically for NHL. Intragumtornchai and colleagues [57] in Thailand studied 155 patients with aggressive NHL undertaking the first course of chemotherapy. They found a 39% incidence of ANC $< 500/\mu L$ and 33% incidence of febrile neutropenia. Serum albumin, serum LDH, and bone marrow involvement were significant risk factors in predicting the development of febrile neutropenia.

Voog et al. [58] studied the value of tumor necrosis factor TNF-2 levels to estimate treatment-induced myelosuppression and resulting febrile neutropenia in previously untreated patients. In 101 patients using combination chemotherapy, 67 had an absolute neutrophil count (ANC) less than $500/\mu L$ (WHO grade IV), which persisted for more than 5 days in 22 patients. There were 37 cases of febrile neutropenia with and 23 patients had documented infections including one death. They found that the type of chemotherapy, the use of hematopoietic colony stimulating factors, performance status, and levels of TNF were predictive of the severity of neutropenia and its complications.

AUTOPSY DATA

Worldwide, several groups reported on autopsy data in patients with hematological malignancies [59–62]. Although these cases encompassed a variety of hematological malignancies and treatment regimes, the patterns in infection were surprisingly consistent. Bacterial infections predominate, and fungal infections comprise approximately 30% of the cases, most of these were discovered antemortem. Srivastava et al. [60] in India analyzed 72 patients in India. They found infections in 51% (37/72), bacterial 27% (20/72), gram-negative infections 18% (10/72), gastrointestinal candidiasis (10/72), Aspergillus (10/72), CMV (3/72), and polymicrobial 15% (11/72). Nosari et al. [59] in Milan found a similar pattern in the 95 autopsies they evaluated. Infections were found in 63% of the patients; bacterial ones comprised 43%, fungal infections 28%, viral 9%, mycobacterial 7%, and polymicrobial 7%.

SUMMARY

The main infectious risk to patients with NHL is treatment-related neutropenia. Combination chemotherapy for the aggressive NHL produces 30–80% neutropenia in at least one treatment cycle, febrile neutropenia in 30%, and microbiologically documented infections in 18–27%. The most common organism is bacterial, chiefly gram-positive infections, although gram-negative infections are found also. In addition, as most of these regimes include corticosteroids, there is an additional risk of developing fungal infections. Opportunistic infections are generally rare. Hemopoietic growth factors decrease the degree and duration of the neutropenia and allow timely delivery of each chemotherapy cycle.

The purine analogs such as fludarabine are used singly and in combination in the therapy of the indolent NHL. These regimes demonstrate an increased risk of opportunistic infections, especially PCP and herpes zoster, although the degree of risk is less than that seen in the treatment of CLL and hairy cell leukemia. It is recommended that PCP prophylaxis be utilized during treatment.

The unconjugated anti-CD 20 antibody, rutuximab, and the radio-immunoconjugates such as Bexxar and Zevalin, show efficacy and markedly less neutropenia. When used as single agents, the neutropenia in mild, mainly Grade I/II. There are similar numbers of fevers and infections, but these are mild also. There is an increase in herpes zoster and herpes simplex.

REFERENCES

1. Baris D, Zahm SH. Epidemiology of lymphomas. Current Opinion in Oncology 2000; 12:383–394.
2. Clarke CA, Glaser SL. Changing incidence of non-Hodgkin lymphomas in the United Sates. Cancer 2002; 94(7):2015–2023.
3. Harris NL, Jaffe ES, Diebold J, Flandrin G, Muller-Hermelink K, Vardiman J, Lister TA, Bloomfield CD. World Health Organization classification of neoplastic diseases of the hematopoietic and lymphoid tissues; report of the Clinical Advisory Committee meeting, Airlie House, Virginia, U.S.A. November 1997. J Clin Oncol 1999; 17:3835–3849.
4. The non-Hodgkin's lymphoma classification project. A clinical evaluation of the International Lymphoma Study Group classification of non-Hodgkin's lymphoma. Blood 1997; 89:3909–3918.

5. Giamarellou H. Infectious complications of febrile leukopenia. Infect Dis Clin North Am 2001; 15:457–482.
6. Talcott JA, Siegel RD, Finberg R, Goldman L. Risk assessment in cancer patients with fever and neutropenia: a prospective, two-center validation of a prediction rule. J Clin Oncol 1992; 10:316–322.
7. Bow EJ. Infection risk and cancer chemotherapy: the impact of the chemotherapeutic regimen in patients with lymphoma and solid tissue malignancies. J Antimicrob Chemother 1998; 41:1 5.
8. Safdar A. Infectious morbidity in critically ill patients with cancer. Crit Care Clin 2001; 17:531–570.
9. Bodey GP, Buckley M, Sathe YS, Freireich EJ. Quantitative relationships between circulating leukocytes and infection in patients with acute leukemia. Ann Internal Med 1966; 64:328–340.
10. Pizzo P. Fever in immunocompromised patients. N Engl J Med 1999; 341:893–900.
11. Heussel CP, Kauczor HU, Heussel GU, Fischer B, Begrich M, Mildenberger P, Thelen M. Pneumonia in febrile neutropenic patients and in bone marrow and blood stem-cell transplant recipients: use of high-resolution computed tomography. J Clin Oncol 1999; 17:796–805.
12. Hughes WT, Armstrong D, Bodey GP, Brown AE, Edwards JE, Feld R, Pizzo P, Rolston K, Shenep JL, Young LS. Guidelines for the use of antimicrobial agents in neutropenic patients with unexplained fever. Clinical Infectious Diseases 1997; 25:551–573.
13. Kim SK, Demetri GD. Chemotherapy and neutropenia. Hem Onc Clinics North Am 1996; 10:377–395.
14. Klein NC. Infections associated with steroid use. Infect Dis Clin North Am 2001; 15:423–432.
15. Chrischilles E, Delgado D, Stolshek S, Lawless G, Fridman M. Impact of age and colony-simulating factor use on hospital length of stay for febrile neutropenia in CHOP related non-Hodgkin's lymphoma. Cancer Control 2002; 9(3):203–211.
16. Shaklai S, Bairey O, Blickstein D. Severe myelotoxicity of oral etoposide in heavily pretreated patients with non-Hodgkin's lymphoma or chronic lymphatic leukemia. Cancer 1996; 77:2313–2317.
17. Bastion Y, Blay JY, Divine M, Brice P, Bordessoule D, Sebban C, Blanc M, Tilly H, Lederlin P, Deconinck E, Salles B, Dumontet C, Briere J, Coiffier B. Elderly patients with aggressive non-Hodgkin's lymphoma: disease presentation, response to treatment, and survival—a Groupe d'Étude des Lymphomes de l'Adulte study on 453 patients older than 69 years. J Clin Oncol 1997; 15(8):2945–2953.
18. Brice P, Bastion Y, Lepage E, Brousse N, Haioun C, Moreau P, Straetmans N, Tilly H, Tabah I, Solal-Celigny P. Comparison in low-tumor-burden follicular lymphomas between an initial no-treatment policy, prednimustine, or interferon alpha: a randomized study from the Groupe d'Étude des Lymphomes Folliculaires. J Clin Oncol 1997; 15:1110–1117.

19. Johnson PW, Rohatiner AZ, Whelan JS, Price CG, Love A, Lim J, Matthews J, Norton AJ, Amess JA, Lister TA. Patterns of survival in patients with recurrent follicular lymphoma: a 20-year study from a single center. J Clin Oncol 1995; 13:140–147.

20. Cabanillas F, Horning S, Kaminski M, Champlin R. Managing indolent lymphomas in relapse: working our way through a plethora of options. Hematology 2000; 166–179.

21. Brandt L, Kimby E, Nygren P, Glimelius B. A systematic overview of chemotherapy effects in indolent non-Hodgkin's lymphoma. Acta Oncologica 2001; 40:198–212.

22. Cheson BD. Infectious and immunosuppressive complications of purine analog therapy. J Clin Oncol 1995; 13(9):2431 2448.

23. Lazzarino M, Orlandi E, Baldanti F, Furione M, Pagnucco G, Astori C, Arcaini L, Viglio A, Paulli M, Gerna G, Bernasconi C. The immunosuppression and potential for EBV reactivation of fludarabine combined with cyclophosphamide and dexamethasone in patients with lymphoproliferative disorders. British Journal of Haematology 1999; 107(4):877–882.

24. Flinn IW, Byrd JC, Morrison C, Jamison J, Diehl LF, Murphy T, Piantadosi S, Seifter E, Ambinder RF, Vogelsang G, Grever MR. Fludarabine and cyclophosphamide with filgrastim support in patients with previously untreated indolent lymphoid malignancies. Blood 2000; 96:71–75.

25. Foran JM, Oscier D, Orchard J, Johnson SA, Tighe M, Cullen MH, de Takats PG, Kraus C, Klein M, Lister TA. Pharmacokinetic study of single doses of oral fludarabine phosphate in patients with low-grade non-Hodgkin's lymphoma and B-cell chronic lymphocytic leukemia. J Clin Oncol 1999; 17:1574.

26. Hochster HS, Kim KM, Green MD, Mann RB, Neiman RS, Oken MM, Cassileth PA, Stott P, Ritch P, O'Connell MJ. Activity of fludarabine in previously treated non-Hodgkin's low-grade lymphoma: results of an Eastern Cooperative Oncology Group study. J Clin Oncol 1992; 10:28–32.

27. Redman JR, Cabanillas F, Velasquez WS, McLaughlin P, Hagemeister FB, Swan F Jr, Rodriguez MA, Plunkett WK, Keating MJ. Phase II trial of fludarabine phosphate in lymphoma: an effective new agent in low-grade lymphoma. J Clin Oncol 1992; 10:790–794.

28. Pigaditou A. Fludarabine in low-grade lymphoma. Semin Oncol 1993; 20(5 suppl 7):24–27.

29. Whelan JS, Davis CL, Rule S, Ranson M, Smith OP, Mehta AB, Catovsky D, Rohatiner AZ, Lister TA. Fludarabine phosphate for the treatment of low grade lymphoid malignancy. British Journal of Cancer 1999; 64(1):120–123.

30. Solal-Celigny P, Brice P, Brousse N, Caspard H, Bastion Y, Haioun C, Bosly A, Tilly H, Bordessoule D, Sebban C, Harousseau JL, Morel P, Dupas B, Plassan F, Vasile N, Fort N, Leporriei M. Phase II trial of fludarabine monophosphate as first-line treatment in patients with advanced follicular lymphoma: a multicenter study by the Groupe d'Étude des Lymphomes de l'Adulte. J Clin Oncol 1996; 14:514–519.

31. Flinn IW, Byrd JC, Morrison C, Jamison J, Diehl LF, Murphy T, Piantadosi S,

Seifter E, Ambinder RF, Vogelsang G, Grever MR. Fludarabine and cyclophosphamide with filgrastim support in patients with previously untreated indolent lymphoid malignancies. Blood 2000; 96:71 75.

32. Velasquez DL, et al. SWOG 95-01: A phase II trial of a combination of fludarabine and mitoxantrone (FN) in untreated advanced low grade lymphoma. An effective, well tolerated therapy. Proceedings of the American Society of Clinical Oncology, 1999:18–27.

33. Zinzani PL, Magagnoli M, Moretti L, De Renzo A, Battista R, Zaccaria A, Guardigni L, Mazza P, Marra R, Ronconi F, Lauta VM, Bendandi M, Gherlinzoni F, Gentilini P, Ciccone F, Cellini C, Stefoni V, Ricciuti F, Gobbi M, Tura S. Randomized trial of fludarabine versus fludarabine and idarubicin as frontline treatment in patients with indolent or mantle-cell lymphoma. Journal of Clinical Oncology 2000; 18(4):773–779.

34. Hochster HS, Oken MM, Winter JN, Gordon LI, Raphael BG, Bennett JM, Cassileth PA. Phase I study of fludarabine plus cyclophosphamide in patients with previously untreated low-grade lymphoma: results and and long-term followup–a report from the Eastern Cooperative Oncology Group. J Clin Oncol 2000; 18:987–994.

35. McLaughlin P, Hagemeister FB. Fludarabine, mitoxantrone, and dexamethasone: an effective new regimen for indolent lymphoma. J Clin Oncol 1996; 14:1262–1268.

36. McLaughlin P, Grillo-Lopez AJ, Link BK, Levy R, Czuczman MS, Williams ME, Heyman MR, Bence-Bruckler I, White CA, Cabanillas F, Jain V, Ho AD, Lister J, Wey K, Shen D, Dallaire BK. Rituximab chimeric anti-CD20 monoclonal antibody therapy for relapsed indolent lymphoma: half of patients respond to a four-dose treatment program. J Clin Oncol 1998; 16:2825–2833.

37. Davis TA, Grillo-López AJ. Rituximab anti-CD20 monoclonal antibody therapy in non-Hodgkin's lymphoma: safety and efficacy of re-treatment. J Clin Oncol 2000; 18:3135–3143.

38. Sweetenham J, Hieke K, Kerrigan M, Howard P, Smart PF, McIntyre A, Townshend S. Cost-minimization analysis of CHOP, fludarabine and rituximab for the treatment of relapsed indolent B-cell non-Hodgkin's lymphoma in the U.K. British Journal of Haematology 1999; 106:47–54.

39. Kaminski MS, Zelenetz AD, Press OW, Saleh M, Leonard J, Fehrenbacher L, Lister TA, Stagg RJ, Tidmarsh GF, Kroll S, Wahl RL, Knox SJ, Vose JM. Pivotal study of Iodine I 131 tositumomab for chemotherapy-refractory low-grade or transformed low-grade B-cell non-Hodgkin's lymphomas. J Clin Oncol 2001; 19:3918–3928.

40. Witzig TE, Gordon LI, Cabanillas F, Czuczman MS, Emmanouilides C, Joyce R, Pohlman BL, Bartlett NL, Wiseman GA, Padre N, Grillo-López AJ, Multani P, White CA. Randomized controlled trial of yttrium-90-labeled ibritumomab tiuxetan radioimmunotherapy versus rituximab immunotherapy for patients with relapsed or refractory low-grade, follicular, or transformed B-cell non-Hodgkin's lymphoma. J Clin Oncol 2002; 20:2453–2463.

41. The International Non-Hodgkin's Lymphoma Prognostic Factors Project. A

predictive model for aggressive non-Hodgkin's lymphoma. N Engl J Med 1993; 329:987–994.

42. Kimby E, Brandt L, Ngyren P, Glimelius B. A systematic overview of chemoherapy effects in aggressive non-Hodgkin's lymphoma. Acta Oncologica 2001; 40:213–223.

43. Fisher RI, Gaynor ER, Dahlberg S, Oken MM, Grogan TM, Mize EM, Glick JH, Coltman CA, Miller TP. Comparison of a standard regimen (CHOP) with three intensive chemotherapy regimens for advanced non-Hodgkin's lymphoma. N Engl J Med 1993; 328:1002–1006.

44. Coiffier B. Fourteen years of high-dose CHOP (ACVB regimen): preliminary conclusions about the treatment of aggressive-lymphoma patients. Annals of Oncology 1995; 6:211–217.

45. Coiffier B, Lepage E, Brière J, Raoul Herbrecht R, Tilly H, Bouabdallah R, Morel P, Van Den Neste E, Salles G, Gaulard P, Reyes F, Lederlin P, Gisselbrecht C. CHOP chemotherapy plus rituximab compared with CHOP alone in elderly patients with diffuse large-B-cell lymphoma. N Engl J Med 2002; 346:235–242.

46. Hoskins PJ, Le N, Gascoyne RD, Klasa R, Shenkier T, O'Reilly S, Connors JM. Advanced diffuse large-cell lymphoma treated with 12-week combination chemotherapy: natural history of relapse after initial complete response and prognostic variables defining outcome after relapse. Annals of Oncology 1997; 8:1125–1132.

47. Gutierrez M, Chabner BA, Pearson D, Steinberg SM, Jaffe ES, Cheson BD, Fojo A, Wilson WH. Role of a doxorubicin-containing regimen in relapsed and resistant lymphomas: an 8-year follow-up study of EPOCH. J Clin Oncol 2000; 18:3633–3642.

48. Ozer H, Armitage JO, Bennett CL, Crawford J, Demetri GD, Pizzo PA, Schiffer CA, Smith TJ, Somlo G, Wade JC, Wadè JL III, Winn RJ, Wozniak AJ, Somerfield MR. 2000 update of recommendations for the use of hematopoietic colony-stimulating factors: evidence-based, clinical practice guidelines. J Clin Oncol 2000; 18:3558–3585.

49. Gisselbrecht C, Haioun C, Lepage E, Bastion Y, Tilly H, Bosly A, Dupriez B, Marit G, Herbrecht R, Deconinck E, Marolleau JP, Yver A, Dabouz-Harrouche F, Coiffier B, Reyes F. Placebo-controlled phase III study of lenograstim (glycosylated recombinant granulocyte colony-stimulating factor) in aggressive non-Hodgkin's lymphoma influencing chemotherapy administration. Leuk Lymphoma 1997; 25:289–300.

50. Bennett CL, Weeks JA, Somerfield MR, Feinglass J, Smith TJ. Use of hematopoietic colony-stimulating factors: comparison of the 1994 and 1997 American Society of Clinical Oncology surveys regarding ASCO clinical practice guidelines. J Clin Oncol 1999; 17:3673–3681.

51. Zinzani PL, Pavone E, Storti S, Moretti L, Fattori PP, Guardigni L, Falini B, Gobbi M, Gentilini P, Lauta VM, Bendandi M, Gherlinzoni F, Magagnoli M, Venturi S, Aitini E, Tabanelli M, Leone G, Liso V, Tura S. Randomized trial with or without granulocyte colony-stimulating factor as adjunct to induction

VNCOP-B treatment of elderly high-grade non-Hodgkin's lymphoma. Blood 1997; 89:3974–3979.

52. Pettengell R, Gurney H, Radford JA, Deakin DP, James R, Wilkinson PM, Kane K, Bentley J, Crowther D. Granulocyte colony-stimulating factor to prevent dose-limiting neutropenia in non-Hodgkin's lymphoma: a randomized controlled trial. Blood 1992; 80:1430–1436.

53. Gerhartz HH, Engelhard M, Meusers P, Brittinger G, Wilmanns W, Schlimok G, Mueller P, Huhn D, Musch R, Siegert W. Randomized double-blind, placebo-contolled phase III study of recombinant human granulocyte-macro-phage colony-stimulating factor as adjunct to induction treatment of high-grade malignant non-Hodgkin's lymphomas. Blood 1993; 82:2329–2339.

54. Bergmann L, Karakas T, Knuth A, Lautenschlager G, Mitrou PS. Recombi-nant human granulocyte-macrophage colony stimulating factor after combined chemotherapy in high-grade non-Hodgkin's lymphoma a randomized pilot study. Eur J Cancer 1995; 31:2164–2168.

55. Klastersky J, Paesmans M, Rubenstein EB, Boyer M, Elting L, Feld R, Gallagher J, Herrstedt J, Rapoport B, Rolston K, Talcott J. The Multinational Association for Supportive Care in Cancer Risk Index: a multinational scoring system for identifying low-risk febrile neutropenic cancer patients. J Clin Oncol 2002; 18:3038–3051.

56. Blay JY, Chauvin F, Le Cesne A, Anglaret B, Bouhour D, Lasset C, Freyer C, Philip T, Biron P. Early lymphopenia after cytotoxic chemotherapy as a risk factor for febrile neutropenia. J Clin Oncol 1996; 14:636–643.

57. Intragumtornchai T, Sutheesophon J, Sutcharitchan P, Swasdiul D. A predic-tive model for life-threatening neutropenia and febrile neutropenia after the first course of CHOP chemotherapy in patients with aggressive non-Hodgkin's lymphoma. Leuk Lymphoma 2000; 37(3–4):351–360.

58. Voog E, Bienvenu J, Warzocha K, Moullet I, Dumontet C, Thieblemont C, Monneret G, Gutowski M, Coiffier B, Salles G. Factors that predict chemo-therapy-induced myelosuppression in lymphoma patients: role of the tumor necrosis factor ligand-receptor system. J Clin Oncol 2000; 325–331.

59. Nosari A, Barberis M, Landonio G, Magnani P, Majno M, Oreste P, Sozzi P. Infections in haematologic neoplasms: autopsy findings. Haematologica 1991; 76(2):135–140.

60. Srivastava VM, Krishnaswami H, Srivastava A, Dennison D, Chandy M. In-fections in haematological malignancies: an autopsy study of 72 cases. Trans-actions of the Royal Society of Tropical Medicine and Hygiene 1996; 90(4):406–408.

61. Doran HM, Sheppard MN, Collins PW, Jones L, Newland AC, van der Walt JD. Pathology of the lung in leukaemia and lymphoma: a study of 87 autopsies. Histopathology 1991; 18(3):211 219.

62. Jandrlic M, Kalenic S, Labar B, Nemet D, Jakic-Razumovic J, Mrsic M, Plecko V, Bogdanic V. An autopsy study of systemic fungal infections in patients with hematologic malignancies. European Journal of Clinical Micro-biology and Infectious Diseases 1995; 14(9):768–774.

11

Infections Unique to Hodgkin's Disease

Karla Richards and John N. Greene
University of South Florida School of Medicine
and Moffitt Cancer Center and Research Institute
Tampa, Florida, U.S.A.

"Hodgkin's disease (HD) is a localized or disseminated malignant prolifer-ation of tumor cells arising from the lymphoreticular system, primarily involving lymph node tissue and the bone marrow." It is diagnosed by the presence of Reed–Sternberg cells present in the lymph nodes as well as the liver, bone marrow, or other parenchymal tissue [1]. Hodgkin's disease usually presents with a bimodal age distribution that peaks between 15 and 34 and again after age 60. The disease is classified into one of four varieties, nodular sclerosis 67%, mixed cellularity 25%, lymphocyte depleted 5%, and lymphocyte predominant 3% [1]. The last is the most aggressive form and usually occurs in young men [2]. Staging is dependent upon lymph node involvement and whether dissemination to local or distant nodes or organs has occurred. Stage 1 has one lymph node and stage 4 involves the bone marrow, lungs, or liver.

The American Cancer Society estimates that in 2003 about 7,600 new cases of Hodgkin's disease will be diagnosed in the United States. This number has not changed significantly in several years, although the prognosis has dramatically improved. In general, Hodgkin's has a 1 year survival rate of 95%, a 5 year survival of approximately 84%, and a 10 year at 75%. Although

Hodgkin's disease-related deaths have decreased, overall mortality remains above that of the general population largely because of the development of congestive heart failure and secondary malignancy ("treatment toxicities") [2]. Secondary cancers developing after treatment for Hodgkin's disease are acute myelogenous leukemia (AML) 3.6%, non-Hodgkin's lymphomas 1.3%, and solid tumors 8.3% [3]. The risk increases with the more aggressive treatment regimens for primary Hodgkin's disease.

Treatment of HD is primarily dependent upon its stage regardless of its cellularity. It typically consists of various combinations of chemotherapy, with radiation therapy, depending upon stage and type. The chemotherapy combinations are MOPP (mechlorethamine + vincristine + procarbazine + prednisone) and a newer one ABVD (doxorubicine + bleomycin + vinblastine + dacarbazine). Many studies have been done to determine the best way to administer chemotherapy with the least side effects. At 10 years, the relative risk of developing acute leukemia with MOPP was approx 3%, while the risk associated with ABVD was less than 1% [3].

Out of 70 patients with HD in a study of infections in lymphomas, 70% were due to bacteria, 13% were viral, 4% fungal, and 11% mixed infections [4]. It was noted that Hodgkin's disease patients have an increased susceptibility to mycobacteria or cryptococcus infections related to their loss of cellular immunity. Antibody formation was retained in patients until the illness was well advanced [5], as most infections have occurred in the last quarter of their illness [4].

INFECTIONS RELATED TO CELL-MEDIATED IMMUNODEFICIENCY

Hodgkin's disease cells are Reed–Sternberg cells that are usually CD 15 and CD 30 T cells. T cell mediated immunity is critical for controlling many viral infections as well as nonviral intracellular pathogens such as listeria, mycobacterium, leishmania, and toxoplasma [6]. It would seem intuitive that infections prominent in patients with other T cell disorders such as HIV are also present in patients with Hodgkin's disease.

Pneumocystis carinii pneumonia (PCP) was first reported to occur in patients with malnutrition, acute lymphocytic leukemia (ALL), and HD. Opportunistic bacterial infections that may occur in patients with HD include *Nocardia*, *Mycobacterium tuberculosis*, and nontuberculous *Mycobacterium* (*M. avium complex*, *M. kansasii*, *M. fortuitum*, *M. chelonae*, and *M. abscessus*). These infections usually involve the lung, but brain and skin dissemination may occur.

Fungal infections include *Candida* species and *Aspergillus* species, especially during periods of prolonged neutropenia. In addition, radiation therapy to the lungs and mediastinum and prolonged corticosteroids may predispose to pulmonary Aspergillosis. Cryptococcal pneumonia, meningitis, cellulitis, or disseminated infection may occur in HD patients due to cellular immunodeficiency. A review of 54 patients with HD who developed crypto-coccosis noted several common features. The presence of HD for more than 12 months, stage IV disease, absolute lymphopenia, and extensive chemo-therapy regimens predisposed HD patients to the development of Crypto-coccal infections [7]. Endemic mycosis has also been reported in patients with HD, namely, Blastomycosis [8] and Histoplasmosis [4].

INFECTIONS RELATED TO SPLENECTOMY AND HUMORAL IMMUNODEFICIENCY

In the diagnosis and staging of HD a splenectomy is often required. Asplenics are susceptible to sepsis from those bacteria that contain a capsule such as *Streptococcus pneumoniae*, and *Haemophilus influenzae*, in addition to gram-negative bacilli such as *E. coli* and *Pseudomonas aeruginosa* [9]. Other causes of sepsis are *N. meningitides*, the third most common cause of postsplenec-tomy sepsis (PSS), and *Capnocytophaga canimorsis*, a gram-negative that one obtains from dog bites and scratches. Also, parasitic infections such as malaria and protozoa are more dangerous in asplenic patients.

There have been many cases of infections with *Streptococcus pneumo-niae* and *Haemophilus influenzae* in splenectomized patients with Hodgkin's disease [10]. Sepsis occurring with streptococcal infections is much more common in splenectomized patients, with the risk decreasing with increasing age. The risk of infection in adults was equal to that of the general population, but the risk of death due to sepsis was increased 58 times in the asplenic population [9]. *S. pneumoniae* is the causative agent in 50 to 90% of cases of postsplenectomy sepsis. The second most common infection is that of *H. influenzae*, which typically occurs in children under 15 years of age (86%). Therefore all patients undergoing a splenectomy should have *H. influenzae* vaccine as well as pneumococcal vaccine 2 weeks prior to surgery. To em-phasize this point, a 13 year old girl with stage IV B Hodgkin's disease under-went MOPP chemotherapy and was in complete remission after 6 cycles. Six months later she developed a fatal case of *Hemophilus influenzae* sepsis be-lieved to result from immune changes due to the splenectomy, rather than the Hodgkin's disease [11]. However, *H. influenzae* (type B) sepsis is very uncom-mon in the present era of widespread *H. influenzae* type B (HIB) vaccination.

In a randomized trial that included 92 patients with HD that had undergone splenectomy, the most common infection developing in the remission period was due to *Varicella zoster* virus (VZV), occurring in 22 of the 92 patients studied (24%) [10]. Being female and under 30 years old were found to be risk factors for VZV infection. Other infections also reported during the remission period were due to *S. pneumoniae*.

INFECTIONS RELATED TO NEUTROPENIA

Treatment of HD frequently results in neutropenia for 1 to 3 weeks, especially following stem cell transplantation. Neutropenia can result in a variety of infections that changes as the duration increases. Patients with HD are at the same risk for neutropenia-related infections as patients with leukemia and non-Hodgkin's lymphoma and are covered in the chapter called Infections Related to Stem Cell Transplantation.

CONCLUSION

In conclusion, infections occurring in patients with Hodgkin's disease develop in response to the nature of the immunodeficiency, such as T cell deficiency, humoral immune dysfunction from splenectomy, and neutropenia. Recognizing the duration of HD, prior number of chemotherapy cycles, asplenia, and current immunosuppressive medications such as corticosteroids allows one to predict the opportunistic pathogens likely to be causing infections in patients with Hodgkin's disease.

REFERENCES

1. Beers Mark H, Berkow Robert, eds. The Merck Manual. 17th ed. Westpoint, PA: Merck Research Laboratories, 1999.
2. Diehl V, Sextro M. Franklin J, Hansmann ML, Harris N, Jaffe E, Poppema S, Harris M, Fransilla K, van Krieken J, Marafioti T, Anagnostopoulos I, Stein H. Clinical presentation, course, and prognostic factors in lymphocyte-predominant Hodgkin's disease. J Clin Oncol 1999; 17(3): 776–783.
3. Valagussa P, Santoro A, Fossati-Bellani F, Banfi A, Bonadonna G. Second acute leukemia and other malignancies following treatment for Hodgkin's disease. J Clin Oncol 1986; 4(6):830–836.
4. Casazza AR, Duvall CP, Carbone PP. Infection in lymphoma. Histology treatment and duration in relation to incidence and survival. JAMA 1966; 197:710.
5. Aisenberg AC, Leskowitz S. Antibody formation in Hodgkin's disease. NEJM 1963; 268:1269–1272.
6. Mandell Gerald L, Bennett JE, Dolin R. Principles and Practice of Infectious Diseases. 5th ed. Vol. 1. Philadelphia: Churchhill Livingstone USA, 2000.
7. Korfel A, Menssen HD, Schwartz S, Thiel E. Cryptococcosis in Hodgkin's disease: description of two cases and review of the literature. Ann Hematol 1998; 76(6):283–286.

8. Winquist Eric W, Walmsley Sharon, Berinstein Neil L. Reactivation and dissemination of Blastomycosis complication of Hodgkin's disease: a case report and review of the literature. Amer J Hematol 1993; 43:129–132.
9. Sumaraju V, Smith L, Smith S. Infectious complications in asplenic hosts. IDCNA 2001; 15(2):551–565.
10. Schimpff SC, O'Connell MJ, Greene WH, Wiernik PH. Infections in 92 splenectomized patients with Hodgkin's disease. American J Med 1975; 59:695–701.
11. Nixon DW, Aisenberg A. Fatal hemophilus influenzae sepsis in an asymptomatic splenectomized Hodgkin's disease patient. Ann Int Med 1972; 77:69–71.

12

Infectious Complications in Stem Cell Transplant Recipients

John N. Greene
University of South Florida School of Medicine
and Moffitt Cancer Center and Research Institute
Tampa, Florida, U.S.A.

PRETRANSPLANTATION PHASE (DAY −30–0)

Prior to stem cell transplantation, the host immunity is relatively intact, except for those patients with active progressive cancer, prolonged neutropenia, or chronic steroid use. Those without these risk factors are prone to the same infections as the general population at large. The predominant pathogens are community-acquired viruses that mostly affect the respiratory tract, such as influenzae, respiratory syncytial virus, parainfluenzae, adenovirus, coronavirus, and the newly discovered metapneumovirus.

The predominant bacterial pathogens also affect the respiratory tract and are *S. pneumoniae*, *H. influenzae*, and *Moraxella catarrhalis*. The illnesses caused by these pathogens are similar to those of the noncancer patient and are primarily upper and lower respiratory tract infections.

Central venous catheter infections can occur, especially when the large-bore stem-cell-harvesting catheters are used. Gram-positive skin flora such as coagulase-negative *Staphylococci*, *S. aureus*, and *Corynebacteria* species predominate. Catheter removal in addition to antibiotics is occasionally necessary for cure of the infection. The patients with risk factors for opportunistic infections will be discussed later in the chapter.

EARLY TRANSPLANTATION PHASE (DAY 0–30)

Neutropenia is the predominant defect in host immunity during this phase. Neutropenia can be divided into three distinct periods; short-term (less than 1 week), midterm (1 to 2 weeks) and long-term (over 2 weeks), with different infections occurring at each time. Because of the predominance of gram-negative bacilli (GNB) infections with significant morbidity and mortality during neutropenia, prophylactic antimicrobials were explored. After tri-methoprim–sulfamethoxazole (TMP/SMZ) prophylaxis significantly reduced GNB infections, the anti-Pseudomonal flouroquinolones were studied. The fluoroquinolones were more successful at reducing GNB infections than TMP/SMZ, especially *Pseudomonas aeruginosa* infections. There was no difference in overall or infection-related mortality with the prophylactic use of flouroquinolones for febrile neutropenia. However, they are widely used for this purpose, especially in the SCT patient. The result of this practice is the increasing occurrence of gram-positive cocci (GPC) infections, namely, coag-ulase-negative *Staphylococci*, alpha hemolytic *Streptococci*, and *S. aureus*.

SHORT-TERM NEUTROPENIA (DAY 0–7)

Bacteria Infections

Because of the frequent use of the flouroquinolones for prophylaxis, the predominant infections are GPC. Coagulase-negative *Staphylococci* are most common and result in bacteremia frequently related to a central venous catheter infection. Usually, catheter removal is not required, and the infection rapidly clears with the addition of vancomycin. Alpha hemolytic *Streptococci* (AHS) (sometimes referred to as viridians *Streptococci*) are second in frequency to coagulase negative staphylococcus bacteremia, with a higher mortality (4–22%) [1]. Septic shock, adult respiratory distress syndrome, and multiorgan dysfunction have been described in neutropenic patients with AHS bacteremia. Mucositis, especially that induced by cytarabine, is the major risk factor, along with quinolone prophylaxis. *S. aureus*, including methicillin-resistant strains, can cause bacteremia and CVC-related infections and are the third, most common cause of GPC infections during this period.

Breakthrough GNB infections while on quinolone prophylaxis during the first week of neutropenia is highly unlikely. In the absence of quinolone prophylaxis, however, GNB causing bacteremia, urinary tract infection, or pneumonia would occur more commonly. Most transplant centers use cefepime and vancomycin intravenously when febrile neutropenia develops while receiving quinolone prophylaxis. In the majority of cases, no source of infection is found, and the fever tends to disappear. Antibiotic treatment is continued until resolution of neutropenia and fever. One hypothesis for fever during neutropenia with negative cultures is that of endotoxin from GNB translocating across the GI tract. Blood cultures remain negative because the reticuloendothelial clearance or the antibiotics being infused prevent microbial growth. Other causes of fever include progressing tumor, medications, especially antibiotics (β-lactam is most common), and granulocyte colony stimulating factor (GCSF) or granulocyte monocyte colony stimulating factor (GMCSF).

Anerobic infections, namely neutropenic enterocolitis (NE) and oral ulcers with submandibular or cervical lymphadenopathy can occur while receiving flouroquinolones, cephalosporins, or vancomycin because of their lack of anaerobic coverage [2]. NE is caused primarily by *Clostridium septicum* and aerobic GNB [3,4]. Right lower quadrant rebound tenderness with diarrhea and possibly ileus is suggestive of NE. The onset is toward the end of the first week of neutropenia. Metronidazole begun early has significantly lowered the morbidity from this infection. Piperacillin/tazobactam, a carbapenem, and clindamycin also have good anaerobic activity. The oral ulcers with lymphadenopathy are due to *Capnocytophaga ochracea* or *Fusobacterium* species and respond to the aforementioned antibiotics used for NE. The diagnosis is clinical and definitive when blood cultures are positive for the offending pathogen. However, bacteremia occurs in the minority of cases.

Fluconazole prophylaxis is commonly given during this period. Fungal infections are rare in the first week of neutropenia even when fluconazole prophylaxis is not given. The next two periods of neutropenia are the high risk periods of invasive fungal infections, namely *Candida* species and *Aspergillus* species.

The primary viral infection during this period is reactivation of herpes simplex virus (HSV) 1 or 2, occurring in up to 80% of allogeneic SCT recipients and 60% of leukemia patients who are not receiving SCT [5]. With the universal use of acyclovir for prophylaxis in seropositive patients, this infection has been virtually eliminated. Resistance to acyclovir does not occur during this period but can develop later on when graft versus host disease (GVHD) is present. Oral, genital, or perianal HSV infections cause morbidity but do not directly cause mortality. However, the mucosal induced ulcers allow for an increase incidence of AHS bacteremia and *Candida* species fungemia, which can cause serious illness or death [5]. Cytomegalovirus (CMV) and *Varicella zoster* virus (VZV) occur later in the course of transplantation.

MIDTERM NEUTROPENIA (DAY 7–14)

This second period of neutropenia, from 7 to 14 days, is a transition period; predominant pathogens are also found in the short- and long-term periods. The potential infections that develop are dependent on the empirical antimicrobial being used. Assuming the patient is receiving vancomycin, cefepime, acyclovir, and fluconazole at this time, the major infections are due to bacteria and fungi.

Bacteria

Resistant GNB from the production of inducible B lactamases, namely *Serratia marcescens, Pseudomonas aeruginosa,* indole-positive *Proteus vulgaris, Citrobacter* species, and *Enterobacter* species (SPICE) are the major concern. Two other GNB, *Klebsiella* pneumonia and *E. coli* can develop resistance by producing extended spectrum β lactamase (ESBL). These GNB are more likely to occur when ceftazidime, piperacillin/tazobactam, ticarcillin/clavulanate, or aztreonam are used as monotherapy. They occur less likely with cefepime because of its stable structure in the presence of these enzymes. The drug of choice for these "resistant" GNB is a carbapenem (imipenem/cilastatin or meropenem).

While receiving vancomycin, the GPC infections at this period would be vancomycin-resistant *Enterococcus* species. Treatment with linezolid or quinupristin/dalfopristin is indicated. Ampicillin can be used if susceptible. *Leuconostoc, Pediococcus,* and *Lactobacillus* (a gram-positive rod) are vancomycin resistant and can cause bacteremia/CVC infection, but are very rare [6]. Penicillin, clindamycin, or a carbapenem are the treatment of choice. Anaerobic bacterial infections are primarily NE or oral mucositis, as mentioned previously. The antibiotics discussed in that section such as metronidazole would provide effective coverage. *Clostridium difficile* could cause colitis at any time when antibiotics are given.

Fungi

Fungal infections during this period depend on the antifungal agent administered, if any. When no antifungal drug is used, *Candida albicans* causing mucocutaneous, urinary tract, CVC site, or bloodstream infection predominates. If fluconazole is used, nonalbicans *Candida* infections predominate, such as *C. glabrata, C. krusei, C. tropicalis,* and rarely others [7]. The yeast Trichosporin species can cause infection when no antifungal drug is given, but is rare. The molds, especially *Aspergillus,* begin to emerge during this period as a serious infection risk. Because of the lack of mold coverage with fluconazole, other drugs have been used during this period. Itraconazole can be used, but breakthrough mold infections have been reported. Amphotericin B or lipid formulations of Amphotericin B can be used, but they are nephrotoxic, and the latter are expensive. Voriconazole, which has excellent mold coverage and nonalbicans (as well as albicans) *Candida* activity, is being used during this period with increasing success. Caspofungin can also be used at this time, with good activity against *Aspergillus* and *Candida* species infections.

LATE NEUTROPENIA (DAY 14–ENGRAFTMENT)

The pathogens mentioned during midterm neutropenia take on an increasing significance as the duration of neutropenia increases. The most common infections will depend on the antimicrobials in use. SPICE organisms, GNB that make ESBLs, VRE, *Candida* non*albicans* more so than *C. albicans* and molds predominate. *Acinetobacter* species and *Alcaligenes* species may rarely cause infections and tend to be multidrug resistant. Carbapenems are the drug of choice. *Stenotrophomonas maltophilia* bacteremia, pneumonia, or urinary tract infection can occur, especially when carbapendemas are being given. The drugs of choice are TMP/SMZ, ticarcillin/clavulanate, or a flouroquinolone.

Breakthrough *Candida* species are usually nonalbicans species found in the bloodstream or urine. The drugs of choice include amphotericin B, lipid formulations of amphotericin B, and caspofungin possibly in combination with 5-flucytosine. Mold infections besides *Aspergillus* species include *Fusarium* species [8], *Scedosporium* species [9], *Paecilomyces* species [10], and Zygomycetes [11]. Antifungals used alone or in combination include itraconazole, voriconazole, caspofungin, or lipid formulations of amphotericin B.

POSTENGRAFTMENT PHASE

Early (Engraftment–100 days)

The postengraftment phase following allogeneic stem cell transplantation can be divided into early (engraftment to 100 days) and late (over 100 days) periods with similar pathogens but different levels of risk for some organisms (Table 1). The primary immune defect during the early phase is cell mediated (T cell/macrophage/monocyte) from the use of cyclosporin A and corticosteroids or similar medications used to prevent or treat GVHD.

Viral infections during this period include HSV CMV, human herpes virus 6, (HHV6) and community-acquired respiratory viruses. Mucocutaneous herpes simplex virus infections occur sporadically. HSV infection readily responds to antiviral therapy such as acyclovir or one of its analogs. Esophagitis, hepatitis, pneumonia, and encephalitis due to HSV are rare.

TABLE 1 Periods of Risk for Infectious Complications Following Allogeneic SCT

Host immunity	Neutropenia	Cellular immunodeficiency	Cellular and humoral immunodeficiency
Viruses	HSV, CMV	CMV, HHV-6, EBV, community-acquired respiratory viruses (Table 2)	CMV, HHV-6, VZV, EBV, community-acquired respiratory viruses (Table 2)
Bacteria	GPC (Table 3), GPR (Table 4), GNR, anaerobes	GPC (Table 3), GPR (Table 4), MDR-GNR (Table 5), Nocardia, MOTT (Table 6)	GPC (Table 3), GPR (Table 4), MDR-GNR (Table 5), Nocardia, MOTT (Table 6)
Fungi	*Candida albicans*, non*albicans Candida*, *Aspergillus*, *Fusarium*	Non*albicans Candida*, *Aspergillus*, *Fusarium*, *Scedosporium*, *Zygomycosis*, endemic mycosis	Non*albicans Candida*, *Aspergillus*, *Fusarium*, *Scedosporium*, *Zygomycosis*, endemic mycosis
Protozoa		PCP	PCP
Parasites		Strongyloidiasis	Strongyloidiasis
Days following SCT	0	30	100 365

HSV = herpes simplex virus, CMV = cytomegalovirus, HHV6 = human herpes virus 6, EBV = Epstein–Barr virus, GPC = gram-positive cocci, GPR = gram-positive rods, GNR = gram-negative rods, MDR = multidrug resistant, MOTT *Mycobacterium* other than tuberculosis, PCP = pneumocystis carinii pneumonia.

Acyclovir-resistant HSV infections are uncommon and usually occur in the setting of prolonged high-dose immunosuppressive therapy for chronic GVHD. Prolonged use of low-dose acyclovir or its analogs may also select out the thymidine-kinase-deficient strains of HSV that are acyclovir resistant.

Weekly serum CMV antigen detection screening has virtually eliminated CMV disease. Preemptive ganciclovir or valganciclovir effectively prevents

TABLE 2 Community-Acquired Respiratory Viruses

Influenzae
Parainfluenzae
RSV
Adenovirus

TABLE 3 Gram-Positive Cocci

Staphylococcus aureus
Coagulase-negative *Staphylococcus*
Pediococcus
Leuconostoc
Stomatococcus

active infection. Ganciclovir-resistant CMV is uncommon, like acyclovir-resistant HSV, and occurs in a similar setting of immunosuppression. Both resistant viral infections are treated with foscarnet. CMV-induced pneumonia, esophagitis, gastroenteritis, retinitis, hepatitis, encephalitis, and hemorrhagic cystitis have all been reported but remain rare in the setting of weekly CMV screening.

HHV-6 can reactivate and result in pancytopenia (failure or loss of engraftment), pneumonia (interstitial), encephalitis, or viremia resulting in fever of unknown origin. Routine screening for HHV-6 is not done as this infection remains rare. Treatment consists of ganiciclovir (or valganciclovir) or foscarnet.

Other less common viral infections include BK virus, a polyoma virus, causing hemorrhagic cystitis and rarely renal insufficiency [12]. No effective treatment exists except to improve host immunity by reducing immunosuppressive therapy when possible. Adenovirus also can cause hemorrhagic cystitis. Ribavirin has been used successfully in a few cases. The community-acquired respiratory viruses can cause significant morbidity and mortality and occasionally cause outbreaks among SCT recipients [13,14]. The most common include influenzae, RSV, adenovirus, and parainfluinzae [15]. Therapy once pneumonia occurs is not very effective for any of the respiratory viruses. RSV immunoglobin with or without inhaled ribivirin can be used for RSV infections. Rimantadine or oseltamivir may be used to treat influenzae. The use of interferon with any of these viruses is reasonable, but effectiveness remains unknown.

Following engraftment, the primary route of bacterial invasion of the bloodstream is from CVCs and the gastrointestinal tract, especially when

TABLE 4 Gram-Positive Rods

Corynebacterium JK (vs. non-*JK*)
Bacillus species
Lactobacillus species

TABLE 5 Gram-Negative
Bacilli

Serratia
Pseudomonas aeruginosa
Acinetobacter
Citrobacter
Enterobacter
Klebsiella
Escherichia coli
Alcaligenes
Stenotrophomonas

GVHD is present. The predominant organisms will be CVC-related GPC (previously mentioned) and gram-positive rods (GPR) such as *Corynebacterium* (JK and non-JK species) and *Bacillus* species. GNB can also cause CVC-related bacteremia, especially when the patient assumes care of their CVC as an outpatient (usually without neutropenia) [16].

Pneumonia may develop after engraftment, especially while receiving therapy for GVHD with corticosteroids, cyclosporine A, and other immunosuppressive drugs. The predominant pathogens include GNB and molds such as *Aspergillus*, *Fusarium*, and *Zygomycetes*. The latter is a special concern when iron overload (ferritin greater than 2 gms/dL) is present from frequent transfusions of packed red blood cells. The overall one-year survival rate for patients infected with molds following SCT is 20%, with an increase over the last decade of nonfumigatus *Aspergillus* species, *Fusarium*, and *Zygomycetes* [17,18]. *Legionella* [19], *Nocardia* [20], *Mycobacterium* (nontuberculous) [21], endemic mycosis (*Histoplasma*, *Blastomyces*, *Coccidioidomyces*), and PCP can rarely cause pneumonia especially when corticosteroids are used. High-resolution CT scan of the lungs will help to delineate the aforementioned infections as well as evaluate noninfectious causes such as idiopathic interstitial pneumonia, bronchiolitis obliterans with organizing pneumonia (BOOP), diffuse alveolar hemorrhage (DAH), and chemoradiation-therapy induced pneumonitis [22].

TABLE 6 Mycobacterium

M. avium–intracellular complex
M. abscessus/chelonae/fortuitum (rapid growers)
M. kansasii

Late (Over 100 Days)

During the late period following SCT, the primary immune defect is cell-mediated immunodeficiency, especially if chronic GVHD is present (with its inherent treatment with corticosteroids, cyclosporine A, etc.). In addition, humoral immunity is also defective during this period. The primary viral infections of concern during this period include CMV, VZV, and community-acquired respiratory viral pathogens. Because of the frequent use of acyclovir or one of its analogs for HSV treatment or prophylaxis in the first 100 days following SCT, VZV infections occur primarily during the late period. Other rare causes of viral infections include HHV-6, BK virus, or acyclovir-resistant HSV, CMV, or VZV.

The most common bacterial infections are the CVC-related gram-positive organisms followed by GNB. The GNB infections include CVC-associate bacteremia pneumonia and UTI with multidrug resistance found more frequently [23]. Other opportunistic infections that can occur during this period include *Nocardia*, PCP, nontuberculous *Mycobacterium*, and fungi. *Aspergillis* is the most frequent fungal infection along with *Candida* (frequently non*albicans* species). Zygomycete infections occur most commonly during the late period, especially in the presence of iron overload. Endemic mycosis is rare but does occur during this period; it involves the lung or skin or is disseminated.

With the use of CMV antigen detection on a weekly basis, and prophylactic voriconazole or itraconazole when corticosteroids are used for GVHD, the incidence of CMV and *Aspergillus* infections is expected to decline. Whether emerging fungal infections that are resistant to the aforementioned antifungal agents will increase remains to be seen. Awareness of the host immunity at any given period following SCT allows for a more accurate prediction of the next infection likely to develop. Therefore future progress in managing infectious complications following SCT will include early pathogen detection (like CMV), effective prophylactic therapy (especially for the molds), and less immunosuppressive regimens for the treatment of GVHD.

REFERENCES

1. Cordonnier C, Buzyn A, Leverger G. Epidemiology and risk factors for gram-positive coccal infections in neutropenia: toward a more targeted antibiotic strategy. Clin Infect Dis 2003; 36:149–158.
2. Dominguez ER, Greene JN, Sandin RL. Capnocytophaga: a case series and review. Infect in Med 1996; 13:165–166.
3. Brokamp K, Greene JN, Sandin RL, Vincent AL, Arnold SR. Clostridial bacteremia in a cancer hospital: a 6.5 year experience. Infect Med 1995; 12:587–591.

4. Nadiminti U, Greene JN, Vincent AL, Sandin RL. Typhlitis in neutropenic patients: an analysis of thirty-nine patients in a cancer hospital. Infect Dis Clin Pract 2000; 9:153–158.
5. Fitzmorris KL, Greene JN, Sandin RL, Field T. Recognition and management of herpes simplex mucositis in neutropenic patients. Infect Med 2000; 17:413–416.
6. Shah S, Vincent AL, Greene JN, Sandin RL, Gompf S. Rare gram-positive infections in cancer patients: study and literature review. Infect Dis Clin Pract 2000; 9:141–147.
7. Sanders SL, Greene JN, Sandin RL. Disseminated candidiasis complicating treatment of acute leukemia. Infect Med 1999; 16:403–405, 409–410, 413–416.
8. Poblete SJ, Greene JN, Sandin RL. Disseminated Fusarium in the immuno-compromised host. Infect Dis Clin Pract 1998; 7:339–344.
9. Strickland LB, Greene JN, Sandin RL, Hiemenz JW. *Scedosporium* species infections in cancer patients: three cases and a review of the literature. Infect Dis Clin Pract 1998; 1:4–11.
10. Gompf SG, Paredes A, Quilitz R, Greene JN, Hiemenz JW, Sandin RL. Paecilomyces lilacinus osteomyelitis in a bone marrow transplant patient. Infect Med 1999; 16:766–770.
11. Venkattaramanabalaji GV, Foster D, Greene JN, Muro-Cacho CA, Sandin RL, Saez R, Robinson L. Mucormycosis associated with deferoxamine therapy after allogeneic bone marrow transplantation. Cancer Control 1997; 3:168–171.
12. Greene JN, Sandin RL, Fields KK, Moscinski LC, Beatty A, Pow-Sang J, Elfenbein GJ. Hemorrhagic cystitis in bone marrow transplant patients: is it an infection or chemotherapy toxicity? Cancer Control 1994; 4:411–415.
13. Ljungman P. Respiratory virus infections in bone marrow transplant recipients: the European perspective. Am J Med 1997; 102(3A):44–47.
14. Wendt CH, Weisdorf DJ, Jordan MC, Balfour HH, Hertz MI. Parainfluenza virus respiratory infection after bone marrow transplantation. N Engl J Med 1992; 326:921–926.
15. Bowden RA. Respiratory virus infections after marrow transplant: the Fred Hutchinson Cancer Research Center Experience. Am J Med 1997; 102(3A):27–30.
16. Greene JN. Catheter-related complications of cancer therapy. Infect Dis Clin North Amer 1996; 10(2):255–295.
17. Marr KA, Carter RA, Crippa F, Wald A, Corey L. Epidemiology and outcome of mould infections in hematopoietic stem cell transplant recipients. Clin Infect Dis 2002; 34:909–917.
18. Baddley JW, Stroud TP, Salzman D, Pappas PG. Invasive mould infections in allogeneic bone marrow transplant recipients. Clin Infect Dis 2001; 32:1319–1324.
19. Tsambiras BM, Tsambiras PE, Greene JN, Sandin RL, Vincent AL, Gompf S. Legionella pneumophila pneumonia in cancer patients: a case report and review. Infect Dis Clin Pract 2000; 9:261–268.
20. Watkins A, Greene JN, Sandin RL, Vincent AL. Nocardial infections in cancer

patients: our experience and a review of the literature. Infect Dis Clin Pract 1999; 8:294–300.

21. Kourbeti IS, Maslow MJ. Nontuberculous Mycobacterial infections of the lung. Cur Infect Dis Rep 2000; 2:193 200.

22. Somboonwit C, Greene JN. Diagnostic methodologies for invasive fungal infections in hematopoietic stem-cell transplant recipients. Sem Resp Infect 2002; 17:151 157.

23. Saavedra S, Jarque I, Sanz GF, Moscardo F, Jiménez C, Martin G, Plume G, Regadera A, Martinez J, De La Rubia J, Acosta B, Peman J, Perez-Belles C, Gobernado M, Sanz MA. Infectious complications in patients undergoing unrelated donor bone marrow transplantation: experience from a single institution. Clin Microbiol Infect 2002; 8:725–733.

13

Infections in Patients with Brain Tumors

Christoph Michael Stoll
Städtisches Klinikum
Karlsruhe, Germany

Albert L. Vincent
University of South Florida and
Moffitt Cancer Center and Research Institute
Tampa, Florida, U.S.A.

PREDISPOSING FACTORS

Depending on size, location, and invasiveness, intracranial tumors may produce concurrent neurologic deficits, predisposing to infectious disease. The most significant deficits include reduced levels of consciousness with absent protective reflexes, immobility, and loss of sensation. After initial treatment, patients with brain tumors may show cognitive changes (80%), hemi- or tetraparesis (78%), sensory loss (38%), bladder and bowel dysfunction (37%), cranial nerve palsy (29%), or dysphagia (26%) [1]. Prolonged hospitalization and stays in nursing homes predispose to colonization with potentially pathogenic and often multiresistant microorganisms. Neurosurgical wounds and devices such as tracheal tubes, central lines, indwelling catheters, or intracranial pressure transducers further increase the probability of infections.

Intracranial tumors themselves can cause impaired cell-mediated immunity and alterations in humoral immunity. In glioma patients a significant decrease in the absolute number of circulating T lymphocytes, especially of CD4 + (T-helper/inducer) lymphocytes, is a frequent finding, even without immunosuppressive drug therapy [2,3]. Glioma-induced apoptosis of activated T cells may be the cause of T lymphocytic destruction [3]. Perhaps as a result of the CD4 lymphopenia, patients show diminished B cell function, weakened lymphocyte responsiveness to antigens, and cutaneous anergy [2,4,5].

Therapy regimens such as cytoreductive chemotherapy, radiation, and corticosteroid treatment further compromise host defense. Long-term corticosteroid treatment, e.g., with daily doses of 4 to 24 mg dexamethasone, is often necessary to control vasogenic edema surrounding unresectable tumors. A decrease in lymphocyte count is common in brain tumor patients receiving steroids. CD4 + and CD8 + T lymphocytes were more affected than B lymphocytes, though IgG levels were also reduced [6]. Further, an increase of neutrophils and monocytes and a decrease in eosinophils have been reported. In addition, anticonvulsants are thought to contribute to immunodeficiency [5]. Neurosurgery itself may decrease lymphocytes and IgG levels [6].

PNEUMONIA

Pneumonia is one of the most common infectious complications in patients with altered consciousness. In brain tumor patients, protective pulmonary clearance is often impaired by reduced vigilance, depressed swallowing, cough, and gag reflexes, immobility, and poor respiratory effort, all leading to retention of secretions. Among all cancer patients, those with brain tumors are at special risk for development of aspiration pneumonia [7]. Seizures, impaired levels of consciousness, and dysphagia all favor aspiration and the subsequent development of pneumonitis. Dysphagia is a frequent finding in brain tumor patients, with an incidence of 14 to 26% [1,8]. It may be caused by oropharyngeal paresis, reduced pharyngeal sensation, or by failure of integration with oral apraxia. The responsible lesions can be unilateral and supratentorial, as well as within the brain stem. Food aspiration, continuous silent aspiration of oropharyngeal secretions, or aspiration of gastric contents, all can lead to pneumonitis. The resulting pneumonia is directly related to the colonization patterns of the source of the aspirated material. The upper airways (oropharynx and trachea) with their indigenous and nosocomially acquired flora represent the most important reservoir of pathogens causing lower respiratory tract colonization and infection [9]. Gastric juice, as the evident source of infection, seems to be unusual in neurosurgical patients [10]. Gastric overgrowth with gram-negative bacteria is favored by a lower gastric acidity (pH >4), as with stress ulcer prophylaxis. Aspiration of gastric juice can be facilitated by seizures, protracted emesis with increased intracerebral pressure, and nasogastric tubes, which cause cardiac sphincter insufficiency with reflux. Finally, colonization of the tracheobronchial tree with enteric flora results in an increased risk of nosocomial pneumonia in long-term ventilated patients [11].

NEUROSURGICAL ICU AND VENTILATOR-ASSOCIATED PNEUMONIA

Endotracheal intubation is an iatrogenic risk factor for pneumonia, causing extension of oropharyngeal flora into the tracheobronchial tree. Tubes allow leakage of oropharyngeal secretions into the tracheobranchial tree and impair cough [12,13]. Dauch et al. [14] retrospectively investigated lower respiratory tract infections in 289 patients requiring intensive care after brain tumor surgery. They found an 11% incidence of symptomatic bronchitis and a 21% incidence of pneumonia. Freedom from postoperative infection decreased exponentially with length of time intubated, with a half-life of 3.5 days. Postoperative nosocomial infections of the lower respiratory tract seem to occur almost exclusively in brain tumor patients with severe depression of T helper cells secondary to corticosteroid usage [6]. Increased risk for lower respiratory tract infections after surgery was identified for the following independent variables: preoperative corticosteroid therapy, preoperative disturbances of consciousness, cardiac insufficiency, age of 60 years or older, and meningioma tumor type. Patients with transsphenoidal resection of pituitary tumors showed a reduced risk [14].

Early onset pneumonia (within the first 4 days) is frequent in neurosurgical patients and is caused mainly by *Staphylococcus aureus* (33%), *Haemophilus* spp. (23%), and *Streptococcus pneumoniae* (about 20%) [9,15]. These organisms reflect the early oropharyngeal, and later tracheobronchial, colonization by pathogens that has been shown in mechanically ventilated patients with traumatic and medical head injuries [9]. Initial tracheobronchial colonization is associated with early onset pneumonia [9]. Nasal carriers are at high risk for *S. aureus* pneumonia. Tracheal colonization with *S. aureus* led to ventilator-associated pneumonia in 21% of cases [16,17]. Previous short-term antibiotics are protective against colonization of the tracheobronchial tree with *S. aureus*, *Streptococcus pneumoniae*, and *Haemophilus* spp., but they seem to be a risk factor for colonization with other gram-negative pathogens [9].

In patients with neurologic disorders a high incidence of isolating anaerobes in early-onset ventilator-associated pneumonia is reported. Most frequently isolated were *Bacteroides* spp., *Prevotella melaninogenica*, *Fusobacterium nucleatum*, and *Veillonella parvula* [18,19]. While gram-negative bacilli other than *Haemophilus* are responsible for only 19% of early onset pneumonia in ventilated neurosurgical patients, they account for late-onset pneumonia [15]. Once more, these findings reflect the oropharyngeal and tracheal colonization pattern; the increase of bacterial load after day two of intubation is due mainly to increased colonization by *Pseudomonas* spp., *Acinetobacter* spp., *Klebsiella* spp., and other gram-negative enteric pathogens. Their count is significantly higher from day six forward [9]. After 7 days of ventilation, *Pseudomonas aeruginosa* is the most frequently isolated microorganism in ventilator-associated pneumonia [20]. Tracheobronchial colonization with gram-negative pathogens, duration of mechanical ventilation, and prolonged (>24 h) antibiotic treatment are predictors of late-onset pneumonia after day four of ventilation [9]. Multiresistant microorganisms are common in late-onset pneumonia. Teoh and coauthors [21] found that early tracheostomy in neurosurgical patients with poor Glaskow Coma Scale Scores was associated with reduced incidence of tracheobronchial colonization by multiple pathogens, improvement in lung infections, and rapid weaning from ventilatory support.

NON-ICU-RELATED ASPIRATION PNEUMONIA

The microbial etiology of aspiration pneumonia depends on the setting in which the aspiration occurs. In community acquired disease the indigenous oral flora usually account for aspiration pneumonia: anaerobes (primarily *Porphyromonas*, *Bacteroides oris*, *B. buccae*, *Fusobacterium nucleatum*, and *Peptostreptococcus*), viridans streptococci, *Moraxella catarrhalis*, and *Eikanella corrodens*. In hospital or nursing home settings one finds other typical nosocomially acquired pathogens such as *S. aureus*, *Streptococcus pyogenes*, and various gram-negative bacilli (*P. aeruginosa*, *K. pneumoniae*, *Enterobacter*, *Serratia*, *E. coli*, and *Proteus*) [13]. Infections are often polymicrobial, and aerobes are mixed with anaecobes.

Beside typical symptoms of pneumonitis, aspiration pneumonia often presents subacutely with malaise, low-grade fever, cough, weight loss, and anemia. The dependent segments of the lung (posterior segments of the upper lobes and the superior segments of the lower lobes) are most frequently involved. Necrotizing pneumonia, lung abscess, and empyema can follow after 1 to 2 weeks of ongoing aspiration pneumonia. Foul-smelling discharge indicates the involvement of anaerobes [13].

Initial empirical antibiotic therapy should be adjusted to the patient's setting and known oropharyngeal colonization. Upper airway colonization is an independent predictor of follow-up tracheobronchial colonization of nosocomially acquired pathogens [9]. Hence organisms causing pneumonia are often the same as those isolated from swab and sputum cultures. In any case, differentiation of infection and colonization is difficult. Absence of pathogens such as *S. aureus* or gram-negative bacilli in cultures of upper airway secretions and sputum makes their involvement in pneumonitis unlikely. It is often necessary to give a prolonged antibiotic course, which should be guided by definitive bacteriological diagnosis. Rapid and appropriate specimens for aerobic and anaerobic cultures can be obtained by bronchoscopy with protected specimen brush or by bronchoalveolar lavage, transtracheal aspiration, or pleural fluid aspiration [13].

While about 14.5% complain of dysphagia, most patients with brain tumors are unaware of their actual level of swallowing dysfunction [8] and are unaware of silent aspiration. These patients should be evaluated for dysphagia and aspiration by a speech-language pathologist using videofluorography, to judge the critical pharyngeal stage of glutition. Delayed initiation of the swallowing reflex, reduced pharyngeal peristalsis, and insufficient laryngeal closure are associated with aspiration [22]. The level of alertness correlates with the severity of aspiration [8]. Swallowing rehabilitation should be pursued, and in some patients alternate methods of feeding, e.g., gastrostomy tube placement, may be indicated to prevent food aspiration. Oral hygiene should be encouraged to reduce oropharyngeal bacterial load. High risk patients should be monitored for early signs of pneumonia.

PNEUMOCYSTIS CARINII PNEUMONIA (PCP)

This life-threatening pneumonitis is caused by the unicellular eukaryote *pneumocystis carinii* and represents an opportunisic infection in the immunocompromised host. Among cancer patients, brain tumor patients are at special risk for PCP [23,24]. Predispositions include long-term corticosteroid therapy and the resulting CD4 lymphopenia, often aggravated by cytoreductive chemotherapy. In a retrospective study with 587 brain tumor patients, 1.7% developed PCP [25]. In 64 brain tumor patients receiving corticosteroids and radiation, an incidence of 6% has been reported [26].

Twenty-five cases of PCP in patients with primary brain tumors have been reviewed quantitatively [25–27]. The mean duration of dexamethasone treatment until the onset of PCP was 14.5 weeks (first onset after 5 weeks), with a mean dexamethasone dose of 11.3 mg (1–60 mg) per day at date of onset. Only one-third developed PCP while receiving a stable dose of steroids, while two-thirds of the cases became symptomatic during steroid taper. Steroids are a known adjunct therapy for PCP. Perhaps in the majority of cases, steroid taper unmasks an ongoing pulmonary inflammation from PCP that had initially developed under immunosuppressive therapy [27]. In contrast to HIV patients with a more gradual onset of symptoms over a few weeks, HIV-negative patients with PCP are hospitalized earlier and present with a more acute disease. There are higher respiratory rates (34/min versus 22/min) and lower arterial pO_2 values (52 mmHG versus 69 mmHG) [27,28]. The mean onset of symptoms was 10 days before diagnosis of PCP. Patients presented with fever, a usually nonproductive cough, dyspnea, hypoxia, and alveolar or interstitial bilateral infiltrates. Recurrence of PCP appeared in two patients. Mortality was high (28%), despite appropriate antibiotic therapy. Most of the patients had received additional cytoreductive chemotherapy, radiotherapy, or both. Many patients had absolute lymphopenia and leukopenia.

Brain tumor patients on steroid treatment or with lymphopenia who present with unexplained fever or respiratory symptoms should be evaluated for PCP and may be presumptively treated [27]. In suspicious patients with negative chest x-ray a high-resolution CT scan of the lung is indicated. Identification of *Pneumocystis* can be made with sputum induced by nebulized saline or bronchoalveolar lavage samples.

Treatment of PCP is intravenous trimethoprim-sulfamethoxazole (TMP-SMX) followed by the oral form when stable for a total of 3 weeks. Prophylactic TMP-SMX one tablet daily thrice weekly should be given for 6 months. Side effects are more frequent in HIV-positive patients than in others (12%). Alternative drugs are dapsone, pentamidine, atovaquone, or clindamycin. In brain tumor patients given steroid treatment for more than 5 weeks, TMP-SMX is effective prophylaxis [24] and is especially indicated in patients with further risk factors such as cytoreductive chemotherapy or radiation, CD4 lymphopenia, or steroid taper.

URINARY TRACT INFECTION (UTI)

Urinary incontinence is a frequent finding in patients with altered levels of consciousness. Management with indwelling catheters is a common cause of urinary tract infection in these patients. Frequency of UTI in stroke patients is reported at 15 to 30% during both acute hospitalization and rehabilitation [29,30]. On admission to inpatient rehabilitation, 24% of 1029 stroke patients had a foley catheter [29]. Early alterations of the skin flora in hospitalized neurologic patients [31] and catheterization both change the urethral colonization from gram-positive cocci, diphtheroids, and lactobacilli to urinary pathogens. Indwelling catheters damage uroepithelium, induce inflammation, and lead to tissue invasion. The most common bacteria causing UTI in these patients are *E. coli*, *Enterococci*, *Enterobacter* spp., *Klebsiella* spp., *Pseudomonas* spp., *Citrobacter* spp., *Proteus* spp., *S. aureus*, streptococci, and yeasts [19]. Duration of indwelling urethral catheterization should be minimized, as it is the most prevalent risk indicator for UTI. Silver alloy catheters have a lower risk of infection [32].

Neurogenic bladder with incomplete bladder emptying is another important risk factor for UTIs in brain tumor patients. Tumors can interrupt all neural pathways modulating the storage or voiding mechanisms of the bladder and urethra. A 41% incidence of urinary dysfunction with retention has been reported in children with spinal tumors [33]. In patients with brain tumors the incidence of neurogenic bladder was found to be 18%, with the highest incidence seen in those with pontine tumors [34].

Neuroanatomical organization of bladder control is complex. The sacral micturition center is the most distal part of the central nervous system, with its afferent and efferent innervation of the lower urinary tract. In pontine micturition, neurons in the dorsal tegumentum of the pons control detrusor and distal sphincter activity and coordinate them to storage and voiding modes. Lesions in this area can lead to detrusor sphincter dysfunction or a fixed unrelaxing distal sphincter, which is responsible for incomplete bladder emptying. Higher centers, especially the mesial frontal lobes, modulate the neural programs of the pontine micturition centers. They seem to mediate a voluntary inhibition on neural micturition programs. Lesions can lead to detrusor hyperreflexia and urge incontinence [35]. As a consequence, depending on tumor localization two types of urinary symptoms in patients with CNS tumors can be differentiated [36]:

1. Irritative symptoms (frequency, nocturia, urgency, urge incontinence) are often found in patients with frontal tumors, even in the absence of intellectual or moral deterioration [37]. Incontinence management with indwelling catheters is the main risk factor for UTIs in these patients. A therapeutic option for incontinence with detrusor hyperreflexia would be an anticholinergic drug like oxybutynin.

2. Obstructive symptoms (hesitancy, poor stream, terminal dribbling, retention) are observed in patients with tumors in an area extending from the pons to the cauda equina. In patients with pontine tumors, urinary retention and difficulty in voiding are reported to occur in 71% [38], while in patients with frontal tumors obstructive symptoms are rare [37].

As the normal washout effect is diminished, microorganisms have a better opportunity to multiply and propagate in the stagnant residual urine. Consequently, lower urinary tract colonization is frequent. *E. coli, Pseudomonas, Klebsiella, Proteus, Serratia, Providencia*, enterococci, and staphylococci are found in urine of spinal cord injured patients with neurogenic bladder [39]. Mucosal ischemia with bladder overdistension and high pressure voiding can facilitate tissue invasion. Elevated bladder pressures favor vesicourethral reflux and access of urinary pathogens to the kidneys. Serious complications such as pyelonephritis, perinephric abscess [40], septicemia, and compromised renal function [41] may result. Urosepsis rather than renal failure has now become the most common cause of death relating to the urinary tract in patients with neurogenic bladder [41]. These complications can be avoided by adequate bladder drainage with minimal residual urine volume and low pressure voiding to maintain unrestricted urine flow from the kidneys. All patients with a brain tumor should be evaluated for incomplete bladder emptying by simple and inexpensive ultrasound measurement of the post-micturition residual volume. Values of more than 100 mL are abnormal. Bladder management with intermittent catheterization has been shown to lower the UTI rate related to a neurogenic bladder [32,39]. The best treatment option for emptying the bladder and avoiding infections are suprapubic catheters [32], which cause significantly lower rates of infections than does intermittent catheterization [42].

For purposes of antibiotic therapy, lower urinary tract colonization should be differentiated from inflammation with tissue invasion. In immunocompetent patients with neurogenic bladder even significant bacteriuria should only be treated with antibiotics if associated with symptoms (e.g., fever, chills, nausea or vomiting, increased sweating, abdominal discomfort, costovertebral angle pain) or pyuria (10^4/white blood cells per mL), a sign of invasion [39,41]. On the other hand, infection may occur with bacterial counts less than 10^5 cfu/mL, which warrants treatment. Indwelling catheters should be removed when possible and antibiotic treatment should last at least 7 days. With recurrent UTIs, the duration of antibiotic use should be at least 7 to 14 days [39]. Organism-specific therapy in accordance with culture susceptibility is preferred, as the variety of organisms is broader than in uncomplicated cases. These complicated UTIs are often polymicrobial and frequently include Candida spp. [39].

A meta-analysis of 15 trials showed that antimicrobial prophylaxis for urinary tract infection in patients with spinal cord injury did not significantly decrease the incidence of symptomatic infections and even doubled the emergence of resistant strains of bacteria [43]. Therefore general prophylaxis with antibiotics is not recommended [39,43], though it may be considered with recurrent UTIs. Patients with recurrent symptomatic urinary tract infections should be reevaluated for inadequate bladder emptying, obstruction, calculi, and compromised immune status. Facultative urease-positive organisms predisposing for renal calculi are *Proteus, Pseudomonas, Serratia, Morganella, Providencia, Klebsiella, Staphylococci, Ureaplasma,* and *E. coli* [41].

DECUBITUS ULCERS

Pressure sores are a frequent finding in neurological patients, as their mobility is often impaired due to paresis or reduced consciousness. Deterioration of sensation may contribute to ischemic necrosis within decubiti. The incidence of decubitus ulcers in stroke patients in rehabilitation is reported to be 21% during hospital admission and about 3 to 12% during rehabilitation [30,44]. Because of their localization (sacrum in 52% of cases, ischial tuberosities in

29%, heels 13%, trochanteric regions 12%, and buttocks 12% [45]), most pressure sores are colonized by a number of pathogens. Fecal microbes such as *Enterococci, Enterobacteriaceae,* anaerobic *Streptococci,* and *Bacteroides* species are often found in addition to nosocomially acquired pathogens such as *Pseudomonas* species and *S. aureus* [46]. Bacterial skin flora of patients with spinal cord injury has been shown to change soon after hospitalization. Within two or three days after admission, diverse often multidrug-resistant gram-negative bacilli can be found [31].

In immunocompetent patients with ulcers without acute infection, the routine use of antibiotics is not recommended [47]. Basic therapy is pressure relief, surgical debridement of necrotic material, general wound care, nutritional support, and later perhaps coverage with a skin graft. The use of local anti-infectives is controversial. Antibiotics are required in patients with extensive purulence or cellulitis, suspected osteomyelitis of the underlying bone, or bacteremia. Especially if bone is visible within the ulcer, osteomyelitis should be assumed and proven by biopsy and culture [48]. Bacteremia with decubitus ulcers may be polymicrobial; the most common species isolated are *Bacteroides fragilis, Proteus mirabilis, S. aureus,* and *E. coli.* When present, sepsis has a poor outcome [45]. Debridement is frequently associated with transient bacteremia [49] and should only be done with antibiotic coverage.

In immunocompromised patients, instituting antibiotic treatment early is recommended. As decubitus ulcers are polymicrobic, extended spectrum penicillins (piperacillin-tazobactam, ticarcillin-clavulanate), imipenem, or ciprofloxacin plus clindamycin may be reasonable choices for initial therapy [50]. Further antibiotic therapy should be guided by culture and susceptibility results. An increasing incidence of multidrug-resistant microbes such as methicillin-resistant *Staphylococcus aureus* (MRSA), vancomycin-resistant *Enterococcus* (VRE), and multidrug-resistant gram-negative bacilli are cultured from these wounds [51].

INFECTIONS SUPERIMPOSED ON BRAIN TUMORS

Bradytrophic tissues, which are areas of necrosis and cysts within brain tumors, are vulnerable to superinfection. In addition, local suppression of inflammatory leukocytes within brain tumors has been observed and may favor bacterial and viral growth [52]. The source of infection causing a brain abscess is either direct extension from an adjacent infection such as sinusitis and meningitis, hematogenous spread, or more commonly contiguous spread from the wound from recent neurosurgery.

The majority of brain abscesses that result from the direct extension of a paranasal sinusitis are found with sellar or parasellar tumors (pituitary tumors or craniopharyngeomas). Microorganisms found are those colonizing the oropharynx: *S. aureus, Pneumococcus, nonhemolytic streprococci, Bacteroides*, and *Corynebacterium striatum*. Cases with *E. coli, S. epidermidis, S. albus*, and *Mycobacterium tuberculosis* have also been reported [53–57]. Three cases of brain tumors with secondary meningitis are found in the literature [53]: two craniopharyngeomas and one ependymoma; bacteria isolated were *Pneumococcus* and *Meningococcus*.

Bacteremia as a source of an abscess developing within a brain tumor is rather rare. Alterations within the blood–brain barrier and open gaps between the capillary endothelial cells in tumor tissue, as documented for meningomas [58], may be the predisposing mechanism. Enterobacteriaceae are the most common pathogens found with hematogenous spread. *Salmonella* in particular has a known tendency to infect tumorous tissues [59]. Reports include a malignant astrocytoma and a craniopharyngioma superinfected with *Salmonella typhi*, a brain metastasis of testicular carcinoma with *Salmonella enteritidis* group D, a meningioma with *Proteus mirabilis*, and a meningioma with *E. coli* [53,59,60]. Further, a glioblastoma multiforme with *S. aureus*, a CNS lymphoma with *Streptococcus*, a meningioma with *Bacteroides oralis*, and a pituitary adenoma with abscess formation after tooth extraction have been documented. [53,59,61,62]. Several cases of herpes simplex encephalitis within malignant astrocytromas are documented in the literature [63,64].

Though abscesses in brain tumors are rare, any patient with no other explanation of fever or neurological deterioration, and with consistent radiological findings, this diagnosis must be taken into account. Preoperative diagnosis and differentiation from noninfected necrotic areas are difficult. CSF gram stain and cultures are often negative. Combined MR diffusion and perfusion imaging [65], gallium-67 scan, or unlabeled autologous white blood cell scan [55] may be helpful, but only histopathological examination and culture can confirm the diagnosis. As prognosis with infected brain tumors is rather poor, and aggressive treatment with antibiotics and surgical drainage of abscesses is indicated. In sellar processes a transsphenoidal approach is recommended to prevent contamination of the CSF [55]. There are reports of patients with brain tumors in whom regression or cure of the tumor appeared to be temporally related to an CNS infection [66,67], but the cause and effect remain unclear.

Besides tumor progression, infections are the leading cause of mortality in patients with brain tumors. Early recognition of the unique infections found in patients with brain tumors is essential. Prompt institution of appropriate antimicrobials and surgical drainage when indicated can improve survival in these patients. With more treatment modalities available that cause longer and more profound immunosuppression, infectious complications are expected to increase.

REFERENCES

1. Mukand JA, Blackinton DD, Crincoli MG, Lee JJ, Santos BB. Incidence of neurologic deficits and rehabilitation of patients with brain tumors. Am J Phys Med Rehabil 2001; 80:346–350.
2. Bhondeley MJ, Mehra RD, Mehra NK, Mohapatra AK, Tandon PN, Roy S, Bijlani V. Imbalances in T cell subpopulations in human gliomas. J Neurosurg 1988; 68:589–593.
3. Morfold LA, Dix AR, Brooks WH, Roszman TL. Apoptotic elimination of peripheral T lymphocytes in patients with primary intracranial tumors. J Neurosurg 1999; 91(6):935 946.
4. Roszman TL, Brooks WH, Steele C, Elliott LH. Pokeweed mitogen-induced immunoglobulin secretion by peripheral lymphocytes from patients with primary intracranial tumors. Characterization of T helper and B cell function. J Immunol 1985; 134(3):1545–1550.
5. Neuwelt EA, Kikuchi K, Hill S, Lipsky P, Frenkel EP. Immune responses in patients with brain tumors. Factors such as anticonvulsants that may contribute to impaired cell-mediated immunity. Cancer 1983; 51(2):248–255.
6. Dauch WA, Krex D, Heymanns J, Zeithammer B, Bauer BL. Peri-operative changes of cellular and humoral components of immunity with brain tumor surgery. Acta Neurochir (Wien) 1994; 126(2–4):93–101.
7. Rolston KVI. The spectrum of pulmonary infections in cancer patients. Current Opinion in Oncology 2001; 13:218–223.
8. Newton HB, Newton C, Pearl D, Davidson T. Swallowing assessment in primary brain tumor patients with dysphagia. Neurology 1994; 44:1927–1932.
9. Ewig S, Torres A, El-Ebiary M, Fabregas N, Hernandez C, Gonzales J, Nicolas JM, Soto L. Bacterial colonization patterns in mechanically ventilated patients with traumatic and medical head injury; incidence, risk factors and association with ventilator-associated pneumonia. Am J Respir Crit Care Med 1999; 159: 188–198.
10. Reusser P, Zimmerli W, Scheidegger D, Marbet GA, Buser M, Gyr K. Role of gastric colonization in nosocomial infections and endotoxemia: a prospective study in neurosurgical patients on mechanical ventilation. J Infect Dis 1989; 160(3):414–421.
11. Tryba M, Cook DJ. Gastric alkalization, pneumonia, and systemic infections: the controversy. Scand J Gastroenterol Suppl 1995; 210:53–59.
12. Ding R, Logemann JA. Pneumonia in stroke patients: a retrospective study. Dysphagia 2000; 15:51–57.
13. Finegold SM. Aspiration pneumonia. Reviews of Infectious Diseases 1991; 13 (suppl 9):737 742.
14. Dauch WA, Landau G, Krex D. Prognostic factors for lower respiratory tract infections after brain-tumor surgery. J Neurosurg 1989; 70:862–868.
15. Berrouane Y, Daudenthun I, Riegel B, Emery MN, Martin G, Krivosic R, Grandbastien B. Early onset pneumonia in neurosurgical intensive care unit patients. J Hosp Infect 1998; 40(4):275-280.
16. Bergmans D, Bonten M, Gaillard C, de Leeuw P, van Thiel F, Stobbering E, van

der Geest S. Clinical spectrum of ventilator-associated pneumonia caused by methicillin-sensitive Staphylococcus aureus. Eur J Clin Microbiol Inf Dis 1996; 15(6):437–445.

17. Campell W, Hendrix E, Schwalbe R, Fattom A, Edelman R. Head-injured patients who are nasal carriers of Staphylococcus aureus are at high risk for Staphylococcus aureus pneumonia. Crit Care Med 1999; 27(4):798–801.

18. Dore P, Robert R, Grollier G, Rouffineau J, Lanquetot H, Charriere JM, Fauchere JL. Incidence of anaerobes in ventilator-associated pneumonia with use of a protected specimen brush. Am J Resp Crit Care Med 1996; 153:1292–1298.

19. Dettenkofer M, Ebner W, Els T, Babikir R, Lücking C, Pelz K, Rüden H, Dashner F. Surveillance of nosocomial infections in a neurology intensive care unit. J Neurol 2001; 248:959–964.

20. Boque MC, Bodi M, Rello J. Trauma, head injury, and neurosurgery infections. Semin Respir Infect 2000; 15(4):261–263.

21. Teoh WH, Goh KY, Chan C. The role of early tracheostomy in critically ill neurosurgical patients. Ann Acad Med Singapore 2001; 30(3):234–238.

22. Horner J, Massey EW, Riski JE, Lathrop DL, Chase KN. Aspiration following stroke: clinical correlates and outcome. Neurology 1988; 38:1359–1362.

23. Sepkowitz KA, Brown AE, Telzak EE, Gottlieb S, Armstrong D. *Pneumocystis carinii* pneumonia among patients without AIDS at a cancer hospital. JAMA 1992; 267(6):832–837.

24. Wen PY, Marks PW. Medical management of patients with brain tumors. Curr Opin Oncol 2002; 14(3):299–307.

25. Henson JW, Jalai JK, Walker RW, Stover DE, Fels AO. *Pneumocystis carinii* pneumonia in patients with primary brain tumors. Arch Neurol 1991; 48(4):406–409.

26. Slivka A, Wen PY, Shea WM, Loeffler JS. *Pneumocystis carinii* pneumonia during steroid taper in patients with primary brain tumors. Am J Med 1993; 94(2):216–219.

27. Schiff D. Pneumocystis pneumonia in brain tumor patients: risk factors and clinical features. Journal of Neuro-Oncology 1996; 27:235–240.

28. Kovacs JA, Hiemenez JW, Macher AM, Stover D, Murray HW, Shelhamer J, Lane HC, Urmacher C, Honig C, Longo DL. Pneumocytis carinii pneumonia: a comparison between patients with acquired immunodeficiency syndrome and patients with other immunodeficiencies. Ann Intern Med 1984; 100:663–671.

29. Roth EJ, Lovell L, Harvey RL, Heinemann AW, Semik P, Diaz S. Incidence of and risk factors for medical complications during stroke rehabilitation. Stroke 2001; 32:523–529.

30. Langhorne P, Stott DJ, Robertson L, Mac Donald J, Jones L, McAlpine C, Dick F, Taylor GS, Murray G. Medical complications after stroke. Stroke 2000; 31:1223–1229.

31. Fawcett C, Chawla JC, Quoraishi A, Stickler DJ. A study of the skin flora of spinal cord injured patients. J Hosp Infect 1986; 8(2):149–158.

32. Biering-Sorensen F. Urinary tract infection in individuals with spinal cord lesion. Curr Opin Urol 2002; 12(1):45–49.

33. Dincer F, Dincer C, Baskaya MK. Results of combined treatment of paediatric intraspinal tumors. Paraplegia 1992; 30:718–728.
34. Ueki K. Disturbances of micturition observed in some patients with brain tumors. Neurol Med Chir 1960; 2:25–33.
35. Fowler CJ. Investigation of the neurogenic bladder. J Neurol Neurosurg Psychiatry 1996; 60(1):6–13.
36. Soler D, Borzyskowski M. Lower urinary tract dysfunction in children with central nervous system tumors. Arch Dis Child 1998; 79:344–347.
37. Maurice-Williams RS. Micturition in frontal tumors. J Neurol Neurosurg Psychiatry 1974; 37:431–436.
38. Renier WO, Gabreels FJM. Evaluation of diagnosis and non-surgical therapy in 24 children with a pontine tumor. Neuropediatrics 1980; 11:262–271.
39. Biering-Sorensen F, Bagi P, Hoilby N. Urinary tract infections in patients with spinal cord lesions: treatment and prevention. Drugs 2001; 61(9):1275 1287.
40. Deck AJ, Yang CC. Perinephric abscesses in the neurologically impaired. Spinal Cord 2001; 39:477–481.
41. Stover SL, Lloyd LK, Waites KB, Jackson AB. Neurogenic urinary tract infection. Neurol Clin 1991; 9(3):741 755.
42. Noll F, Russe O, Kling E, Botel U, Schreiter F. Intermittant catherization versus percutaneous suprapubic cystostomy in the early management of traumatic spinal cord lesions. Paraplegia 1988; 26(1):4–9.
43. Morton SC, Shekelle PG, Adams JL, Bennett C, Dobkin BH, Montgomerie J, Vickrey BG. Antimicrobial prophylaxis for urinary tract infection in persons with spinal cord dysfunction. Arch Phys Med Rehabil 2002; 83(1):129–138.
44. Daveport RJ, Dennis MS, Wellwood I, Warlow CP. Complications after acute stroke. Stroke 1996; 27(3):415–420.
45. Bryan CS, Dew CE, Reynolds KL. Bacteremia associated with decubitus ulcers. Arch Intern Med 1983; 143:2093–2095.
46. Bello YM, Phillips TJ. Recent advances in wound healing. JAMA 2000; 283 (6):716–718.
47. O'Meara SM, Cullum NA, Majid M, Sheldon TA. Systemic review of antimicrobial agents used for chronic wounds. Br J Surg 2001; 88(1):4–21.
48. Senet P, Meaume S. Decubitus sores in geriatric medicine. Local and general treatment of pressure sores in the aged. Presse Med 1999; 28(33):1840–1845.
49. Glenchur H, Patel BS, Pathmarajah C. Transient bacteremia associated with debridement of decubitus ulcers. Military Med 1981; 146:432–433.
50. Richardson JD. Diagnosis and management of systemic infections and fever in neurologic patients. Seminars in Neurology 2000; 20(3):387–391.
51. Mylotte JM, Kahler L, Graham R, Young L, Goodnough S. Prospective surveillance for antibiotic-resistant organisms in patients with spinal cord injury admitted to an acute rehabilitation unit. Am J Infect Control 2000; 28(4):291 297.
52. Black KL, Chen K, Becker DP, Merrill JE. Inflammatory leukocytes associated with increased immunosuppression by glioblastoma. J Neurosurg 1992; 77:120–126.

53. Nassar SI, Haddad FS, Hanbali FS, Kanaan NV. Abscess superimposed on brain tumor: two case reports and review of the literature. Surg Neurol 1997; 47:484–488.

54. Zorub DS, Martinez AJ, Nelson PB, Lam MT. Invasive pituitary adenoma with abscess formation: case report. Neurosurgery 1979; 5:718–722.

55. Jadhav RN, Dahiwadkar HV, Palande DA. Abscess formation in invasive pituitary adenoma: case report. Neurosurgery 1998; 43:616–619.

56. Sharma MC, Vaish S, Arora R, Gaikwad S, Sarkar C. Composite pituitary adenoma and intrasellar tuberculoma: report of a rare case. Pathol Oncol Res 2001; 7(1):74–76.

57. Gazioglu N, Ak H, Öz B, Seckin MS, Kuday C, Sarioglu AC. Silent pituitary tuberculoma associated with pituitary adenoma. Acta Neurochirurgica 1999; 141(7):785–786.

58. Long DM. Vascular ultrastructure in human meningeomas and schwannomas. J Neurosurg 1973; 38:401–419.

59. Rodriguez RE, Valero V, Watanakunakorn C. Salmonella focal intracranial infections: review of the world literature (1884–1984) and report of an unusual case. Reviews of Infectious Diseases 1986; 8:31–41.

60. Eisenberg MB, Lopez R, Stanek AE. Abscess formation within a parasaggital meningeoma. J Neurosurg 1998; 88:895–897.

61. Kroppenstedt SN, Liebig T, Mueller W, Gräf KJ, Lanksch WR, Unterberg AW. Secondary abscess formation in pituitary adenoma after tooth extraction. J Neurosurg 2001; 94:335–338.

62. Kano M, Watanabe M, Maeda M. Primary CNS lymphoma associated with streptococcal abscess: an autopsy case. Brain Tumor Pathol 1999; 16(2):92–97.

63. Benjamin SP, McCormack LJ, Chatty ME, Dohn DF. Coexistent herpes simplex encephalitis and malignant astrocytoma, a clinicopathologic study of three cases. Cleveland Clinic Quarterly 1972; 39(4):135–143.

64. Sheleg SV, Nedzved MN, Nezved AM, Klichkovskaya IV. Contamination of glioblastoma multiforme with type 1 herpes simplex virus. J Neurosurg 2001; 95:721.

65. Chan JH, Tsui EY, Chau LF, Chow KY, Chan MS, Yuen MK, Chan TL, Cheng WK, Wong KP. Discrimination of an infected brain tumor from a cerebral abscess by combined MR perfusion and diffusion imaging. Comput Med Imaging Graph 2002; 26(1):19–23.

66. Kapp JP. Microorganisms as antineoplastic agents in CNS tumors. Arch Neurol 1983; 40:637–642.

67. Bowles AP, Perkins E. Long-term remission of malignant brain tumors after intracranial infection: a report of four cases. Neurosurgery 1999; 44:636–643.

14

Infections in Patients with Head and Neck Cancer

Charurut Somboonwit
and John N. Greene
University of South Florida School of Medicine
Moffitt Cancer Center and Research Institute
Tampa, Florida

Carcinomas of the head and neck arise from the epithelial lining and are usually squamous cell in origin, except for tumors of the salivary glands. Head and neck cancers include tumors of the paranasal sinuses, oral cavity, nasopharynx, oropharynx, hypopharynx, larynx, and salivary gland. In the United States, approximately 40,000 people develop cancer of the head and neck each year, accounting for 5% of cancers in adults. They usually develop after the age of 50. Alcohol and tobacco use are the most common risk factors in the United States. Smokeless tobacco is also a risk factor for cancer of the oral cavity. Other potential risk factors are marijuana use, textile fibers, woodworking, and dietary habits. Nasopharyngeal carcinoma in the Mediterranean area and the Far East is frequently associated with Epstein-Barr virus (EBV) infection. Premalignant lesions include leukoplakia and erythroplakia.

Infections in patients with head and neck cancer can develop from direct tumor invasion, but more commonly occur as a consequence of specific cancer treatment. Comorbidities, especially alcohol consumption and tobacco use, may contribute to the risk of infection.

Smoking is directly related to an increased risk of *Streptococcus pneumoniae* and *Hemophilus influenzae* sinopulmonary infection. Patients with head and neck cancer have an increased risk of penicillin-resistant pneumococcal infections compared to other malignancies [1]. These patients also have a defect in the fibronectin lining of the respiratory tract, which increases colonization of gram-negative bacilli, especially *Pseudomonas aeruginosa*. Chronically ill patients with frequent hospitalizations are also at risk for methicillin-resistant *Staphylocuccus aureus* (MRSA) colonization and infection. The risks for MRSA colonization and infection include prolonged hospitalization, intensive-care stay, prolonged antimicrobial therapy, surgery, and close proximity to patients with MRSA infection, both in the hospital and via household contact [2]. Patients colonized with MRSA are at risk for MRSA wound infections.

Infections frequently coexist with malignances of the head and neck. In addition, early presentations of cancer of the head and neck can mimic an infection. Infections contiguous to the tumor site can develop, such as sinusitis, parotitis, mandibular skull osteomyelitis, and oral ulcers. Less common infections include retropharyngeal abscess, brain abscess, and meningitis.

SINUSITIS

Anatomical disruption of the sinus or surrounding structures due to tumor invasion or surgery can result in sinus obstruction, which can lead to sinusitis. Rhinovirus, influenza virus, and parainfluenza virus are common viral causes of sinusitis in adults, with or without cancer [3]. Viral sinusitis damages the sinonasal cilia and increases mucous production, which can lead to acute bacterial sinusitis. *S. pneumoniae* and *H. influenzae* are the major causes of bacterial sinusitis in the community. Other leading causes are other α-hemolytic streptococci, *Moraxella catarrhalis*, *S. aureus*, aerobic gram-negative bacilli, and anaerobic bacteria [4–6]. Causes of chronic sinusitis lasting more than 30 days include *S. pneumoniae*, *H. influenzae*, *M. catarrharlis*, *S. aureus* (including MRSA), *P. aeruginosa*, anaerobes and other gram-negative bacteria [5–7]. Patients with head and neck cancer, especially following radiation therapy, will be more likely to harbor the latter four pathogens found in chronic sinusitis.

Although rare, progression of the underlying malignancy, chemotherapy, radiation therapy, and prolonged antibiotic use predispose patients with head and neck cancer to fungal sinusitis. Fungal pathogens that can cause sinusitis include Zygomycetes, *Aspergillus* spp., *Fusarium* spp., *Pseudallesche-*

ria boydii, *Scedosporium* spp., *Alternaria* spp., *Bipolaris* spp., *Cladosporium* spp., and *Curvularia* spp. [8].

PAROTITIS

Local tumor invasion of the salivary duct can result in obstruction and suppurative parotitis. More commonly it develops in the chronically ill, malnourished, dehydrated, and postoperative patient. Radiation therapy frequently reduces saliva production and can predispose a patient to develop suppurative parotitis. Patients present with acute painful, firm, and erythematous swelling at the pre- and postauricular area. Progression of the infection may lead to massive swelling of the neck, respiratory depression, contiguous spread of the infection to adjacent facial structures and sepsis. The most common bacterial pathogens are *S. aureus* (including MRSA), Enterobacteriaceae, and anaerobes. Treatment is decompression and drainage of the affected glands along with appropriate antibiotics [9,10].

MUCOSITIS

Leukoplakia and erythroplakia are premalignant lesions that can resemble infections. Chronic ulcers of the oral cavity, including those caused by chronic trauma, can lead to squamous cell carcinoma. Secondary bacterial infections of oral ulcers include *Streptococcus viridans*, anaerobic *Streptococcus*, *Prevotella* spp., and *Fusobacterium* spp. Herpes stomatitis is frequently reactivated in patients with head and neck cancer from radiation therapy and can be misdiagnosed as radiation mucositis. Refractory aphthous ulcers of the oral cavity can be confused with herpes stomatitis. They usually respond to topical corticosteroids and rarely require thalidomide or systemic steroids. Finally, *Candida* can cause white pseudomembranous plaques or diffuse erethema throughout the oropharynx.

MANDIBULAR OSTEOMYELITIS

The mandible has a relatively thinner cortex and poorer blood supply than the maxillary bone. Therefore, mandibles are more susceptible to develop osteomyelitis. Most cases of mandibular osteomyelitis are associated with preexisting odontogenic infection. However, local tumor invasion, radiation therapy, chemotherapy, and steroid use predispose patients to mandibular osteomyelitis. Severe mandibular pain is the most common symptom and may be accompanied by paresthesia of the affected area. Osteoradionecrosis and actinomycosis can cause a variant form of mandibular osteomyelitis called chronic sclerosing osteomyelitis. This presents with a localized hard, non-tender swelling over the mandible. Organisms involved in mandibular osteomyelitis include *S. aureus* (including MRSA), *S. viridans*, anaerobic bacteria, and, less commonly, gram-negative bacilli. Treatment includes surgical debridement, systemic antibiotics, smoking cessation, and possibly hyperbaric oxygen in resistant cases [10,11].

BASILAR SKULL OSTEOMYELITIS

Base of the skull osteomyelitis is classically seen in diabetic patients with untreated otitis externa and is usually caused by *P. aeruginosa*. Other underlying conditions that predispose to basilar skull osteomyelitis include cell-mediated immunodeficiency, prior radiation therapy, and underlying malignancy. The common pathogens that cause basilar skull osteomyelitis are *P. aeruginosa*, *S. aureus*, and rarely *Aspergillus* spp. [12]. Acute infection leads to progressive osteolytic bone destruction, sclerosis, and granulomatous formation. Complications of spreading infection include cranial nerve palsies, vertebral instability (especially at the craniovertebral junction), meningitis, dural sinus septic thrombophlebitis, and brain abscess [13,14]. Diagnosis of basilar skull osteomyelitis is challenging because there is neither a pathognomonic physical finding nor a characteristic radiographic finding. Thus surgical intervention is needed to rule out underlying malignancy, to obtain a clinical specimen for microbiology testing and histopathology examination, and to adequately remove dead bone. When surgery is not an option, chronic suppressive antibiotics may prevent further spread of infections for a time. Oral ciprofloxacin, clindamycin, amoxicillin/clavulanate, and doxycycline are frequently used in combination.

OTHER SITES OF INFECTION

In patients with head and neck cancer, local tissue destruction and inflammation may be related to tumor invasion and/or infection. As a consequence, life-threatening infections can develop and be difficult to diagnose and distinguish from progression of the malignancy. From the initial cancer site, infection may extend along the fascial planes into deep cervical spaces or vascular compartments. Airway obstruction and contiguous infection of the mediastinum or carotid sheath may result. Other infectious complications include parameningeal infections, retropharyngeal abscess, carvernous sinus thrombosis, suppurative jugular thrombophlebitis, and metastatic abscesses [10,15,16].

Most patients with nasopharyngeal carcinoma present with an advanced stage with metastatic cervical nodes. A retropharyngeal abscess can be a rare presenting feature [17]. Owing to the proximity of the retropharyngeal space to the nasopharynx, the tumor can spread into the retropharyngeal space, as can infection. The organisms usually involved are upper respiratory flora including anaerobes, gram-negative bacteria, S aureus, and Candida spp. [15].

ASPIRATION PNEUMONIA

Aspiration is a common complication of head and neck surgery, especially following laryngectomy. Aspiration pneumonitis can lead to necrotizing pneumonia and lung abscess. Organisms causing aspiration pneumonia include anaerobes (Bacteroides spp., Fusobacterium spp., Actinomyces spp., microaerophilic streptococci), S. pneumoniae, H. influenzae, S. aureus, and Enterobacteriaceae. However, several studies showed no anaerobic growth in lung abscess culture specimens [18–21]. In chronically ill patients or institutionalized patients, P. aeruginosa and methicillin-resistant S. aureus (MRSA) have increased significance. Because of the variety of organisms causing aspiration pneumonia, especially when complicated by necrotizing pneumonia and lung abscess, bronchoscopy is an essential tool. A poor prognosis is associated with the presence of lung abscess, isolation of S. aureus, P. aeruginosa, or Klebsiella pneumoniae, and advanced age. Although some authors have reported satisfactory results from an aggressive surgical approach, most infections are treated with antibiotics alone. Since the predisposing factor of the pneumonia (i.e., the tumor) in most cases cannot be removed, complete resolution of the pneumonia by antibiotics alone is difficult to attain [21,22]. The most important intervention to prevent aspiration is preoperative and postoperative training and counseling by speech therapy in supraglottic swallowing, breathing, and coughing. Finally, tracheostomy may be required to prevent recurrent aspiration of oropharyngeal secretions.

SURGICAL WOUND INFECTION

Because of the abundance of microorganisms in the oval cavity, surgical wound infection is relatively common after head and neck surgery. The major determinant of surgical wound infection is the degree of contamination of the wound. Other comorbid conditions (diabetes mellitus, nutritional deficiency, excessive tobacco use or alcohol intake, poor oral hygiene), stage and location of the tumor, prior cancer treatment (chemotherapy, radiation therapy, tracheotomy), type of surgical procedure, preoperative antibiotics, and postoperative factors (wound care, postoperative metabolic status) contribute to an increased risk of a surgical wound infection [23]. The current recommendation for perioperative antibiotic prophylaxis of major head and neck surgeries is cefazolin, 2 g intravenously, one dose, or clindamycin, 600–900 mg intravenously, single dose, with or without gentamicin 1.5 mg/kg single dose. Despite appropriate antibiotic prophylaxis, the rate of postoperative wound infection is still high [24].

Salivary leak is a complication of total larygectomy. It can lead to wound infection. The first sign of salivary leak is a small loculated wound infection. About 9% to 21% of salivary leaks are complicated with fistula formation, especially in patients who received radiation. When a pharyngocutaneous fistula develops, appropriate antibiotics, good local wound care, and nothing per mouth are indicated. Generally, fistulas should heal in 1 to 2 weeks. If a fistula persists, a mucocutaneous flap or free-tissue transfer for closure should be considered [25].

Neck dissection is often done in conjunction with laryngectomy in the treatment of laryngeal cancer. Sacrificing both internal jugular veins leads to chronic lymphedema and venous stasis. Lymphedema will predispose to skin and soft-tissue infections particularly from group A *Streptococcus* and *S. aureus*. Sometimes a chyle leak develops and provides a portal of entry for bacterial superinfection. With massive drainage of chyle (more than 600 ml/day), surgical exploration and repair is warranted [26].

INFECTIOUS COMPLICATIONS OF RADIATION THERAPY

Radiotherapy of head and neck cancer frequently causes pain and odynophagia, which may result in inadequate oral intake. Malnutrition has a major impact on host defenses against infection and wound healing. Moreover, radiation destruction of salivary glands results in xerostomia and mucositis. Mucositis allows local invasion of oral microflora and other pathogens, including gram-negative bacilli, *S. aureus*, and *Candida* spp. Radiation therapy increases the risk of reactivation of herpes simplex virus [27,28].

Postoperative wound infections commonly occur when the incision areas were previously exposed to radiotherapy. The common organisms are group A *Streptococcus*, *S. aureus*, and gram-negative bacilli. Melaney's synergistic gangrene can occur in the radiated area with mixed aerobic and anaerobic organisms. It is advised to wait at least 3 weeks after radiotherapy before surgery to prevent wound dehiscence and infection [29,30].

Osteoradionecrosis is a well-documented complication of radiotherapy of the head and neck region. It predisposes to cellulitis of the overlying soft tissue and osteomyelitis underneath. The organisms commonly involved include *S. aureus*, *Candida* spp., and gram-negative bacilli [31,32].

Cerebral injury from radiotherapy, especially in the treatment of nasopharyngeal carcinoma, has been increasingly recognized. Patients present with neurological deterioration and sometimes with fever with an unidentifiable source. Magnetic resonance imaging shows a wide range of findings, including mild subclinical cortical changes, cystic lesions, abscess with ring enhancement, or large confluent areas with necrosis and vasogenic edema. Ventriculitis due to a ruptured cyst or abscess is rare [33].

INFECTIOUS COMPLICATIONS ASSOCIATED WITH CHEMOTHERAPY

Chemotherapy, usually cisplatin and fluorouracil, plays a large role in treatment of head and neck cancer. The major side effects are gastrointestinal symptoms, including nausea, vomiting, diarrhea, and mucositis, which is more commonly found in patients receiving concomitant chemoradiotherapy [26,34]. Myelosuppression is another complication of chemotherapy and is a major dose-limiting toxicity. Neutropenia can lead to life-threatening infections. The primary site of infection often includes the gastrointestinal tract, where chemotherapy-induced mucosal damage allows invasion of colonizing pathogens. Because of the high incidence of disruption of the mucous membranes of the oropharynx in patients with head and neck cancer, translocation of oral flora into the bloodstream is a concern when neutropenia develops. The predominant pathogens are *S. viridans*, gram-negative, bacilli, and *Candida* spp. Empirical antimicrobial therapy for febrile neutropenia for head and neck cancer is the same for all solid malignancies [35,36].

CONCLUSION

Infectious complications of head and neck cancer are usually related to the underlying cancer and its therapy. Understanding the common pathogens in patients with head and neck cancer may lead to more rapid diagnosis and earlier institution of appropriate therapy. The increasing trend of resistant pathogens found in patients receiving treatment for head and neck cancer warrants a more judicious use of antibiotics. Antimicrobial coverage of MRSA and *P. aeruginosa* is becoming increasingly necessary in the postoperative patient with head and neck cancer.

REFERENCES

1. Gill JK, Field T, Vincent AL, Greene JN, Sandin RL, Sinnot JT. Antiobitic susceptibility among penicillin-resistant pneumococcal isolates. Infections in Medicine 2003; 439–444.

2. Salgado CD, Farr BM, Calfee DP. Community-acquired methicillin-resistant *Staphylococcus aureus*: a meta-analysis of prevalence and risk factors. Clin Infect Dis 2003; 36, 131 139.
3. Gwaltney JM. Sinusitis. In: Mandell GL, Bennett JE, Dolin R, eds. Principles and Practice of Infectious Diseases. 5th ed. Philadelphia: Churchill Livingstone, 2000, 676–686.
4. Hamory BH, Sande MA, Sydnor A Jr, et al. Etiology and antimicrobial therapy of acute maxillary sinusitis. J Infect Dis 1979; 139:197–202.
5. Gwaltney JM Jr, Scheld WM, Sande MA, Sydnor A. The microbial etiology and antimicrobial therapy of adults with acute community-acquired sinusitis: a fifteen-year experience at the university of Virginia and review of other selected studies. J Allergy Clin Immunol 1992; 90:457–462.
6. Mra Z, Roach JC, Brook AL. Infectious and neoplastic diseases of the sphenoid sinus—a report of 10 cases. Rhinology 2002; 40(1):34–40.
7. Winther B, Vickery CL, Gross CW, et al. Microbiology of the maxillary sinus in adults with chronic sinus disease. Am J Rhinol 1996; 10:347–350.
8. Mitchell TG. Overview of basic medical mycology. Otolaryngol Clin North Am 2000; 33:237–249.
9. Goldberg MH. Infections of the salivary glands. In: Topazian RG, Goldberg MH, eds. Oral and Maxillary infections. 2nd ed. Philadelphia: WB Saunders, 1987, 239.
10. Chow AW. Infections of the oral cavity, neck and head. In: Mandell GL, Bennett JE, Dolin R, eds. Principles and Practice of Infectious Diseases. 5th edition. Philadelphia: Churchill Livingstone, 2001, 689–702.
11. Taher AA. Osteomyelitis of the mandible in Teharan, Iran: analysis of 88 cases. Oral Surg Oral Med Oral Pathol 1993; 76:28–31.
12. Shelton JC, Antonelli PJ, Hickett R. Skull base fungal osteomyelitis in an immunocompetent host. Otolaryngol Head Neck Surg 2002; 126:76–78.
13. Dudic Y. Management of osteomyelitis of the anterior skull base and cranio-vertebral junction. Otolaryngol Head Neck Surg 2003; 128:39–42.
14. Rowlands RG, Lekakis GK, Hinton AE. Masked pseudomonal skull base osteomyelitis presenting with a bilateral Xth cranial nerve palsy. J Laryngol Otol 2002; 116:556–558.
15. Olarinde O. Candidal abscess in a second primary neoplasm of the neopharynx. J Laryngol Otol 2000; 114:974–975.
16. Chow AW. Life-threatening infections of the head and neck. Clin Infect Dis 1992; 14:991–1004.
17. Pak MW, Chan KL, van Hasselt CA. Retropharyngeal abscess: a rare presentation of nasopharyngeal carcinoma. J Laryngol Otol 1999; 113:70–72.
18. Marik PE. Aspiration pneumonitis and aspiration pneumonia. N Engl J Med 2001; 344:665–671.
19. Marik PE, Careau P. The role of anaerobes in patients with ventilator-associated pneumonia and aspiration pneumonia: a prospective study. Chest 1999; 115:178–183.
20. Mier L, Dreyfuss D, Darchy B, et al. Is penicillin G an adequate initial treatment

for aspiration pneumonia? A prospective evaluation using a protected specimen brush and quantitative cultures. Intens Care Med 1993; 19:279–284.

21. Tseng Y. Surgery for lung abscess in immunocompetent children. J Pediatr Surg 2001; 36:470–473.

22. Hoffer FA. Lung abscess versus necrotizing pneumonia: implications for interventional therapy. Pediatr Radiol 1999; 29:87–91.

23. Coskun H, Erisen L, Basut O. Factors affecting wound infection rates in head and neck surgery. Otolaryngol Head Neck Surg 2000; 123:328–333.

24. Nichols RL. Preventing surgical site infection: a surgeon perspective. Emerg Infect Dis 2001; 7:220–224.

25. Hiler M, Black MJ, Lafond G. Pharyngo-cutaneous fistulas after total laryngectomy: incidence, etiology and outcome analysis. J Otolaryngol 1993; 22:164.

26. Weissler MC. Management of complications resulting from laryngeal cancer treatment. Otolaryngol Clin North Am 1997; 30:269–278.

27. Nikoskelainen J. Oral infections related to radiation and immunosuppressive therapy. J Clin Periodontal 1990; 17:504–507.

28. Redding SW, Zellars RC, Kirkpatrick WR, McAtee RK, Caceres MA, Fothergill AW, Lopez-Ribot JI, Bailey CW, Rinaldi MG, Patterson TF. Epidemiology of orapharyngeal candida colonization and infection in patients receiving radiation for head and neck cancer. J Clin Microbiol 1999; 37:3896–3900.

29. Hom DB, Adams GL, Monyak D. Irradiated soft tissue and its management. Otolaryngol Clin North Am 1995; 28(5):1003–1019.

30. Moore MJ. The effect of radiation on connective tissue. Otolaryngol Clin North Am 1984; 17:389–399.

31. Jereczek-Fossa BA, Orecchia R. Radiotherapy-induced mandibular bone complications. Cancer Treat Rev 2002; 28(1):65–74.

32. Celik N, Wei FC, Chen HC, et al. Osteoradionecrosis of the mandible after oromandibular cancer surgery. Plast Reconstr Surg 2002; 109(6):1875–1881.

33. Wong WC, Cheng PW, Chan FL, et al. Improved diagnosis of a temporal lobe abscess in a post-irradiated nasopharyngeal carcinoma patient using diffusion-weighted magnetic resonance imaging. Clin Radiol 2002; 57(11):1040–1043.

34. Vokes EE. Head and neck cancer. In: Braunwald E, Hauser SL, Fauci AS, Longo DL, Kasper DL, Jameson JL, eds. Harrison's Principles of Medicine. 15th ed. New York: McGraw-Hill, 2001, 559–562.

35. Hughes WT, Armstrong D, Bodey GP, et al. 2002 guideline for the use of antimicrobial agents in neutropenic patients with cancer. Clin Infect Dis 2002; 34:730–751.

36. DeMarie S, Van den Broek PJ, Willemze R, et al. Strategy for antibiotic therapy in febrile neutropenic patients on selective antibiotic decontamination. Eur J Clin Microbiol Infect Dis 1993; 12:897–906.

15

Infections in Patients with Lung Cancer

Charurut Somboonwit
University of South Florida College of Medicine
and Moffitt Cancer Center and Research Institute
Tampa, Florida, U.S.A.

Charles Craig
St. Joseph Mercy Health System
Ann Arbor, Michigan, U.S.A.

John N. Greene
University of South Florida School of Medicine
and Moffitt Cancer Center and Research Institute
Tampa, Florida, U.S.A.

Primary lung cancer is the leading cause of cancer death of both men and women in the United States. The peak incidence of lung cancer is between 55 and 65 years of age, with increasing incidence occurring in women [1]. Most lung cancers are caused by carcinogen and tumor promoters inhaled through cigarette smoking. Chronic obstructive pulmonary disease (COPD), which is also a smoking-related disease, will further increase the risk of lung cancer. Signs and symptoms of lung cancer are caused by local tumor growth, invasion of adjacent structures, lymphatic spread, distant metastasis, and paraneoplastic syndromes. Infections related to lung cancer are infections that occur in the background of COPD, tumor growth, bronchial obstruction, and extension along lymphatics. Infectious complications related to lung cancer treatment are due to surgery, chemotherapy-induced neutropenia and mucositis, and radiation therapy.

INFECTIONS RELATED TO CHRONIC OBSTRUCTIVE PULMONARY DISEASES

Cigarette smoking is the single most important risk factor of both COPD and lung cancer. It impairs mucociliary clearance, which is the primary defense mechanism of the respiratory system. Damaged respiratory tract epithelium decreases ciliary mucous clearance. Viral infections cause release of inflammatory mediators, increase local permeability, and predispose the airway to bacterial colonization. *Haemophilus influenza* especially produces substrate to impair ciliary function, increase mucous production, and destroy local immunoglobulin and impair neutrophil fuction. Acute tracheobronchitis preceding acute exacerbations of COPD and community-acquired pneumonia invariably occur in patients with lung cancer. Most COPD exacerbations are caused by bacterial infections or viral tracheobronchitis superinfected by bacterial pathogens. Community-acquired pneumonia in COPD patients is generally caused by *Streptococcus pneumoniae*, *H. influenzae*, and *Moraxella catarrhalis* [2]. Patients present with cough (more than 90%), dyspnea, sputum production, and pleuritic chest pain [3,4]. Sometimes, pneumonia itself is the first presentation of lung cancer, especially unresolving pneumonia despite appropriate treatment. Severe community-acquired pneumonia is increased in patients with underlying COPD and malignancy, with a higher risk of respiratory failure and mortality. The important pathogens are *S. pneumoniae*, *Legionella pneumophila*, *H. influenzae*, *Staphylococcus aureus*, and less commonly gram-negative enteric pathogens [5]. Bacteremia is a more common presentation when multilobar pneumonia is present. Regardless of the pathogen, bacteremia is not an indicator of disease severity. However, the yield of a blood culture is higher in patients with severe pneumonia, and the result of identifying the pathogen will facilitate appropriate antibiotic selection [5,6]. Patients with severe COPD are also at risk for nontuberculous mycobacterial infections. The common pathogens are *Mycobacterium avium* complex (MAC), *Mycobacterium kansasii*; less commonly, *M. abscessus*, *M. chelonae*, *M. malmonense*, and *M. xenopi* [7]. Presentations of nontuberculous mycobacterial infections resemble tuberculosis with fever, weight loss, hemoptysis, and progressive dyspnea. Radiographic findings are cavitary lesions, pulmonary nodules, bronchiectasis, and infiltrates. MAC infection in patients with COPD and lung cancer rarely disseminates outside the lung [7,8].

INFECTIONS RELATED TO LOCAL TUMOR GROWTH

Postobstructive pneumonia, necrotizing pneumonia and lung abscess are possible complications of lung cancer. The most common mechanism for developing pneumonia is aspiration of secretions with oral flora. Intrinsic and extrinsic obstruction of the bronchus can result in atelectasis, lung collapse, and pneumonia. In more severe cases, destruction of lung parenchyma results in the formation of fluid filled cavities. Some authors differentiate necrotizing pneumonia from lung abscess by the size of cavities, <2 cm or >2 cm, respectively [9]. Organisms causing postobstructive pneumonia include oral anaerobes (*Bacteroides*, *Prevotella*, *Fusobacterium*, *Actinomyces*, microaerophilic streptococci), *S. pneumoniae*, *H. influenzae*, *S. aureus*, and *Enterobacteraciae*. In chronically ill patients or institutionalized patients, *Pseudomonas aeruginosa* and methicillin-resistant *S. aureus* (MRSA) have increased significance. However, several studies demonstrated no anaerobic growth in lung abscess culture specimens, thus downplaying the significance of anerobes in this setting [10–12]. Fungal pathogens, especially *Aspergillus*, are occasionally isolated from bronchial aspirates and can invade locally or form a fungus ball if a cavity is present. The variety of causative organisms causing postobstructive pneumonia, especially those complicated by necrotizing pneumonia and lung abscess, make bronchoscopy an essential tool. It not only provides an adequate specimen collection but also delineates the contribution by tumor invasion. A poorer prognosis is associated with the presence of a lung abscess, the presence of *S. aureus*, *P. aeruginosa*, or *Klebsiella pneumoniae*, and advanced age. Some authors have reported satisfactory results from an aggressive surgical approach, since the predisposing factor of the pneumonia, namely obstruction and lack of adequate drainage, in most cases cannot be removed. Complete resolution of the pneumonia by antibiotics alone is difficult to attain, especially when obstruction persists [13,14].

INFECTIOUS COMPLICATIONS OF SURGICAL RESECTION OF LUNG CANCER

Surgical resection of lung cancer offers the best chance of cure for non–small cell lung cancer. Overall, major complications following pulmonary resection are 17 to 27%, with postoperative mortality 3.7 to 5.7% [15–17]. Postoperative wound infections are usually caused by *S. aureus* (including methicillin-resistant isolates) and coagulase negative *Staphylococci*. Leakage of anastomostic sites can lead to bronchopleural fistula formation, pneumonia, and empyema. These infections are usually polymicrobial and consist of gram-negative bacilli, anaerobes, and Candida species in addition to the aforementioned *Staphylococci* species. Chest tube drainage, and sometimes intrapleural fibrinolysis or decortications, are needed.

Postoperative pneumonia can develop from atelectasis or retention of secretions, or it can be aggravated by postoperative pain, sedatives, and analgesia as well as phrenic nerve injury. In one study, postoperative pneumonia after lung resection developed in 2.5% of patients with an increased risk of mechanical ventilation, and ICU stay [18]. Gram-negative bacilli colonizing the digestive tract and upper respiratory tract during the preoperative period are the primary pathogens. Pneumonia caused by *P. aeruginosa* or *Acinetobacter* spp. have a 40% attributed mortality with a relative risk of death of 2.5 [19]. There are multiple risk factors for developing nosocomial pneumonia after lung resection. These include the duration of hospital stay, the duration of mechanical ventilation (especially if more than 7 days), previous antibiotic therapy, the presence of potentially drug-resistant pathogens (especially methicillin-resistant *S. aureus* and *P. aeruginosa*), structural lung disease, and prior steroids use. Prompt institution of antibiotics should include those with antipseudomonal activity such as antipseudomonal penicillins, antipseudomonal cephalosporins, carbapenems, aztreonam with or without an antipsuedomonal fluoroquinolone. If patients are at risk of methicillin resistant *S. aureus*, vancomycin should be added. Linezolid or quinupristin/dalfopristin might serve as an alternative to vancomycin if allergic or intolerant [19,20].

INFECTIOUS COMPLICATIONS OF RADIOTHERAPY OF LUNG CANCER

The extent of radiation damage depends mainly on the volume of tissue irradiated, the total dose delivered, the fraction size, and the intrinsic radiosensitivity of the tissue. Radiation-induced injury can cause pneumonitis, pericarditis, myelitis with irreversible demyelization injury of the spinal cord, esophagitis, and skin changes.

Acute radiation pneumonitis can mimic bacterial pneumonia. It typically presents 4 to 12 weeks after radiation therapy, with low-grade fever, dyspnea, and nonproductive cough. Physical examination is usually normal but can reveal wheezing, pleural rub, or signs of consolidation. Chest radiograph initially shows diffuse haziness of the irradiated areas with loss of clarity of the pulmonary vasculature. When pneumonitis progresses, infiltrates become more patchy or confluent but usually correspond to the shape of the treatment port. Computed tomography is more sensitive in demonstrating early changes such as homogenous attenuation uniformly involving the irradiation port. Later, patchy consolidation at the corresponding port area can develop. Other tests that may support the diagnosis of radiation pneumonitis are magnetic resonance imaging (MRI), nuclear scanning (i.e., gallium scan), and pulmonary function testing [17]. It is important to rule out infectious causes because corticosteroids are the treatment of choice for radiation pneumonitis. Antibiotic therapy should be given in addition to corticosteroids, since radiation pneumonitis can predispose to infection. As radiation damage progresses to chronic pulmonary fibrosis, which usually evolves over a period of 6 months to 2 years after radiotherapy, lower respiratory tract infections are seen more often. Right-sided heart failure can also predispose to recurrent upper respiratory tract infection. Bronchiolitis obliterans with organizing pneumonia (BOOP) is a complication outside the radiation field that can mimic pneumonia. Patients present with low-grade fever, dry cough, and pulmonary infiltrates. The presence of intra-alveolar granulation tissue and an increase in activated CD4 cells in bronchoalveolar larvage specimens favor the diagnosis of BOOP. Dramatic improvement of BOOP occurs after the administration of corticosteroids in most cases [17,21].

Radiation esophagitis is an early complication following radiotherapy. Initially dysphagia develops. The histopathology reveals submucosal fibrosis and mucosal atrophy. Esophageal stenosis and fistula formation lead to serious infectious complications such as abscess formation, mediastinitis, or aspiration pneumonia.

INFECTIOUS COMPLICATIONS ASSOCIATED WITH CHEMOTHERAPY

Chemotherapy for lung cancer can improve both mortality and quality of life. In small cell lung cancer, the response is about 85 to 90% with limited disease, and 65–85% with extensive disease. The overall 5-year survival is only 5% in the latter group [22]. In non–small cell lung cancer, chemotherapy is increasingly being used with palliative care and with neoadjuvant use. The principal adverse effects of chemotherapy that predispose to infections are myelosuppression and chemotherapy-induced mucosal damage.

Myelosuppression is a major dose-limiting toxicity of chemotherapy. Neutropenia is defined by an absolute neutrophil count less than 1000 cell/mm^3. However, there is a significant risk of opportunistic infections if the absolute neutrophil count falls below 500 cells/mm^3. Neutropenia usually occurs 7 to 10 days following chemotherapy. At least 50% of neutropenic patients become febrile, and 20% of patients who have less than 100 cells/mm^3 have bacteremia. The primary site of infection often includes the gastrointestinal tract, where chemotherapy induced mucosal damage allows for the invasion of enteric pathogens. Also, intravascular devices often provide a portal of entry for infections.

According to the Infectious Diseases Society of America, guidelines for the use of antimicrobial agents in neutropenic patients with fever [23], initial antibiotic therapy should be given promptly. Afebrile patients with signs and symptoms compatible with infection should also be treated in like manner. Empiric treatment should include coverage for *Pseudomonas aeruginosa*. Vancomycin may be added to improve coverage of gram-positive cocci. Vancomycin may be discontinued 24 to 48 hours later if no gram-positive infection is identified. Patients at risk for gram-positive infections that necessitate initial empirical therapy with vancomycin are those with suspected intravenous catheter infections, known colonization with methicillin-resistant *S. aureus*, positive blood culture for gram-positive cocci pending identification and susceptibility testing, or evidence of cardiovascular impairment [24].

Granulocyte colony stimulating factor (GCSF) or granulocyte monocyte stimulating factor (GMCSF) is used as adjunctive therapy for febrile neutropenia. However, routine use in uncomplicated cases of fever and neutropenia is not recommended if the duration of neutropenia is expected to be less than 1 week [25]. GCSF or GMCSF is recommended in patients with pneumonia, severe cellulitis or sinusitis, systemic fungal infection, hypotensive episodes, or sepsis with multiorgan dysfunction [23].

SPECIFIC PATHOGENS CAUSING INFECTIONS IN LUNG CANCER PATIENTS

Drug Resistant Pneumococcal Infections

In the past decade, there is a number of *S. pneumoniae* isolates with increasing resistance to β-lactams, macrolides, and trimethoprim-sulfamethoxazole (TMP-SMX). The prevalence of penicillin-resistant pneumococcus varies in each region of the country, with the highest in the Southeast, and the lowest in the New England area [26]. The risk factors of drug-resistant pneumococcal infections are recent hospitalization, extreme ages, attendance at day care centers, presence of underlying diseases, HIV infection, and immunosuppression [27,28]. In patients with lung cancer, the risk is increased not only from the underlying cancer itself but also from hospitalization and cancer treatment causing immunosuppression. Penicillin-resistance of pneumococcus has an impact on the prognosis of meningitis and otitis media but has little effect on the outcome of nonmeningeal infection including community-acquired pneumonia and bacteremia [28]. However, there was evidence of a poor outcome in patients with intermediate susceptibility to penicillin [29]. Pneumococcal pneumonia with high resistance to penicillin was associated with suppurative infection, respiratory failure, and a higher mortality (relative risk

2.1) in another study [28]. General recommendations from the Infectious Diseases Society of America and the Canadian Infectious Diseases Society recommend a macrolide, doxycycline, or an antipneumococcal fluoroquinolone as treatment options of empirical outpatient treatment of community-acquired pneumonia. Fluoroquinolones with pneumococcal activity are preferred in patients with underlying lung disease. For inpatient treatment of community-acquired pneumonia, combination therapy of a β-lactam and a macrolide or fluoroquinolone monotherapy is recommended [2,30]. Pneumococcus can also be resistant to other β-lactam antibiotics, macrolides, TMP-SMX, tetracyclines, and chloramphenicol. There is a correlation between β-lactam resistance and macrolide resistance, which is a major concern because of the common use of macrolides as empiric therapy of respiratory tract infections [31]. As macrolide resistant pneumococcus becomes endemic in North America, treatment failure is expected. However, macrolides remain the drug of choice for mild to moderate pneumonia in patients that do not require hospitalization. An additional benefit of a macrolide is coverage of atypical pathogens such as *Chlamydia* spp., *Mycoplasma pneumonia*, and Legionella. For patients with underlying lung disease such as COPD or lung cancer, an antipneumococcal fluoroquinolone should be considered, which also provides atypical pathogen coverage. In patients with COPD or lung cancer, pneumococcal vaccination should be given. The 23-valent vaccine encompasses most serotypes responsible for both penicillin and macrolide resistance. The vaccine not only reduces nasopharyngeal carriage but also reduces invasive pneumococcal infections.

Legionella Infection

Cigarette smoking, underlying lung disease, and immunosuppression (especially corticosteroids therapy) are risk factors for Legionella infection. Patients with lung cancer are at significant risk. *Legionella pneumophila* is one of the top three causes of community-acquired pneumonia [32]. Although the incidence of nosocomial Legionella infection has gradually decreased owing to the availability of in-house diagnostic tests in many hospitals, it is still a major concern because of the severity of the illness. The modes of transmission are inhalation of contaminated aerosols, contaminated hospital water supply, and, often underrecognized, aspiration of retained secretions in a nasogastric tube. Pneumonia is the major presentation with a wide a range of severity. However, in patients with underlying cancer or immunosuppression, a severe systemic illness is common. Gastrointestinal symptoms, especially diarrhea, are usually prominent. Other common extrapulmonary manifestations are relative bradycardia, hypophosphatemia, or hyponatremia. Legionellosis with concurrent bacteremia has been reported. Diagnosis includes Legionella urinary antigen testing, sputum culture on buffered charcoal yeast extract (BCYE), direct fluorescent antibody staining, serology testing, and nucleic acid amplification. Using urinary antigen detection plus culture is the best diagnostic combination in most instances. The disadvantage of urinary antigen is it is only reliable for detection of *Legionella pneumophila* serogroup 1. Antibiotic therapy of legionella infection includes macrolides, fluoroquinolones, doxcycline, and rifampin. Fluoroquinolones have good intracellular activity and are recommended for use in combination with rifampin in severely ill patients with legionellosis [33].

Nontuberculous Mycobacteria Infection

COPD, immunosuppression (especially steroid use), and lung cancer are risk factors for nontuberculous mycobacteria (NTM) of the lung. The clinical presentation resembles pulmonary tuberculosis, including fever, night sweats, weight loss, and pulmonary symptoms. In the United States, *Mycobacterium avium* complex, followed by *M. kansasii* and *M. abscessus*, are the leading causes of NTM pulmonary infections [34]. Unless severe cell-mediated immunity dysfunction exists, the disease remains localized to the lungs. Radiographic findings are nonspecific, but with high-resolution computed tomography (HRCT) the finding of nodular bronchiectasis in a tree in bud pattern is characteristic of MAC infection. Recovery of the organism in a respiratory specimen is not proof of infection. But in high-risk patients, such as those with lung cancer or COPD, with the appropriate radiographic abnormality and associated symptoms, the initiation of antimycobacterial treatment is warranted. The diagnostic approach includes HRCT of the lungs and a respiratory specimen for acid-fast stain and culture to help confirm the diagnosis. If acid-fast bacilli grow within 7 days, the rapid growers *M. abscessus*, *M. chelonae*, or *M. fortuitum* are likely. Treatment for each species of *Mycobacterium* should be guided by susceptibility testing. Recurrence of disease and treatment failure can occur owing to antimicrobial resistance and the uncorrectable underlying pulmonary abnormality [34–36].

Fungal Infections

Fungal infections can complicate the course of lung cancer owing to the underlying malignancy itself, to steroid use, and to chemotherapy-related neutropenia. Opportunistic fungal infections, especially Aspergillosis, have increasing importance in patients with lung cancer, especially with late stages of cancer. Recovery of *Aspergillus* spp. from a respiratory specimen does not necessarily indicate invasive pulmonary aspergillosis. However, in neutropenic patients, the positive predictive value is 95% for invasive diseases [37]. Prior radiation therapy, the use of corticosteroids, and a cavity increase the risk of invasive pulmonary aspergillosis. The signs and symptoms of aspergillosis include fever, dyspnea, cough, hemoptysis, and pleuritic chest pain. The chest radiograph can be normal, or one can detect the development of pulmonary nodules. Chest computed tomography is sensitive and can provide more diagnostic detail than the chest radiograph. The common computed tomographic findings of invasive fungal infection, especially aspergillosis, is ground glass attenuation early in the process. Consolidation and peripheral nodular infiltrations occur later in the course of the infection. A nodule surrounded by ground-glass attenuation and air (air-crescent sign) is characteristic. Early computed tomographic scanning allows for an earlier diagnosis and empirical therapy [38,39]. These radiographic findings may lead to a more invasive diagnostic workup if necessary. Because of the increasing incidence of *Aspergillus* and other molds, culture and identification of the organism is preferred. Invasive diagnostic procedures such as bronchoscopy or lung biopsy are sometimes indicated to obtain the best sample.

CONCLUSION

Advancement in cancer treatment and an increase survival in patients with lung cancer make the cure of infections a major target to further reduce morbidity and mortality. Increasingly antibiotic-resistant pathogens are prompting new strategies to combat these life-threatening infections. Recognition of early signs and symptoms of infection can lead to a more prompt diagnosis and institution of appropriate empirical therapy.

REFERENCES

1. American Cancer Society. Cancer facets and figures 1996. Atlanta: American Cancer Society.
2. Barlett JG, Dowell SF, Mandell LA, et al. Practice guideline for the management of community-acquired pneumonia in adults. Clin Infect Dis 2002; 31:347–382.
3. Fine MJ, Stone RA, Singer DE, et al. Process and outcome of care for patients with community acquired pneumonia: result from the pneumonia Patient Outcomes Research Team (PORT) cohort study. Arch Intern Med 1999; 159:970–980.
4. Metlay JP, Schulz R, et al. Measuring symptomatic and functional recovery in patients with community-acquired pneumonia. J Gen Intern Med 1997; 12:423–430.
5. Rello J, Bodi M, Mariscal D, et al. Microbiology testing and outcome of patients with severe community acquired pneumonia. Chest 2003; 123:174–180.
6. Cunha B. Severe community acquired pneumonia. Critical Care Clinics 1998; 14:105–118.

7. Kourbeti IS, Maslow MJ. Nontuberculous mycobacterial infections of the lung. Current Infect Dis Reports 2000; 2:193–200.

8. Tanaka K, Amitani R, Niimi A, et al. Yield of computed tomography and bronchoscopy for the diagnosis of mycobacterium avium complex pulmonary diseases. Am J Respir Crit Care Med 1997; 155:2041–2046.

9. Finegold SM. Lung abscess. In: Mandell GL, Bennett JE, Dolin R, eds. Principle and Practice of Infectious Diseases. Philadelphia: Churchill Livingston, 2000:751–755.

10. Marik PE. Aspiration pneumonitis and aspiration pneumonia. N Eng J Med 2001; 344:665–671.

11. Marik PE, Careau P. The role of anaerobes in patients with ventilator-associated pneumonia and aspiration pneumonia: a prospective study. Chest 1999; 115:178–183.

12. Mier L, Dreyfuss D, Darchy B, et al. Is penicillin G an adequate initial treatment for aspiration pneumonia? A prospective evaluation using a protected specimen brush and quantitative cultures. Intensive Care Med 1993; 19:279–284.

13. Tseng Y. Surgery for lung abscess in immunocompetent children. J Ped Surg 2001; 36:470–473.

14. Hoffer FA. Lung abscess versus necrotizing pneumonia: implications for interventional therapy. Pediatr Radiol 1999; 29:87–91.

15. Dealauriers J, Ginsberg RJ, Fournier B. Prospective assessment of 30-day postoperative morbidity for surgical resection of lung cancer. Chest 1994; 106:329–339.

16. Ginsberg RJ, Hill LD, Eagan RT, et al. Modern thirty-day operative mortality for surgical resection in lung cancer. J Thorac Cardiovasc Surg 1983; 86:654–658.

17. Ah-See MW, Spiro SG. Evaluation and management of complications of lung cancer treatment. Seminars Respir Crit Care Med 2000; 21:451–462.

18. Nagasaki F, Flehinger BJ, Martini N. Complications of surgery in the treatment of carcinoma of the lung. 1982; 82:25–29.

19. Höfferken G, Niegerman MD. Nosocomial pneumonia. The importance of a de-escalating strategy for antibiotic treatment of pneumonia in the ICU. Chest 2002; 122:2183–2196.

20. Donowitz GR, Mandel GL. Acute pneumonia. In: Mandell GL, Bennett JE, Dolin R, eds. Principle and Practice of Infectious Diseases. Philadelphia: Churchill Livingston, 2000:717–743.

21. Prakash UBS. Radiation-induced injury in the non-radiated lung. Euro Respir J 1999; 13:715–717.

22. Smith EF, Postmus PE. Chemotherapy of small-cell lung cancer. In: Carney DN, ed. Lung Cancer. London: Edward Arnold, 1995:156–172.

23. Hughes WT, Armstrong D, Bodey GP, et al. 2002 guideline for the use of antimicrobial agents in neutropenic patients with cancer. Clin Infect Dis 2002; 34:730–751.

24. Centers for Diseases Control and Prevention. Recommendations for preventing the spread of vancomycin resistance: recommendations of the Hospital Infection

Control Practice Advisory Committee (HICPAC). MMWR Morb Mortal Wkly Rep 1995; 44(R–12):1–13.

25. Ozer H, Armitage JO, Bennett CL, et al. 2000 update of recommendations for the use of hematopoietic colony-stimulating factors: evidence-based clinical practice guideline. J Clin Oncol 2000; 18:3358–3385.

26. Thornsberry C, Sahm DF, Kelly LJ, et al. Regional trends in antimicrobial resistance among clinical isolates of *Streptococcus pneumoniae*, *Haemophilus influenza* and *Moraxella catarrhalis* in the United States: results from the TRUST surveillance program, 1999-2000. Clin Infect Dis 2002; 34(suppl 1):S4–16.

27. Campbell GD, Silberman R. Drug-resistant *Streptococcus pneumoniae*. Clin Infect Dis 1998; 26:1188–1195.

28. File TM. Appropriate use of antimicrobials for drug-resistant pneumonia: focus on the significance of β-lactam-resistant *Streptococcus pneumoniae*. Clin Infect Dis 2002; 34(suppl 1):S17–26.

29. Heffelfinger JD, Dowell SF, Jorgensen JH, et al. Management of community-acquired pneumonia in the era of pneumococcal resistance: a report from the Drug-Resistant *Streptococcus pneumoniae* Therapeutic Working Group. Arch Intern Med 2000; 160:1399–1408.

30. Mandell LA, Marrie TJ, Grossman RF, et al. Canadian guidelines for the initial management of community acquired pneumonia: an evidence-based update by the Canadian Infectious Diseases Society and the Canadian Thoracic Society. Clin Infect Dis 2000; 31:383–421.

31. Whitney CG, Farley MM, Hadler J, et al. Increasing prevalence of multidrug-resistant *Streptococcus pneumoniae* in the United States. N Engl J Med 2000; 343:1917–1924.

32. Stout JE, Yu VL. Legionellosis. N Eng J Med 1997; 337:682–687.

33. Tan MJ, Tann JS, File TM. Legionnaires disease with bacteremia coinfection. Clin Infect Dis 2002; 35:533–539.

34. Wallace RJ Jr, Cook JL, Glassroth J, et al. Diagnosis and treatment of disease caused by nontuberculous mycobacteria. American Thoracic Society Statement 1997; 156(suppl):S1–25.

35. Brown BA, Wallace RJ Jr. Infections due to nontuberculous mycobacteria. In: Mandell GL, Bennett JE, Dolin R, eds. Principle and Practice of Infectious Diseases. Philadelphia: Churchill Livingston, 2000:2630–2636.

36. Kourbeti IS, Maslow MJ. Nontuberculous mycobacterial infections of the lung. Current Infect Dis Reports 2000; 2:193–200.

37. Wald A, Leisenring W, Burik J, et al. Epidemiology of Aspergillus infection in a large cohort of patients undergoing bone marrow transplantation. J Infect Dis 1997; 175:1459–1466.

38. Stevens DA, Han VL, Judson MA, et al. Practice guideline for diseases caused by *Aspergillus*. Clin Infect Dis 2000; 30:696–709.

39. Calliot D, Casasnovas O, Bernard A, et al. Improved management of invasive pulmonary aspergillosis in neutropenic patients using early thoracic computed tomographic scan and surgery. J Clin Oncol 1997; 15:139–147.

16

Infections Complicating Breast Cancer and Its Treatment

Julia E. Richards
University of Tennessee Medical Center
Knoxville, Tennessee, U.S.A.

Larry M. Baddour
Mayo Clinic, College of Medicine
Rochester, Minnesota, U.S.A.

INTRODUCTION

Infections that are seen in patients with breast cancer today are largely complications of surgical procedures used in disease treatment and in breast reconstruction. Rarely is untreated breast cancer complicated by infection in developed countries with better access to advanced health care. Nevertheless, malignancy can induce inflammatory changes that lead to an incorrect diagnosis of infection in some patients. This chapter addresses breast cancer and infection in four phases: (1) untreated (and usually undiagnosed) breast cancer; (2) early surgical site infections in patients after excisional biopsy, lumpectomy, or mastectomy; (3) delayed infection following surgical intervention; and (4) infection that complicates breast reconstruction, which can include implant infection. While a variety of infections have been described that complicate breast cancer and its treatment (Table 1), it is anticipated that

TABLE 1 Infectious Syndromes Complicating
Breast Cancer

Infections in untreated breast cancer
  Infected malignant breast and chest wall ulcers
  Pseudoinfectious syndromes
    Inflammatory breast cancer
    Paget's disease
    Cancer en cuirasse
    Adenosarcoma
    Lymphoma
    Primary squamous cell carcinoma
Early infections following surgery
  Surgical site infections
Delayed infections following surgery
  Cellulitis
    Breast
    Ipsilateral upper extremity
  Breast abscess
  Septic arthritis - ipsilateral shoulder
  Sternal wound infection
    Following coronary artery bypass graft surgery
Infections complicating reconstructive surgery
  Surgical site infections
  Tissue expander infections
  Implant infections

---

newer syndromes will be added to the list as novel medical, surgical, and radiation therapy interventions are adopted in the future.

INFECTIONS IN UNTREATED BREAST CANCER

Two clinical scenarios should be considered in patients with untreated (and usually undiagnosed) breast cancer. First, whether breast cancer, through its production of skin ulceration, soft tissue necrosis or lymphatic obstruction, can predispose to secondary infection. Second, certain clinical signs and symptoms of breast cancer can mimic those of infection and result in a delay in tumor diagnosis because of a clinical impression that infection is present.

    Infection complicating untreated breast cancer is uncommonly seen in clinical practice today. Relatively early breast cancer detection and treatment in developed countries likely accounts for the lack of infections seen in untreated breast cancer patients. Nevertheless, patients with infected malignant breast and chest wall ulcers are seen [1] among populations with limited access to medical care. Systemic spread of infection did not occur in 33 patients given chemotherapy in one survey, although purulence was seen at the ulcer site. Ulcers healed in 18 patients whose tumors responded to chemotherapy.

Untreated breast cancer mimicking infection has been well described [2–8] and linked to inflammatory breast cancer, Paget's disease, cancer en cuirasse, adenosarcoma, lymphoma (Figure 1), and primary squamous cell carcinoma of the breast. Several case reports [2–4] describe inflammatory breast cancer or carcinoma erysipeloids presenting as breast cellulitis or abscess. In each case, multiple courses of antibiotics were administered before tissue biopsy was performed. Thus appropriate treatment with chemotherapy and/or irradiation was delayed.

Primary squamous cell carcinoma of the breast, an uncommon malady [7], has also been confused as infection in at least five reported cases. In three cases, tumor presented as breast abscess [7,8], and in the remaining two cases [8], a palpable mass with inflammatory skin changes were described. Repetitive surgical drainage procedures were performed for treatment of presume abscess, but relapse occurred. Tissue biopsy showed squamous cell carcinoma with secondary ulceration, necrosis and acute inflammation. Squamous cell carcinoma was the exclusive oncological diagnosis in two cases [8], and mixed infiltrating ductal carcinoma with squamous cell carcinoma was present in the remaining three cases [5,7,8].

Nguyen and coworkers [6] used breast ultrasonography to distinguish abscess from tumor. In their retrospective analysis, they found that the

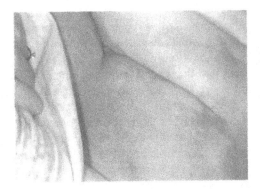

FIGURE 1   Cellulitislike changes to the lateral breast and chest wall due to primary skeletal muscle lymphoma with extension into the skin.

presence of either a hypoechoic wall or adjacent interstitial fluid surrounding the presumed abscess had an overall sensitivity of 55% and a specificity of 100% in the diagnosis of abscess. These two sonographic findings were seen in no cases of breast cancer.

A variety of signs and symptoms that are suggestive of infection have been described in patients with breast cancer masquerading as infection and include both local and systemic findings. Local manifestations include edema, induration, erythema, increased warmth, vesicle or bullae formation, and exfoliation, lymphadenopathy, decreased range of motion of involved joints, and pain. Systemic complaints include low-grade fever, weakness, and anorexia. These findings are likely due, in part, to lymphatic blockage and the presence of inflammatory cells, usually lymphocytes. Some [4] have speculated that because lymphocytes are unable to migrate into the lymphatic and capillary vessels owing to blockage by the tumor, lymphocytes aggregate to produce inflammatory changes.

SURGICAL SITE INFECTIONS FOLLOWING BREAST PROCEDURES

Surgical site infections are a direct result of the surgical procedure and occur at or near the incision within 30 days of the procedure [9–11]. If the surgical procedure requires placement of a prosthesis such as a breast implant, the incubation period for infection to become clinically evident can extend for up to 1 year. Because of the heterogeneous clinical course of surgical site infections based on the presence or not of breast prostheses, only acute ($\leq$30 days) surgical site infections not associated with prosthesis placement will be addressed here (Figure 2). Prosthesis-related infections will be addressed later in this chapter.

Breast biopsy, lumpectomy, and mastectomy represent procedures that are classified as clean wounds based on a widely accepted wound classification system [12–14]. A clean wound is defined as an uninfected operative wound in which no inflammation is present and the wound is closed primarily. The surgical site infection rate should range from 1.3% to 2.9% [12–15]. Data from several investigations [16–20] indicate that the rate of surgical site infection complicating breast procedures is higher than expected. Rotstein and colleagues [16] surveyed a consecutive cohort of patients undergoing surgical procedures for suspected carcinoma of the breast. The overall clean infection rate was 8.7% in 448 patients; the infection rate for each procedure was 2.3% for biopsy, 6.6% for lumpectomy, and 19% for mastectomy. Risk factor analysis was performed but was restricted to univariate testing because either the percentage of infections in each subgroup was too small or zero, or there

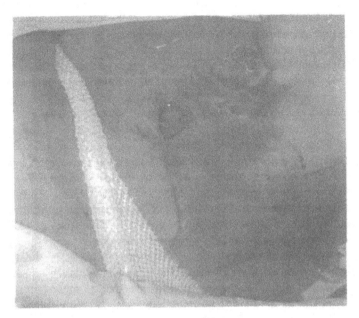

FIGURE 2 Surgical site infection with an area of poor wound healing following mastectomy and local irradiation.

was a lack of statistical significance in univariate testing to warrant multivariate analysis. Factors significantly associated with the development of clean surgical wound infection include the presence of a surgical drain ($P <$ 0.01), closed suction drainage (odds ratio [OR] = 16.5, confidence interval [CI_{95}] = 50–54.7), location of the drain (OR = 3.3, CI_{95} 1.7–6.6), prolonged preoperative stay (OR = 1.2, CI_{95} = 1.0–1.5), length of surgery (OR = 2.2, CI_{95} = 1.7–3.0), and greater mean age (OR = 1.6, CI_{95} = 1.2–2.1). No surgical site infection occurred among patients without surgical drains; 10% of patients with drains developed infection (OR inestimable). Closed suction drain systems were associated with a higher infection risk than open drains (20.1% verses 1.5%, OR = 16.5, CI_{95} = 1.7–6.6). The authors [16] also analyzed data from 14 other studies examining surgical site infection rates among patients who had undergone breast procedures and found infection rates that exceeded the expected (2.9%) maximum for clean surgery in 12 of the 14 surveys.

Because of the high surgical site infection rates associated with procedures used in the management of breast cancer, and because there are few modifiable risk factors identified for breast surgical site infections, the utility of preoperative antibiotic prophylaxis has garnered considerable interest as a means of infection prevention. Bertin and coworkers [18] reported that a single dose of cefazolin sodium given within 1 hour of incision was associated with a decline in surgical site infections, and the decline in rate was statistically significant (0.9% vs. 4%, $P = 0.02$). Additional trials have been conducted, and results have varied regarding the efficacy of antibiotic prophylaxis. The investigations listed in a recent review [17] suggest that there is a benefit to administering preoperative antibiotics to patients undergoing breast surgery when data are collectively examined. Individually, some studies failed to achieve statistical significance in infection rate differences seen in recipients of antibiotic versus placebo. Nevertheless, downward trends in infection rates among antibiotic recipients were evident, and had trials included a larger number of enrollees, then statistical significance in the rates of infection would have been achieved, provided the trends remain constant. One study [19] not included in the review demonstrated no benefit of preoperative amoxycillin-clavulanic acid in reducing surgical site infections in clean elective breast surgery in women undergoing definitive surgery for breast malignancy. There are concerns, however, about the applicability of this study to other populations. First, the infection rates in both antibiotic- and placebo-recipients were unusually high (17.7% and 18.8%, respectively). Second, 98% of patients in both groups had a drain placed, which has previously been shown [16] to be a major risk factor for surgical site infection.

Platt and colleagues [20] compared cefonicid to placebo in certain types of breast surgery (90% of procedures were either lumpectomy or modified radical mastectomy). Not only was the surgical site infection rate reduced by one-half in the cefonicid recipients, but also other benefits were realized. The occurrence of urinary tract infection was reduced, as was the need for postoperative antibiotic therapy, nonroutine visits to a physician for wound healing problems, incision and drainage procedures, and hospital readmission because of wound healing complications. These data indicated that preoperative cefonicid would prevent, for every 1,000 patients undergoing breast surgery, 23 surgical site infections and 16 urinary tract infections. No cost–benefit analysis was conducted.

The investigators [21] further examined the role of preoperative antibiotic prophylaxis in the prevention of surgical site infections by performing a meta-analysis of published data from a randomized trial and an observational data set. A total of 2587 surgical procedures, including excisional biopsy, lumpectomy, mastectomy, reduction mammoplasty, and axillary node dissection, were reviewed. Antibiotic prophylaxis was given in 44% of the procedures and prevented 38% of surgical site infections after controlling for operation type, duration of surgery, and participation in the randomized trial (OR = 0.62; CI_{95} = 0.40–0.95, $P = 0.03$).

DELAYED INFECTIONS

Cellulitis After Axillary Lymph Node Dissection

Cellulitis can complicate axillary lymph node dissection in two patient populations. In one, patients have undergone lymph node dissection as part of surgical intervention with mastectomy [22]. In the other population, patients have had lymph node dissection in conjunction with lumpectomy and radiotherapy as part of the breast-sparing form of treatment of early stage carcinoma known as breast conservation therapy [23–30]. For the former, the anatomical distribution of cellulitis is limited to the ipsilateral upper extremity (Figure 3). For the latter, cellulitis can involve either the ipsilateral upper extremity, which is clinically similar to what is seen among patients who have undergone mastectomy, or the remaining breast in breast conservation therapy patients (Table 2). While the breast is the major area of involvement, some patients may also develop patchy erythema in the anterior upper chest, ipsilateral upper pectoralis, and ipsilateral humeral regions (Figure 4).

Characteristically, the duration between the surgical intervention and the initial episode of cellulitis, the so-called incubation period, is measured in months to years in both the mastectomy group and the lumpectomy patients. Fortunately, the large majority of patients who undergo either form of surgical treatment do not develop cellulitis. Five percent or less do, however,

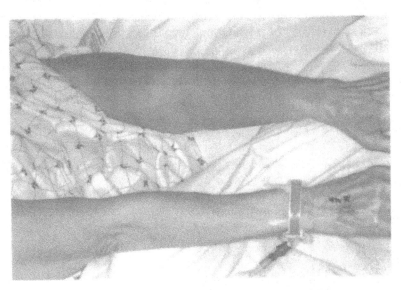

FIGURE 3   Ipsilateral upper extremity cellulitis following axillary lymph node dissection and breast conservation therapy.

TABLE 2   Published Breast Cellulitis Series, 1994–1998

Authors, year [ref]	No. of patients	No. of episodes	No. of patients with recurrences	Mean interval from radiotherapy to initial bout of cellulitis (months)
Rescigno et al., 1994 [23]	11	20	3	10.9
Staren et al., 1996 [24]	10	>11	1	Not mentioned
Hughes et al., 1997 [25]	5	12	3	5.25 (2 patients)
Mertz et al., 1998 [26]	9	13	2	4.9
Miller et al., 1998 [27]	8	8	0	6.75
Total	43	>64	9 (20.9%)	

Source: Reprinted by permission from Baddour LM. Internation J Antimicrob Agents 14:113–116, 2000.

develop cellulitis, often repeatedly. The portion of patients who develop recurrent bouts of cellulitis is dependent upon the length of the follow-up, because recurrences may not occur for years after the initial episode. As a general rule, 20 to 50% of patients who manifest an initial episode of acute cellulitis will develop recurrences.

In one retrospective survey [22] that included patients who had undergone either mastectomy or lumpectomy there were observed differences in the

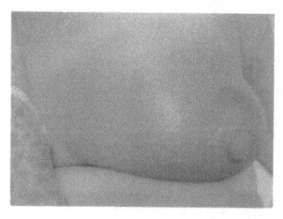

FIGURE 4   Breast cellulitis following breast conservation therapy.

incubation periods for both groups. Six of seven (86%) cellulitis episodes occurred within 1 year of surgery in the lumpectomy group. In contrast, 13 of 19 (68%) bouts of cellulitis among the mastectomy group occurred greater than 1 year postoperatively.

Risk factors for breast cellulitis complicating breast conservation therapy have been analyzed [31]. Seven patients who had developed breast cellulitis were matched to 34 control patients, and potential risk factors were statistically analyzed. Because of a limited sample size, a multiple logistic regression model was not created. Statistical analyses indicated that there were six factors associated with the development of breast cellulitis. These included hematoma formation, postoperative ecchymosis, lymphedema, volume of resected breast tissue, number of previous breast biopsies, and number of breast seroma aspirations. A protective association was found for ecchymosis. Lymphedema was most strongly (10.154 odds ratio; 95% confidence interval, 1.348–208.860) associated with the development of breast cellulitis. The finding that lymphedema was the factor most strongly associated with the onset of cellulitis is consistent with the findings of case-control invetigation [32] of lower extremity cellulitis and a long-held clinical recognition that lymphedema predisposes to the subsequent development of cellulitis. In the case-control study [32] of lower extremity cellulitis–associated risk factors, multivariate analysis was conducted. The odds ratio for lymphedema was 71.2.

A microbiological etiology has not been defined in most cases of cellulitis complicating either mastectomy or lumpectomy, regardless of whether the cellulitic lesion is involving the ipsilateral upper extremity or the remaining breast. Pathogens were identified in only seven of the more than 79 episodes of breast cellulitis described in several case series [29]. Four organisms were identified in 15 episodes of ipsilateral upper extremity cellulitis. Streptococci have been recovered most frequently, including non–group A beta-hemolytic streptococci. Prior work [33] supports the notion that, for as yet undefined reasons, there is an association between venous and lymphatic compromise and cellulitis due to non–group A beta-hemolytic streptococci. Viridans group streptococci have also been isolated from patients with breast and ipsilateral upper extremity cellulitis. This has prompted speculation [28] for an oral source of infection. Viridans group streptococci can colonize skin so that this could also be a source of the organisms. Staphylococci has been recovered less often than streptococci.

Treatment of acute cellulitis is usually empirical because a specific pathogen (Figure 5), as previously outlined, is not identified in the large majority of cases. Antibiotic selection should include coverage of both beta-hemolytic streptococci and *Staphylococcus aureus*. Because these infections are delayed in onset, as compared to what we classically have referred to as postoperative infections (now referred to as surgical site infections), coverage for methicil-

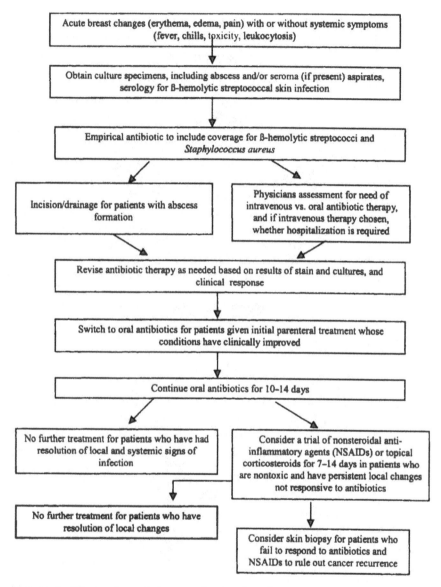

FIGURE 5 Diagnostic and therapeutic algorithm for use in the management of breast cellulitis in patients who have undergone breast conservation therapy. *Source*: Reprinted by permission from Mertz KR et al. Clin Infect Dis 26:481–486, 1998.

lin-resistant strains of *S. aureus* is not required unless there is evidence of prior or current colonization or infection with this organism. Nafcillin or cefazolin are appropriate for use in patients who require parenteral therapy. For those who can be treated with oral agents, cephalexin or dicloxacillin can be used in patients without histories of beta-lactam allergies. Clindamycin is an alternative drug for use in those who cannot be given penicillins or cephalosporins. In addition, clindamycin impacts ribosomal activity of bacteria, and in the case of beta-hemolytic streptococci and *S. aureus*, it limits the production of exotoxins, which are thought to induce host cytokine responses that account for much of the local and systemic signs and symptoms. Surgical intervention may be required if abscess formation complicates breast cellulitis. Abscess formation in the setting of ipsilateral upper extremity cellulitis is unlikely.

Antibiotic therapy is usually administered for 10 to 14 days. Systemic complaints, including fiver, chills, and toxicity, usually resolve within 24 to 48 hours of initiation of appropriate antibiotics. The local cellulitic findings slowly resolve with treatment and may require up to 14 days for complete resolution.

In patients who have persistent local changes of the breast that do not resolve with antibacterial therapy, a limited trial using topical corticosteroids or nonsteroidal anti-inflammatory agents can be employed. Skin biopsy should be considered to evaluate for local breast cancer recurrence.

As previously mentioned, recurrent episodes of cellulitis occur in a considerable portion of patients who develop an initial bout of cellulitis. Thus efforts should be taken to prevent recurrences. Aggressive skin care is mandatory, and treatment of any underlying chronic dermatological diseases such as psoriasis is required. Decongestive lymphatic therapy may be helpful to reduce the severity of lymphedema and possibly the risk of cellulitis recurrence.

Long-term low-dose suppressive therapy with antibiotics can be used for carefully selected patients with frequent and/or severe recurrences. "Preemptive" therapy can also be employed and involves patient-initiated treatment at the earliest sign of cellulitis onset. Numerous factors have to be considered before adopting these choices of therapy, and evaluation by an infectious diseases consultant is advisable.

Winkelmann and colleagues [34] highlighted the clinical features of pseudosclerodermatous panniculitis in four patients who had completed breast conservation therapy. These patients had local breast findings, including edema and erythema, that were attributed to cellulitis. The skin and soft tissue changes developed 1 to 6 months following completion of local radiation therapy and were not associated with systemic findings including fever or toxicity. Antibiotics (either dicloxacillin or erythromycin) were given in each case but had no apparent impact on the local breast changes. Tissue biopsy demonstrated a combination of findings, some of which were radiation-related. There was pronounced lymphocytic dermal and fat infiltration with focal plasma cell deposition. Macrophages were prominent in both dermis and fat tissue. Although the local breast findings decreased over the initial 2 to 5 months, residual signs of inflammation persisted at 6 to 24 months of follow-up.

Other Delayed Infectious Complications

There are additional infection syndromes that can occur months to years following initial surgical intervention for breast cancer. These include breast abscess, septic arthritis of the ipsilateral shoulder, and sternal wound infection following coronary artery bypass graft surgery in patients previously treated for breast cancer.

Keidan and colleagues [35] retrospectively reviewed the charts of 112 patients who had undergone breast conservation therapy at their medical center over 28 months. The median follow-up of patients after surgery was 18 months. Seven (6.25%) patients developed breast abscess from 1.5 to 8 months (median, 5 months) following lumpectomy with axillary lymph node dissection. None of the patients had diabetes mellitus or were immunocompromised. Two of the seven patients did develop abscesses while receiving adjunctive chemotherapy. Four patients had either prior biopsy site infection, skin (incision) edge necrosis, or seromas ($n = 2$) that required aspiration for pain relief. All abscesses occurred in patients seen in the first 12 months of the study period. The risk of abscess formation was statistically associated with the size of the lumpectomy specimen submitted to pathology (152.6 vs. 111.2 cc, mean; 134 vs. 80 cc median; $P = 0.0440$). All patients responded to antibiotics and either surgical drainage of the abscess ($n = 6$) or drainage performed by serial percutaneous aspiration ($n = 1$). Cosmesis was affected in six patients.

Septic arthritis of the ipsilateral shoulder has been described in five patients who had undergone prior mastectomy and radiotherapy [36]. Arthritis symptoms appeared years after mastectomy, and all patients had underlying ipsilateral upper extremity lymphedema. Diagnosis was delayed in all cases with joint destruction ($n = 2$) or movement restriction ($n = 2$) complicating infection. Radionecrosis was considered as the cause of the joint complaints in all five cases rather than infection. Interestingly, non–group A beta-hemolytic streptococci were recovered in two cases. S. aureus ($n = 2$) and S. epidermidis ($n = 1$) were isolated in the remaining three cases.

The risk of sternal wound infection may be increased in patients who undergo coronary artery bypass grafting and have previously had mastectomy or lumpectomy and radiotherapy [37]. In one case-control analysis, the sternal wound infection rate was higher in the breast cancer group than in the control group without previously treated breast cancer (25% vs. 6%, P = 0.027). The mean time interval between breast surgery and subsequent bypass grafting was 15.9 years with a range of from 1 to 32 years. Independent variables that were associated with sternal wound infections by multivariate analysis were radiotherapy (P = 0.018; odds ratio = 10.9) and recent history of myocardial infarction (P = 0.035; odds ratio = 7.4). Patients with a history of right-sided breast cancer had a higher sternal wound complication rate than those with prior left-sided breast cancer (50% vs. 12.5%; P = 0.068, odds ratio = 7). One possible explanation for this difference based on sidedness was that prior radiotherapy-induced devascularization occurred with the right internal mammary artery, and because the left internal mammary artery had been harvested for grafting, the sternum was left in an avascular state, which led to poor wound healing and infection.

INFECTIONS THAT COMPLICATE BREAST RECONSTRUCTION

Infections that complicate breast reconstruction fall into two broad categories. In one, autogenous tissue is used to reconstruct the breast following mastectomy for breast cancer. In the other, a prosthesis is used for implantation to create the breast. A tissue expander is another type of medical device that can become infected. It is used as a temporary device that is ultimately removed and replaced by a permanent implant, or it can itself serve as a permanent implant.

Infections of Autogenous Tissue

As pointed out by Menke and colleagues [38], because of more advanced disease, breast conservation therapy is not a treatment option in approximately 30% of patients with breast cancer, and mastectomy is required. Autogenous tissue, including musculocutaneous latissimus dorsi (LDF), transverse rector abdominis musculocutaneous (TRAM), and deep inferior epigastric perforator (DIEP) flaps have been used for years to create the breast.

In the most recent series reported, Menke et al. [38] retrospectively examined the results of breast reconstruction with LDF at their institution. One hundred twenty-one patients with at least 12 months of follow-up were included in this review at a teaching hospital between 1994 and 1998. The complication rate was low, with the exception of seroma formation (60%), and wound infection occurred in 2% of patients. No flap was lost, and 90% of patients had no complaints with the procedure.

Earlier studies detail the results of TRAM flaps. Jacobsen and colleagues [39] described their experience with 147 consecutive patients who had the procedure performed at the Mayo Clinic between 1981 and 1992. The median duration of follow-up was 29 months, and no TRAM flap infection occurred.

Watterson and coworkers [40] examined their clinical experience with 556 female patients who had undergone TRAM flap breast reconstruction, 89% of whom had a history of breast cancer. The patients had been seen between 1982 and 1992 and had an overall complication rate of 23.7 percent. Complications included partial flap loss, fat necrosis, abdominal hernia, hematoma, wound infection, or a group of miscellaneous events. Wound infection occurred in 5% of patients. Multivariate analysis using stepwise logistic regression indicated that risk factors for overall complications included smoking, history of radiation therapy, obesity, and "significant" abdominal scarring.

Paige and colleagues [41] reviewed the records of all women who had undergone bilateral or unilateral pedicled TRAM flap reconstruction and analyzed cases depending upon whether breast site infection or abdominal infection occurred. In patients with unilateral flaps, the breast and abdominal infection rates were both 2.4 percent. The infection rates for both anatomical sites among patients who underwent bilateral TRAM flap reconstruction was statistically similar to those who underwent unilateral procedures (4.6 and 2.3%, respectively). Breast wound infections were associated with obesity, smoking, diabetes mellitus, and hypertension. Infection at the abdominal-donor site was associated with diabetes mellitus, obesity, prior irradiation, smoking, hypertension, and the presence of two or more comorbid factors.

Infections of Tissue Expanders and Implants

Tissue expanders and implants are used to reconstruct the breast. Tissue expanders can be used temporarily and later replaced with permanent implants or used permanently in place of an implant. Tissue expanders, like implants, are foreign material and magnify the likelihood of infection at the surgical site. In one retrospective analysis [42], immediate reconstruction with tissue expanders at the time of mastectomy was a risk factor for the subsequent development of breast infection. Of the eight (24%) out of 33 patients who underwent reconstructive surgery and developed infection, all eight (53%) were among a subgroup of 15 patients who had immediate reconstruction with a tissue expander. Delayed use of a tissue expander did not increase infection risk. The results of this study may have limited applicability today because patients were seen between 1985 and 1986 and tissue expanders have undergone a number of technical advances since then.

Disa and colleagues [43] reviewed the charts of 770 consecutive patients seen at the Memorial Sloan-Kettering Cancer Center between 1987 to 1997 who had received tissue expanders at the time of mastectomy (90%) or as a secondary procedure (10%). Tissue expansion was generally begun 10 to 14 days following insertion and continued on a weekly basis until completion or removal. Only fourteen (1.8%) patients required premature device removal, and they were removed, on average, 3.2 months following placement. In 7 (50%) cases, premature removal was due to device infection. At least three of these infections were due to *S. aureus*. In one case, *Enterobacter* species was isolated from wound cultures, and in the three remaining cases, wound cultures were negative.

Gabriel and colleagues [44] surveyed the medical records of 749 women who were residents of Olmsted County, Minnesota, and received their first breast implant at the Mayo Clinic between 1964 and 1991. They cataloged complications among the group that led to additional surgical intervention after implantation. Implantation had been done for cosmetic reasons in 532 patients and related to cancer or to prophylactic mastectomy in 125 and 92 patients, respectively. The mean duration of follow-up was 7.8 years among the three groups. Two hundred eight women had 450 additional implant-related surgical procedures. Of these, complications prompted additional surgery in 178 (23.8%) of patients. Infectious complications at the implantation site prompted surgical intervention in 19 women. Overall, the local complication rate varied greatly among the three populations. It was highest for patients who had had implantation after mastectomy for breast cancer (21.8% at 1 year, 34% at 5 years). The rates for patients who had undergone prophylactic mastectomy were 17.3% at 1 year and 30.4% at 5 years. The rates for these two groups were significantly ($P < 0.001$) greater than that seen for patients who had undergone implantation for cosmetic reasons (6.5% at 1 year, 12% at 5 years).

Furey and coworkers [45] reviewed their experience with 112 patients with breast cancer who had undergone mastectomy and immediate breast reconstruction with implants. They found no statistical risk ($P = 0.13$) increase in wound complications among patients who also received early adjunctive chemotherapy as compared to those who did not receive chemotherapy. They therefore concluded that chemotherapy need not be delayed in these patients. The rate of wound complications was approximately 50% higher, however, in the group given chemotherapy (27.8%) than that seen in the group that received no chemotherapy (17.9%). Thus the statistical power of the comparison may have been limited owing to the relatively small number of patients included in the analysis. Also, a greater number of axillary lymph nodes were resected in the chemotherapy group, which could have been reflective of more extensive surgery, and this could have impacted the wound complication rate.

Women who have had mantle irradiation for prior Hodgkin's disease are at risk of developing breast cancer. They make up a unique population of women who often develop bilateral breast cancer at a younger age. Complications following breast reconstruction using tissue expanders and implants were examined in seven patients who had undergone mastectomy and had been previously treated for Hodgkin's disease [46]. Their mean age was 35 years (range, 28 to 42 years). All seven underwent two-stage reconstruction with initial placement of tissue expanders at the time of mastectomy (bilateral in five patients), and later the expanders were replaced with textured surface saline-filled implants. The average follow-up was three years, and in only one case did infection (cellulitis) complicate the postoperative course. No revisions were requested or required. Thus these patients can be considered for breast implant reconstruction, as mantle irradiation did not compromise the results of this procedure.

A variety of microorganisms have been associated with breast implantation infections. The infections vary in onset and can appear days to weeks to months following implantation. This is, in part, related to the virulence of the infecting organism. For less virulent organisms, including coagulase-negative staphylococci, *Corynebacterium* species and *Propionibacterium acnes*, infection is indolent in its presentation. Because clinical signs and symptoms may be subtle, diagnosis of infection can be difficult. For more aggressive pathogens, including *S. aureus* and aerobic gram-negative bacilli, the clinical presentation of infection is acute. Rarely, the more acute presentation following implantation can be complicated by toxic shock syndrome [47]. This complication is not limited to implantation procedures; toxic shock syndrome has also been described as a complication of autogenous tissue breast reconstruction with TRAM and LDF procedures [48,49].

Mycobacterial species [50–54], fungi [55,56], anaerobes [57], *Listeria* [58], and *Enterococcus* species [59] are some of the additional microorganisms that have been described as causes of breast implantation infection. Because of the wide variety of organisms that can produce implant infection, choosing empirical therapy is difficult, and aspiration of periprosthetic fluid should be done to secure an etiological diagnosis to direct antimicrobial therapy.

There are no evidence-based data that address two of the most important issues in treating implant infections. First, an appropriate duration of antimicrobial therapy is undefined. At least two weeks of treatment, usually with parenterally administered drugs, is given, particularly if implant salvage is the goal. Second, factors that necessitate implant removal have not been established. For those patients with implant infection who clinically worsen despite treatment or suffer systemic toxicity, the decision to remove the infected implant is straightforward. Patients with infection caused by nontuberculous mycobacterial species [50–54] should also be considered for device removal because infection is difficult to cure otherwise. For patients who do not fall into these categories, an individualized approach should be adopted in regard to device removal.

REFERENCES

1. Dauphin S, Katz S, El Tamer M, Wait R, Sohn C, Braverman AS. Chemotherapy is a safe and effective initial therapy for infected malignant breast and chest wall ulcers. J Surg Oncol 1997; 66:186–188.
2. Finkel LJ, Griffiths CEM. Inflammatory breast carcinoma (carcinoma erysipeloides): an easily overlooked diagnosis. Brit J Derm 1993; 129:324–326.
3. Meadows, Kappa P, Conleth AG. Vesicular carcinoma erysipelatodes. Acad Derm 1999; 40:805–807.
4. Siegel JM. Inflammatory carcinoma of the breast. AMA Arch Derm and Syphil 1952; 66:710–716.
5. Melamed JB, Schein M, Decker GAG. Squamous carcinoma of the breast presenting as an abscess. S African Med J 1986; 69:771–772.
6. Nguyen SL, Doyle AJ, Symmans PJ. Interstitial fluid and hypoechoic wall: two sonographic signs of breast abscess. J Clin Ultrasound 2000; 28:319–324.
7. Stevenson JT, Graham J, Khiyami A, Mansour EG. Squamous cell carcinoma of the breast: a clinical approach. Ann Surg Oncol 1996; 3:367–374.
8. Wrightson WR, Edwards MJ, McMaster KM. Primary squamous cell carcinoma of the breast presenting as a breast abscess. Am Surg 1999; 65:1153–1155.
9. The Society for Hospital Epidemiology Control, the Association for Practitioners in Infection Control, the Centers for Disease Control, the Surgical Infection Society. Consensus paper on the surveillance of surgical wound infections. Infect Cont Hosp Epidemiol 1992; 20:263–270.
10. Horan TC, Gaynes RP, Martone WJ, Jarvis WR, Emori TG. CDC definitions of nosocomial surgical site infections, 1992: a modification of CDC definitions of surgical wound infections. Infect Cont Hosp Epidemiol 1992; 13:606–608.
11. DHHS and CDC Draft Guidelines for the Prevention of Surgical Site Infection 1998. Fed Regist 1998; 63:33168–33192.
12. Cruse PJ, Foord R. The epidemiology of wound infection. A 10-year prospective study of 62,939 wounds. Surg Clin N Am 1980; 60:27–40.
13. Olson M, O'Connor M, Schwartz ML. Surgical wound infections. A 5-year prospective study of 20,193 wounds at the Minneapolis VA Medical Center. Ann Surg 1984; 199:253 259.
14. Haley RW, Culver DH, Morgan WM, White JW, Emori TG, Hooton TM. Identifying patients at high risk of surgical wound infection. A simple multivariate index of patient susceptibility and wound contamination. Am J Epidemiol 1985; 121:206–215.
15. Culver DH, Horan TC, Gaynes RP, Martone WJ, Jarvis WR, Emori TG, Banerjee SN, Edwards JR, Tolson JS, Henderson TS, Hughes JM, NNIS System. Surgical wound infection rates by wound class, operative procedure, and patient

risk index. National Nosocomial Infections Surveillance System. Am J Med 1991; 91(suppl 3B):152S–157S.

16. Rotstein C, Ferguson R, Cummings M, Piedmonte MR, Lucey J, Banish A. Determinants of clean surgical wound infections for breast procedures at an oncology center. Infect Cont Hosp Epidemiol 1992; 13:207–214.

17. Hall JC, Hall JL. Antibiotic prophylaxis for patients undergoing breast surgery. J Hosp Infect 2000; 46:165–170.

18. Bertin ML, Crowe J, Gordon SM. Determinants of surgical site infection after breast surgery. Am J Infect Cont 1998; 26:61–65.

19. Gupta R, Sinnett D, Carpenter R, Preece PE, Royle GT. Antibiotic prophylaxis for postoperative wound infection in clean elective breast surgery. Europ J Surg Oncol 2000; 26:363–366.

20. Platt R, Zaleznik DF, Hopkins CC, Dellinger EP, Karchmer AW, Bryan CS, Burke JF, Wikler MA, Marino SK, Holbrook KF, Tosteson TD, Segal MR. Perioperative antibiotic prophylaxis for herniorrhaphy and breast surgery. N Engl J Med 1990; 322:153–160.

21. Platt R, Zucker JR, Zaleznik DF, Hopkins CC, Dellinger EP, Karchmer AW, Bryan CS, Burke JF, Wikler MA, Marino SK, Holbrook KF, Tosteson TD. Perioperative antibiotic prophylaxis and wound infection following breast surgery. J Antimicrobial Chemother 1993; 31(suppl B):43–48.

22. Simon MS, Cody RL. Cellulitis after axillary lymph node dissection for carcinoma of the breast. Am J Med 1992; 93:543–548.

23. Rescigno J, McCormick B, Brown AE, Myskowski PL. Breast cellulitis after conservative surgery and radiotherapy. Int J Rad Oncol Biol Phys 1994; 29:163–168.

24. Staren ED, Klepac S, Smith AP, Hartsell WF, Sergretti J, Witt TR, Griem KL, Bines SD. The dilemma of delayed cellulitis after breast conservation therapy. Arch Surg 1996; 131:651–654.

25. Hughes LL, Styblo TM, Thoms WW, Schwatzmann SW, Landry JC, Heaton D, Carsor GW, Wood WC. Cellulitis of the breast as a complication of breast-conserving surgery and irradiation. Am J Clin Oncol 1997; 20:338–341.

26. Mertz KR, Baddour LM, Bell JL, Gwin JL. Breast cellulitis following breast conservation therapy: a novel complication of medical progress. Clin Infect Dis 1998; 26:481–486.

27. Miller SR, Mondry T, Reed RS, Findley A, Johnstone PAS. Delayed cellulitis associated with conservative therapy for breast cancer. J Surg Oncol 1998; 67:242–245.

28. Manian FA. Cellulitis associated with an oral source of infection in breast cancer patients: report of two cases. Scand J Infect Dis 1997; 29:421–422.

29. Baddour LM. Breast cellulitis complicating breast conservation therapy. J Intern Med 1999; 245:5–9.

30. Baddour LM. Cellulitis syndromes: an update. Internat J Antimicrob Agents 2000; 14:113–116.

31. Brewer VH, Hahn KA, Rohrbach BW, Bell JL, Baddour LM. Risk factor

analysis for breast cellulitis following breast conservation therapy. Clin Infect Dis 2000; 31:654–659.

32. Dupuy A, Benchiki H, Roujeau J-C, Bernard P, Vaillant L, Chosidow O, Sassolas B, Guillaume J-C, Groh J-J, Bastuji-Garin S. Risk factors for erysipelas of the leg (cellulitis): case-control study. Brit Med J 1999; 318:1591 1594.

33. Baddour LM, Bisno AL. Non group A beta-hemolytic streptococcal cellulitis. Association with venous and lymphatic compromise. Am J Med 1985; 79:155–159.

34. Winkelmann RK, Grado GL, Quimby SR, Connolly SM. Pseudoscleroder-matous panniculitis after irradiation: an unusual complication of mega voltage treatment of breast carcinoma. Mayo Clin Proceed 1993; 68:122–127.

35. Keidan RD, Hoffman JP, Weese JL, Hanks GE, Solin LJ, Eisenberg BL, Ottery FD, Boraas M. Delayed breast abscesses after lumpectomy and radiation therapy. Am Surg 1990; 56:440–444.

36. Chaudhuri K, Lonergan D, Portek I, McGuigan L. Septic arthritis of the shoulder after mastectomy and radiotherapy for breast carcinoma. J Bone Joint Surg (Br) 1993; 75-B:318–321.

37. Erez E, Eldar S, Sharoni E, Abramor D, Sulkes A, Vidne BA. Coronary artery operation in patients after breast cancer therapy. Ann Thorac Surg 1998; 66: 1312–1317.

38. Menke H, Erkens M, Olbrisch RR. Evolving concepts in breast reconstruction with latissimus dorsi flaps: results and follow-up of 121 consecutive patients. Ann Plast Surg 2001; 47:107–114.

39. Jacobsen WM, Meland NB, Woods JE. Autologous breast reconstruction with use of transverse rectus abdominis musculocutaneous flap: Mayo Clinic experience with 147 cases. Mayo Clin Proceed 1994; 69:635–640.

40. Watterson PA, Bostwick J III, Hester TR Jr, Bried JT, Taylor GI. TRAM flap anatomy correlated with a 10-year clinical experience with 556 patients. Plast Reconstr Surg 1995; 95:1185–1194.

41. Paige KT, Bostwick J III, Bried JT, Jones G. A comparison of morbidity from bilateral, unipedicled and unilateral, unipedicled TRAM flap breast reconstruc-tions. Plast Reconstr Surg 1998; 101:1819–1827.

42. Armstrong RW, Berkowitz RL, Bolding F. Infection following breast recon-struction. Ann Plast Surg 1989; 23:284–288.

43. Disa JJ, Ad-EL DD, Cohen SM, Cordeiro PG, Hidalgo DA. The premature removal of tissue expanders in breast reconstruction. Plast Reconstr Surg 1999; 104:1662 1665.

44. Gabriel SE, Woods JE, O'Fallon WM, Beard CM, Kurland LT, Melton LJ III. Complications leading to surgery after breast implantation. N Engl J Med 1997; 336:677–682.

45. Furey PC, MacGillivray DC, Castiglione CL, Allen L. Wound complications in patients receiving adjunctive chemotherapy after mastectomy and immediate breast reconstruction for breast cancer. J Surg Oncol 1994; 55:194–197.

46. Bacilious N, Cordeiro PG, Disa JJ, Hidalgo DA. Breast reconstruction using

tissue expanders and implants in Hodgkin's patients with prior mantle irradiation. Plast Reconstr Surg 2002; 109:102–107.

47. Holm C, Mühlbauer W. Toxic shock syndrome in plastic surgery patients: case report and review of the literature. Aesth Plast Surg 1998; 22:180–184.

48. Cederna JP. Toxic shock syndrome after transverse rectus abdominis musculoskeletal flap reconstruction. Ann Plast Surg 1995; 34:73–75.

49. Gosain AK, Larson DL. Toxic shock syndrome following latissimus dorsi musculocutaneous flap breast reconstruction. Ann Plast Surg 1992; 29:571–575.

50. Clegg HW, Foster MT, Sanders WE Jr, Baine WB. Infection due to organisms of the *Mycobacterium fortuitum* complex after augmentation mammoplasty: clinical and epidemiologic features. J Infect Dis 1983; 147:427–432.

51. Walsh R, Kliewer MA, Sullivan DC, Hertzberg B, Paulson EK, Soo MS, Saksouk FA, Kornguth PJ. Periprosthetic mycobacterial infection. CT and mammographic findings. Clin Imaging 1995; 19:193–196.

52. Lee D, Goldstein EJC, Zarem HA. Localized *Mycobacterium avium–intracellulare* mastitis in an immunocompetent woman with silicone breast implants. Plast Reconstr Surg 1995; 95:142–144.

53. Eliopoulos DA, Lyle G. *Mycobacterium avium* infection in a patient with the acquired immunodeficiency syndrome and silicone breast implants. South Med J 1999; 92:80–83.

54. Heinstein JB, Mangino JE, Ruberg RL, Bergese JJ. A prosthetic breast implant infected with *Mycobacterium fortuitum*. Ann Plast Surg 2000; 44:330–334.

55. Niazi ZBM, Salzberg CA, Montecalvo M. *Candida albicans* infection of bilateral polyurethane-coated silicone gel breast implants. Ann Plast Surg 1996; 37:91–93.

56. Young YL, Hertl MC, Murray PR, Lambros VS. *Paecilomyces variotii* contamination in the lumen of a saline-filled breast implant. Plast Reconstr Surg 1995; 96:1430–1434.

57. Hunter JG, Padilla M, Cooper-Vastola S. Late *Clostridium perfringens* breast implant infection after dental treatment. Ann Plast Surg 1996; 36:309–312.

58. Gnanadesigan N, Pechter EA, Mascola L. *Listeria* infection of silicone breast implant. Plast Reconstr Surg 1994; 94:531–535.

59. Ablaza VJ, laTrenta GS. Late infection of breast prosthesis with *Enterococcus avium*. Plast Reconstr Surg 1998; 102:227–230.

17

Infectious Complications of Gastrointestinal Cancer

Albert L. Vincent
University of South Florida School of Medicine
Tampa, Florida, U.S.A.

John N. Greene
University of South Florida School of Medicine
and Moffitt Cancer Center and Research Institute
Tampa, Florida, U.S.A.

COLORECTAL CANCER

Among underlying bowel cancers, adenocarcinoma of the colon is most likely to present as a bacteremia, an abscess, or gangrene. Although many infections have been associated with underlying cancer of the large bowel, *Streptococcus bovis* septicemia and *Clostridium septicum* gangrene are the most frequently reported. Infections may spread from the site of the primary neoplasm or metastasize to distant sites from nectrotic tumors during transient bacteremia [1]. These unusual infections may be the first presentation or the sole clue to bowel cancer and should prompt a precautionary colonoscopy. Some recently reported sites of abscesses include the abdominal wall [2,3], retroperitoneum [4] gluteus muscle [5], psoas muscle [6], spleen [7], liver [8], pleural space [9], and eye [10]. Translocation of intestinal bacteria to mesenteric lymph nodes seems to be common in patients with cecal carcinoma, but it has no clinical significance unless other lesions are superimposed [11].

Of 162 cases of atraumatic cases of *C. septicum* reviewed by Kornbluth et al. [12], 44% proved to have an associated colon adenocarcinoma, and most of the rest had a hematological malignancy. In many patients, a portal of entry could be identified in the large bowel. Relatively aerotolerant, *Clostridium septicum* is a major cause of spontaneous nontraumatic gas gangrere in the extremities, solid organs, or retroperitoneum. A colonic carcinoma is often the portal of entry to the bloodstream and a source of metastatis to remote sites. The characteristic presentation includes excruciating pain, swelling of tissue, crepitance, and bullae. Inflammatory cells are characteristically absent, and the majority of patients expire within 24 hours of onset [13]. Clostridial myonecrosis and associated malignancies carry a high risk of mortality, but early diagnosis and treatment may avert unnecessary deaths [14]. "Distant myonecrosis" and gangrene may cause death in 79% of patients, often hours after diagnosis [12]. Myocarditis is rare but was extensive in a case reported by den Bakker et al. [15]. Symptoms may be minimal or nonspecific until just before fulminant toxemia [16]. Patients who develop signs and symptoms of sepsis, especially associated with abdominal pain or acute pain in an extremity, should be treated for presumed clostridial infection and subjected to a thorough search for an underlying colonic malignancy. Asymptomatic bacteremia with Clostridia species should prompt a computerized tomography scan for intra-abdominal abscesses [12]. Diabetic patients are also at risk for occult colon cancer resulting in Clostridial infections and require urgent laparotomy [17]. Ridgeway and Grech [18] reviewed the literature on *C. septicum* as a cause of endocarditis. Colon cancer was frequently identified as the source of infection. In the absence of a history of antibiotic use, *C. difficle*–associated diarrhea may indicate an underlying colonic neoplasm [19].

Streptococcus bovis septicemia is a relatively uncommon finding. These patients are at high risk of harboring undetected colorectal adenocarcinoma or adenomatous polyps. Bacteremia may also be associated with viral or alcoholic liver disease [20]. It is important to differentiate the species of any Group D streptococci isolated from the blood, as *S. bovis* belongs to this group [21]. Patients with positive cultures should be considered for yearly colonoscopy. Interestingly, *S. bovis* does not appear selectively to colonize colorectal neoplasms [22].

Streptococcus bovis bacteremia has long been associated with colon cancer. Colonic polyps with dysplastic change have been reported in 18.2% of patients with *S. bovis* peritonitis. Diagnostic paracentesis, blood culture, and ascitic fluid culture are indicated. The treatment of choice is still intravenous penicillin [23]. The incidence of *S. bovis* endocarditis has increased, especially in the elderly population. A 74-year-old man with intermittent fever over the past two months became afebrile after 3 days administration of penicillin G. A colonofiberoscopy revealed an occult 2 × 2 cm mass that proved to be an adenocarcinoma of the colon [24]. Ballet et al. [25] reviewed a series of *S. bovis* endocarditis cases in a tertiary care cardiology hospital between 1980 and 1991. The mean age was 59 years. Twelve had previously suffered valvular disease, and three had a valvular prosthesis. Forty-three patients (81%) were given a full colon examination, which revealed polyps in 20 and adenocarcinoma in seven. Patients became afebrile after antibiotic treatment, but 11 late deaths were attributed to the underlying malignancy [25]. *S. bovis* endocarditis may be complicated by embolic events or, rarely, osteomyelitis [26]. Also recently reported are brain abscess [27], peritonitis [28], lateral neck abscess [29], splenic abscess [30], septic arthritis [31], and thoracic empyema [32].

Streptococcus salivarius was documented as a cause of fulminant meningitis in an elderly patient. Because exact speciation of streptococci is difficult, investigations for underlying neoplasms are perhaps also warranted by infections with species closely related to *S. bovis* [33]. Presentations which have also pointed to underlying colorectal neoplasms include *S. sanguis* bacteremia [34]. *S. anginosus* spondylodiskitis [35], and *S. milleri* liver abscess [36].

Enterococcus faecalis is another organism that should prompt a search for an underlying carcinoma of the large bowel [37]. A 66-year-old woman with abdominal pain, fever, and chills proved to have a hepatic abscess that responded to percutaneous drainage and intravenous long-term antibiotics. Pus cultures grew *E. faecalis*. Colon cancer was found during the management of the liver abcess. Rare organisms ordinarily of low pathogenicity can cause severe infections in patients with colon cancer. *Staphlococcus cohnii* was isolated from the peripheral blood and central venous catheter of a patient with colon cancer and sepsis [38].

In addition to the association of bacteremia and metastatic infection with colon cancer, infectious complications from local tumor spread can occur. These infections result from obstruction, perforation, or fistula formation. In addition, an advanced colorectal cancer with a necrotic center can communicate with the intestinal lumen and become infected, resulting in abscess or fistula formation. In patients with unresectable bulky tumor with frequent bouts of bacteremia or infectious-related fever, long-term antibiotics directed against enteric flora may reduce or eliminate these complications. However, this approach must be weighed against the development of resistant pathogens.

STOMACH CANCER

Cancer of the stomach usually does not increase the risk of infection unless perforation or obstruction occurs. Lymphoma of the stomach is more likely to perforate, especially following chemotherapy. As the tumor is reduced in size, the wall of the stomach may become thinned, perforate, and lead to peritonitis and/or sepsis. Most infections related to stomach cancer are a result of a postsurgical wound infection, peritonitis, or an intra-abdominal abscess.

There are relatively few reports of infections and sepsis secondary to stomach cancer, but some unusual organisms have been noted. *Candida catenulata*, a contaminant of dairy products, was repeatedly isolated from the blood of a patient who often ate cheese and had multiple gastric ulcers as well as stomach cancer [39]. The protozoan *Entamoeba histolytica*, a pathogen of the colon, was found within a large-cell β lymphoma of the stomach [40]. In contrast to colorectal cancer, stomach cancer is only rarely associated with *Streptococcus bovis* bacteremia [41]. *Citrobacter diversus* was isolated from the blood and bronchioalveolar lavage of a 61-year-old man with a localized gastric tumor and pneumonia [42]. Other streptococcal isolates include bacteremia from Group B *Streptococcus* in a case of adenocarcinoma of the stomach [43], alpha hemolytic streptococci in a liver abscess of a young woman with a gastric leiomyosarcoma [44], and *S. anginosis*, again in a liver abscess [45].

ESOPHAGEAL CANCER

Esophageal cancer is associated with infection when local extension results in mediastinitis, or fistula formation between the trachea, bronchi, pleural, or pericardial space [46–48]. As with colon cancer resulting in *S. bovis* bacteremia, a case of Group G streptococcus bacteremia led to the diagnosis of an occult esophageal carcinoma [49]. Obstruction of the esophagus can result in aspiration pneumonia. However, most infections related to esophageal cancer are postsurgical complications ranging from wound infections to mediastinitis, empyema, and pneumonia. The most common pathogens are oral or enteric flora and represent polymicrobial infection. Radiation therapy can cause radiation esophagitis or result in an infectious esophagitis due to Candida species, herpes simplex virus, or CMV. Dilation of a malignant stricture may be followed by esophageal rupture, mediastinitis, and empyema [50].

In summary, most infections related to gastrointestinal malignancies are due to local tumor extension or postsurgical complications. However, the association of (1) bacteremia and distant foci infection with *S. bovis* and *C. septicum* and (2) occult colon cancer remains a diagnostic and therapeutic challenge.

REFERENCES

1. Panwalker AP. Unusual infections associated with colorectal cancer. Rev Infect Dis 1988; 10(2):347–364.

2. John AK, Gur U, Cade D. Carcinoma of sigmoid colon presenting as abdominal wall abscess. Indian J Gastroenterol 2002; 21(3):117 118.

3. Matsumoto G, Asano H, Kato E, Matsuno S. Transverse colonic cancer presenting as an anterior abdominal wall abscess: report of a case. Surg Today 2001; 31(2):166–169.

4. Lizarralde E, Martinez Odriozola P, Tobalina I, Maniega R, Miguel F. Intra-abdominal abscess as presentation of colonic cancer. An Med Interna 2000; 17(1):32–34. Spanish.

5. Shimizu J, Kinoshita T, Tatsuzawa Y, Takehara A, Kawaura Y, Takahashi S. Gluteal abscess caused by perforating rectal cancer: case report and review of the literature. Tumori 2001; 87(5):330–331.

6. Kobayashi H, Sakurai Y, Shoji M, Nakamura Y, Suganuma M, Imazu H, Hasegawa S, Matsubara T, Ochiai M, Funabiki T. Psoas abscess and cellulitis of the right gluteal region resulting from carcinoma of the cecum. J Gastroenterol 2001; 36(9):623 -628.

7. Nakao A, Iwagaki H, Isozaki H, Kanagawa T, Matsubara N, Takakura N, Tanaka N. Portal venous gas associated with splenic abscess secondary to colon cancer. Aticancer Res 1999; 19(6C):5641–5644.

8. Sarmiento JM, Sarr MG. Necrotic infected liver metastasis from colon cancer. Surgery 2002; 132(1):110–111.

9. Osada T, Nagawa H, Masaki T, Tsuno NH, Sunami E, Watanabe T, Muto T, Shibata Y. Thoracic empyema associated with recurrent colon cancer: report of a case and review of the literature. Dis Colon Rectum 2001; 44(2):291–294.

10. Augsten R, Konigsdorffer E, Strobel J. Endogenous endophthalmitis in severe generalized diseases. Ophthalmologe 1997; 94(6):397–400. In German.

11. Schoeffel U, Pelz K, Haring RU, Amberg R, Schandl R, Urbaschek R, von Specht BU, Farthmann EH. Inflammatory consequences of the translocation of bacteria and endotoxin to mesenteric lymph nodes. Am J Surg 2000; 180(1):65–72.

12. Kornbluth AA, Danzig JB, Bernstein LH. *Clostridium septicum* infection and associated malignancy. Report of 2 cases and review of the literature. Medicine (Baltimore) 1989; 68(1):30–37.

13. Stevens DL, Musher DM, Watson DA, Eddy H, Hamill RJ, Gyorkey F, Rosen H, Mader J. Spontaneous, nontraumatic gangrene due to *Clostridium septicum*. Rev Infect Dis 1990; 12(2):286–296.

14. Fernandez RJ, Gluck JL. *Clostridium septicum* gas gangrene of the gluteus maximus and an ascending colon malignant tumor. A case report. Clin Orthop 1994; (308):178–182.

15. den Bakker MA, Werdmuller RF, Niemans A, Maartense E, Eulderink F. Gas gangrene of ischemic myocardial tissue caused by *Clostridium septicum*. Ned Tijdschr Geneeskd 1996; 140(51):2547–2550. In Dutch.

16. Kolbeinsson ME, Holder WD Jr, Aziz S. Recognition, management, and prevention of *Clostridium septicum* abscess in immunosuppressed patients. Arch Surg 1991; 126(5):642 645.

17. Kudsk KA. Occult gastrointestinal malignancies producing metastatic *Clostridium septicum* infections in diabetic patients. Surgery 1992; 112(4):765–770.

18. Ridgeway EJ, Grech ED. Clostridial endocarditis: report of a case caused by *Clostridium septicum* and review of the literature. J Infect 1993; 26(3):309–313.
19. Heymann TD, Rampton DS. Community-acquired Clostridium difficile–associated diarrhoea in a patient with colonic carcinoma. Int J Clin Pract 1998; 52(2): 132–133.
20. Gonzalez-Quintela A, Martinez-Rey C, Castroagudin JF, Rajo-Iglesias MC, Dominguez-Santalla MJ. Prevalence of liver disease in patients with *Streptococcus bovis* bacteraemia. J Infect 2001; 42(2):116–119.
21. Grieve DA, Chen SC, Chapuis PH, Bradbury R. *Streptococcus bovis* bacteraemia: its significance for the colorectal surgeon. Aust N Z J Surg 1990; 60(7):550–552.
22. Norfleet RG, Mitchell PD. *Streptococcus bovis* does not selectively colonize colorectal cancer and polyps. J Clin Gastroenterol 1993; 17(1):25–28.
23. Vilaichone RK, Mahachai V, Kullavanijaya P, Nunthapisud P. Spontaneous bacterial peritonitis caused by *Streptococcus bovis*: case series and review of the literature. Am J Gastroenterol 2002; 97(6):1476–1479.
24. Ma HM, Shyu KG, Hwang JJ, Huang SH, Hsieh WC, Lien WP. *Streptococcus bovis* endocarditis associated with colonic adenocarcinoma: report of a case. J Formos Med Assoc 1992; 91(8):814–817.
25. Ballet M, Gevigney G, Gare JP, Delahaye F, Etienne J, Delahaye JP. Infective endocarditis due to *Streptococcus bovis*. A report of 53 cases. Eur Heart J 1995; 16(12):1975–1980.
26. Spadafora PF, Qadir MT, Cunha BA. *Streptococcus bovis* endocarditis and vertebral osteomyelitis. Heart Lung 1996; 25(2):165–168.
27. Emiliani VJ, Chodos JE, Comer GM, Holness LG, Schwartz AJ. *Streptococcus bovis* brain abscess associated with an occult colonic villous adenoma. Am J Gastroenterol 1990; 85(1):78–80.
28. Ackerman Z, Eliakim R, Stalnikowicz R. Spontaneous peritonitis caused by *Streptococcus bovis*: search for colonic neoplasia. J Clin Gastroenterol 1995; 21(3):263.
29. Goumas PD, Naxakis SS, Rentzis GA, Tsiotos PD, Papadas TA. Lateral neck abscess caused by *Streptococcus bovis* in a patient with undiagnosed colon cancer. J Laryngol Otol 1997; 111(7):666–668.
30. Genta PR, Carneiro L, Genta EN. *Streptococcus bovis* bacteremia: unusual complications. South Med J 1998; 91(12):1167–1168.
31. Garcia-Porrua C, Gonzalez-Gay MA, Monterroso JR, Sanchez-Andrade A, Gonzalez-Ramirez A. Septic arthritis due to *Streptococcus bovis* as presenting sign of 'silent' colon carcinoma. Rheumatology (Oxford) 2000; 39(3):338–339.
32. Osada T, Nagawa H, Masaki T, Tsuno NH, Sunami E, Watanabe T, Muto T, Shibata Y. Thoracic empyema associated with recurrent colon cancer: report of a case and review of the literature. Dis Colon Rectum 2001; 44(2):291–294.
33. Legier JF. *Streptococcus salivarius* meningitis and colonic carcinoma. South Med J 1991; 84(8):1058–1059.
34. Macaluso A, Simmang C, Anthony T. *Streptococcus sanguis* bacteremia and colorectal cancer. South Med J 1998; 91(2):206–207.

35. Balsam LB, Shepherd GM, Ruoff KL. *Streptococcus anginosus* spondylodiskitis. Clin Infect Dis 1997; 24(1):93 94.
36. Tzur T, Liberman S, Felzenstein I, Cohen R, Rivkind AI, Almogy G. Liver abscesses caused by *Streptococcus milleri*: an uncommon presenting sign of silent colonic cancer. Isr Med Assoc J 2003; 5(3):206–207.
37. Teitz S, Guidetti-Sharon A, Manor H, Halevy A. Pyogenic liver abscess: warning indicator of silent colonic cancer. Report of a case and review of the literature. Dis Colon Rectum 1995; 38(11):1220–1223.
38. Basaglia G, Moras L, Bearz A, Scalone S, Paoli PD. Related articles, Links *Staphylococcus cohnii* septicaemia in a patient with colon cancer. Med Microbiol 2003; 52(pt 1):101 102.
39. Radosavljevic M, Koenig H, Letscher-Bru V, Waller J, Maloisel F, Lioure B, Herbrecht R. *Candida catenulata* fungemia in a cancer patient. J Clin Microbiol 1999; 37(2):475–477.
40. Otrakji CL, Albores-Saavedra J, Martinez AJ. Gastric malignant lymphoma with superimposed amebiasis. Am J Gastroenterol 1990; 85(1):72–75.
41. Friedman E, Elian D, Eisenstein Z. *Streptococcus bovis* bacteremia and underlying gastrointestinal neoplasms. Med Pediatr Oncol 1986; 14(6):313–315.
42. Zuniga J, Gonzalez P, Henriquez A, Fernandez A. Bacteremic pneumonia caused by *Citrobacter diversus*: report of a case. Rev Med Chil 1991; 119(3):303–307. Spanish.
43. Gelfand MS, Hughey JR, Sloas DD. Group B streptococcal bacteremia associated with adenocarcinoma of the stomach. Clin Infect Dis 1994; 19(2):364.
44. Matsutani T, Onda M, Miyashita M, Hao K, Yokoyama S, Matsuda T, Futami R, Takubo K, Sasajima K. Liver abscesses associated with stromal tumour of the stomach in a young woman. Eur J Gastroenterol Hepatol 2001; 13(12):1485 1489.
45. Gil Lasa I, Montalvo Ollobarren II, Mensa Landaburu G, Garcia Bengoechea M, Castiella Eguzquiza A, Arenas Mirave JI. Liver abscess caused by *Streptococcus anginosus*. Rev Esp Enferm Dig 1995; 87(11):821–823. In Spanish.
46. Kaufman J, Thongsuwan N, Stern E, Karmy-Jones R. Esophageal-pericardial fistula with purulent pericarditis secondary to esophageal carcinoma presenting with tamponade. Ann Thorac Surg 2003; 75(1):288 289.
47. Oliaro A, Filosso PL, Casadio C, Ruffini E, Molinatti M, Cianci R, Porrello C, Rastelli M, Leo F, Maggi G. Right post pneumonectomy pleural empyema caused by an esophagopleural fistula due to an esophageal carcinoma. J Cardiovasc Surg (Torino) 1995; 36(6):607–609.
48. Muto M, Ohtsu A, Boku N, Tajiri H, Yoshida S. *Streptococcus milleri* infection and pericardial abscess associated with esophageal carcinoma: report of two cases. Hepatogastroenterology 1999; 46(27):1782 1784.
49. Karlawish JH. Group G streptococcal bacteremia caused by an asymptomatic esophageal carcinoma in an elderly man. South Med J 1994; 87(6):667–678.
50. Hinojar AG, Castejon MA, Hinojar AA. Conservative management of a case of cervical esophagus perforation with mediastinal abscess and bilateral pleural effusion. Auris Nasus Larynx 2002; 29(2):199 201.

18

Infections in Patients with Cancer of the Liver and Biliary Tract

Carlos A. Castillo Albán
Universidad San Francisco de Quito
Quito, Ecuador

John N. Greene
University of South Florida School of Medicine
and Moffitt Cancer Center and Research Institute
Tampa, Florida, U.S.A.

Primary hepatocellular carcinoma (HCC) is responsible for one quarter of a million to one million deaths per year. It is the seventh leading cause of cancer death in men and the ninth in women. HCC has specific and unique geographic, sex, and age distributions.

The incidence of HCC varies widely depending on the geographic area. Its incidence also varies depending on various ethnic groups and regions within the same country. High incidence regions in the world (more than 15 cases per 100,000) are sub-Saharan Africa, Hong Kong, Taiwan, and the People's Republic of China, where over 40% of all cases of HCC occur. The annual incidence rate is 137,000 cases per year. Low-incidence regions of the world (less than 3 cases per 100,000 per year) include North and South America, most of Europe, Australia, and parts of the Middle East [1,2]. The incidence in the United States has increased over the past two decades, in part because of the large amount of people suffering from long-standing chronic hepatitis C. These great differences in the incidence of HCC are possibly due to regional variations in exposure to hepatitis viruses and other environmental pathogens. This can be corroborated by showing that there is a higher incidence of hepatitis B virus carriers in the regions where HCC is found frequently. Conversely, in the regions where the incidence of HCC is low, there is a lower frequency of hepatitis B virus carriers. There are a variety of well-known risk factors for the development of HCC. These include chronic hepatitis B virus infection, chronic hepatitis C virus infection, cirrhosis of almost any cause, hereditary hemochromatosis, and environmental toxins. The incidence of infectious complications in patients with HCC is rare but is significantly increased if there are associated risk factors. Cirrhosis and diagnostic (biopsies) or therapeutic interventions (i.e., embolization) increase the possibility of infection.

Cholangiocarcinomas (CCAs) are rare malignant tumors arising from the extrahepatic bile ducts. Ulcerative colitis is a significant risk factor. The risk of CCAs is also increased in patients with anomalies of the pancreaticocholedachal junction and in patients with choledochal cysts. There is no convincing link with the presence of gallstones or parasites such as *Clonorchis sinensis* or *Opisthorchis viverrini*, in which the risk of cholangiocellular carcinoma (intrahepatic CCA) is increased. In the case of the CCAs, infectious complications are more frequent and increase considerably with the use of diagnostic or therapeutic techniques such as ERCP, papillotomy, and percutaneous cholangiography [3].

IMMUNOLOGICAL FUNCTION OF THE LIVER

The liver is a special organ in many ways. In its anatomy, physiology, and immunology, the liver reacts differently from other organs against some infections. Its portal irrigation comes directly from the enteric area and can be seen as a connection between the intestine and its flora and the rest of the body. As a result of the liver's rich vascularization, microorganisms that travel in the blood have a high possibility of circulating through the liver. Because of this, it is amazing that there are not many more cases of liver abscesses [4].

The strategic position of the Kupffer cells facilitate the clearance of bacteria, viruses, endotoxins, and immune complexes from portal blood. These cells have a significant role not only in the phagocytosis but also in the initiation of the immune response because of their capacity to create and segregate several cytokines, lysosomic enzymes, and arachidonic acid products and their derivates [5]. The frequent association between cirrhosis and HCC, as well as the chemotherapeutic and immunosuppressive treatment of these tumors, alters the immune function of the liver. As a consequence, infectious complications are more common. However, if surgical or endoscopic treatment for the management of HCC is not done, the frequency of infection is low [5].

SPONTANEOUS INFECTIONS IN PATIENTS WITH HCC AND CCAs

The clinical presentation of HCC is variable, depending on associated cirrhosis and progression of the cancer. Intermittent fever and leukocytosis can result from HCC. In a 17-year retrospective study, there were only 10 cases of HCC complicated with pyogenic liver abscess [6]. Tumor necrosis and biliary tract obstruction from the tumor resulted in the development of the abscesses. Pyogenic hepatic abscesses can be the clinical presentation of hepatopancreaticobiliary malignant tumors in their terminal stages and have a very serious prognosis. In one study, 72% of these patients died of biliary sepsis within 6 months after the diagnosis was made. Abscesses communicating with the intrahepatic biliary tract were frequently seen. *Escherichia coli* and *Klebsiella pneumoniae* were the predominant bacteria encountered [7]. There have been a few cases of HCC and associated amebic or tuberculous (TB) pyogenic liver abscesses described in the literature [8]. *Salmonella* spp. can rarely cause hepatic abscesses in association with HCC [9,10].

Cholangitis is frequently associated with benign diseases of the biliary tract such as gallstones. However, cholangitis can result from malignant obstruction by CCAs or by cancer of the papilla of Vater or pancreas. The frequency of cholangitis as a complication of these tumors increases considerably with the use of diagnostic or therapeutic instrumentation techniques of the bile tract. Concomitant hepatolithiasis increases the risk of severe infection [11].

INFECTIOUS COMPLICATIONS FROM THE THERAPEUTIC MANAGEMENT OF HCC

Treatment options for HCC are divided into surgical therapies (i.e., resection, cryoablation, and orthotopic liver transplantation) and nonsurgical therapies (i.e., percutaneous ethanol injection, radio-frequency ablation, transarterial chemoembolization, chemotherapy, and radiation).

Percutaneous Ethanol Injection (PEI)

Before the arrival of radio-frequency ablation (RFA), PEI was the most accepted and minimally invasive method for treating HCC. This technique involved the injection of 95% ethanol into the tumor, inducing necrosis and ultimately reduction in the size of the tumor. Complications of this therapeutic method are rare; less than 5% of patients develop intraperitoneal hemorrhage, bile duct necrosis, biliary fistula, or hepatic infarction. Liver abscess after the use of PEI is also rare. In the literature there is a case report of a patient with a history of cholecystoduodenostomy for congenital dilatation of the bile duct [12]. Pneumobilia was observed in the intrahepatic bile duct prior to PEI. *Klebisella pneumoniae* was isolated from the abscess.

Transarterial Chemoembolization (TACE)

TACE requires the injection of a chemotherapeutic agent, with or without lipidol, into the hepatic artery. TACE is commonly complicated by pain, fever, and elevated aminotransferases; this is known as postembolization syndrome. Sepsis and abscesses are serious complications following TACE. The exact incidence and the necessity for antibiotic prophylaxis for TACE remain undetermined. The reported incidence varies between 1.1 and 4.5% [13,14]. Organisms isolated from these infectious complications demonstrated normal intestinal flora [14]. Prior bilioenteric anastomosis is the major determinant of liver abscess after TACE. Several authors report that the major risk factor that leads to the formation of an abscess after TACE is biliary infection in patients with a prior bilioenteric anastomosis [14–16]. Other studies suggest other risk factors, such as the ischemic destruction of the intrahepatic ducts secondary to occlusion of the peribiliary arterial plexus by lipidol, and/or the direct effects, of anticancer drugs on these vessels [17,18].

In one study of 452 TACE procedures performed over a 2 year period in 289 patients with HCC, four men and one woman with a mean age of 68.4 years were diagnosed as having a liver abscess 1–8 weeks (mean 4.6 weeks) after chemoembolization [13]. The incidence of this complication in this study was 1.1% (5/452). The most common symptoms included fever, chills, and right upper quadrant abdominal pain. Serum aminotransferase, alkaline phosphatase and gamma-glutamyltransferase levels were frequently elevated, as was the leukocyte count. All the abscesses appeared as areas of hypodensity on CT scans and hypoechogenicity on ultrasound. The causative microorganisms most commonly isolated were gram-positive spp. (60%). This is in contrast to the predominance of gram-negative aerobic bacteria encountered in sporadic liver abscess. There is one case report of a lung abscess as a complication of TACE [19]. Prior gastrectomy was a risk factor for bacterial infections following TACE [20].

Liver Transplantation

Liver transplantation for primary HCC has resulted in poor outcomes. Currently, patients with HCC should be offered orthotopic liver transplantation (OLT) only when it is in the context of investigative protocols involving neoadjuvant therapy. Liver transplantation can result in a myriad of infectious complications similar to those of bone marrow transplantation, which are addressed in detail in another chapter.

INFECTIOUS COMPLICATIONS FROM THE THERAPEUTIC MANAGEMENT OF CCAs

The most common clinical manifestations of patients with cholangiocarcinoma are jaundice, pruritus, and right upper quadrant abdominal pain. Occasionally, patients present with the typical signs and symptoms of cholangitis. Infection of the bile duct, before the use of instrumentation, is uncommon with high-grade malignant obstruction. Palliation of jaundice can be accomplished by operative biliary-enteric bypass or endoscopic-percutaneous stenting of the biliary tree [21]. The major problem associated with endoscopic stenting is obstruction of the stent with time. This leads to a recurrence of the pain and jaundice and carries an increased risk for cholangitis [22–24]. Cholangitis is generally caused by enteric flora. More than one organism is isolated in 30 to 87% of the episodes. *E. coli* and *Klebsiella* are the most common microorganisms. Antibiotics should be administered before cholangiography and should cover for Enterobacteriaceae and *Pseudomonas aeruginosa* [25].

Aggressive treatment for malignancies of the biliary tract has resulted in an increased incidence of pyogenic liver abscess. A retrospective study by Kubo et al. demonstrated the risk factors for infection in the biliary-enteric anastomosis [26]. The study was of 45 patients who underwent pancreatoduodenectomy (study group A), 38 patients who underwent liver resection with biliary-intestinal anastomosis (study group B), and 55 patients who underwent biliary intestinal anastomosis alone (study group C) during the period from 1986 to 1999. Liver abscess occurred in six patients in group A and four in group B. No patients developed liver abscess in group C. Pancreatoduodenectomy or liver resection with biliary-intestinal anastomosis, anastomosis with subsegmental bile ducts, and vascular reconstruction are risk factors for refractory liver abscess after biliary intestinal anstomosis.

REFERENCES

1. Kew MC. Tumors of the liver. In: Zakin D, Bayer T, eds. Hepathology: A Textbook of Liver Disease. 3d ed. W.B. Saunders, 1996:1513–1548.
2. Wand JR, Blum HE. Primary hepatocellular carcinoma. N Engl J Med 1991; 325:729–731.
3. Vauthey JN, Blumgart LH. Recent advances in the management of cholangiocarcinoma. Semin Liver Dis 1994; 14:109 114.
4. Nouri-Aria KT, Eddleston AL. Funciones inmunes del Higado. In: Rodés J,

Benhamou JP, Bicker J, McIntyre N, Rizzetto M, eds. Tratado de hepatología clínica. Masson, 1993:114–119.

5. Winwood PJ, Arthur MJ. Kupffer cells: their activation and role in animal models of liver injury and human liver diseases. Semin Liver Dis 1993; 13:50–59.

6. Yeh TS, Jan YY, Jeng LB, Chen TC, Hwang TL, Chen MF. Hepatocellular carcinoma presenting as a pyogenic liver abscess: characteristics, diagnosis and management. Clin Infect Dis 1998; 26(5):1224–1226.

7. Yeh TS, Jan YY, Jeng LB, Hwang TL, Ckao TC, Chien RN, Chen MF. Pyogenic liver abscess in patients with malignant disease: a case report of 52 cases treated at a single institution. Arch Surg 1998; 133(3):242–245.

8. Atoba MA, Otutana BA, Adebajo AO. Primary liver cell carcinoma associated with infective liver disease [abstr]. Trop Geogr Med 1998; 40(3):244–246.

9. Simmers TA, Misnhout GS, Van Meyel JJ. Salmonellosis: an unusual complication of hepatocellular carcinoma [abstr]. Second J Gastroenterol 1997; 32(11):1180–1182.

10. Lee CC, Doom SK, Chen GH. Spontaneous gas-forming liver abscess caused by *salmonella* within hepatocellular carcinoma: a case report and review of the literature. Dig Dis Sci 2002; 47(3):586–589.

11. Yan YY, Yeh TS, Chen MF. Cholangiocarcinoma presenting as pyogenic liver abscess: is its outcome influenced by concomitant hepatolithiasis? [abstr]. Am J Gastroenterol 1998; 93(2):253–255.

12. Okada S, Aoki K, Okazaki N, Nose H, Yoshimori M, Shimada K, Yamamoto J, Takayama T, Kosuge T, Yamasaki S. Liver abscess after percutaneous ethanol injection (PEI) therapy for hepatocellular carcinoma. A case report [abstr]. Hepatogastroenterology 1993; 40(5):496–498.

13. Chen C, Chen PJ, Yang PM, Huang GT, Lai MY, Tsang YM, Chen DS. Clinical and microbiological features of liver abscess after transarterial embolization for hepatocellular carcinoma. Am J Gastroenterol 1997; 92(12):2257–2259.

14. Kim W, Clark TW, Baum RA, Soulen MC. Risk factors for liver abscess formation after hepatic chemoembolization [abstr]. J Vasc Interv Radiol 2001; 12(8):965–968.

15. Ishikawa H, Kanai T, Ono T, Shimoyama Y, Aizawa K, Ishida H, Saitoh Y, Hata H, Aoki A, Okuda S, et al. Analysis of cases with liver abscess following transcatheter arterial chemoembolization (TAE) for malignant hepatic tumors [abstr]. Gan To Kagaku Ryoho 1994; 21(13):2233–2236.

16. Song SY, Chung JW, Han JK, Lima HG, Koh YH, Park JH, Lee HS, Kim CY. [abstr]. Liver abscess after transcatheter oily chemoembolization for hepatic tumors: incidence, predisposing factors, and clinical outcome. J Vasc Interv Radiol 2001; 12(3):313–320.

17. Inoue H, Hori A, Satake M, Kanetsuki I, Ueno K, Nishida H, Ikeda K, Kobayashi H, Nakajo M. Liver abscess formation after treatment of liver cancer by arterial injection using adriamycin/mitomycin C oil suspension (ADMOS) [abstr]. Nippon Igaku Hoshasen Gakkai Zasshi 1992; 52(2):155–163.

18. Hashimoto T, Mitani T, Nakamura H, Hori S, Kozuka T, Kobayashi Y, Nakata A, Tsujimura T. Fatal septic complication of transcatheter chemoembolization

for hepatocellular carcinoma [abstr]. Cardiovasc Intervent Radiol 1993; 16(5): 325–327.

19. Cubiella J, Sans M, Llovet JM, Bustamante J, Ferre A, Caballeria J, Rodes J. Pulmonary abscess as a complication of transarterial embolization of multi-nodular hepatocellular carcinoma. Am J Gastroenterol 1997; 92(10):1942–1943.

20. Chen C, Tsang YM, Hsueh PR, Huang GT, Yang PM, Sheu JC, Lai MY, Chen PJ, Chen DS. Bacterial infections associated with hepatic arteriography and transarterial embolization for hepatocellular carcinoma: a prospective study [abstr]. Clin Infect Dis 1999; 29(1):161 166.

21. Vauthey JN, Blumgart LH. Recent advances in the management of cholangio-carcinomas. Semin Liver Dis 1994; 14:109–114.

22. Smith AC, Dowsett JF, Russell RC, Hatfield AR, Cotton PB. Randomised trial of endoscopic stenting versus surgical bypass in malignant low bileduct obstruction. Lancet 1994; 344:1655–1660.

23. Speer AG, Cotton PB, Russell RC, Mason RR, Hatfield AR, Leung JW, MacRae KD, Houghton J, Lennon CA. Randomized trial of endoscopic vs. percutaneous stent insertion in malignant obstructive jaundice. Lancet 1987; 2:57–62.

24. Prat F, Chapat O, Ducot B, Ponchon T, Pelletier G, Fritsch J, Choury AD, Buffet C. A randomized trial of endoscopic drainage methods for inoperable malignant strictures of the common bile duct. Gastrointest Endosc 1998; 47:1–7.

25. Motte S, Deviere J, Dumonceau JM, Serruys E, Thys JP, Cremer M. Risk factors for septicemia following endoscopic biliary stenting. Gastroenterology 1991; 101(5):1374–1381.

26. Kubo S, Kinoshita H, Hirohashi K, Tanaka H, Tsukamoto T, Kanazawa A. Risk factors for and clinical findings of liver abscess after biliary-intestinal anastomosis. Hepatogastroenterology 1999; 46(25):116–120.

19

Infections in Patients with Neuroendocrine Tumors

John N. Greene
University of South Florida School of Medicine
and Moffitt Cancer Center and Research Institute
Tampa, Florida, U.S.A.

Neuroendocrine tumors can be divided into two large categories: small cell carcinomas of the lung with neuroendocrine differentiation and tumors related to the gastrointestinal (GI) tract such as carcinoid, pancreatic islet cell tumors (gastrinoma, insulinoma, glucagonoma, VIPoma, somatostatinoma), paragangliomas, and pheochromocytomas. Other neuroendocrine tumors include thyroid carcinoma and Merckel cell tumors. Infections related to small cell lung cancer primarily develop in the setting of myelosuppression from chemotherapy, corticosteroid therapy for metastasis to the central nervous system, and postobstructive pneumonia. These complications are covered in other chapters. Infections occurring in patients with neuroendocrine tumors of the GI tract are primarily due to treatment of liver metastasis, namely hepatic artery chemoembolization, radio frequency ablation, cryoablation, surgical resection of the tumor or its metastasis, liver transplant, and rarely chemotherapy.

HEPATIC ARTERY CHEMOEMBOLIZATION (HAC)

The predominant site of metastatic spread of neuroendocrine tumors of the GI tract is the liver. For patients with liver metastasis who are candidates for partial liver resection, hepatic artery occlusion or embolization is an alternative treatment. The principles behind HAC is that the blood supply to the tumor is from the hepatic artery, whereas the hepatocytes derive blood from the portal venous circulation. Theoretically, this allows for killing of the tumor while sparing the areas of normal liver. Gelfoam powder with or without antineoplastic agents such as doxorubicin, cisplatin, or streptozocin (termed chemoembolization) is infused into the hepatic artery through an angiography catheter.

The response rates to HAC are over 50%, with a duration of response ranging from 4 to 24 months [1]. In patients with symptomatic metastatic carcinoid tumors, HAC can reduce symptoms of flushing and diarrhea, with a response that lasts 1 to 18 months [2,3]. The complications of HAC include fever, leukocytosis, severe abdominal pain, rise in serum aminotransferase values, infection, and death [4]. Infections related to HAC include liver abscess, cholangitis, and subphrenic abscess [5,6].

RADIOFREQUENCY ABLATION (RFA) AND CRYOABLATION

Other forms of treatment of liver metastasis include the use of radio frequency ablation (RFA) and cryoablation (CA), either alone or in conjunction with surgical debulking. A series of 31 symptomatic patients with metastatic carcinoid [20], islet cell tumor [10], and medullary thyroid cancer [1] who were refractory to conventional therapy, underwent resection, CA and/or RFA [7,8]. After a medium follow-up of 26 months, symptoms were eliminated in 27 (87%), and 16 had progression or recurrent disease. These procedures appear to have less risk of complication than liver metastasis resection or HAC. Infections associated with this procedure include liver abscess, cholangitis, peritonitis, and surgical wound infection.

SURGICAL RESECTION OF LIVER METASTASIS

Palliation of symptoms from hormonal hypersecretion of neuroendocrine tumors can be achieved for awhile with surgical resection of hepatic metastasis [9]. In one series of 74 patients undergoing hepatic resection for liver metastasis, symptomatic relief occurred in over 90% of patients and the four+ year survival rate was over 70% [10]. Infection complications from surgical resection of liver metastasis are liver abscess, cholangitis, peritonitis, and surgical wound infection. The predominant pathogens include *Staphy-*

lococcus aureus (including methicillin-resistant *S. aureus* [MRSA]), aerobic gram-negative bacilli, Enterococcus species, and anaerobes. Vancomycin combined with pipercillin/tazobactam or imipenem/cilastatin would cover the above-mentioned organisms. Surgical drainage of the abscess when possible is usually indicated.

Differentiation of liver necrosis from HAC, RFA, and CA from liver abscess is frequently difficult. CT-directed aspiration of the area in question for cytology, gram stain, and culture may be necessary. Neuroendocrine tumors are rare to begin with. Infections from the treatment of these malignancies are rarer still.

REFERENCES

1. Eriksson BK, Larsson EG, Skogseid BM, Lofberg AM, Lorelius LE, Oberg KE. Liver embolizations of patients with malignant neuroendocrine gastrointestinal tumors. Cancer. 1998 Dec 1; 83(11):2293 2301.
2. Maton PN, Camilleri M, Griffin G, Allison DJ, Hodgson HJ, Chadwick VS. Role of hepatic arterial embolisation in the carcinoid syndrome. Br Med J (Clin Res Ed) 1983 Oct 1; 287(6397):932 935. PMID: 6412893 [PubMed-indexed for MEDLINE].
3. Caplin ME, Buscombe JR, Hilson AJ, Jones AL, Watkinson AF, Burroughs AK. Carcinoid tumor. Lancet 1998 Sep 5; 352(9130):799 805. Review. PMID: 97373902 [PubMed-indexed for MEDLINE].
4. Modlin IM, Lye KD, Kidd M. A 5-decade analysis of 13,715 carcinoid tumors. Cancer 2003 Feb 15; 97(4):934–959.
5. Yokoi Y, Suzuki S, Sakaguchi T, Okumura T, Kurachi K, Konno H, Nakamura S. Subphrenic abscess formation following superselective transcatheter chemo-embolization for hepatocellular carcinoma. Radiat Med 2002; 20:45 49.
6. McCallion K, Wilson RH, Mellrath E, Rowlands BJ. Hepatic abscess formation following embolisation of a carcinoid metastasis. Ulster Med J 1995; 64:185–190.
7. Chung MH, Pisegna J, Spirit M, Guiliano AE, Ye W, Ramming KP, Bilchik AJ. Hepatic cytoreduction followed by a novel long-acting somatostatin analog: a paradigm for intractable neuroendocrine tumors metastatic to the liver. Surgery 2001 Dec; 130(6):954–962.
8. Berber E, Flesher N, Siperstein AE. Laparoscopic radiofrequency ablation of neuroendocrine liver metastasis. World J Surg 2002 Aug; 26(8):985 990. Epub 2002 May 21. PMID: 12016479 [PubMed-indexed for MEDLINE].
9. McEntee GP, Nagorney DM, Kvols LK, Moertel CG, Grant CS. Cytoreductive hepatic surgery for neuroendocrine tumors. Surgery 1990 Dec; 108(6):1091 1096. PMID: 1701060 [PubMed-indexed for MEDLINE].
10. Que F, Nogorney D, Batts KP, Linz LJ, Kvols LK. Hepatic resection for metastatic neuroendocrine carcinomas. Am J Surg 1995 Jan; 169(1):36–42; discussion 42 3. PMID: 7817996 [PubMed-indexed for MEDLINE].

20

Infections in Patients with Bladder and Kidney Tumors

Kadry R. Allaboun
Bradenton, Florida, U.S.A.

Renal cell tumors represent a heterogeneous group of tumors ranging from benign to malignant neoplasms. Renal cell carcinoma is the most common malignant tumor arising from the kidney and accounting for 90% of renal malignant neoplasms. The male to female ratio is 2:1. It generally presents in late middle age with hematuria, flank pain, abdominal mass, weight loss, and anemia. The risk is increased with cigarette smoking, obesity, Von Hippel–Lindau syndrome (VHL), tuberous sclerosis, and polycystic kidney disease. Patients with kidney tumors are susceptible to develop recurrent urinary tract infection [1], clostridial infection [2], salmonellosis [3], xanthogranulomatous pyelonephritis [4], emphysematous pyelonephritis [5], malakoplakia [6], renocolic fistula [7], renal abscess [8], psoas abscess [9], urinary sepsis [10], purulent cholecystitis [11], and interstitial pneumonia [12]. Bladder cancer accounts for more than 90% of urinary tract malignancies. The male to female ratio is 3:1.

Transitional cell carcinoma is the most common cancer in the urinary bladder; 8% develop in the renal pelvis and 2% in the ureter or urethra. Less common types are 7% squamous cell carcinoma and 2% adenocarcinoma. The risk factors for bladder cancer are cigarette smoking, schistosoma haematobium, high fat diet, exposure to aniline dye, cyclophosphamide, phenacetin, and external-beam radiation. Infections that can be associated with bladder cancer are salmonellosis [13], gonococcal cystitis [14], and psoas abscess [15].

OPPORTUNISTIC INFECTIONS

Opportunistic infections are a major cause of morbidity and mortality in cancer patients. They can be acquired from the endogenous flora, hospital environment, and general environment with greater severity in immunocompromised patients. The risk factors to develop opportunistic infections depend on the virulence of microorganisms, length of hospital stay, overuse of antibiotics, indwelling devices, and the immune system of the patient. The immune system can be influenced by chronic underlying illnesses (the cancer itself, diabetes, and chronic renal failure), the use of immunosuppressive agents, radiation therapy, malnutrition, and the age of patient. The immune defenses of cancer patients are compromised in several ways. Opportunistic pathogens may occur in the genitourinary tract of cancer patients after the use of chemotherapy and other modalities of treatment. Infectious complications after chemotherapy in patients with urogenital cancer are pyelonephritis, acute prostatitis, bacteremia, and pneumonia. These infections are more likely to develop in patients with urinary diversion, hydronephrosis, and neutropenia [16]. Severe neutropenia can be a rare side effect of intravesical thiotriethylenethiophosphoramide (TEPA) leading to sepsis [17,18].

The use of BCG immunotherapy in patients with urinary bladder cancer lowers the resistance to intracellular pathogens such as Listeria monocytogenes in a mouse model [19]. Cell-mediated immunity is also impaired in patients with urinary bladder cancer associated with schistosomiasis [20]. Disseminated *Nocardia caviae* has been reported in patients with renal cell carcinoma [21]. Treatment of renal cell carcinoma with interleukin-2 (IL-2) can be associated with fever, chills, malaise, bone marrow suppression, neutropenia, increased incidence of bacteremia, sepsis, catheter-related infections, urinary tract infections, respiratory infections, and skin and muscle infections. Interleukin-2-related infections are more frequent in patients with vascular access catheters, open wounds, biliary obstruction, and coexisting infections [22–24].

Development of fungal infections is mainly due to *Candida* spp. Candida adhers to epitheliod cells infiltrated by cancer more avidly than normal cells [25]. Disseminated fungal infections with unusual pathogens such as fusarium oxysporum may occur and be fatal in patients with chemotherapy-induced neutropenia as occurred in a child with Wilms tumor of the kidney [26]. Viral infections such as herpes simplex virus (HSV) and cytomegalovirus

(CMV) may cause multiple mouth ulcers in patients with renal cancer [27]. Also, the polyoma virus JC virus was identified using immunohistochemical staining in nontumorous renal tissue in patients with renal cancer [28].

RENAL ABSCESS

Renal tumors may present with renal and perirenal abscesses [29,30]. The microorganisms responsible for renal abscesses are usually *Staphylococcus aureus* and gram-negative bacilli. Patients with bulky necrotic renal tumor masses following invasive procedures may develop anaerobic infections such as *Clostridium perfringens* and *Bacteroides fragilis* due to favorable conditions of low oxygen tension in the tumor mass [31–33]. Renal and perirenal abscesses can be formed by other unusual pathogens such as nocardia [34], salmonella [35], and tuberculosis [36] or as a complication of transcatheter arterial embolization (TAE) treatment [37]. Because the symptoms and radiological appearance of renal abscess are similar to renal cancer, a high index of suspicion is required in patients with large necrotic tumors and fever of unknown origin. Intravenous pyelography (IVP) and arteriography are helpful diagnostic procedures to differentiate between them.

COMPLICATIONS OF BCG IMMUNOTHERAPY

Bacillus Calmette–Guerin (BCG), a viable attenuated strain of *Mycobacterium bovis*, was identified by Calmette and Guerin in 1921. The efficacy of BCG in the treatment of superficial bladder cancer was first reported by Morales in 1976 with a success rate varying between 63 and 100 percent [38,39]. The U.S. Food and Drug Administration approved the use of BCG in 1990 [40]. BCG immunotherapy has been clinically successful in the treatment and prophylaxis of superficial bladder cancer and carcinoma in situ. The benefits of BCG therapy are attributed to nonspecific immune stimulation, increased production of lymphokines including interleukin-2 (IL-2), and the severe inflammatory response to BCG therapy that results in local ischemia that destroys tumor cells and delays their progression [41,42].

BCG therapy is more effective than most chemotherapeutic agents. It improves survival and progression rates in patients who have moderate-risk and high-risk tumors. But the therapy has its own risks. It is a live-attenuated strain of *Mycobacterium bovis* that can persist in the urinary tract for at least 16.5 months and inhibit certain immune functions. Local and potentially fatal systemic infections may result after the completion of intravesical instillation therapy (Table 1) [43–45].

Local complications such as influenzalike syndrome, cystitis, hematuria, ureteral obstruction, pyelonephritis [46], prostatitis [47], balanitis [48],

TABLE 1 Complications of BCG Immunotherapy

Local complications	Frequency (%)	Systemic complications	Frequency (%)
Cystitis	90	Fever 103°F	3.9
Granulomatous prostatitis	0.9	Pneumonitis/hepatitis	0.7
Epididymitis/orchititis	0.4	Sepsis	0.4
Ureteral obstruction	0.3	Arthralgia/arthritis	0.5
Contracted bladder	0.2	Cytopenia	0.1
Renal abscess	0.1	Hypotension	0.1

Source: Data from Refs. 79 and 84.

epididymo-orchitis [49], regional lymphadenitis [50], tuberculous enteritis [51], skin eruption [52], and prevesical and inguinal abscess may occur after BCG therapy [53].

Systemic complications including fatal sepsis [54], disseminated infection [55], rhabdomyolysis [56], pulmonary complications (interstitial pneumonitis [57], miliary lung disease [58], empyema, and diffuse alveoloar damage [59]), granulomatous hepatitis [60], granulomatous renal masses [61], peritonitis [62], bone marrow granuloma [63], osteomyelitis [64], arithritis [65], Reiter's disease [66], prostatic abscess [67], psoas abscess [68], mycotic vascular infections (aortic arch [69], abdominal aorta [70], iliac artery [71], and femoral artery [72]), endophthalmitis [73], iritis [74], uveitis [75], infections of indwelling foreign devices (osteomyelitis of hip arthoplasty [76], prosthetic total knee infection [77], and infection of an automated implantable cardiac defibrillator (AICD) [78]).

Infections following intravesical BCG therapy are related to strain virulence of BCG, coexisting urinary tract infection, previous history of tuberculosis, immune status of the patient, and bladder epithelium disruption (traumatic catheterization, bladder biopsy, and transurethral resection of bladder tumors). Instillations in inflamed bladder and intralesional injection of BCG will result in systemic absorption, because most of the bladder tumors are well vascularized. Mycobacterium bovis (BCG) DNA was isolated from patients using polymerase chain reaction (PCR) and pulsed field gel electrophoresis when Ziehl–Neelsen staining was negative [79–81]. Treatment options depend on the severity of BCG toxicity from withholding instillations to treatment with antituberculous drugs for at least 6 to 12 months and possibly corticosteroids. The organism is sensitive to several antituberculous agents other than pyrazinamide. Systemic complications may be prevented by prophylactic isoniazid (INH) for 3 days with each BCG treatment [82–84].

UROLOGICAL INSTRUMENTATION AND TRANSURETHRAL RESECTION OF BLADDER TUMORS

Since patients with bladder cancer are frequent candidates for catheterization, diagnostic instrumentation, and surgery, they have a greatly increased risk of infections. Urinary tract infection (UTI) is a major complication after urological procedures and a main cause of postoperative morbidity. Bacteriuria after endoscopic procedures in patients with bladder cancer is higher than those with benign conditions because of the tumor effect on the immune host defense mechanisms [85].

One of the treatment options for bladder cancer is transurethral resection. It is the treatment of choice for low-grade, low-stage bladder tumors and patients who are not good candidates for cystectomy. The main complications of this procedure are bladder perforation, infection, hemorrhage, and postoperative death. Infections include pyelonephritis and peritonitis and intra-abdominal abscess when the procedure is complicated with perforation. The source of urinary infection after transurethral resection originates from the bacteria present within the tumor (where the tumor acts as a privileged site for bacterial growth) or from perioperative manipulation [86,87].

COMPLICATIONS OF CYSTECTOMY

Radical cystectomy combined with urinary diversion is the procedure of choice for the treatment of invasive transitional cell carcinoma of the bladder. The procedure is associated with early and late complications. Early postoperative complications are pyelonephritis, wound infection, pulmonary complications, vascular complications, ileus, dehiscence of the intestinal anastomosis, and postoperative death. Postoperative urinary bacterial infections in patients with bladder cancer after cystectomy are mainly caused by gram-negative bacilli [88]. Late complications are ileus, ureterointestinal obstruction, urethrogluteal fistula [89], ileourethral fistula [90], intestinal fistula [91], ureteroileal fistulas [92], rectal fistula [93], renal abscess [94], splenic abscess [95], and pelvic abscess [96].

Wound infection is the most common complication after cystectomy, and ileus is the most common cause of prolonged hospital stay. The risk of postoperative infection is higher in the elderly and neonates and with preoperative pelvic irradition, prolonged hospitalization, immunosuppressive therapy, indwelling catheters, malnutrition, and advanced bladder cancer [97–99]. The incidence of postoperative complications can be lowered by meticulous perioperative care, improved nutritional status, careful and conservative use of catheters, early antibiotic therapy, and early ambulation after surgery.

In summary, infections in patients with kidney and bladder tumors are incrasing in frequency as the surgical and chemotherapeutic options are becoming more intensive. In addition, resistant pathogens are becoming more prevalent and now require unique antimicrobial therapy. Finally, profound immunosuppression induced by immunotherapy predisposes to opportunistic infections that are difficult to diagnose and require prolonged therapy for patients with bladder or kidney tumors.

REFERENCES

1. Boustead GB, Beard RC, Liston TL, Wright ED. Renal cell carcinoma as a source of recurrent urinary tract infections. British Journal of Urology 1995; 76:670.
2. Graham BS, Johnson AC, Sawyers JL. Clostridial infection of renal cell carcimona. J Urol 1986; 135:354–355.
3. Wolfe Martin S, Armstrong Doland, Louria Doland B, Blevins Anne. Salmonellosis in patients with neoplastic disease. Arch Intern Med 1971; 128:546–554.
4. Goulding Frederick J, Moses Anthony. Xanthogranulomatous pyelonephritis with associated renal cell carcinoma. Urology 1984; 23:385–386.
5. Wang Ming-Cheng, Tseng Chin-Chung, Lan Rong-Rue, Lin Ching-Yuan, Chen Fen-Fen, Huang Jeng-Jong. Double cancers of the kidney and ureter complicated with emphysematous pyelonephritis within the parenchyma of the renal tumour. Scand J Urol Nephrol 1999; 33:420–422.
6. Lew S, Siegal A, Aronheim M. Renal cell carcinoma with malakoplakia. Eur Urol 1988; 14:426–428.
7. Soriano Pastor G, Orobitg Huguet J, Olazabal Zudaire A, Cadafalch Arpa J. Clostridium perfringens sepsis and hypernephroma. Med Clin (Barc) 1988; 91(5): 197. In Spanish.
8. Perimenis P. Pyonephrosis and renal abscess associated with kidney tumours. British Journal of Urology 1991; 68:463–465.
9. Miyata Y, Fujii Y, Kitade K, Hara M. A case of psoas abscess due to renal pelvic carcinoma complicated with non-ketotic hyperosmolar diabetic coma. Nippon Ronen Igakkai Zasshi 1991; 28(5):688–692. In Japanese.
10. Perez Cespedes M, Lopez Costea MA, Riera LL, Armora J, Blancafort JM, Camps N, Serrallach N. Urinary sepsis as manifestation of a renal angiomyolipoma. Actas Urol Esp 1992; 16(5):422–425. In Spanish.
11. Skotnicka B, Martula M. Case of purulent cholecystitis associated with renal carcinoma. Wiad Lek 1971; 24(5):463–466. In Polish.
12. Al Shaalan M, Law BJ, Israels SJ, Pianosi P, Lacson AG, Higgins R. Mycobacterium fortuitum interstitial pneumonia with vasculitis in a child with Wilms' tumor. Pediatr Infect Dis J 1997; 16(10):996–1000.
13. Sinkovics Joseph G, Smith Julian P. Salmonellosis complicating neoplastic diseases. Cancer 1969; 24:631–636.

14. Blackwell AL, Barrow J. Carcinoma of the bladder presenting as gonococcal cystitis. Br J Vener Dis 1980; 56(2):105–106.
15. Masters JG, Cumming JA, Jennings P. Psoas abscess secondary to metastases from transitional cell carcinoma of the bladder. Br J Urol 1996; 77(1):155–156.
16. Matsumoto T, Takahashi K, Tanaka M, Kumazawa J. Infectious complications of combination anticancer chemotherapy for urogenital cancers. Int Urol Nephrol 1999; 31(1):7 14.
17. Bruce Daniel W, Edgcomb John H. Pancytopenia and generalized sepsis following treatment of cancer of the bladder with instillations of Triethylene Thiophosphoramide. J Urol 1967; 97:482.
18. Watkins Wilfred E, Kozak John A, Flanagan Malachi J. Severe pancytopenia associated with the use of intravesical Thio-TEPA. J Urol 1967; 98:470–471.
19. Wing EJ. Bacillus Calmette–Guerin (BCG) decreases resistance to Listeria monocytogenes infection in mice. Immunology 1981; 44(3):509–515.
20. Raziuddin S, Shetty S, Ibrahim A, Patil K. Activated CD4-positive T-lymphocytes and impaired cell-mediated immunity in patients with carcinoma of the urinary bladder with schistosomiasis. Cancer 1990; 65(4):931–939.
21. Arroyo JC, Nichols S, Carroll GF. Disseminated Nocardia caviae infection. American Journal of Medicine 1977; 62:409–412.
22. Escudier B, Lethiec JL, Angevin E, Andremont A, Cosset-Delaigue MF, Antoun S, Leclercq B, Nitenberg G. Totally implanted catheters to reduce catheter-related infections in patients receiving interleukin-2: a 2-year experience. Support Care Cancer 1995; 3(5):297 300.
23. Pockaj BA, Topalian SL, Steinberg SM, White DE, Rosenberg SA. Infectious complications associated with interleukin-2 administration: a retrospective review of 935 treatment courses. J Clin Oncol 1993; 11(1):136–147.
24. Hardy JR, Moore J, Lorentzos A, Ellis E, Jameson B, Gore ME. Infectious complications of interleukin 2 therapy. Cytokine 1990; 2(4):311.
25. Skoutelis AT, Lianou PE, Votta E, Bassaris HP, Papavassiliou JT. Adherence of Candida albicans to epithelial cells from normal and cancerous urinary bladders. Int Urol Nephrol 1994; 26(5):519–522.
26. Neumeister B, Bartmann P, Gaedicke G, Marre R. A fatal infection due to Fusarium oxysporum in a child with Wilms' tumour. Case report and review of the literature. Mycoses 1992; 35(5–6):115–119.
27. Takagi M, Ishikawa G. Double viral infection of the mouth in the cancer patient. Bull Tokyo Med Dent Univ 1977; 24(3):233–238.
28. Aoki N, Kitamura T, Tominaga T, Fukumori N, Sakamoto Y, Kato K, Mori M. Immunohistochemical detection of JC virus in nontumorous renal tissue of a patient with renal cancer but without progressive multifocal leukoencephalopathy. J Clin Microbiol 1999; 37(4):1165–1167.
29. Perimenis P. Pyonephrosis and renal abscess associated with kidney tumours. British Journal of Urology 1991; 68:463–465.
30. Chintapalli K, Lawson TL, Foley WD, Berland LL. Perinephric abscess with renal cell carcinoma. Urol Radiol 1981; 3(2):113–115.

31. Lenkey JL, Reece GJ, Herbert DL. Gas abscess transformation of a huge hypernephroma. AJR 1979; 133:1174–1175.

32. Graham Barney S, Johnson AC, Sawyers John L. Clostridial infection of renal cell carcinoma. J Urol 1986; 135:354–355.

33. Bogucki MS, August DA, Andriole VT. Clostridial infection of a locally recurrent renal cell carcinoma with sepsis. Cancer 1990; 66(3):601–603.

34. Arroyo JC, Nichols S, Carroll GF. Disseminated Nocardia caviae infection. American Journal of Medicine 1977; 62:409–412.

35. Olson ES, Asmussen T, Vicca AF, Osborn DE. Case report of renal abscess caused by Salmonella virchow phage type 1 associated with a papillary renal cell carcinoma. J Infect 1999; 38(1):56–57.

36. Steyn JH, Logie NJ. Coincident tuberculous perinephric abscess and carcinoma of the kidney. Br J Urol 1966; 38:7–8.

37. Koga F, Goto S, Suzuki S. Retroperitoneal abscess formation accompanied by intraabdominal free air, a rare complication of transcatheter arterial embolization of renal tumor: a case report. Hinyokika Kiyo 1996; 42(6):443–446. In Japanese.

38. Witjes JA, van der meijden APM, Debruyne FMJ. Use of intravesical bacillus Calmette–Guerin in the treatment of superficial transitional cell carcinoma of the bladder: an overview. Urol Int 1990; 45:129–136.

39. Morales A, Eidinger D, Bruce AW. Intracavitary Bacillus Calmette–Guerin in the treatment of superficial bladder tumor. J Urol 1976; 116:180–183.

40. US Food and Drug Administration. FDA Drug Bulletin, October 1990; 3–4.

41. Moss JT, Kadmon D. BCG and the treatment of superficial bladder cancer. DICP: Ann Pharmacother 1991; 25:1355–1366.

42. Haaff EO, Catalona WJ, Ratliff TL. Detection of interleukin 2 in the urine of patients with superficial bladder tumors after treatment with intravesical BCG. J Urol 1986; 136(4):970–974.

43. Lamm DA, Steg A, Boccon-Gibod L, Morales A, Hanna MG Jr, Pagano F, Alfthan O, Brosman S, Fisher HA, Jakse G, et al. Complications of bacillus Calmette-Guerin immunotherapy: review of 2602 patients and comparison of chemotherapy complications. Prog Clin Biol Res 1989; 310:335–355.

44. Morales A. Long term results and complications of intracavitary bacillus Calmette–Guerin therapy for bladder cancer. J Urol 1984; 132:457–459.

45. Bowyer L, Hall RR, Reading J, Marsh MM. The persistence of bacille Calmette Guerin in the bladder after intravesical treatment of bladder cancer. Br J Urol 1995; 75:188–192.

46. Kondratowicz GM. BCG pyelonephritis following intravesical BCG. British Journal of Urology 1989; 64:649–656.

47. Rifkin MD, Tessler FN, Tublin ME, Ross JS. US case of the day Granulomatous prostatitis resulting from BCG therapy. Radiographics 1998; 18(6):1605–1607.

48. Erol A, Ozgur S, Tahtali N, Akbay E, Dalva I, Cetin S. Bacillus Calmette–Guerin (BCG) balanitis as a complication of intravesical BCG immunotherapy: a case report. Int Urol Nephrol 1995; 27(3):307–310.

49. Truelson T, Wishnow KI, Johnson DE. Epididymo-orchitis developing as a late

manifestation of intravesical bacillus Calmette Guerin therapy and masquerading as a primary testicular malignancy: a report of 2 cases. J Urol 1992; 148(5): 1534–1535.

50. Ali-El Dein B, Nabeeh A. Tuberculosis iliac lymphadenitis: a rare complication of intravesical bacillus Calmette Guerin and cause of tumor over staging. J Urol 1996; 156(5):1766–1767.

51. Nemoto R, Nakamura I, Honjyo I, Takahashi M, Abe C. Tuberculous enteritis after intravesical bacillus Calmette–Guerin therapy: a case of mistaken identity. J Urol 1998; 159(6):2091 2092.

52. Honl BA, Keeling JH, Lewis CW, Thompson IM. A pityriasis rosea like eruption secondary to bacillus Calmette–Guerin therapy for bladder cancer. Cutis 1996; 57(6):447 450.

53. Martínez-Caceres Pedro, Rubio-Briones José, Palou Juan, Salvador José, Vicente José. Prevesical and inguinal abscess following intravesical BCG instillation. Scan J Urol Nephrol 1998; 32:409–410.

54. Izes JK, Bihrle W, Thomas CB. Corticosteriod-associated fatal mycobacterial sepsis occurring 3 years after instillation of intravesical bacillus Calmette–Guerin. J Urol 1993; 150:1498 1500.

55. Elkabani M, Greene JN, Vincent AL, Vanhook S, Sandin RL. Disseminated mycobacterium bovis Calmette–Guerin treatment for bladder cancer. Cancer Control 2000; 7(5):476–481.

56. Armstrong RW. Complications after intravesical instillation of bacillus Calmette Guerin: rhabdomyolysis and metastatic infection. J Urol 1991; 145(6):1264–1266.

57. Israel-Biet D, Venet A, Sandron D, Ziza JM, Chretien J. Pulmonary complications of intravesical bacille Calmette–Guerin immunotherapy. Am Rev Respir Dis 1987; 135:763–765.

58. Jasmer RM, McCowin MJ, Webb WR. Miliary lung disease after intravesical bacillus Calmette–Guerin immunotherapy. Radiology 1996; 201:43 44.

59. Kesten S, Title L, Mullen B, Grossman R. Pulmonary disease following intravesical BCG treatment. Thorax 1990; 45:709 710.

60. Leebeek FWG, Quwendijk RJ Th, Kolk AHJ, Dees A, Meek J Ch E, Nienhuis JE, Dingemans-Dumas AM. Granulomatous hepatitis caused by bacillus Calmette–Guerin (BCG) infection after BCG bladder instillation. Gut 1996; 38(4): 616–618.

61. Stanisic TH, Brewer ML, Graham AR. Intravesical bacillus Calmette–Guerin therapy and associated granulomatous renal masses. J Urol 1986; 135:356–358.

62. Kim IY, Smith C, Olivero J, Lapin SL. Bacillus Calmette Guerin induced peritonitis in a patient on dialysis. J Urol 2000; 163(1):237.

63. Dederke B, Riecken EO, Weinke T. A case of BCG sepsis with bone marrow and liver involvement after intravesical BCG instillation. Infection 1998; 26(1): 54–57.

64. Morgan MB, Iseman MD. Mycobacterium bovis vertebral osteomyelitis as a complication of intravesical administration of bacillus Calmette Guerin. Am J Med 1996; 100:372 373.

65. Devlin M, Deodhar A, Davis M. Arthritis as a complication of intravesical BCG vaccine. BMJ 1994; 308(6944):1638.

66. Hogarth MB, Thomas S, Seifert MH, Tariq SM. Reiter's syndrome following intravesical BCG immunotherapy. Postgrad Med J 2000; 76(902):791–793.

67. Matlaga BR, Veys JA, Thacker CC, Assimos DG. Prostate abscess following intravesical bacillus Calmette–Guerin treatment. J Urol 2002; 167(1):251.

68. Hakim S, Heaney JA, Heinz T, Zwolak RW. Psoas abscess following intravesical bacillus Calmette–Guerin for bladder cancer: a case report. J Urol 1993; 150:188–189.

69. Izes JK, Bihrle W 3rd, Thomas CB. Corticosteriod-associated fatal mycobacterial sepsis occurring 3 years after instillation of intravesical bacillus Calmette–Guerin. J Urol 1993; 150:1498 1500. Review.

70. Woods JM IV, Schellack J, Stewart MT, Murray DR, Schwartzman SW. Mycotic abdominal aortic aneurysm induced by immunotherapy with bacille Calmette -Guerin vaccine for malignancy. J Vasc Surg 1988; 7:808–810.

71. Deresiewicz RL, Stone RM, Aster JC. Fatal disseminated mycobacterial infection following intravesical bacillus Calmete–Guerin. J Urol 1990; 144:1331–1334.

72. Bornet P, Pujade B, Lacaine F, Bazelly B, Paquet JC, Roland J, Huguier M. Tuberculosis aneurysm of the femoral artery: a complication of bacille Calmette -Guerin vaccine immunotherapy: a case report. J Vasc Surg 1989; 10:688–692.

73. Lester Harriet, Erdey Richard A, Fastenberg David M, Schwartz Peter L, Rosenhaus Jay B. Bacillus Calmette–Guerin (BCG) endophthamitis. Retina 1988; 8:182–184.

74. Price GE. Arithritis and iritis after BCG therapy for bladder cancer. J Rheumatol 1994; 21:465 564.

75. Wertheim M, Astbury N. Bilateral uveitis after intravesical BCG immunotherapy for bladder carcinoma. Br J Ophthalmol 2002; 86(6):706.

76. Guerra Carmen E, Betts Robert F, O'Keefe Regis J, Shilling Jack W. Mycobacterium bovis Osteomyelitis involving a hip arthroplasty after intravesicular bacille Calmette–Guerin for bladder cancer. Clinical Infectious Diseases 1998; 27:639–640.

77. Chazerain P, Desplaces N, Mamoudy P, Leonard P, Ziza JM. Prosthetic total knee infection with a bacillus Calmette–Guerin (BCG) strain after BCG therapy for bladder cancer. Journal of Rheumatology 1993; 20:2171–2172.

78. Stone RD, Estes NAM, Klempner MS. Mycobacterium bovis infection of an implantable defibrillator following intravesical therapy with bacille Calmette–Guerin. Clin Infect Dis 1993; 16:825–826.

79. Lamm DL, Stogdill VD, Stogdill BJ, Crispen RG. Complications of bacillus Calmette -Guerin immunotherapy in 1,278 patients with bladder cancer. J Urol 1986; 135:272–274.

80. Talbot EA, Williams DL, Frothingham R. PCR identification of mycobacterium bovis BCG. J Clin Microbiol 1997; 35:566–569.

81. Kristjansson M, Green P, Manning HL, Slutsky AM, Brecher SM, von Reyn CF, Arbeit RD, Maslow JN. Molecular confirmation of bacillus Clamette–Guerin as

the source of pulmonary infection following urinary tract instillation. Clin Infect Dis 1993; 17:228 230.

82. van der Meijden AP. Practical approaches to the prevention and treatment of adverse reactions to BCG. Eur Urol 1995; 27(suppl 1):23–28.

83. Stassar MJ, Vegt PD, Steerenberg PA, van der Meijden AP, Meiring HD, Dessens-Kroon M, Geertzen HG, Denotter W. Effects of isoniazid (INH) on the BCG-induced local immune response after intravesical BCG therapy for superficial bladder cancer. Urol Res 1994; 22:177 184.

84. Lamm DL, van der Meijden PM, Morales A, Brosman SA, Catalona WJ, Herr HW, Soloway MS, Steg A, Debruyne FM. Incidence and treatment of complications of bacillus Calmette–Guerin intravesical therapy in superficial bladder cancer. J Urol 1992; 147:596–600.

85. Cox CE, Cass AS, Boyce WH. Bladder cancer. A 26-year review. J Urol 1969; 101:550–558.

86. Goldwasser B, Bogokowsky B, Nativ O, Sidi AA, Jonas P, Many M. Urinary infections following transurethral resection of bladder tumors, rate and source. J Urol 1983; 129:1123–1124.

87. Appell RA, Flynn JT, Paris AMI, Blandy JP. Occult bacterial colonization of bladder tumors. J Urol 1980; 124:345–346.

88. Vodvarka P, Jancova J. Bacterial infection of urine in patients with bladder cancer. Neoplasma 1988; 35(2):243–250.

89. Tasca A, Aragona F, Piazza R, Calabro A, Artibani W. Urethrogluteal fistula occurring after radical cystectomy for bladder cancer. Eur Urol 1987; 13(3):213–214.

90. Hertz M, Goldwasser B, Rubinstein ZJ, Lindner A, Feivel M. Ileourethral fistula following cystectomy: a rare complication. Urol Radiol 1984; 6(3–4):187–189.

91. Herranz Amo F, Diez Cordero JM, Verdu Tartajo F, Bueno Chomon G, Leal Hernandez F, Bielsa Carrillo A. Abdominal pain in patients undergoing radical cystectomy for bladder cancer. Arch Esp Urol 1998; 51(4):342–346. In Spanish.

92. Sullivan JW, Grabstald H, Whitmore WF Jr. Complications of ureteroileal conduit with radical cystectomy: review of 336 cases. J Urol 1980; 124(6):797 801.

93. Skinner DG, Crawford ED, Kaufman JJ. Complications of radical cystectomy for carcinoma of the bladder. J Urol 1980; 123(5):640–643.

94. Bergman B, Knutson F. Renal infection after ileal conduit urinary diversion. An autopsy study. Acta Pathol Microbiol Scand [A] 1978; 86(3):245–250.

95. Reinberg Y, Moore LS, Lange PH. Splenic abscess as a complication of percutaneous nephrostomy. Urology 1989; 34(5):274–276.

96. Montie JE, Wood DP Jr. The risk of radical cystectomy. Br J Urol 1989; 63(5): 483–486.

97. Freiha FS. Complications of cystectomy. J Urol 1980; 123(2):168–169.

98. Chang SS, Baumgartner RG, Wells N, Cookson MS, Smith JA Jr. Causes of increased hospital stay after radical cystectomy in a clinical pathway setting. J Urol 2002; 167(1):208–211.

99. Childs Stacy J. Infections in patients with advanced bladder cancer. Urol 1988; 31(suppl 2):22–28.

21

Infections in Patients with Gynecological Malignancies

Masoumeh Ghayouri and Cuc Mai
James A. Haley Veterans Hospital
Tampa, Florida, U.S.A.

Albert L. Vincent
University of South Florida School of Medicine
Tampa, Florida, U.S.A.

Infections in patients with gynecological malignancies occur frequently and are the cause of death in 50 to 60% of the cases. The patient with cancer is a compromised host with an increased susceptibility to infection due to malignancy itself on the one hand and to therapeutic modalities, like extensive surgical procedures, radiation and cytotoxic chemotherapy on the other. Etiologically these infections are mostly due to a disruption of anatomical structures that normally prevent the invasion of the endogenous or exogenous microorganisms, or to obstructive processes or tumor necrosis. Septicemia can result from propagation of such a localized infection beyond the site of the tumor. The causative pathogens infecting the compromised host are mostly members of the indigenous microbial flora of the genital tract, which is influenced by surgery, irradiation, and chemotherapy. Postoperatively in the vaginal vault the number of most potentially pathogenic aerobic and anaerobic bacterial species is higher; polymicrobial mixed infections are frequent. Neither intracavitary radiation therapy with radium or iridium-192 (after loading) nor external high-voltage therapy decreases the number of pathogenic bacterial species in the uterus or the vagina of patients with cervical or endometrial cancer. The symptoms of infection in cancer patients can be masked. Infections following radical hysterectomy, irradiation, and/or cytotoxic chemotherapy: such as pelvic abscesses, peritonitis, pneumonia, and septicemia, can be fatal. Urinary tract, wound, and vaginal vault infections occur frequently, but are rarely severe [1]. This chapter will review of the most common infections seen in gynecological oncology.

URINARY TRACT INFECTIONS

Urinary tract infection is the most common microbiologically confirmed infection in gynecological oncology patients. Multiple infections are common especially after radical pelvic procedures, including total pelvic exenteration, radical vulvectomy, and radical hysterectomy. The most common organism is *E. coli* and other *Enterobacteriaceae* with *Pseudomonas aeruginosa* and Enterococcus less frequent [2].

PROGRESSIVE NECROTIZING WOUND INFECTIONS

Progressive gangrenous wound infections are described in patients who received whole pelvic irradiation prior to surgery for genital tract cancer [3]. The wounds that provide the portal of infection are closed with wire in the Smead–Jones fashion. All the wound infections began during the first week following surgery. The area of the wound was neither painful nor was there visible evidence of local reaction or inflammatory response. Once infection began, rapid dissolution of the abdominal tissues ensued. The patients never appeared sick and did not exhibit a febrile response during the infection. All patients had either *Bacteroids* species *B. fragilis* or *E. coli* in their wounds as well as a variety of gram-negative rods and, less frequently, gram-positive cocci. In each patient, the infected gangrenous wound was excised from the skin through the peritoneum. The area of excision was carried back to normal bleeding tissue as soon as the diagnosis was made and the defect covered with Marlex Mesh. The mesh was tailored to the defect and then sutured to the fascia. In each case so treated, the infection was controlled.

In addition, radiation may play a role in the initiation of the gangrenous process. Radiation injury is a progressive one and the end result is obliterative endarteritis followed by fresh thin-walled vessels that develop similarly to telangiectasia of the skin. Treatment of a gangrenous postoperative wound infection is based on the rapid recognition of the gangrenous process and the immediate wide and full-thickness debridement of the abdominal wall, reaching back to viable bleeding margins.

SYNERGISTIC BACTERIAL GANGRENE FOLLOWING ABDOMINAL HYSTERECTOMY

Synergistic bacterial gangrene is an infection that occurs due to the combined activity of aerobic and anaerobic bacteria in the destruction of skin and subcutaneous tissue. Involvement of muscle and fascia may occur secondarily in some cases. There are different types of synergistic bacterial gangrene. Differentiation must be made from gas gangrene, stereptococcal gangrene, Meleney's cellulites, and necrotizing fasciitis. Meleney's synergistic gangrene and necrotizing fasciitis are probably variants of the same entity.

Gas gangrene is particularly rare following elective gynecologic surgery [4]. It is usually seen following traumatic wounds. The most common cause is *Clostridium welchii*. The infection is of rapid onset from 12 to 72 hours postoperatively. There is severe local pain and restlessness and tachycardia out of proportion to the fever present. The classic clinical sign of crepitus occurs late in abdominal wall infections making the diagnosis sometimes difficult.

Acute hemolytic streptococcal gangrene is an extremely rapid process resulting in most cases from a synergistic reaction between anaerobic streptococci and *Staphylococcus aureus*. Occasionally a gram-negative organism such as *E. coli* may be found. The affected areas become swollen, hot, red, and tender with areas of acute inflammation spreading in all directions. The skin shows a progressive ischemia turning from red to purple and finally to blue. Blisters and bullae then begin to form. In the later stages the patient may develop pulmonary symptoms and metastatic abscesses in other parts of the body. Cultures for anaerobic as well as aerobic bacteria are essential in addition to a gram stain from the wound. Antibiotics should be given in high doses, but surgery is the mainstay of therapy. Hyperbaric oxygenation may be used if available and has been shown to be bacteriostatic.

Meleney's cellulitis is slower in its rate of growth than acute streptococcal gangrene. It typically begins at a suture or ostomy site as a wound infection, but it slowly develops the typical picture of Meleny's ulcer with a central necrotic zone, an intermediate purple zone, and an outer erythematous zone fading into normal skin. These lesions are very painful and not anesthetic as is acute hemolytic streptococcal gangrene. The lesion usually appears 7 to 14 days following surgery.

NECROTIZING FASCIITIS FOLLOWING DIAGNOSTIC LAPAROSCOPY

A case of necrotizing fasciitis of the abdominal wall, following an uneventful diagnostic laparoscopy in an elderly diabetic patient, is reported [5]. The prevailing characteristic of the bacterial isolate is the proteolytic toxin production by a single bacterium (streptococcus, staphylococcus, or pseudomonas) or by the synergistic association of multiple bacteria (anaerobic bacteria including Bacteroides spp. with facultative anaerobes). The disease is usually associated with injury, frequently a trivial one, but in the majority of reported instances the necrotizing fasciitis occurred postsurgically. The extremities and the abdomen are the most common sites of the initial lesion.

Immediate total debridement of the skin and subcutaneous tissue until it can no longer be separated from deep fascia is mandatory to decrease mortality. Aggressive parenteral antibiotic therapy should include high doses of penicillin and clindamycin when group A streptococci are suspected. Anaerobic and gram-negative bacilli coverage is needed when polymicrobial infection is considered.

PERITONITIS AND INTRA-ABDOMINAL ABSCESS

Bacterial peritonitis is a possible complication associated with catheters implanted for intraperitoneal chemotherapy in patients with extensive ovarian carcinoma [6]. In addition, the tumor can compromise the integrity of the vaginal wall and allow seeding of the endogenous vaginal flora into the pelvic and peritoneal cavities. Previous antibiotics, radiation therapy, and the tumor itself may alter the normal genital flora. Peritonitis, with or without abscess formation, may occur postoperatively after hysterectomy or with bowel injury.

The diagnosis of peritonitis is usually made on clinical grounds. Radiological investigation is generally required to diagnose an abscess. A sonogram, computed tomography (CT) scan, or magnetic resonance image (MRI) of the abdomen may show the collection. The microbiological diagnosis in each of these syndromes requires culture for aerobes and anaerobes. Acute generalized peritonitis usually requires urgent surgery to irrigate the peritonium and repair any perforation. Broad spectrum antibiotic coverage of enteric flora is generally effective for these polymicrobial infections.

COLITIS

Altered bowel function in an oncology patient is common. Functional changes associated with bowel resection, alterations of diet, and stress of anticipated therapy may cause diarrhea. Management often includes dietary manipulation or the use of antiperistaltic drugs. In the presence of *C. difficile* colitis, antiperistaltic agents may actually aggravate the degree of bowel inflamation by slowing the transit of toxins through the colon.

Symptomatic relapse of patients with *C. difficile* toxin associated colitis occurred in three patients with ovarian cancer [7]. Although it is often associated with previous antibiotic use, *C. difficile* toxin associated colitis may occur as an opportunistic infection complicating leukemia, diabetes mellitus, chronic renal failure, cancer chemotherapy, and immunosuppression.

Management should include adequate hydration, correction of the electrolyte abnormalities, and institution of appropriate enteric precautions. If broad spectrum antibiotics were implemented before the onset of diarrhea, they should be discontinued as soon as possible. Although various treatment regimens involving metronidazole, cholestyramine, and bacitracin have been proposed, several authorities continue to regard vancomycin as the preferred drug for patients who are seriously ill.

LYMPHATIC ASCITIS

Lymphatic ascitis has rarely been described following gynecological procedures. Over a period of four years, seven patients have been identified with symptomatic lymphatic ascitis following either pelvic or para-aortic lymph node dissection [8]. The ascitis is associated with abdominal distention, pain and prolonged paralytic ileus, which resulted in significant patient morbidity and prolonged hospitalization. The diagnosis should be considered in any patient with prolonged paralytic ileus and abdominal distention following a pelvic or para-aortic lymphadenectomy.

LACTOBACILLUS SEPTICEMIA

A case of severe Lactobacillus septicemia in a patient treated with chemotherapy because of metastatic choriocarcinoma is described [9]. Chemotherapy used in the treatment of disseminated choriocarcinoma frequently induces bone marrow depression including granulocytopenia. During this period, infections, especially septicemia, can occur, originating mostly from the gastrointestinal tract. Most causative microorganisms are gram-negative bacteria. However, in patients with choriocarcinoma in whom necrotic tumor is present in the uterus, attention should be paid to the infections caused by microorganisms present in the female genital tract such as lactobacilli.

RECURRENT CELLULITIS

Cellulitis is a common infection of the skin extending to the dermis and subcutaneous tissue caused by Group A Streptococcus or *Staphylococcus aureus.* Episodes are usually isolated, frequently following a small break in the skin or trauma. Cellulitis also has a strong tendency to recur in the same place in association with lymphatic or venous compromise and to exacerbate existing lymphatic damage. Predisposing factors for recurrent cellulitis include deep venous thrombosis, venous stasis, congenital absence of lymphatic ducts, filiariasis, cancer resections with lymph node dissections, radiation therapy, and saphenous venectomies associated with coronary artery bypass grafts [10]. Each episode of cellulitis requires evaluation of risk factors contributing to the recurrence, management of the acute episode of cellulitis, and prophylactic therapy to prevent recurrences.

Most reports of recurrent cellulitis involve surgical patients, patients with breast or gynecological carcinomas. In a study by Simon et al., [11], six of the 273 patients (2.2%) with axillary lymph node dissections for breast cancer developed recurrent cellulitis. Likewise, Dankert and Bouma [12] found two cases in 66 patients (3.0%) with hysterectomies and pelvic lymphadenectomies, as well as three cases among 270 patients (1.1%) given radical hysterectomies and pelvic lymphadenectomies. These percentages were low when compared to the 21 cases of cellulitis among 126 patients (17.5%) with a history of radical vulvectomy [13]. Although radical vulvectomies involve surgical interruption of both venous and lymphatic systems, statistical evidence ($p = 0.10$) does not show a significantly higher proportion of recurrence with this procedure compared to radical hysterectomies. In radical hysterectomy patients, impaired lymphatic drainage due to pelvic lymphadenectomy and postoperative irradiation is thought to be responsible for the onset of lymphedema and cellulitis [13]. The high frequency in patients following radical vulvectomy may be due to both the impaired venous drainage caused by excision of the proximal part of the saphenous veins and the impaired lymphatic drainage caused by the dissection of the inguinal lymph nodes [13]. Irradiation may also enhance the impairment of the vascular drainage.

As noted in Table 1, many risk factors have been suggested for recurrent cellulitis, but few have been quantitatively documented. Nevertheless, lymph node dissection and radiation therapy are strong risk factors for recurrent cellulitis. In a study of cellulitis after axillary lymph node dissection for carcinoma of the breast, 15 of 273 patients who developed single or recurrent episodes also manifested lymphedema [11]. The pathogenesis of lymphedema is complex, and experimentally induced lymphedema requires much more tissue damage than that created by breast cancer treatments [14]. Cellulitis and lymphedema can form a vicious cycle, one exacerbating the other. This interrelationship is clearly illustrated in Neto's study [15] where 23.2% of patients developed lymphangitis as the precipitating factor in the onset of arm edema, while 52.1% with existing baseline edema had exacerbation of edema after subsequent episodes of lymphangitis. Lymph fluid is a rich medium for

TABLE 1   Predisposing Conditions for Recurrent Cellulitis

Removal of saphenous vein for coronary artery bypass grafting.
Surgery with lymph node dissection
Prior radiation therapy
Chronic lymphedema
Dermatophytosis, i.e., tinea pedis
Colonization of upper respiratory system, vagina, cervix
Congestive heart failure
Varicose veins
Parasitic infections, i.e., filiariasis
Congenital absence of lymphatics
Venous insufficiency
Obesity

bacterial growth, infection, and inflammation of the soft tissue; this in turn precipitates more occlusive damage to the lymphatics.

A break in the skin is an obvious portal of entry for pathogens that cause cellulitis. A case control study of 167 patients, 23% with recurrence, admitted for cellulitis by Dupuy et al., showed that the most significant factors for cellulitis, acute and recurrent, were toe web intertrigo and preexisting lymphedema [16]. Tinea pedis is a common cutaneous fungal infection. Up to 70% of the general population has, at one point in their lifetime, this infection. In a report of nine patients with cellulitis after coronary artery bypass grafting, all also had coexisting mild to severe tinea pedis. After treatment with antifungals and antibiotics for the cellulitis, these patients had no recurrences. Besides lymphedema and toe-web intertrigo, Table 1 lists other apparent risk factors including venous insufficiency and obesity. Patients with positive cultures for beta hemolytic streptococcus taken from the upper respiratory tract, the vagina, or the cervix 1 day prior to radical vulvectomy were also at higher risk of developing recurrent cellulitis [13]. Ellison and McGregor [17] also reported an association between Group B vaginal colonization and recurrent postcoital cellulitis of the legs. Again, many of these risk factors have not been substantiated by controlled studies. Diabetes and alcohol abuse were not confirmed as significant risk factors in one analysis [16], while another found only a small difference in cellulitis recurrence rates between patients with and without diabetes [18].

The diagnosis of cellulitis is predominantly a clinical one. Patients with cellulitis most commonly present with complaints of erythema, swelling, pain, malaise, fevers, and chills. The rash has indistinct borders compared to erysipelas, where the border is well defined and raised. However, deep venous thrombosis and cancer recurrence can mimic cellulitis. In one study, 8.5% of patients with arm edema after treatment for breast cancer had concomitant axillary venous thrombosis [19]. Five percent of those patients with worsening arm edema were found to have cancer recurrence in a 6 month follow-up period [19] (Table 2).

Management of recurrent cellulitis is based on first the correct diagnosis and treatment of the presenting episode and secondly on preventing recurrences. Since cases yield no demonstrable organisms, antibiotic regimens should provide coverage for both beta hemolytic *streptococcus* and *Staphylococcus aureus*. Amoxicillin/clavulanate, cephalexin, dicloxacillin, and clindamycin are the oral drugs of choice. Ampicillin/sulbactam, cephalexin, oxacillin, and clindamycin are the intravenous drugs of choice. It is also important to consider methicillin-resistant *S. aureus*, requiring treatment with vancomycin. If cellulitis is known to be of streptococcal origin, treatment with penicillin or erythromycin is adequate. In most case reports of recurrent cellulitis, patients treated with penicillin improved within 24 hours, with total resolution within 5 to 7 days. The choice of oral versus intravenous delivery of antibiotics should depend on the severity of the acute episode and comorbid medical conditions such as diabetes mellitus. Some general improvement should be expected within 24 to 48 hours. However, resolution of the erythematous lesion may take several more days. The total length of antibiotic treatment and intravenous versus oral dosage is not fixed but should be based on symptomatic improvement and on the tendency to recur.

Various prophylactic antibiotic regimens have also been suggested. Kremer et al. [20] studied 36 patients who had suffered two or more episodes of erysipelas or cellulitis. The study patients received erythromycin base 250 mg tid for 18 months and none experienced recurrences. In contrast, half of the patients in the untreated group relapsed. Wang et al. [18] studied the role of penicillin as a prophylactic agent, giving the experimental group benza-

TABLE 2 Differential Diagnosis for Cellulitis

Deep venous thrombosis
Cancer recurrence
Radiation changes
Perioperative wound infection
Acute allergic contact dermatitis
Giant urticaria
Angioedema
Erythema nodosum
Early herpes zoster

thine penicillin G, at a dosage of 1.2 million units per month for 1 year. The difference in recurrence rates between the experimental and control groups, however, was not statistically significant. Interestingly, they simultaneously studied the role of potential "predisposing factors" such as diabetes mellitus, deep venous thrombosis, liver cirrhosis, obesity, congestive heart failure, varicose veins, and previous operation of the legs on the effectiveness of penicillin prophylaxis. All patients in the experimental group who had recurrences also had one or more of the risk factors. The authors suggest that increasing the dosage to 3.6 to 4.8 million units or shortening the interval to 2 weeks might improve this regimen. In addition, patients should be referred for the appropriate management of lymphedema. Current therapies to control lymphedema include compression stockings, physical therapy, massage therapy, diuretics, and surgery. Recurrences have been reduced by combined physiotherapy. Foldi [19] studied 150 women with a prior history of at least three episodes of cellulitis. After phase I of combined physiotherapy, 63.3% of the patients had no further episodes of cellulitis for the 2 year follow-up.

Studies by Dupuy et al. [16] and Greenberg et al. [21] have documented the role of tinea pedis in recurrent cellulitis. The application of a topical antimycotic once or twice daily for about 4 weeks can treat interdigital tinea pedis, if onychomycosis is not involved. If so, the patient may be treated with 12 weeks of terbinafine 250 mg per day, itraconazole 200 mg per day, or itraconazole pulse therapy. Intermittent fluconazole at a dose of 150 to 300 mg once weekly for 6 months is also effective. Consider the use of emollients with lactic acid if there is extensive hyperkeratosis [22].

Finally, one must also consider colonization of various sites in patients with recurrent lower extremity cellulitis. Streptococcal colonization of the upper respiratory tract, vagina, or cervix prior to radical vulvectomy may be a risk factor for cellulitis [13]. Colonization of the vagina appeared to be a factor in case summaries by Ellison and McGregor [17]. Vaginal colonization with Group B streptococcus was associated with postcoital development of cellulitis. Recognition and prevention of infection of the vagina prior to intercourse prevented recurrences in both patients.

The approach to the patient with recurrent cellulitis is more comprehensive than the simple antibiotic regimens given for isolated episodes of cellulitis. One must consider various underlying processes, including deep vein thrombosis and recurrent cancer. Identification and good management of predisposing factors can prevent most recurrences. The role of lymphedema and tinea pedis in recurrent cellulitis has been particularly well documented. Although studies have shown the benefit of prophylactic penicillin and erythromycin, some cases are refractory to a variety of antibiotics. In these cases, novel therapies must combine the use of effective antibiotics with good intracellular and tissue penetration, reduction of lymphedema, eradication of cutaneous fungal infections, and control of other skin diseases.

REFERENCES

1. Klin W. Infections in patients with gynelogic malignancy. Wonchenscher 1983; 95(20):708–718.
2. McNeely SMD Jr, Hopkins M, Ehlerova B, Roberts J. Infection on a gynecologic oncology service. Gynecologic Oncologic 1990; 37:183–187.
3. Daly JW, Facog C, King CR, Monif GR. Progressive necrotizing wound infections in postirradiated patients. Obstetrics and Gynecology 1978; 52(suppl 1).
4. Henderson WH, Facog. Obstetrics and Gynecology 1977; 49(suppl 1).
5. Sotrel G, Hirsch E, Edelin KC. Necrotizing fasciitis following diagnostic laparascopy. Obstetrics and Gynecology 1983; 62(suppl 3).
6. Sepkowitz KA, Hemsell DL, Armestrong D. Management of infections in gynecologic cancer patients. Principles and Practice of Gynecologic Oncology. 2d ed. 1997:487–505.
7. Satin AJ, Harrison CR, Hancock KC, Zahn CM. Relapsing clostridium difficile toxin-associated colitis in ovarian cancer patients treated with chemotherapy. Obstetrics and Gynecology 1989; 74(3). Part 2.
8. Krishnan CS, Grant PT, Robertson G, Hacker NF. Lymphatic ascites following lymphadenectomy for gynecological malignancy. IGCS International Journal of Gynecological Cancer 2001; 11:392–396.
9. Andriessen MP, Mulder JG, Sleijfer DT. Lactobacillus septicemia, an unusual complication during the treatment of metastatic choriocarcinoma. Gynecologic Oncology 1991;40(1):87–89.
10. Woodruff A, Olivero J. Recurrent cellulitis complicating chronic lymphedema. Hospital Practice 1995; 87:91.
11. Simon M, Cody R. Cellulitis after axillary lymph node dissection for carcinoma of the breast. American Journal of Medicine 1992; 93:543–548.
12. Dankert J, Bouma J. Recurrent acute leg cellulitis after hysterectomy with pelvic lymphadnectomy. British Journal of Obstetrics and Gynaecology 1987; 94:788–790.
13. Bouma J, Dankert J. Recurrent acute leg cellulitis in patients after radical vulvectomy. Gynecologic Oncology 1988; 29:50–57.
14. Mortimer P. The pathophysiology of lymphedema. Cancer 1998; 83(suppl 12 American):2798–2802.
15. Neto HJ. Arm edema after treatment for breast cancer. Lymphology 1998; 83(suppl 12 American):2798 2802.
16. Dupuy A, Benchikhi H, Roujeau J, et al. Risk factors for erysipelas of the leg (cellulitis) case-control study. BMJ 1999; 318:1591–1594.
16a. Foldi E. Prevention of dermatolymphangioadenitis by combined physiotherapy of the swollen arm after treatment for breast cancer. Lymphology 1996; 29:48–49.

17. Ellison R, McGregor J. Recurrent postcoital lower-extremity streptococcal erythoderma in women. JAMA 1987; 257:3260–3262.

18. Wang J, Liu Y, Cheng D, Yen MY, Chen YS, Wang JH, Wann SR, Lin HH. Role of benzathine penicillin G in prophylaxis for recurrent streptococcal cellulitis of the lower legs. Clin Infect Dis 1997 Sep; 25(3):685–689.

19. Foldi E. Prevention of dermatolymphangioadenitis by combined physiotherapy of the swollen arm after treatment for breast cancer. Lymphology 1996; 29:48–49.

20. Kremer M, Zuckerman R, Avraham Z, et al. Long-term antimicrobial therapy in the prevention of recurrent soft-tissue infections. Journal of Infection 1991; 22:37–40.

21. Greenberg J, DeSanctis R, Mills R. Vein-donor-leg cellulitis after coronary artery bypass surgery. Annals of Internal Medicine 1982; 97:565–566.

22. Elewski B. Tinea pedis and tinea manuum. Clinical Dermatology 1999; 3:17–19.

22

Infections Related to the Management and Treatment of Sarcomas

Wendy W. Carter and Douglas Letson
Moffitt Cancer Center and Research Institute
Tampa, Florida, U.S.A.

INTRODUCTION

There are multiple histological subtypes of sarcomas, with various clinical presentations, but all with a common mesenchymal origin. Soft tissue sarcomas invade locally but also have a high incidence of distant metastasis and local recurrence despite treatment. Approximately 50 to 60% of all sarcomas present in the extremities; 40% present in the lower limbs, 25% present in the retroperitoneal and visceral cavity, 15% in truncal and thoracic areas, and 5% in the head and neck region [1]. In the United States, 6000 cases of sarcoma are diagnosed and treated annually [2]. The approach to management often involves surgical intervention. Advances in technology have led to the addition of adjuvant and neoadjuvant chemotherapy, immunotherapy, radiation therapy, and even hyperthermic isolated limb perfusion (HILP) therapy in selected cases [3]. These therapies, unfortunately, also have the associated risk of infections.

Surgical intervention is often the cornerstone of treatment for osteosarcoma or soft tissue sarcoma. There are multiple different surgical approaches to the various types of sarcoma, and each patient will have a surgery tailored to their particular presentation and management needs. However, with surgery comes the risk of infection. Infection of the surgical wound, infection of the prosthesis, seroma formation, cellulitis, and recurrent cellulitis can develop.

WOUND AND SOFT TISSUE INFECTIONS

Patients with sarcoma are at increased risk for a surgical wound infection when any surgical procedure is undertaken. However, wound infections in these patients can have devastating consequences, especially if deep infection occurs that can affect an indwelling prosthesis or graft. This can lead to reoperation, graft, or prosthesis removal and occasionally amputation of the involved limb or entire hindquarter [4–6].

The process of wound healing is complex and multifaceted. Many opportunities for contamination and subsequent infection occur from the time of the first incision until full wound healing. Multiple factors affect the healing process. Nutrition should be maximized to an appropriate caloric intake with attention to vitamins A, B, D, and E, zinc, and proteins, in particular, arginine and glutamine. Postoperative oxygen tension should be maintained at a high level by keeping the hemoglobin above 8 gm/dL as this allows for perfusion of oxygen into the fresh wound. In addition, hypothermia causes vasoconstriction, which inhibits both oxygen delivery and the delivery of antibiotics. Therefore attention to normothermia becomes essential to decreasing risk of postoperative infection [7]. In a study by Kurz et al. [8], 200 patients undergoing colorectal surgery were randomized to receive either standard postoperative care (hypothermic group) or additional postoperative warming (normothermic group). All other postanesthesia care, as well as perioperative antibiotics, was identical. Nineteen percent of the hypothermic group had a surgical wound infection, but only 6% of the normothermic group developed a surgical wound infection. In addition, the normothermic group had suture removal one day prior and discharge from the hospital 2.6 days prior when compared to the hypothermic group [8]. Elimination of dead space after bulky tumor resection is imperative to prevent seroma formation, which can result in an abscess or cellulitis. Lastly, timing of the antibiotic is important. The antibiotic that is present at the time of incision is trapped in the fibrin clot as it forms in the fresh wound. The antibiotic can then exert a local effect on the surrounding tissue. If an antibiotic is given later, it is much more difficult to have diffusion of the antibiotic into the fibrin clot and may have little effect on the fresh wound. Therefore the recommendation remains that preoperative antibiotics be given 30 minutes to 1 hour prior to first incision [7].

In addition to the risk of wound infection associated with any surgery, patients with sarcomas may have additional risks due to the size of the necessary tissue resection and other therapies used for treatment such as chemotherapy or radiation therapy. For example, preoperative radiation therapy may be targeted to the tumor, enabling the size of the mass to decrease and therefore allowing for a smaller resection at the time of surgery. Some studies have shown that preoperative radiation is associated with higher rates of postoperative complications, particularly with wound healing and skin flap necrosis. Postoperative radiation is associated with fewer wound complications but exposes a greater area to radiation, and there are long-term effects of this treatment, namely fibrosis and muscle contracture [9]. However, one small study recently published showed that the site of the sarcoma, the radiation field size, the surgical resection volume, the grade of acute radiation toxicity, diabetes, vascular disease, and smoking were not predictive of wound complications following preoperative radiotherapy [10]. Whether radiation is given preoperatively or postoperatively, the 5-year survival is the same. If chemotherapy is given, the immunosuppression that results directly impacts the ability to heal wounds and increases the chance of local wound infection as well as systemic infections related to immunosuppression [9]. However, one retrospective study did not show any increase in postoperative morbidity in patients with soft tissue sarcoma who were treated with neoadjuvant chemotherapy versus those patients who underwent surgery prior to any chemotherapy treatments [11].

Some patients with sarcoma undergo limb salvage procedures that include placement of prosthetic joints or grafts. Infection rates in these procedures vary widely (5–20%), and unfortunately many of these patients develop deep tissue infections necessitating removal of hardware, long courses of antibiotics, and in some cases amputations [4–6,12].

Wound infections in all patients undergoing surgery are an unfortunate complication. The organisms most often associated with wound infections and prosthetic implant infections are *Staphylococcus aureus* and coagulase-negative staphylococci and gram-negative bacilli. Perioperative antibiotics should be tailored to the specific surgery that the patient is to undergo. In addition, empirical antibiotics should cover the most likely infecting organism(s) based on the clinical scenario, until culture results are returned [13]. Consideration for resistant organisms is necessary in cancer patients. Many patients with neoplastic disease have prior hospitalizations or outpatient facility visits and exposure to selective antibiotics prior to surgery, which places them at higher risk for resistant organism colonization and infection. Empirical vancomycin and cefepime are effective antibiotics for treatment of these infections until culture results are available.

SEROMAS

A seroma is a collection of serum and lymph that develops after a surgical procedure. They often cause swelling and pain under a surgical incision.

Unlike an abscess, a seroma usually lacks warmth and erythema on physical exam. Seromas are a complication associated with surgical removal of sarcomas as well as other surgeries. Seromas are less likely than hematomas to become infected, but a seroma may become inoculated with bacteria with therapeutic aspiration attempts [15]. The literature regarding seromas in patients with sarcoma is scarce. However, studies have been done in relation to breast cancer, and seroma development in relation to operative procedure which can be applied to the patient with saroma.

The pathophysiology of seroma formation is unknown. We have yet to find a unique cause or a treatable process for the development of a seroma. Proposed factors that may influence the formation of seromas are the amount of postoperative activity, closure of anatomic dead space, use of closed suction drainage, use of preoperative radiation or chemotherapy, and use of electrocautery [16–18]. Although seroma is not a life-threatening complication, it does add to the recovery time, delay other treatments, and increase the health care dollars spent on postoperative care. Postoperative rates of seroma development in breast cancer patients vary from 3 to 60% [16,17]. Woodworth et al. showed that seroma was increased in patients who received neoadjuvant chemotherapy for breast cancer. There also was an increased incidence of seroma formation in patients who had core needle biopsy and breast preservation surgery over those with open biopsy [16]. The standard for treatment of a seroma is drainage, by either aspiration or closed suction drain. Both methods have risks of infection, and patients should be watched for signs or symptoms of infection. The studies done with breast cancer patients can be applied to the care and management of sarcoma patients. These patients undergo similar courses of therapy that often include surgery, radiation, and chemotherapy. Therefore the risks are similar, and in our clinical experience, the development of seromas in sarcoma patients is not uncommon.

CELLULITIS

Cellulitis is an acute infection of skin and soft tissue. Cellulitis and recurrent cellulitis are syndromes that again are shared by patients with breast cancer and patients with sarcomas. It is a frequently diagnosed syndrome that in some cases may become recurrent and in both instances causes significant morbidity.

The most common pathogen associated with cellulitis is β-hemolytic streptococci and *Staphylococcus aureus*. Both Lancefield group A (*S. pyogenes*) and non–group A (B, C, F, G) β-hemolytic streptococci have been associated with cellulitis [19]. In patients with venous and lymphatic compromise and cellulitis, the non–group A streptococci are often the pathogen [20]. Patients often show other factors that influence the organisms that may cause cellulitis. For example, an immunocompromised patient may have deficits in number or function of neutrophils, humoral immune dysfunction with lowered antibody levels and decreased complement activity, or inadequate cellular immune function with loss of lymphocytes, natural killer cells, or immature macrophages. In the immunocompromised patient, other bacteria and fungi as well as viruses and parasites must be considered when evaluating cellulitis. Other bacteria of concern that cause cellulitis in a neutropenic host includes *Pseudomonas aeruginosa*, *Stenotrophomonas maltophilia*, and methicillin-resistant *Staphylococcus aureus* [21]. Although β-hemolytic streptococci and *S. aureus* will cause the majority of cellulitis, patients with sarcoma need to be evaluated individually for any immune defects that would increase the risk of an unusual pathogen.

Clinical observation over the years resulted in the recognition that lymphatic and venous compromise is often present when cellulitis and particularly recurrent cellulitis develops. Because of medical advances, lymphatic and venous compromise have increased from more intensive surgical interventions. Two such cases are saphenous venectomy for coronary artery bypass grafting and breast conservation therapy for early-stage breast cancer [20,22–24]. This is similar to the surgical interventions that patients with sarcoma undergo. Radiation therapy and chemotherapy also interplay with both the breast cancer population and the sarcoma population in this clinical scenario.

Two case control studies have proven the association of lymphedema and an increased incidence of cellulitis [25,26]. How lymphedema predisposes patients to recurrent cellulitis is unknown. It is commonly believed that the extra fluid rich in protein and deficient in local immune responses provides the perfect environment for bacterial growth and subsequently clinical cellulitis [27]. Other risk factors that are statistically associated with the development of cellulitis include skin barrier disruptions (ulcers, tinea pedis, dermatosis and wounds), venous insuffiency, leg edema, and being overweight [23].

Treatment for cellulitis is targeted for either acute or chronic management strategies. In patients with acute cellulitis, the most common pathogens (β-hemolytic streptococci and *S. aureus*) should be covered by empirical antibiotic therapy. Parenteral antibiotics include ampicillin/sulbactam, cefazolin or nafcillin. Appropriate oral therapy includes cephalexin, amoxicillin/clavulanate, dicloxacillin, or clindamycin. An advantage of clindamycin therapy is the drug's ability to decrease virulence factor production including pyrogenic toxins, M protein, and capsular polysaccharide containing hyaluronic acid from group A streptococci [19]. Broader antibiotic coverage will depend on the epidemiology of the patient. Therapy for recurrent cellulitis (two or more cases in the same anatomic location) is directed at decreasing associated risk factors. Tinea pedis must be treated, as must any other wounds or dermatological conditions until full healing. Attention to the reduction of lymph-edema is necessary. Patients must also have meticulous skin and nail care to avoid breaks in the protective barrier. For patients who have as many risk factors decreased or eliminated as possible and continue to suffer from bouts of cellulitis, daily chronic suppressive therapy may be considered.

SUMMARY

Patients with sarcomas have multiple clinical presentations that result in various medical interventions, each one with its own risk of infection. Infections related to these patients vary and are often related to the morbidity of the treatments necessary for survival. If clinicians are aware of the commonly occurring syndromes and the pathogens likely to be related to them, patients with infections related to sarcomas may have improved outcomes.

REFERENCES

1. Dirix LY, Van Oosterom AT. Soft tissue sarcoma in adults. Curr Opin Oncol 1999; 11(4):285–295.
2. Lewis JJ, Leung D, Espat J, Woodruff JM, Brennan MF. Effect of reresection in extremity soft tissue sarcoma. Ann Surgery 2000; 231(5):655–663.
3. Bramwell VHC. Osteosarcomas and other cancers of bone. Curr Opin Oncol 2000; 12(4):330–336.
4. Lietman SA, Tomford WW, Gebhardt MC, Springfield DS, Mankin HJ. Complications of irradiated allografts in orthopaedic tumor surgery. Clin Orthop Rel Research 2000; 375:214–217.
5. Malawer MM, Chou LB. Prosthetic survival and clinical results with use of large-segment replacements in the treatment of high-grade bone sarcomas. J Bone Joint Surg 1995; 77A(8):1154–1165.
6. Ozaki T, Hoffman C, Hillman A, Gosheger G, Lindner N, Winkelmann W. Implantation of hemipelvic prosthesis after resection of sarcoma. Clin Orthop Rel Research 2002; 396:197–205.
7. Hunt TK, Hopf HW. Wound healing and wound infection: what surgeons and anesthesiologists can do. Surg Clin N Am 1997; 77(3):587–606.
8. Kurz A, Sessler DI, Lenhardt R. Perioperative normothermia to reduce the incidence of surgical-wound infection and shorten hospitalization. N Eng J Med 1996; 334(19):1209–1215.
9. Moley JF, Eberlein TJ. Soft-tissue sarcomas. Surg Clin N Am 2000; 80(2):687–708.
10. Kunisada T, Ngan SY, Powell GN, Choong PFM. Wound complications following pre-operative radiotherapy for soft-tissue sarcoma. Euro J Surg Onc 2002; 28:75–79.
11. Meric F, Milas M, Hunt KK, Hess KR, Pisters PWT, Hildebrandt G, Patel SR, Benjamin RS, Plager C, Papadopolous NEJ, Burgess MA, Pollock RE, Feig

BW. Impact on neoadjuvant chemotherapy on postoperative morbidity in soft tissue sarcomas. J Clin Onco 2000; 189–190:3378–3383.

12. Harrington KD, Johnston JO, Kaufer HN, Luck JV, Moore TM. Limb salvage and prosthetic joint reconstruction for low-grade and selected high-grade sarcomas of bone after wide resection and replacement by autoclaved autogeneic grafts. Clin Ortho Rel Res 1986; 211:180–214.

13. Guideline for prevention of surgical site infection. Centers for Disease Control and Prevention (CDC) Hospital Infection Control Practices Advisory Committee. Am J Infect Control 1999; 27:250–278.

14. Sakai C, Satoh Y, Ohkusu K, Kumagai K, Ishii A. Outbreak of methicillin-resistant *Staphylococcus aureus* (MRSA) infection or colonization among patients with neoplastic disease: a clinico-epidemiological study of 11 cases. J Japanese Assoc Infect Dis 2001; 75(11):940–945.

15. Angood PB, Gingalewski CA, Andersen DK. Surgical complications. In: Towsend CM, Beauchamp RD, Evers BM, Mattox KL, eds. Sabiston Textbook of Surgery. Philadelphia: W.B. Saunders, 2001:198 225.

16. Woodworth PA, McBoyle MF, Helmer SD, Beamer RL. Seroma formation after breast cancer surgery: incidence and predicting factors. Am Surg 2000; 66:444–451.

17. Porter KA, O'Connor S, Rimm E, Lopez M. Electrocautery as a factor in seroma formation following mastectomy. Am J Surg 1998; 176:8–11.

18. Bonnema J, van Geel AN, Ligtenstein DA, Schmitz PIM, Wiggers T. A prospective randomized trial of high versus low vacuum drainage after axillary dissection for breast cancer. Am J Surg 1997; 173:76–79.

19. Baddour LM. Cellulitis syndromes: an update. Intern J Antimicrob Agents 2000; 14:113–116.

20. Baddour LM, Bisno AL. Recurrent cellulitis after saphenous venectomy for coronary bypass surgery. Ann Intern Med 1982; 97:493–496.

21. Lopez FA, Sanders CV. Dermatologic infections in the immunocompromised (non-HIV) host. Infect Dis Clin N Am 2001; 15(2):671–702.

22. Baddour LM. Recent considerations in recurrent cellulitis. Curr Infect Dis Rep 2001; 3:461–465.

23. Baddour LM. Breast cellulitis complication breast conservation therapy. J Int Med 199; 245:5 9.

24. Mertz KR, Baddour LM, Bell JL, Gwin JL. Breast cellulitis following breast conservation therapy: a novel complication of medical progress. Clin Infect Dis 1998; 26:481–486.

25. Brewer VH, Hahn KA, Rohrbach BW, Bell JL, Baddour LM. Risk factor analysis for breast cellulitis complicating breast conservation therapy. Clin Infect Dis 2000; 31:654–659.

26. Dupuy A, Benchikhi H, Roujeau JC, Bernard P, Vaillant L, Chosidow O, Sassolas B, Guillaume JC, Grob JC, Bastuji-Garin S. Risk factors for erysipelas of the leg (cellulitis): case-control study. BMJ 1999; 318:1591 1594.

27. Rockson SG. Lymphedema. Am J Med 2001; 110:288–295.

23

Infections Associated with Cutaneous Malignancy

John S. Czachor
Wright State University School of Medicine
and Miami Valley Hospital
Dayton, Ohio, U.S.A.

INTRODUCTION

Skin is the major interface between humans and their environment, in part functioning as a primary physical barrier against infection. When broached, local infection ensues. Dissemination of the infectious process is dependent upon the depth of the infection, access to vascular/lymphatic channels, and host defense deficits. Infections cross into deeper tissues when the integrity of the stratum corneum is disturbed. The hair follicle may also serve as a portal of entry to these subepithelial regions for bacteria residing on the skin surface. The rich plexus of capillaries beneath the dermal papillae may provide access to the general circulation. Additionally, the skin and its structures may be the receptacle of infection, as pathogens disseminate from the bloodstream, lymphatics, or direct contact with infected areas.

Microbes are found on nearly all skin surfaces, which under the appropriate circumstances form the nidus of infection. Resident flora is permanent and must be able to attach to epithelial skin cells. These microorganisms must constantly repopulate the tissue surface in order to avoid removal during the normal desquamative process. Transient flora is often dislodged from adjacent skin surfaces or from the environment. These organisms do not adhere well, are generally short-term inhabitants, and do not survive for prolonged periods. Temporary flora resides on the skin owing to changes in the environment or in the population of permanent residents. These bacteria do attach to the epithelium and multiply, but they are usually not longstanding in their residence.

The skin itself has several intrinsic properties that limit the spread of microbes beyond the surface [1]. Bacteria can only adhere to the epithelial cell surface by coupling with antigen-specific binding sites. This specificity restricts general attachment of bacteria to the epithelium and decreases the number and variety of potential pathogens. The intact stratum corneum forms a barricade to deeper tissues, and along with its inherent dryness it discourages the growth of microbes. Regular shedding also reduces the number of surface dwellers. Resident flora on the epithelium generate acidic compounds via the metabolism of lipids from sebum, which decreases the local pH and hence bacterial growth. These permanent microbes may further inhibit skin colonization through interference, by occupying bacterial binding sites, exhausting available nutrients, and/or elaborating antimicrobial substances.

The host immune system obviously plays a vital role in conjunction with the skin. Clearly, intact humoral immunity is necessary. Although less frequently involved, an active cell-mediated response may assist in preventing infection. Finally, IgA and IgG antibody secretion into sweat provides added local activity directed against surface microbes.

ASSOCIATIONS OF INFECTION AND NEOPLASM

Cutaneous malignancies contribute to the genesis of infection. Direct effects include the disruption of the protective skin barrier, which allows resident and temporary flora to penetrate and become infective when given the opportunity. These surface cancers may also provide access to deeper tissues and to the bloodstream and lymphatic channels. The cutaneous neoplasms may have immunosuppressive or immunomodulating characteristics that lessen the host's ability to combat infection, though this is a minor contribution. Indirect effects, generated by the modalities employed to treat skin cancers, play a substantial role in the formation of infection. For instance, indwelling vascular access devices, which are implanted to administer different therapies, create a direct route through the skin into the underlying tissues and vascular structures. Chemotherapy, radiation therapy, immunotherapy, and glucocorticosteroids all reduce host immunity in various ways. In addition to its systemic effects, chronic steroid administration will cause thinning and atrophy of the skin, resulting in poor healing [1]. Minor trauma may be enough to disrupt the skin surface and create ready access for microbes to initiate infection. Tumor excision and resection create skin defects that enhance the possibility of pathogens via postoperative infection, although wound infections following excisions of superficial cancers occur no more frequently than after other clean surgical procedures [2]. The direct and indirect effects combine to produce a variety of infectious complications associated with cutaneous malignancies.

To complicate matters further, skin cancers may be confused with infectious processes, and vice versa. Neoplastic tumors that have resembled infections include skin squamous cell carcinoma from fingers mimicking abscess [3], chronic paronychia [4], and verruca vulgaris [5]; mycosis fungoides presenting as dissecting cellulitis of the scalp [6]; metastatic rectal carcinoma in the inguinal region masquerading as cellulitis [7]; malignant fibrous histiocytoma resembling mycetoma [8]; and malignant melanoma presenting as paronychia [9], panniculitis [10], and zosteriform metastases [11]. Infections that have been confused with cutaneous malignancies include both chronic varicella zoster infection [12] and disseminated cryptococcus [13] being mistaken for basal cell carcinoma; mycetoma pedis simulating malignant

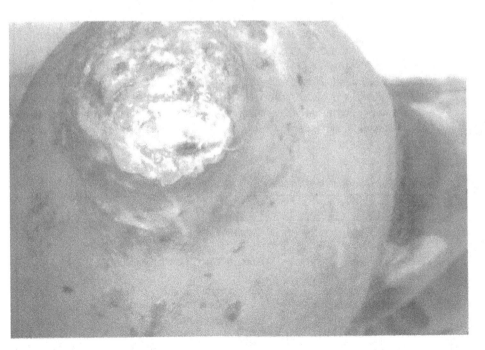

FIGURE 1   Infection surrounds superficial carcinoma on the scalp. Photo courtesy of Hari Polenakovik, M.D.

TABLE 1a   Infections and Cutaneous Neoplasms

Neoplasm	Infectious agent	Ref.
Kaposi's sarcoma	Human herpesvirus 8	1, 21
Posttransplant cutaneous B cell lymphoma	Epstein–Barr virus	1, 22
Invasive squamous cell carcinoma of skin	Human papillomavirus 11, 16, 18	1, 23–26

melanoma [14]; and bilateral tinea nigra plantaris mimicking melanoma [15] (Figure 1).

Cutaneous malignancies and infection may be linked in other ways. Skin neoplasms have developed at the prior site of a healed infection. Basal cell carcinoma has been documented at the site of a gumma [16], as well as forming on the skin following recurrent erysipelas and chronic lymphedema of the leg [17]. There have also been reports of skin carcinoma isolated from the location of previous *Herpes simplex* infection [18,19], while T cell lymphoma has infiltrated a prior varicella zoster dermatome [20]. There are a number of infectious diseases that cause or are suspected of causing skin cancers. See Tables 1a,b. Furthermore, infectious diseases may affect the development of cutaneous neoplasms. For example, repetitive episodes of infection associated with elevated body temperature reduce the risk of malignant melanoma [34]. Even though human immunodeficiency virus (HIV) infected patients possess the same risk factors for developing skin cancers, there is no correlation with the actual number of cancers nor the formation of squamous cell carcinoma and the degree of immunosuppression [35]. However, surface neoplasms grow more rapidly and are more invasive in

TABLE 1b   Speculative Associations

Neoplasm	Infectious agent	Ref.
Cutaneous T cell lymphoma	*Chlamydia pneumoniae*	27,28
Cutaneous T cell lymphoma	Human T lymphotrophic virus I/II	29
Basal cell carcinoma, mycosis fungoides	*Mycobacterium leprae*	30,31
Malignant melanoma of the sinonasal region	Epstein–Barr virus	32
Squamous cell carcinoma of head and neck	*Streptococcus anginosus*	33

AIDS patients than in the general population [36]. Patients who have idiopathic CD_4 (+) T cell lymphocytopenia without HIV infection are also known to have various dermatological findings, including basal cell carcinomas [37].

INFECTIONS AND SQUAMOUS CELL CARCINOMA (SCC)

The incidence of SCC has steadily increased over the past two decades [1,38]. Interestingly, relatively few associations with infection beyond the physical disruption of the skin resulting in infection have been documented. Most problems have been linked to the treatment of the cancer itself, such as active cutaneous tuberculosis [39] and opportunistic cutaneous myiasis [40] following SCC therapy. Larger skin squamous cell cancers are often surgically removed, and in one study of patients with postoperative infection, 12.5% of those who were infected were patients with SCC [2]. On occasion, systemic chemotherapy may be employed in highly advanced cases of skin SCC (also in basal cell carcinoma). Classic chemotherapeutic agents utilized include retinoids, interferon-alpha, cisplatin, and bleomycin; but significant infectious complications are seldom encountered [41–43].

INFECTIONS AND BASAL CELL CARCINOMA (BCC)

Basal cell carcinoma is the most common malignant skin neoplasm found in humans, and as with SCC, there is an ever-increasing number of cases [1,38]. The infectious complications, aside from the potential surface infectious caused by the invading tumor, are related to the treatments rendered against BCC. Because of the propensity to send finger-like projections of tumor into the underlying supporting tissues, Mohs micrographic surgery (MMS) is a treatment option. Thirteen of 24 wound infections in one study were noted following excision of BCC, 12 of which were using the Mohs technique [2]. Five of these postoperative infections were related to surgeries performed on the ear. The overall infection rate with MMS was 2.45%, but when considering just the ear procedures, the rate ballooned to 12.5% (6/48), and 83.3% (5/6) of the infections occurred in BCC patients [2]. Furthermore, tumors with a greater mean area of residual defect after MMS seem to be at greater risk for infection. In addition to the typical pathogens, unusual microorganisms such as yeast, *Pseudomonas aeruginosa*, and *Mycobacterium chelonae* have been cultured from postexcision wound infections in patients undergoing surgery for BCC [2,44].

INFECTIONS AND MALIGNANT MELANOMA (MM)

An increasing number of cases of malignant melanoma has been reported over the past 20 years [1,38]. Unlike SCC and BCC, melanoma has a propensity for metastasis, thus requiring more aggressive interventions. Surgical excision, chemotherapy, immunotherapy, and radiation therapy (alone or in combination) are common treatments. Immunotherapy with bacille Calmette–Guerin (BCG) injected directly into the lesion to alter the course of MM has spawned the complications of primary inoculation tuberculosis [45], distant cutaneous tuberculous granuloma [46], and systemic tuberculous infection [47]. Although postoperative wound infection is infrequent, Papachristou and Fortner documented 40 of 211 patients (18.96%) with infection following MM excision [48]. The authors also sought to evaluate whether these postexcision infections could affect the course of MM, as BCG does. Even though the incidence of local melanoma recurrence in the group of patients who were infected was significantly lower ($p < 0.01$), there was no survival benefit or disease-free interval benefit [48].

INFECTIONS AND CUTANEOUS T CELL LYMPHOMA (CTCL)

Cutaneous T cell lymphoma remains the most commonly encountered primary lymphoma of the skin. CTCL, along with its variants, mycosis fungoides (MF) and Sézary syndrome (SS), has a predisposition toward infection because of its widespread disruption of the skin surface by lymphomatous infiltration, as well as potential systemic immunosuppressive effects. Infection frequently is the cause of death in this patient group, ranging from 27–60% in various studies [49–54].

The skin plays a most prominent role in the formation of infection in this malignancy. The lymphoma involving the skin layers often breaks down the surface epidermis, creating lesions that invariably become colonized and subsequently infected [49,51,55,56]. Invasive surgical procedures, indwelling vascular access devices, radiation therapy, and chemotherapy augment the skin disruption to provide further pathways of entry for cutaneous microorganisms [49,51]. Traditional skin organisms, for example Staphylococcus aureus and ß-hemolytic streptococcus, are readily cultured from these surface infections. Recurrent skin infections have been documented, but they appear related to the development of extracutaneous lymphoma and not the degree of malignant skin involvement [49,57]. Disseminated cutaneous Herpes virus infection due to H. simplex [49,58] and H. varicellazoster [49,59] have been reported, while a small number of patients have manifested herpes infection via Kaposi's varicelliform eruption [49,60,61]. Fungal infections of the skin caused by histoplasmosis [62], Cryptococcus [63,64] and various Candida species [49,65] have also been identified.

Besides being the origination of local infection, the surface lesions double as the source from which infection disseminates [49,51,56]. Staphylococcus aureus is the most common pathogen isolated from the bloodstream, but gram-negative organisms including *Pseudomonas aeruginosa* are also recovered from septicemic episodes [49,51,57]. Secondary nosocomial colonization of skin lesions by Enterobacteriaceae and *Pseudomonas aeruginosa* during *S. aureus* septicemia may be the mechanism behind the gram-negative infective episodes [49,51]. Multiagent chemotherapy has been found to be an independent risk factor for these bacteremic events [49]. Since only 9.5% (2/21) of the patients were neutropenic during its administration, chemotherapy may just be a marker for a group of patients with poor prognosis rather than a potent inducer of infection and an actual risk factor.

Bacterial pneumonia diagnosed in patients with CTCL is an important infectious complication. Third in order of frequency behind skin and bloodstream infections, it is nonetheless a major infectious cause of death in this population [49–53,66,67]. The majority of these lung infections are acquired nosocomially, as is the case for septicemia. Of interest is that when pulmonary infiltrates are radiographically delineated, they are not invariably pneumonia and may have a noninfectious etiology, including the malignancy itself [49,68–70]. In 60% of CTCL patients, a pulmonary focus of malignancy was the first documentation of an extracutaneous focus of tumor. Fiberoptic bronchoscopy, bronchoalveolar lavage with or without biopsy, thoracoscopy with biopsy, or open lung biopsy may be necessary to establish the correct diagnosis.

It is difficult to delineate the exact role CTCL and its relative immunosuppression has upon the infectious process. There is a progressive fall in the absolute numbers of normal circulating T cells, coupled with an increase in the CD_4/CD_8 ratio because of the expanded malignant CD_4 (+) cell population, and a decreased normal CD_8(+) T cell count [54,71,72]. Delayed type hypersensitivity, however, remains intact until the later stages of the disease [73–77], while serum immunoglobulin levels [74,75] and B cell number and function [78,79] are not diminished. In two separate studies of infection and CTCL, there appeared to be little, if any, association of cell mediated immunity (CMI) deficit and infection [49,51]. Scattered reports demonstrating infections with *Pneumocysitis carinii* [80], Cryptococcus [64,81], Aspergillus [49,50], cytomegalovirus [50,55,56], and Toxoplasma [49,50] exist, suggesting that the defect in CMI has a limited contribution toward infectious diseases in patients with CTCL.

CONCLUSION

Infections associated with cutaneous malignancies are generally localized to the skin, but on occasion they may expand beyond the surface into underlying structures. Epidermal defects caused by the cancers remain the main mechanism for development of infection, although necessary surgical procedures and common cancer treatments may provide microorganisms with access into the deeper tissues, lymphatics, and bloodstream. Infections in patients with cutaneous T cell lymphoma may disseminate more widely than in patients with basal cell carcinoma or squamous cell carcinoma, but this may be a function of the widespread skin involvement and the oftentimes more aggressive treatments directed against CTCL, rather than any intrinsic immunosuppressive nature of the malignancy itself. Meticulous attention to sterile technique during procedures, and limiting inpatient hospitalization, may help to reduce or eliminate infectious complications. In addition, aggressive therapy of skin infections should prevent the dissemination of an infection.

REFERENCES

1. Johnson RA. The immune compromised host in the twenty-first century: management of mucocutaneous infections. Seminars in Cutaneous Medicine and Surgery 2000; 19:19–61.
2. Futoryan T, Grande D. Postoperative wound infection rates in dermatologic surgery. Dermatol Surg 1995; 21:509–514.
3. O'Sullivan ST, O'Donoghue JM, Hayes D, O'Shaughnessy M. Squamous cell carcinoma of the finger masquerading as an abscess. Scand J Plast Reconstr Surg Hand Surg 2000; 34:91–92.
4. Betti R, Vergani R, Inselvini E, Tolomino E, Crosti C. Guess what! Subungual squamous cell carcinoma mimicking chronic paronychia. Eur J Dermatol 2000; 10:149–150.
5. Kouskoukis CE, Scher RK, Kopf AW. Squamous-cell carcinoma of the nail bed. J Dermatol Surg Oncol 1982; 8:853–855.
6. Gilliam AC, Lessin SR, Wilson DM, Salhany KE. Folliculotropic mycosis fungoides with large-cell transformation presenting as dissecting cellulitis of the scalp. J Cutan Pathol 1997; 24:169–175.
7. Graham BS, Wong SW. Cancer cellulitis. South Med J 1984; 77:277–278.
8. Soohoo L, Elewski BE. Malignant fibrous histiocytoma resembling mycetoma. J Am Acad Dermatol 1993; 29:318–321.
9. Ware JW. Sub-ungual malignant melanoma presenting as subacute paronychia following trauma. Hand 1977; 9:49–51.
10. Cotton J, Armstrong DJ, Wedig R, Hood AF. Melanoma-in-transit presenting as panniculitis. J Am Acad Dermatol 1998; 39:876–878.
11. North S, Mackey JR, Jensen J. Recurrent malignant melanoma presenting with zosteriform metastases. Cutis 1998; 62:143–146.
12. Tsao H, Tahan SR, Johnson RA. Chronic varicella zoster infection mimicking a basal cell carcinoma in an AIDS patient. J Am Acad Dermatol 1997; 36:831–833.
13. Murakawa GJ, Mauro TM, Egbert B. Disseminated cutaneous Cryptococcus clinically mimicking basal cell carcinoma. Dermatol Surg 1995; 21:992–993.

14. Sommer TC, Carter JB. Mycetoma pedis: report of a case simulating malignant melanoma. J Am Podiatry Assoc 1982; 72:353 355.
15. Tseng SS, Whittier S, Miller SR, Zolar GL. Bilateral tinea nigra plantaris and tinea nigra plantaris mimicking melanoma. Cutis 1999; 64:265 268.
16. Narouz N, Wade AAH, Allan PS. Can basal cell carcinoma develop on the site of a healed gumma? Int J STD AIDS 1999; 10:623–625.
17. Lotem M, Tamir G, Loven D, David M, Hauben D. Multiple basal cell carcinomas of the leg after recurrent erysipelas and chronic lymphedema. J Am Acad Dematol 1994; 31:812–813.
18. Caron GA. Carcinoma at the site of Herpes simplex infection. JAMA 1980; 243:2396.
19. Gecht ML. Carcinoma at the site of Herpes simplex infection. JAMA 1980; 244:1675.
20. Paydas S, Sahin B, Yavuz S, Tuncer I, Gonlusen G. Lymptomatous skin infiltration at the site of previous varicella zoster virus infection in a patient with T-cell lymphoma. Leuk Lymphoma 2000; 37:229–232.
21. Gao SJ, Kingsley L, Hoover DR, Spira TJ, Rinaldo CR, Saah A, Phair J, Detels R, Parry P, Chang Y, Moore PJ. Seroconversion to antibodies against Kaposi's sarcoma–associated Herpesvirus-related latent nuclear antigens before the development of Kaposi's sarcoma. N Engl J Med 1996; 335:233 241.
22. McGregor JM, Yu CC, Lu QL, Cotter FE, Levinson DA, MacDonald DM. Posttransplant cutaneous lymphoma. J Am Acad Dermatol 1993; 29:549–554.
23. Solivan GA, Smith KJ, James WD. Cutaneous horn of the penis: its association with squamous cell carcinoma and HPV-16 infection. J Am Acad Dermatol 1990; 23:969–972.
24. Jenson AB, Geyer S, Sundberg JP, Ghim S. Human papillomavirus and skin cancer. J Investig Dermatol Symp Proc 2001; 6:203–206.
25. Cohen LM, Tyring SK, Rady P, Callen JP. Human papillomavirus type 11 in multiple squamous cell carcinomas in a patient with subacute cutaneous lupus erythematosis. J Am Acad Dermatol 1992; 26:840–845.
26. Moy RL, Eliezri YD, Nuovo G, Zitelli JA, Bennett RG, Silverstein S. Human papillomavirus type 16 DNA in periungual squamous cell carcinoma. JAMA 1989; 261:2669–2673.
27. Abrams JT, Vonderheid EC, Kolbe S, Appelt DM, Akring EJ, Balin BJ. Sezary T-cell activating factor is a *Chlamydia pneumoniae* associated protein. Clin Diagn Lab Immunol 1999; 6:895–905.
28. Abrams JT, Balin BJ, Vonderheid EC. Association between Sezary T-cell-activating factor, *Chlamydia pneumoniae*, and cutaneous T-cell lymphoma. Ann NY Acad Sci 2001; 941:69–85.
29. Pancake BA, Zucker-Franklin D, Coutavas EE. The cutaneous T cell lymphoma, mycosis fungoides, is a human T cell lymphotrophic virus-associated disease. A study of 50 patients. J Clin Invest 1995; 95:547–554.
30. Ratoosh SL, Cohen PR, Troncoso P. Cutaneous malignancy and leprosy. Report of a patient with *Mycobacterium leprae* and basal cell carcinoma concurrently present in the same lesion. J Dermatol Surg Oncol 1994; 20:613–618.

31. Grossman D, Rapini RP, Osborne B, Duvic M. Emergence of leprosy in a patient with mycosis fungoides. J Am Acad Dermatol 1994; 30:313–315.
32. Shinokuma A, Hirakawa N, Tamiya S, Oda Y, Komiyama S, Tsuneyoshi M. Evaluation of Epstein–Barr virus infection in sinonasal small round cell tumors. J Cancer Res Clin Oncol 2000; 126:12–18.
33. Shiga K, Tateda M, Saijo S, Hori T, Sato I, Tateno H, Matsuura K, Takasaka T, Miyagi T. Presence of Stretpococcus infection in extra-orophyngeal head and neck squamous cell carcinoma and its implication in carcinogensis. Oncol Rep 2001; 8:245–248.
34. Kölmel KF, Pfahlberg A, Mastrangelo G, Niin M, Botev IN, Seebacher C, Schneider D, Lambert D, Shafir R, Kokoschka EM, Kleeberg UR, Henz BM, Gefeller O. Infections and melanoma risk: results of a multicentre EORTC case-control study. Melanoma Research 1999; 9:511–519.
35. Lobo DV, Chu P, Grekin RC, Berger TG. Nonmelanoma skin cancers and infection with the human immunodeficiency virus. Arch Dermatol 1992; 128:623–627.
36. Wang CY, Brodland DG, Su WP. Skin cancers associated with acquired immunodeficiency syndrome. Mayo Clin Proc 1995; 70:766–772.
37. Ohashi DK, Crane JS, Spira TJ, Courrege ML. Idiopathic CD$_4$+ T-cell lymphocytopenia with verrucae, basal cell carcinomas and chronic tinea corporis infection. J Am Acad Dermatol 1994; 31:889–891.
38. Phillips TJ, Dover JS. Recent advances in dermatology. N Engl J Med 1992; 326:167–178.
39. Barnadas MA, Baselga E, Curell R, Margall N, de Moragas JM. Active cutaneous tuberculosis after therapy of squamous cell carcinoma of the skin, a PCR study. Int J Dermatol 1996; 35:221–222.
40. Phillips WG, Marsden JR. Opportunistic cutaneous myiasis following radio-therapy for squamous cell carcinoma of the left temple. Br J Dermatol 1993; 129:502–503.
41. Lippman SM, Parkinson DR, Itri LM, Weber RS, Schantz SP, Ota DM, Schusterman MA, Krakoff IH, Gutterman JU, Hong WK. 13-cis-retinoic acid and interferon alpha-2a: effective combination therapy for advanced squamous cell carcinoma of the skin. J Natl Cancer Inst 1992; 19:235–241.
42. Lentz SR, Raish RJ, Orlowski EP, Marion JM. Squamous cell carcinoma in epidermolysis bullosa. Treatment with systemic chemotherapy. Cancer 1990; 66:1276–1278.
43. Denic S. Preoperative treatment of advanced skin carcinoma with cisplatin and blemycin. Am J Clin Oncol 1999; 22:32–34.
44. Saluja A, Peters NT, Lowe L, Johnson TM. A surgical wound infection due to Mycobacterium chelonae successfully treated with clarithromycin. Dermatol Surg 1997; 23:539–543.
45. Caplan SE, Kauffman CL. Primary inoculation tuberculosis after immuno-therapy for malignant melanoma with BCG vaccine. J Am Acad Dermatol 1996; 35:783–785.
46. Moff SL, Corey GR, Gottfredsson M. Distant cutaneous granulomas after

bacille Calmette–Guerin immunotherapy for malignant melanoma: case for direct infection. Clin Infect Dis 1999; 29:1569–1570.

47. Rosenberg EB, Kanner SP, Schwartzman RJ, Colsky J. Systemic infection following BCG therapy. Arch Intern Med 1974; 134:769–770.

48. Papachristou DN, Fortner JG. Effect of postoperative wound infection on the course of stage II melanoma. Cancer 1979; 43:1106–1111.

49. Axelrod PI, Lorber B, Vonderheid EC. Infections complicating Mycosis fungoides and Sézary Syndrome. JAMA 1992; 267:1354–1358.

50. Epstein EH Jr, Levin DL, Croft JD Jr, Lutzner MA. Mycosis fungoides: survival, prognostic features, response to therapy, and autopsy findings. Medicine 1972; 15:61–72.

51. Posner LE, Fossieck BE, Eddy JL, Bunn PA. Septicemic complications of the cutaneous T-cell lymphomas. Am J Med 1981; 71:210–216.

52. Rappaport H, Thomas LB. Mycosis fungoides: the pathology of extra-cutaneous involvement. Cancer 1974; 34:1198–1229.

53. Cohen SR, Stenn KS, Braverman IM, Beck GJ. Mycosis fungoides: clinicopathologic relationships, survival and therapy in 59 patients with observations on occupation as a new prognostic factor. Cancer 1980; 46:2654–2666.

54. Dalton JA, Yag-Howard C, Messina JL, Glass LF. Cutaneous T-cell lymphoma. Int J Dermatol 1997; 36:801–809.

55. Block JB, Edgcomb J, Eisen A, Van Scott EJ. Mycosis fungoides: natural history and aspects of its relationship to other malignant lymphomas. Am J Med 1963; 34:228–235.

56. Cassazza AR, Duvall CP, Carbone PP. Infection in lymphomas: history, treatment, and duration in relation to incidence and survival. JAMA 1966; 197:118–124.

57. Tsambiros PE, Patel S, Greene JN, Sandin RL, Vincent AL. Infectious complications of cutaneous T-cell lymphoma. Cancer Control 2001; 8:185–188.

58. Goldgeier MH, Cohen SR, Braverman IM, Stenn KS. An unusual and fatal case of disseminated cutaneous *Herpes simplex*. Infection in a patient with cutaneous T-cell lymphoma (mycosis fungoides). J Am Acad Dermatol 1981; 4:176–180.

59. Vonderheid EC, Van Voorst Vader PC. *Herpes zoster-varicella* in cutaneous T-cell lymphomas. Arch Dermatol 1980; 116:408–412.

60. Taulbee KS, Johnson SC. Disseminated cutaneous *Herpes simplex* infection in cutaneous T-cell lymphoma. Arch Dermatol 1981; 117:114–115.

61. Segal RJ, Watson W. Kaposi's varicelliform eruption in mycosis fungoides. Arch Dermatol 1978; 114:1067–1069.

62. Pinkus H. Mycosis fungoides and histoplasmosis. Arch Dermatol 1968; 98:323–325.

63. Narayan S, Batta K, Colloby P, Tan CY. Cutaneous cryptoccus infection due to *C. albidus* associated with Sézary syndrome. Br J Dermatol 2000; 143:632–634.

64. Frieden TR, Bia FJ, Herald PW, Eisen RN, Patterson TF, Edelson RL.

Cutaneous cryptococcus in a patient with cutaneous T-cell lymphoma receiving therapy with photopheresis and methotrexate. Clin Infect Dis 1993; 17:776–778.

65. Alteras I, David M, Feurerman EJ, Morojonski G. Widespread cutaneous candidiasis and tinea infection masking mycosis fungoides. Mycopathologia 1982; 80:83–88.

66. Fuks ZY, Bagshaw MA, Farber EM. Prognostic signs and the management of mycosis fungoides. Cancer 1973; 32:1385–1395.

67. Cyr DP, Geokas MC, Worsley GH. Mycosis fungoides: hematologic findings and terminal course. Arch Dermatol 1966; 94:558–573.

68. Foster GH, Eichenhorn MS, VanSlyck EJ. The Sézary syndrome with rapid pulmonary dissemination. Cancer 1985; 56:1197–1198.

69. Rubin DL, Blank N. Rapid pulmonary dissemination of mycosis fungoides simulating pneumonia: a case report and review of the literature. Cancer 1985; 56:649–651.

70. Stoker LM, Vonderheid EC, Abell E, Diamond LW, Rosen SE, Goldwein MI. Clinical manifestations of intrathoracic cutaneous T-cell lymphoma. Cancer 1985; 56:2694–2702.

71. Kim YH, Hoppe RT. Mycosis fungoides and the Sézary syndrome. Semin Oncol 1999; 26:276–289.

72. Heald P, Yan SL, Edelson R. Profound deficiency in normal circulating T cells in erythrodermic cutaneous T-cell lymphoma. Arch Dermatol 1994; 130:198–203.

73. Seitz LE, Golitz LP, Weston WL, Aeling JE, Dustin RD. Defective monocyte chemotoxis in mycosis fungoides. Arch Dermatol 1977; 113:1055–1057.

74. Winkleman RK. Clinical studies of T-cell erythroderma in the Sézary syndrome. Mayo Clin Proc 1974; 49:519–525.

75. Blaylock WK, Clendenning WE, Carbone PP, Van Scott EJ. Normal immunologic reactivity in patients with the lymphoma mycosis fungoides. Cancer 1966; 19:233–236.

76. Lutzner M, Edelson R, Schein P, Green I, Kirkpatrick C, Ahmed A. Cutaneous T-cell lymphomas: the Sézary syndrome, mycosis fungoides and related disorders. Ann Intern Med 1975; 83:534–552.

77. Clendenning WE, Van Scott EJ. Skin autografts and homografts in patients with the lymphoma mycosis fungoides. Cancer Res 1965; 25:1844–1853.

78. Brouet JC, Flandrin G, Seligmann M. Indications of the thymus-derived nature of the proliferating cells in 6 patients with the Sézary syndrome. N Engl J Med 1973; 289:341–344.

79. Schechter GP, Bunn PA Jr, Fischmann AB, Matthews MJ, Guccion J, Soehnlen F, Munson D, Minna JD. Blood and lymph node T-lymphocytes in cutaneous T-cell lymphoma: evaluation by light microscopy. Cancer Treat Rep 1979; 63:571–574.

80. Jacobs JB, Vogel C, Powell RD, DeVita VT. Needle biopsy in *Pneumocystitis carinii* pneumonia. Radiology 1969; 93:525–530.

81. Slevin NJ, Blair V, Todd IDH. Mycosis fungoides: response to therapy and survival patterns in 85 cases. Br J Dermatol 1987; 116:47–53.

24

Central Nervous System Infections in Cancer Patients

Daniel Ginn and John N. Greene
University of South Florida School of Medicine
Moffitt Cancer Center and Research Institute
Tampa, Florida, U.S.A.

Of the potential complications arising during cancer treatment, central nervous system (CNS) infections in a patient pose some of the greatest risks. Ling and Hanley explain that "pathogens can infect the CNS but, more commonly, do not directly invade [it], but instead initiate inflammatory or metabolic disturbances which in turn impair CNS function" [1]. There exists wide variation in the nature of CNS infections. They may be viral, bacterial, or fungal and can be diffuse or focal, as in bacterial meningitis or brain abscess, respectively. Early recognition of these infections is crucial in the care of the cancer patient because failure swiftly to diagnose and treat them can be fatal or result in irreversible neurologic damage [1]. Here, meningitis and brain abscess will each be examined with specific attention given to postoperative wound infection etiology, pathogenicity of infectious agents, clinical features for diagnosis, modes of treatment and management, and prevention.

MENINGITIS

Meningeal inflammation can be viral, bacterial, or fungal in origin—the latter two being of concern in the treatment of cancer patients. Neurosurgical patients face particular risk factors predisposing them to postoperative wound infection: cerebrospinal fluid (CSF) leakage, concurrent non-CNS infection, and perioperative antibiotic therapy. Additional, less significant, risk factors include paranasal sinus entry, placement of a foreign body, and use of a postoperative drain [2]. While relatively rare overall, postoperative wound infections, classified as either deep or superficial, occur more frequently following craniotomy (4.9%) than following spinal (0.9%) or other clean neurosurgery with the level of infection risk varying 11-fold depending upon the type of procedure performed [3]. Immunocompromised patients frequently suffer from nosocomial meningitis because of extended neutropenia or following a transplant [4]. Patients with a history of alcohol abuse or diabetes stand at increased risk of infection [5].

For cancer patients, the cause of postoperative meningitis is usually a bacterial or fungal pathogen. Viral infections leading to meningitis tend to be community-acquired and do not pose any unique threat to cancer patients [6]. There are three bacterial species that are widely considered the most common agents of bacterial meningitis: *Haemophilus influenzae*, *Neisseria meningitidis*, and *Streptococcus pneumoniae*. While most cases of meningitis in neonates are caused by *Escherichia coli* and *Streptococcus agalactiae*, pathogens other than the five noted here should be considered rare, acting opportunistically in patients with surgical and immunological abnormalities [4]. Table 1 lists the most common bacterial and fungal causes of meningitis.

TABLE 1   Common Etiology of Meningitis

Bacterial organisms [5,7]	Fungal organisms [17]
Haemophilus influenzae	*Cryptococcus* species
Neisseria meningitidis	*Coccidioides* species
Streptococcus pneumoniae	*Histoplasma* species
Streptococcus agalactiae	*Blastomyces* species
Staphylococcus epidermidis	*Sporothrix* species
Staphylococcus aureus	*Candida* species
Klebsiella species	*Aspergillus* species
Pseudomonas species	*Zygomycetes* species
Escherichia coli	Dematiaceous fungi
Enterobacter aerogenes	*Pseudallescheria* species
Listeria monocytogenes	
Clostridium species	
Bacteroides species	

Gram-negative bacillary CNS infections are rare in adults but are more common among patients with head trauma, impaired host defenses, and those following neurosurgery. Two-thirds of the 0.5% of neurosurgical patients that develop meningitis do so because of gram-negative bacilli [4]. Gram-negative bacillary meningitis (GNBM) can be difficult to identify at onset because its symptoms resemble typical postoperative reactions—particularly fever, variations in consciousness ranging from confusion to coma, and hypoglycorrhacia [4,8]. Standard treatment for GNBM of chloramphenicol has been replaced by cephalosporins and carbapenems, including ceftazidime, cefepime, and meropenem. These antibiotics have been very effective against gram-negative pathogens, and they enter the CSF in high bactericidal concentrations. Parenteral and intrathecal (possibly intraventricular) gentamicin or tobramycin can be used in combination with the aforementioned antibiotics. Aztreonam, and trimethoprim-sulfamethoxazole (TMP-SMX) have good CSF penetration and high microbiological cure rates and should be considered as additional viable treatment options for GNBM [4,7,9].

Chemical, or aseptic, meningitis generally presents almost identically to bacterial meningitis. This less aggressive postoperative complication is often associated with intrathecal chemotherapy. Distinguishable from its bacterial counterpart by CSF examination, chemical meningitis is more uniquely characterized by polymorphonuclear leukocytes and the absence of organisms on staining and culture of the CSF, and it can be treated with corticosteroids [9–11].

Despite perioperative and postoperative efforts to prevent it, shunt and reservoir infection is common. These infections are caused almost exclusively by *Staphylococcus epidermidis* and *S. aureus* [4,12]. Since implanted CSF reservoirs, Ommaya reservoirs in particular, are internal devices that are repeatedly punctured percutaneously, up to 15% incidence of infection is shown. Kaufman et al. put forth four mechanisms by which shunts may become infected: (1) "retrograde" infection from the distal end; (2) breakdown of the skin covering a surgical wound; (3) hematogenous seeding and infection, although it is infrequent; (4) colonization at the time of surgery, which is probably the most frequent [13]. While both meningitis and abscess are possible clinical manifestations of shunt infection, other presenting symptoms include wound dehiscence, drainage of purulent material, erythema, and pain [12]. Ommaya reservoir and shunt infections have been successfully treated with intravenous or intraventricular administration of antibiotics without removal of the device, or both. However, removal is the ideal course of action since cancer patients are especially vulnerable to opportunistic infections [4,14,15]. Meningitis results 30% of the time from shunt and reservoir infection [13]. Once a staphylococcal infection is established, appropriate antistaphylococcal therapy should commence such as vancomycin or linezolid [16].

Severely immunocompromised patients, notably patients with leukemia and lymphoma, especially while neutropenic, are susceptible to opportunistic fungal infections [4]. Cellular host defenses are necessary to withstand fungal infection of the CNS. Neutropenia can predispose the CNS to infection from *Candida* and molds. Corticosteriods can predispose patients to cryptococcal meningitis [17]. Prolonged neutropenia is the major risk for *Candida* species infection, and it is likely that this will be the most common fungal infection in cancer centers and similar institutions with a high volume of cancer patients [17,18]. While a combination of amphotericin B and flucytosine is generally the most effective therapy for candida meningitis, granulocyte transfusions may be helpful as well [18]. Newer antifungals such as voriconazole, caspofungin, and lipid formulations of amphotericin B may also have a role.

BRAIN ABSCESS

Brain abscess is a focal suppurative condition within the brain parenchyma and is the most common CNS infection that frequently requires surgical intervention. Brain abscess presents characteristically at the extremes of age—in neonates and the elderly. As with postoperative meningitis, patients who are immunosuppressed while undergoing chemotherapy are at risk to develop bacterial or fungal brain abscess. Abnormalities in cell-mediated immunity such as T lymphocyte or mononuclear phagocyte defects caused by lymphocytic leukemia, lymphoma, and bone marrow transplantation make these patients susceptible to *Toxoplasma gondii*, *Nocardia asteroides*, *Cryptococcus neoformans*, *Listeria monocytogenes*, and *Mycobacterium* species. Likewise, neutropenic patients may develop brain abscess as a result of infection by aerobic gram-negative bacteria, *Aspergillus* species, *Fusarium* species, *Scedosporium* species, *Zygomycetes*, and *Candida* species. Prolonged neutropenia along with chronic corticosteroid use and graft versus host disease are the major risk factors for fungal brain abscess [20]. Diagnosing a brain abscess can be difficult because the most common presenting symptoms of headache, fever, and focal neurological deficit can mimic progressing malignancy [20,21]. Diagnosis of brain abscess utilizing CT and MR imaging is possible in the early stages of abscess formation when peripheral borders are well-defined and hypodense. Later, however, the lesion's borders show poor definition with irregular areas of enhancement making diagnosis less obvious [21].

There is no standardized guideline for management of the patient with a brain abscess [20]. *Candida* is a rare cause of brain abscess and is usually seen in the setting of leukemia and neutropenia [22]. As with *Candida* meningitis, treatment includes a prolonged course of amphotericin B, alone or in combination with flucytosine. The newer antifungals previously mentioned may also be useful.

Following neurosurgery, a bacterial abscess most likely originates from bacteria entering the brain during the procedure. This is followed by a long latency period and colonization of the site of tumor resection. The use of a BCNU wafer will increase the risk of brain abscess substantially. The usual pathogens isolated include *S. aureus, S. epidemedis, P. aeruginosa,* and *enterobacteriacea.* The antibiotics used for postneurosurgical meningitis are likewise indicated for brain abscess developing after neurosurgery.

Although CNS infections are rare in cancer patients, higher morbidity and mortality is expected than in noncancer patients. Early recognition of the pathogens that occur with a given immune defect will result in the prompt institution of appropriate antimicrobials that have good CSF penetration. Improvement of the host defenses is necessary for control of the infection.

REFERENCES

1. Ling GSF, Hanley DF. Neurocritical care of CNS infections. In: Scheld WM, Whitley RJ, Durack DT, eds. Infections of the Central Nervous System. Vol. 49. 2d ed. Philadelphia: Lippincott-Raven, 1997:973–979.
2. Mollman HD, Haines SJ. Risk factors for postoperative neurosurgical wound infection. J Neurosurg 1986; 64:902–906.
3. Tenney JH, Vlahov D, Salcman M, Ducker TB. Wide variation in risk of wound infection following clean neurosurgery: implications for perioperative antibiotic prophylaxis. J Neurosurg 1985; 62:243–247.
4. Wood M, Anderson M. Neurological Infections. London: W. B. Saunders, 1988.
5. Roos KL, Tunkel AR, Scheld WM. Acute bacterial meningitis in children and adults. In: Scheld WM, Whitley RJ, Durack DT, eds. Infections of the Central Nervous System. Vol. 21. 2d ed. Philadelphia: Lippincott-Raven, 1997:335–401.
6. Rotbart HA. Viral meningitis and the aseptic meningitis syndrome. In: Scheld WM, Whitley RJ, Durack DT, eds. Infections of the Central Nervous System. Vol. 3. 2d ed. Philadelphia: Lippincott-Raven, 1997:23–46.
7. Fotopoulos TN, Greene JN, Sandin RL, Vincent AL. Successful therapy of postneurosurgical meningitis caused by a resistant strain of *Enterobacter aerogenes.* Cancer Control 1997; 4(3):270–273.
8. Lu C-H, Chang W-N, Chuang Y-C, Chang H-W. Gram-negative bacillary meningitis in adult post-neurosurgical patients. Surg Neurol 1999; 52:438–444.
9. Foracs P, Geyer CA, Freidberg SR. Characterization of chemical meningitis after neurological surgery. Clinical Infectious Diseases 2001; 32:179–185.
10. Ross D, Rosegay H, Pons V. Differentiation of aseptic and bacterial meningitis in postoperative neurosurgical patients. J Neurosurg 1988; 69:669–674.
11. Fukushima T, Sumazaki R, Koike K, Tsuchida M, Okada Y, Maki T, Hamano, K. A magnetic resonance abnormality correlating with permeability

of the blood–brain barrier in a child with chemical meningitis during central nervous system prophylaxis for acute leukemia. Ann Hematol 1999; 78:564–567.

12. Kaufman BA. Infections of cerebrospinal fluid shunts. In: Scheld WM, Whitley RJ, Durack DT, eds. Infections of the Central Nervous System. Vol. 29. 2d ed. Philadelphia: Lippincott-Raven, 1997:555–577.

13. Kaufman BA, Tunkel AR, Pryor JC, Dacey RG. Meningitis in the neurosurgical patient. Infectious Disease Clinics of North America 1990; 4(4):677–701.

14. Obbens EAMT, Leavens ME, Beal JW, Lee Y-Y. Ommaya reservoirs in 387 patients: a 15-year experience. Neurology 1985; 35:1274–1278.

15. Papadakis KA, Vartivarian SE, Vassilaki ME, Anaissie EJ. *Stenotrophomonas maltophilia* meningitis: report of two cases and review of the literature. J Neurosurg 1997; 87:106–108.

16. Jensen AG, Espersen F, Skinhøj P, Rosdahl VT, Frimodi-Moller N. *Staphylococcus aureus* meningitis: a review of 104 nationwide, consecutive cases. Arch Intern Med 1993; 153:1902–1908.

17. Perfect JR, Durack DT. Fungal meningitis. In: Scheld WM, Whitley RJ, Durack DT, eds. Infections of the Central Nervous System. Vol. 38. 2d ed. Philadelphia: Lippincott-Raven, 1997:721–739.

18. McCullers JA, Vargas SL, Flynn PM, Razzouk BI, Shenep JL. Candidal meningitis in children with cancer. Clinical Infectious Diseases 2000; 31:451–457.

19. Greenlee JE, Carroll KC. Cerebrospinal fluid in CNS infections. In: Scheld WM, Whitley RJ, Durack DT, eds. Infections of the Central Nervous System. Vol. 46. 2d ed. Philadelphia: Lippincott-Raven, 1997:899–922.

20. Wispelwey B, Dacey RG, Scheld WM. Brain abscess. In: Scheld WM, Whitley RJ, Durack DT, eds. Infections of the Central Nervous System. Vol. 25. 2d ed. Philadelphia: Lippincott-Raven, 1997:463–493.

21. Bizakis JG, Prassopoulos P, Doxas P, Papadakis CE, Skoulakis CE, Kyrmizakis DE, Helidonis ES. Frontal lobe abscess secondary to head trauma and nasal polyposis. Auris Nasus Larynx 2000; 27:367–370.

22. Tweddle DA, Graham JC, Shankland GS, Kernahan J. Cerebral candidiasis in a child 1 year after leukaemia. British Journal of Haematology 1998; 103:795–797.

23. Biermann C, Fries G, Jehnichen P, Bhakdi S, Husmann M. Isolation of *Abiotrophia adiacens* from a brain abscess which developed in a patient after neurosurgery. J Clin Microbiol 1999; 37:769–771.

25

Pulmonary Infections in Cancer Patients

Charurut Somboonwit
University of South Florida, School of Medicine
Tampa, Florida, U.S.A.

John N. Greene
University of South Florida, School of Medicine
and Moffitt Cancer Center and Research Institute
Tampa, Florida, U.S.A.

Pulmonary infections are the major complications in cancer patients and have negative impacts on survival, duration of hospitalization, and cost of medical care. Cancer patients are susceptible to pulmonary infections because of underlying comorbidities, anatomic impact from the cancer itself, and cancer-treatment-induced immunodeficiency. Evaluation of pulmonary infections or new pulmonary infiltrates in cancer patients is a challenge for clinicians. The differential diagnosis is broad, including a variety of infectious and noninfectious causes. The evaluation of pulmonary infections in cancer patients includes special attention to (1) host factors: the underlying cancer, immunological status, previous therapy, and duration of disease; (2) clinical presentation: rate of deterioration of pulmonary status, the pattern on chest radiograph, and extrapulmonary manifestations; and (3) sensitivity and specificity of computed tomography, bronchoscopy, and open lung biopsy.

COMMUNITY-ACQUIRED PNEUMONIA

The pathogens which cause community-acquired pneumonia (CAP) are the same in normal hosts as in nonneutropenic cancer patients. Most cases are caused by *Streptococcus pneumoniae*, *Hemophilus influenza* or *Moraxella catteralis*; and to a lesser extent by *Mycoplasma pneumoniae*, *Legionella pneumophila*, or *Chlamydia pneumoniae*. Staphylococcal pneumonia is uncommon in both normal hosts and in cancer patients and when present usually follows viral pneumonia such as influenza. In a normal host, polymicrobial pneumonia is rare, except for aspiration pneumonia. In cancer patients with pneumonia, isolation of more than one pathogen is frequent. Immunosuppressed patients have higher rates of oropharyngeal colonization by enteric gram-negative bacilli. Bacteremia from pneumonia is a relatively early manifestation of CAP and is not a poor prognostic indicator [1–6].

NOSOCOMIAL PNEUMONIA

Cancer patients are susceptible to nosocomial pulmonary infections, especially ventilator-associated pneumonia. As in the normal host, gram-negative bacilli are the most common cause of nosocomial pneumonia in cancer patients. *Pseudomonas aeruginosa*, *Klebsiella pneumoniae*, and *Enterobacter* spp. are the most common. Bacteremia associated with nosocomial pneumonia may occur more commonly in cancer patients. However *P. aeruginosa* bacteremia is more commonly found in patients with solid organ tumors than neutropenic patients because of the more frequent use of empirical antibiotics with the latter group [7]. *Legionella* spp., respiratory syncytial virus, and *Aspergillus* spp. have caused outbreaks of nosocomial pneumonia in cancer patients related to a contaminated environmental source.

CAUSES OF PULMONARY INFILTRATES ASSOCIATED WITH ALTERED HOST DEFENSE

1. Short-term neutropenia (duration less than 1 week): gram-negative bacilli, *Staphylococcus aureus*, rarely.
2. Prolonged neutropenia (duration more than 1 week): molds (i.e., *Aspergillus* spp., *Fusarium* spp., *Scedosporium* spp.), rarely *Candida* spp.
3. Cellular immune defect: *Mycobacterium* spp., *Nocardia* spp., *Legionella* spp., *Pneumocystis carinii*, *Cryptococcus* spp., molds (i.e., *Aspergillus* spp., *Fusarium* spp., *Scedosporium* spp., Zygomycetes), endemic mycosis (i.e., histoplasmosis, blastomycosis, coccidioidimycosis), virus, especially RSV, parainfluenza, influenza, adenovirus)

4. Humoral immune defect: encapsulated bacteria (*S. pneumoniae, H. influenza*) and viral (RSV, parainfluenza, influenza, adenovirus)

PULMONARY INFECTIONS IN NEUTROPENIC PATIENTS

Pulmonary infiltrates in neutropenic patients can be classified as early, refractory, and late infiltrations [8–10]. Early pulmonary infiltrates occurring with the onset of fever are usually caused by *Pseudomonas aeruginosa*, *Klebsiella* spp., and other *Enterobacteraciaceae*. It is well known that these bacteria are harbored in the gastrointestinal tract and colonize the oropharynx of hospitalized patients. Chemotherapy-induced mucositis and intercurrent illness may allow an increase of gram-negative bacilli adherence to the respiratory epithelium, which can result in subsequent pneumonia [8]. Unlike CAP, bacteremic pneumonia in neutropenic patients implies a poor outcome. It is the major cause of death in neutropenic patients, especially by *P. aeruginosa*, *E. coli*, and *S. pneumoniae* [9]. Indwelling catheters are a risk factor for Staphylococcal pneumonia. But oropharyngeal colonization of *Staphylococcus* spp., mucositis, and aspiration increase the risk for pneumonia. Refractory pulmonary infiltrates are early pulmonary infections that do not respond clinically to initial empirical antimicrobial treatment. The causes include resistant gram-negative bacilli and other less common gram-positive and anaerobic organisms. These include *Stenotrophomonas maltophila*, *Alcaligenes xylosoxidans*, *Bacillus* spp., *Corynebacterium* spp., and *Bacteroides fragilis*. Moreover it can be caused by *Legionella* spp., *Mycobacterium* spp., *Nocardia* spp., *Cryptococcus* spp., dimorphic fungi, and possibly molds. Late pulmonary infiltrates, occurring after 7 days of empirical antibiotic treatment, for febrile neutropenia develop more frequently, the longer the duration of the neutropenia. Causative organisms are resistant gram-negative bacteria, molds, cytomegalovirus, *Pneumocystis carinii*, *Legionella* spp., *Nocardia* spp., and Mycobacteria (*M. kansasii*, MAI, and rapidly-growing mycobacteria). The earliest cause of invasive fungal infections is *Candida* spp. Fungemia usually arises from an indwelling catheter or the GI tract disrupted by chemotherapy and rarely results in pneumonia. *Candida pneumonia* is variable and can present with diffuse patchy infiltrates, lobar consolidation, occasionally pleural effusion, and frequently with lower lobe 1–2 cm nodules. In patients with prolonged neutropenia, molds become extremely important. *Aspegillus* spp. represent about 30 to 60% of fungal causes of pulmonary infection, especially in patients with hematological malignancies or following bone marrow transplantation.

In bone marrow transplant patients, the incidence in allograft recipients is higher than in autograft recipients [8,10,11]. The lung is the most common site of invasive aspergillosis, although other sites, including sinuses, the central nervous system, the heart, and the skin, are possible. Pulmonary aspergillosis commonly presents with peripleural nodular infiltrates in patients with persistent febrile neutropenia despite antibiotics. The clinical features of invasive pulmonary aspergillosis include fever, dyspnea, dry cough, wheezing, pleuritic chest pain, and occasional hemoptysis. Invasive pulmonary aspergillosis with transbronchial invasion leads to pulmonary vascular thrombosis and pulmonary parenchyma infarction. Chest radiograph findings may be nonspecific, but cavitary diseases can be seen. Other invasive mycoses, such as *Fusarium* spp., *Pseudoallerscheria boydii*, Zygomycetes (such as *Mucor* spp.), *Scedosporum* spp., *Penicillum marneffei* (in its endemic area), Phaeohyphomycoses (*Curvularia, Bipolaris, Exserohilum*, and *Alternaria*), *Trichosporon* spp., and *Malassezia furfur*, can produce nonspecific pulmonary infiltrates as well as widely disseminated disease, and the presentation is indistinguishable from that of invasive aspergillosis [12–15]. Tracheobronchial aspergillosis can present as chronic cough, dyspnea, and hemoptysis A CT scan of chest reveals wall thickening of large bronchi with minimal infiltration of lung parenchyma. Bronchoscopy is necessary for a definitive diagnosis with white "styrofoam" exudate attached to the bronchial wall frequently seen.

PULMONARY INFECTIONS IN PATIENTS WITH CELLULAR IMMUNE DEFECTS

Cellular immune dysfunction exists in patients with chronic lymphocytic leukemia, Hodgkin's disease, non-Hodgkin's lymphoma, corticosteroid use, and bone marrow transplantation. These patients have impaired immunity to intracellular pathogens including bacteria, fungi, and viruses.

Cancer patients with latent tuberculosis are at risk of reactivation from chemotherapy, radiation, or the underlying disease itself. Tuberculosis in cancer patients commonly involves the lung with upper lobe infiltration, scarring, and cavitary lesions. Mass lesions are occasionally seen and can be confused with lung cancer. Extrapulmonary tuberculosis including meningitis, brain abscess, pericarditis, perinephric abscess, empyema, osteomyelitis have also been reported in cancer patients. A pulmonary infiltrate that fails to resolve in a reasonable time frame should be assessed for tuberculosis, and for fungal and other opportunistic infections. Finding acid-fast bacilli in a sputum sample should prompt consideration of tuberculosis until organism identification. However, nontuberculous mycobacteria (NTM), which are ubiquitous in the environment, are more common in cancer patients than tuberculosis. The isolation of NTM from respiratory specimens requires distinguishing true infection from colonization. The most common NTM, such as mycobacterium avium complex (MAC), *M. kansasii*, and rapid-growing mycobacteria (*M. chelonei, M. fortuitum*, and *M. abscessus*) can colonize the respiratory tract or cause progressive pulmonary infiltration. A mixed infection between tuberculosis and NTM can occur in cancer patients, making it difficult to determine the contribution of each organism to the worsening clinical illness.

Actinomycosis is a gram-positive obligate or facultative anaerobe that normally inhabits the oral mucosa. Rarely a pulmonary infection can result, usually in combination with other organisms such as anaerobic streptococci, *Hemophilus* spp., gram-negative bacilli, and fusiform bacilli [17]. The clinical presentation usually consists of chest pain, fever, weight loss, hemoptysis, and a pulmonary mass lesion. Clinical and radiographic findings (the combination of pulmonary consolidation, pleural involvement, and adenopathy) may be confused with tuberculosis, nocardiosis, blastomycosis, and coccidiodimycosis. Pulmonary actinomycosis is sometimes confused with lung cancer, and generally histopathology is required for the diagnosis. Like cancer, actinomycosis spreads across tissue plains, which is unusual for most bacteria, which follow tissue plains without crossing them. Chronic actinomycosis produces the characteristic sulfur granules, finding which leads to a definitive diagnosis, especially since the organism is difficult to grow in culture. The infection can spread to contiguous bone, through fascial planes, or develop draining sinuses. Pulmonary actinomycosis may extend across fissures into the pleural space, producing an empyema. Miliary actinomycosis has been reported [18].

Nocardia spp. are saprophytic gram-positive filamentous bacteria that form branching mycelial structures that grow extremely slowly, and at a wide range of temperature. Nocardia should not be considered a contaminant. The two species that cause most human infections are *Nocardia asteroides* (accounts for 80%), and *Nocardia brasillensis* (15%). The primary site of nocardiosis is the lung, but one-third of patients have no evidence of pulmonary involvement. Pulmonary nocardiosis is characterized by necrotizing abscesses with poor encapsulation, but granuloma formation may be found depending on the degree of cell-mediated immunity. Presentations (i.e., fever, night sweats, and cough) are varied depending on the degree of immunosuppression. Extrapulmonary involvement includes the central nervous system (33% of cases), skin, and soft tissue and bone.

Radiological manifestations are varied. Usually a lung nodule with distinct borders is seen in the lung parenchyma. Irregular nodules and areas of consolidation with or without cavitation are common. There is no predilection for the upper lobes of the lung, as in tuberculosis, or lower lobes, as in actinomycosis. Since cerebral involvement is common, most authorities recommend CT or MRI of the head even in the absence of focal neurological findings [1,10,17].

Legionella pneumophila can cause pneumonia in both community and hospital settings. Patients with community-acquired *legionella* pneumonia commonly have a more severe illness and frequently need admission to an intensive care setting [19,20]. Cell-mediated immunity is still the primary defense mechanism against the intracellular pathogens such as *Legionella* spp. The disease can be acquired by the inhalation of aerosols containing *Legionella* or the aspiration of water contaminated with *Legionella*. Pneumonia is the predominant clinical syndrome, although nonspecific manifestations vary from mild respiratory symptoms and low-grade fever to respiratory and multiorgan failure. Slightly productive cough, pleuritic chest pain, hemoptysis, and systemic manifestations such as headache, high fever, diarrhea, and relative bradycardia are common. Radiographic findings can present with bilateral infiltrates, pleural effusion, or cavitary lesions [19,20]. Progression of pulmonary infiltrates despite appropriate treatment is common. Extrapulmonary legionellosis is rare, but if found it is usually severe and most commonly involves the heart. Other extrapulmonary sites of disease include sinusitis, cellulitis, pancreatitis, peritonitis, pyelonephritis, and bacteremia.

Besides AIDS, *Pneumocystis carinii* pneumonia (PCP) can develop in patients with acute or chronic lymphocytic leukemia, lymphoma, after bone marrow transplant, and prolonged corticosteroid use especially when tapered. Patients usually become ill for several days before seeking medical advice, but when clinical symptoms begin they progress rapidly. PCP commonly presents as fever, dry cough, and tachypnia. At presentation, most patients have hypoxia and hypocapnia, with increased oxygen alveolar-arterial gradient. Chest radiographs are characterized by bilateral interstitial infiltrates with a ground glass appearance and progress to an alveolar pattern. Rarely normal radiographic findings or cavitary lesions can occur [21,22].

Cryptococcus neoformans, Histoplasma capsulatum, and *Coccidioides immitis* can produce nonspecific infiltrates with pulmonary nodules. The initial presentation is usually nonspecific with fever, dry cough, and pleuritic chest pain. Pleural effusions are not commonly seen. Extrapulmonary manifestations includes pericarditis and arthritis in histoplasmosis, erythema nodosum in histoplamosis, coccidioidomycosis, and meningitis in coccidioidomycosis, and more importantly, in cryptococcosis [23,24]. Disseminated diseases can occur with any of the three fungal pathogens, but cyptococcal meningitis can occur with any extent of pulmonary involvement.

Viral pneumonia in cancer patients most commonly develops from reactivation of the Herpesviridae (HSV, CMV, VZV, and HHV-6). They are more common in bone marrow transplant patients during the postengraftment phase, except for HSV, which usually reactivates during the pre-engraftment phase along with neutropenia. Varicella pneumonia or disseminated varicella is caused by the uncontrolled reactivation of the virus; skin lesions can be minimal or absent. Pneumonia is usually interstitial or nodular, and multiorgan involvement is common. CMV causes severe interstital pneumonia with mortality rates up to 90% in post-bone-marrow-transplant patients. CMV interstital pneumonia occurs in patients with positive serology for CMV or is acquired during transplantation. Reactivation of CMV may cause serious morbidity especially those who have multiple organ system failure [10,25]. Prophylaxis of CMV disease during the early post-bone-marrow-transplant phase has significantly reduced the incidence of CMV pneumonia. However, CMV pneumonia is still a problem in the late post-transplant phase, with an increased risk in patients with chronic graft-versus-host disease and those who received T cell–depleted transplants [26]. Detection of CMV viremia or antigenemia has been useful in predicting the risk of CMV disease. The institution of appropriate preemptive treatment for CMV, when CMV is detected by these new techniques, has almost eliminated CMV disease in transplant patients.

HHV-6 causes a number of diseases, particularly in patients after bone marrow transplants. It causes an interstitial pneumonia with fever and rash, encephalitis, and myelosuppression; and it enhances graft-vs.-host disease [27–30]. Improving the methods of viral culture and identification helps to identify the specific virus causing the pneumonia. Adenovirus, influenza virus, and parainfluenza virus causing pneumonia have been reported especially in stem cell transplant recipients [30].

PULMONARY INFECTION IN PATIENTS WITH HUMORAL IMMUNE DEFECT

Causes of humoral immune impairment include multiple myeloma, Waldentrom's macroglobulinemia, chronic lymphocytic leukemia, and postsplenectomy. Patients with these conditions are susceptible to encapsulated bacteria, particularly *Streptococcus pneumoniae*, *Haemophilus influenza*, and *Klebsiella pneumoniae*. In particular, pneumococcal infection in patients with splenic dysfunction or following splenectomy can present with overwhelming sepsis [2,10].

LUNG ABSCESS AND NECROTIZING PNEUMONIA

The common mechanism of lung abscess is the aspiration of normal flora from the upper respiratory tract. Host factors that can lead to a lung abscess are bronchiectasis, pulmonary emboli, and extrinsic or intrinsic bronchial obstruction often caused by a pulmonary neoplasm.

Microbes responsible for lung abscesses in patients without cancer include oral anaerobes like Bacteroides, Fusobacterium, Actinomyces, aerophillic and microaerophillic cocci, and community acquired pathogens such as *Haemophilus influenza* and *Streptococcus pneumoniae*.

In cancer patients, besides the above, enteric gram-negative aerobes, especially *Pseudomonas* spp., *Legionella* spp., *S. aureus*, *Nocardia* spp., and fungi can be the causative organisms. Factors associated with a poorer prognosis are larger size of the abscess or the presence of multiple abscesses, right lower lobe involvement, the presence of *S. aureus*, *K. pneumoniae*, or *P. aeruginosa*, and advanced age. Mortality is up to 30% in patients with a lung abscess secondary to an extensive surgical approach to resect the obstructing cancer, laser therapy, or radiation therapy [31–33].

NONINFECTIOUS CAUSES OF PULMONARY INFILTRATES

1. Congestive heart failure (CHF). CHF can be a preexisting condition in cancer patients. Decompensation of cardiac function may cause diffuse bilateral infiltrates and mimic an infectious process, especially with the fluid overload common in patients receiving intensive chemothrapy. Assessment of hemodynamic status by using a Swan–Ganz catheter, an echocardigram, or a multigated uptake (MUGA) scan can help to establish the diagnosis.

2. Acute respiratory distress syndrome (ARDS). ARDS is a clinical syndrome involving impaired oxygenation resulting from lung injury. The increase of fluid in the interstitial and alveolar space causes a decrease in compliance, hypoxemia, and pulmonary infiltration that can rapidly progress to bilateral interstitial involvement. The overall mortality of ARDS is greater than 50%, depending on the underlying and precipitating cause [34].

3. Drug-induced pneumonitis. Cancer treatment itself can cause pulmonary complications. The most frequent offenders are busulfan, bleomycin, and BCNU. Busulfan can cause fever, dry cough, dyspnea, and interstitial pulmonary infiltrates. Progressive restrictive pulmonary infiltration can be seen even after discontinuation of the drug. Bleomycin and BCNU can cause dose-related interstitial fibrosis, especially where there is underlying pulmonary disease. Methotrexate pneumonitis is not dose related. Fever, dry cough, and dyspnea are clinically apparent manifestations and are often associated with eosinophilia. Cytosine arabinoside can precipitate noncardiogenic pulmonary edema, which often is mistaken for ARDS. Interleukin-2 can result in both noncardiogenic pulmonary edema and a direct cardiotoxic effect causing cardiogenic pulmonary edema. The effect is not dose related and can cause both obstructive and restrictive patterns demonstrated in pulmonary fuction testing. Other chemotherapeutic agents that can cause pneumonitis less frequently are cyclophosphamide, mitomycin, 6-mercaptopurine, semustine, vinblastine, and etoposide [10,35].

4. Diffuse alveolar hemorrhage (DAH). DAH is described in patients after both autologous and allogenic bone marrow transplant. This syndrome

is characterized by the sudden onset of progressive dyspnea, nonproductive cough, fever, and hypoxemia. Hemoptysis is rare. A chest radiograph shows diffused consolidation, and bronchoalveolar lavage (BAL) demonstrates progressive blood return from the alveolar fluid aspiration. This syndrome usually occurs around 10 days after transplant. Patients with advanced age, solid malignancy, prior total body irradiation, severe mucositis, renal insufficiency, and bone marrow engraftment have an increase risk of this syndrome. It is important to recognize DAH because of the high mortality (more than 50%) and the benefit of early institution of high-dose corticosteroid therapy [36].

5. Radiation pneumonitis. Radiation therapy of the chest causes pneumonitis, which generally presents with insidious onset of cough and dyspnea with diffuse bilateral interstitial infiltrates. The incidence is related to the total dose of the radiation and the volume of the affected lung, as well as the underlying lung disease and prior radiation exposure. Radiation pneumonitis can progress to pulmonary fibrosis with a severe restrictive component.

6. Pulmonary embolism and infarction. Thrombosis is a common event in patients with cancer. Pulmonary embolism cannot be excluded in patients with thrombocytopenia. Cancer is a well-known cause of a hypercoagulable state. There is an even greater risk of thrombosis from immobilization in these patients. The diagnosis of pulmonary embolism is difficult, and chest radiography is notoriously insensitive. Ventilation-perfusion scans used to evaluate for a pulmonary embolism can be abnormal from lung cancer or pneumonia. Advances in pulmonary angiography or CT angiography have precluded the need for a pulmonary angiogram in some cases to exclude an embolism.

7. Idiopathic pneumonia syndrome (IPS). IPS is a diffuse lung injury following allogenic bone marrow transplantation in which an infectious etiology has not been identified. It is characterized by a mononuclear infiltration associated with DAH on a histopathological exam of the lung approximately 6 weeks after bone marrow transplantation. Fever, nonproductive cough, dyspnea, hypoxemia and diffuse pulmonary infiltrates herald the onset of IPS. Patients with low performance status, prior total body irradiation, or graft-versus-host disease are at increased risk for IPS. There is no specific treatment, and mortality is high usually from the commonly associated superimposed infections such as gram-negative bacilli, molds, and CMV [37–40].

8. Bronchiolitis obliterans with or without organizing pneumonia (BOOP or BO). BO/BOOP is a serious complication following bone marrow transplantation beginning with dyspnea, cough, and wheezing. Progressive respiratory failure can ensue in a subacute fashion. Chronic graft-versus-host disease is commonly present. High-dose corticosteroids usually bring rapid improvement in symptoms, with recurrence commonly seen when tapering corticosteroid therapy, which requires subsequent induction therapy.

9. Neoplasm. Recurrence of a pulmonary neoplasm, metastatic cancer to the lung, lymphangitic spread of cancer within the lung, and pulmonary leukosrasis (associated with acute myelogenous leukemia and chronic myelogenous leukemia that have a white blood cell count greater than 100,000/μL) can present as pulmonary infiltration that mimicks an infectious process. A lung biopsy is required to confirm the diagnosis with these conditions.

DIAGNOSTIC APPROACH

The initial approach of a respiratory symptom with or without evidence of radiographic infiltrates is important because infection can be rapid and even fatal. Moreover there is no single diagnostic test that is universally applicable or has adequate sensitivity or specificity to establish the diagnosis. Clinical presentation, a thorough history, and the physical manifestation will guide one to the appropriate diagnostic test. Any diagnostic delay can be catastrophic.

Considerations should include

1. Underlying malignancy, other underlying medical problems, modality and temporal relation of cancer treatment, exposure to an ill person, animal contact, travel, vaccination, history of tuberculosis exposure, and extrapulmonary sign of dissemination
2. Severity of the patient's illness and rapidity of progression; some patients may need empirical treatment before diagnosis is made
3. Pattern of pulmonary infiltrates
4. The impact on treatment and outcome if an invasive procedure is indicated

CHEST RADIOGRAPH

The chest radiograph (CXR) is a simple and useful diagnostic tool along with history and physical findings. Acute focal pulmonary infiltration is caused by bacterial pneumonias, pulmonary embolism, whereas subacute focal infiltrates are caused by aspergillosis, nocardiosis, cryptococcoma, tuberculosis/MAI, reactivation of systemic mycoses, and noninfectious process, such as primary or metastatic carcinoma. Acute bilateral diffuse pulmonary infiltrates are the characteristics of PCP pneumonia, with a differential diagnosis of congestive heart failure, ARDS, or diffuse alveolar hemorrhage. Diffuse alveolar infiltrates with an insidious onset are caused by viral pneumonias (including CMV and HHV-6), miliary tuberculosis, and noninfectious causes such as drug-induced pneumonitis, radiation-induced pneumonitis, lymphagitic spread of malignancy, and BOOP [1,10,12]. Cavitary lung lesions caused by bacterial pneumonias (*S. aureus*, *P. aeruginosa*, *K. pneumoniae*, septic pulmonary emboli) usually have a rapid onset. Slowly progressing pulmonary cavitary lesions are caused by tuberculosis/atypical mycobacteria, nocardiosis, fungal pneumonias, melioidosis, and paragonimiasis [39]. Spontaneous pneumothorax is more suggestive of PCP than of invasive fungal infection. Pleural effusion is more common in bacterial pneumonia. Mediastinal lymphadenopathy is associated with lymphoma as well as mycobacterial and fungal infection [1,10,12,40].

COMPUTED TOMOGRAPHY

Computed tomography (CT) has advanced the ability to diagnose and treat pulmonary infection. Conventional CT has shown usefulness for the diagnosis of pulmonary infiltrates in cancer patients, but high-resolution CT (HRCT) and spiral CT allow for even earlier detection. It is extremely important to avoid unnecessary invasive procedures in immunocompromised patients because of the higher rate of complications. The timing of CT scanning is somewhat controversial. It helps to identify subtle infiltrates and to suggest more invasive procedures. CT of the chest can reduce mean time for the diagnosis of invasive aspergillosis, compared to CXR, from 7 to 2 days, with reduction of overall mortality from 50% to 20% [41]. CT scanning can detect six times as many patients with pneumonia as did CXR, and can detect on average five days earlier. An area of consolidation and poorly defined nodules are the most reliable signs of pneumonia, and poorly defined linear opacification and cavitation also suggest infections. Ground-glass opacities are nonspecific and are seen both in infectious (especially viral pneumonias and PCP) and noninfectious processes [42]. CXR is not very sensitive in detecting cavitary lesions, especially at the apices, lung bases, and paramediastinal or retrocardiac regions. CT scanning helps to delineate cavities hidden on CXR.

Lobar and lobular pneumonia due to bacteria appear as increased lung density as a result of air space filling. An air bronchogram is usually seen in lobar pneumonia in both plain CXR and CT. In contrast, lobular pneumonia involves larger airways. Patients may have multifocal areas of increased density. In invasive fungal infection, early disease shows ground-glass attenuation followed by consolidation, peripheral nodular infiltration, and occasionally hilar lymphadenopathy. The nodule with its surrounding halo of ground-glass attenuation (the air crescent sign) that occurs late in the course of pulmonary aspergillosis is characteristic (but it also occurs in other invasive mycoses such as mucormycosis and fusariosis). Candidiasis can cause parenchymal lung diseases with patchy, bilateral airspace consolidation or multiple lung nodules; the halo sign is rarely seen. HRCT demonstrates a diffuse miliary pattern, septal thickening, and nodularity of interlobular fissures with histoplasmosis. With PCP, most advocates emphasize that the distribution of ground-glass opacity is patchy, with spared adjacent lobules (mosaic pattern) by HRCT.

Viral pneumonias such as CMV pneumonitis usually show small nodules surrounded with ground glass appearance and sometimes airspace consolidation.

CT is a useful tool in the evaluation of tuberculosis. It not only detects pulmonary parenchymal involvement but also helps to evaluate hilar and mediastinal adenopathy. HRCT is useful for early diagnosis of miliary TB, which cannot be detected by plain CXR until about 6 weeks after presentation [1,10,12,40-44].

FIBEROPTIC BRONCHOSCOPY, BRONCHOALVEOLAR LAVAGE, AND TRANSBRONCHIAL BIOPSY

Fiberoptic bronchoscopy is the least invasive procedure that directly samples the airway and alveolar spaces. Generally this procedure can be performed safely even in thrombocytopenic patients if preceded by platelet transfusion. It can precipitate respiratory failure 2%, minor bleeding less than 1%, and postprocedural fever 10%. Transbronchial biopsy modestly increases the sensitivity of BAL; because of its false negativity, patients may still require open lung biopsy. The incidence of complications varies by institution and patient population. Compared to brochoscopy with BAL, it increases the risk of major complications including significant bleeding 3%, pneumothorax 5%, and death 0.2%. The specimen obtained usually influences therapy; sometimes bronchoscopic findings help in making a diagnosis (such as herpes tracheobronchitis, *aspergillus*-associated tracheobronchitis, or bronchial obstruction leading to postobstructive pneumonia), although the impact on survival may not be altered in some patient groups [10,36,45-47].

After obtaining the specimen, it should be sent for gram stain and bacterial culture, fungal culture, AFB smear and culture, Nocardia smear and culture, *Legionella* direct fluorescent antigen and culture, respiratory viral culture, direct fluorescent antibody for HSV, influenza virus, adenovirus, respiratory syncytial virus, adenovirus, and parainfluenza virus, CMV DFA and shell vial culture, cytology, and Gomori's methenamine silver stain or direct fluorescent staining for *P. carinii*. BAL may not be very helpful in diagnoses of noninfectious processes, particularly drug-induced pneumonitis, GVHD, BOOP, and idiopathic interstitial pneumonitis, which usually require clinical correlation and lung biopsy [36,45,48,49].

LUNG BIOPSY

Transthoracic needle aspiration biopsy is rarely used in diagnoses of pulmonary infiltrates, but does have a role in evaluating peripheral masses. The sensitivity is approximately 70% for focal lesions. Complications including hemoptysis and pneumothorax can occur about 10 to 15% of the time, and hemoptysis about 3% [10,36].

Video-assisted thoracoscopic wedge resection of the lung (VAT) was limited until the recent advent of miniaturized video cameras placed at the tip of a flexible thoracoscope. It is useful in selected patients, especially those with peripheral lesions, small lesions (less than 3 cm), or interstitial lung diseases. Patients with large, irregular nodules should undergo thoracotomy. Complications of VAT are minimal in most cases [50].

Open-lung biopsy is the most invasive but standard diagnostic procedure to diagnose pulmonary infiltrates and pulmonary focal lesions in cancer patients. The risk of life-threatening hemoptysis may outweigh the benefit for lesions near the hilum or great vessels, despite the sensitivity ranges between 60 and 80%. Complications include bleeding, pneumothorax, wound infection, and respiratory failure. The mortality related to this procedure is less than 1% [36,50].

The complications of invasive procedures should be taken into consideration when deciding on the diagnostic approach.

MICROSCOPY AND CULTURE

1. Sputum and other respiratory fluid examination. In general sputum examination is safe, rapid, and noninvasive. Unfortunately, oropharyngeal contamination is problematic, especially with *Candida* spp., and gram-negative bacteria. Gram stain of the specimen should contain less than 25 epithelial cells per low-power field before further investigation under a high-power field. Phase-contrast microscopy is helpful to visualize fungal elements. Histoplasma, Coccidioides, and Blastomyces are not colonizing organisms, especially in immunocompromised patients. Although *Aspergillus* spp. may colonize the oropharynx, in high-risk patients such as febrile neutropenic patients antifungal therapy is indicated to prevent invasive sinopulmonary aspergillosis [51]. PCP can be detected by Gomori methenamine silver stain, but indirect immunofluorescent stain increases the sensitivity and specificity [52]. Immunofluorescent staining is also useful for the detection of *Legionella pneumophila*. Culture will enhance the sensitivity and specificity of stains, except for PCP.

2. Blood culture. Blood culture helps to identify invasive/disseminated infections, but negative blood culture does not rule them out. Bacteremia can be detected when patients present with respiratory symp-

toms and new pulmonary infiltrates. Gram-negative bacteremia along with pneumonia requires more aggressive treatment. Blood cultures for invasive fungal infections (candidiasis, fusariosis, paecilomycosis) are diagnostic about half the time. Aspergillosis is rarely detected by blood culture. *Aspergillus fungemia* does not predict deep-seated infection or clinical outcome, because it usually presents after diagnosis and treatment have already been established [53].

SEROLOGY, ANTIGEN DETECTION, AND PCR

Serology and PCR are important parts of the workup for pulmonary infiltrates in cancer patients. Examination fluids and aspirates from infected lesions may be examined by the serological method. It helps not only in diagnosis but also in assessing the risk, if the patients require preemptive treatment. Moreover, it helps to follow the response to the treatment. *Legionella* urinary antigen is a relatively inexpensive test, with a sensitivity of 70% and a specificity of nearly 100%. The drawback of this test is that it detects only the *Legionella* serogroup 1; and while it is useful for diagnosis, it is not for follow-up, since the test will remain positive for weeks after treatment [19]. PCR or DNA probe is helpful to diagnose tuberculosis and atypical mycobacteria, and it can directly detect the organism in sputum, respiratory aspirates, and even tissue specimens.

In bone marrow transplant patients, recipients with positive CMV antibody will have a risk of reactivation of CMV disease. The follow-up of CMV viremia/antigenemia is useful for preemptive treatment. Utilization of CMV antigenemia detection (such as detection of pp65, pp67, CMV DNA by PCR) markedly decreases the incidence of CMV disease posttransplant [10,16,54]. PCR is useful in detecting viral etiology of pneumonias in cancer patients including HHV-6 (detects circulating DNA), parainfluenza virus, RSV, rhinovirus, influenza virus, enterovirus, and corona virus (reparatory specimen) [55].

For the detection of pulmonary fungal infection, currently one can use latex agglutination, enzyme-linked immunosorbent assay, and detection of $(1{\rightarrow}3)$-β-D glucan (BDG). Latex agglutination is specific but not very sensitive. An enzyme-linked immunosorbent assay has acceptable sensitivity and specificity. The detection of BDG seems very promising, though validation and availability are still underway. In many studies, PCR is useful for early detection of invasive fungal infections. Detection of fungal DNA from the blood would be most helpful, because respiratory specimens may contain spores or may be contaminated with colonized mold [56–61]. Detection of fungal antigenemia correlated with treatment response and prognosis in a small study [62].

CONCLUSION

Pulmonary infections in cancer patients are a major cause of morbidity and mortality. Knowledge of the underlying malignancy, cancer-treatment status, and immunosuppression status is important in predicting the predominant pathogens. Newly developed diagnostic techniques may help to decrease the use of invasive procedures. Awareness of early signs and symptoms guide one to prompt diagnostic strategies as well as appropriate empirical or preemptive therapy. The approach has to be individualized, following intervention strategies that are the least invasive and the most likely to yield the diagnosis of these potentially life-threatening pulmonary complications.

REFERENCES

1. Cunha BA. Pneumonia in the compromised host. Infect Dies Clint North Am 2001; 15:591–609.
2. Cunha BA. Severe community-acquired pneumonia. Crit Care Clin 1998; 14: 105–118.
3. Neiderman MS, Mandell LA, Anzueto A, Bass JB, Broughton WA, Campbell GD, Dean N, File T, Fine MJ, Gross PA, Martinez F, Marrie TJ, Plouffe JF, Ramirez J, Sarosi GA, Torres A, Wilson R, Yu VL. Guideline for the management of adults with community-acquired pneumonia. Am J Respir Crit Care Med 2001; 163:1730–1754.
4. Bonoan JT, Cunha BA. *Staphyllococcus aureus* as a cause of community acquired pneumonia in patients with diabetes mellitus. Infect Dis Clin Practice 1999; 8:319–321.
5. Sheagren JN. Commentary: *Staphyllococcus aureus* is almost never a cause of community-acquired pneumonia. Infect Dis Clin Practice 1999; 8:321–322.
6. Mundy LM, Auwaerter PG, Oldach D, Warner ML, Burton A, Vance E, Gaydos CA, Joseph JM, Gopalan R, Moore RD, et al. Community-acquired pneumonia: impact of immune status. Am J Respir Crit Care Med 1995; 152:1309–1315.
7. Chatzinikolaou I, Abi-Said D, Bodey GP, Rolston KV, Tarrand JJ, Samonis G. Recent experience with *Pseudomonas aeruginosa* bacteremia in patients with cancer. Arch Intern Med 2000; 160:501–509.
8. Shelhamer JH, Toews GB, Masur H, Suffredini AF, Pizzo PA, Walsh TJ, Henderson DK. Respiratory diseases in the immunocompromised patient. Ann Intern Med 1992; 117:415.
9. Carratala J, Roson B, Fernandez-Sevilla A, Alcaide P, Gudiol F. Bacteremic pneumonia in neutropenic patients with cancer. Arch Intern Med 1998; 158:868–872.
10. Bergen GA, Shelhamar JH. Pulmonary infiltrates in the cancer patient, new approaches to an old problem. Infect Dis Clin North Am 1996; 10:297–325.
11. Marr KA, Carter RA, Crippa F, Wald A, Corey L. Epidemiology and outcome of mould infections in hematopoietic stem cell transplant recipients. Clin Infect Dis 2002; 34:909–917.

12. Walsh TJ. Management of immunocompromised patients with evidence of an invasive mycosis. Hematol Oncol Clin North Am 1993; 7:1003.
13. Cigorna C, Armstrong D. Mucormycosis inpatients with cancer. Infect Med 1994; 11:562.
14. Vartivarian SE, Anaissie EJ, Bodey GP. Emerging fungal pathogens in immunocompromised patients: classification, diagnosis, and management. Clin Infect Dis 1993; 17(suppl 2):S487–S491.
15. Denning DW. Invasive aspergillosis. Clin Infect Dis 1998; 26:781–805.
16. Leather HL, Wingard JR. Infection following hematopoietic stem cell transplantation. Infect Dis Clin N Am 2001; 15:483–519.
17. Conant EF, Wechsler RJ. Actinomycosis and nocardiosis of the lung. J Thorac Imaging 1992; 7(4):75–84.
18. Kinnear WJM, MacFarlane JT. A survey of thoracic actinomycosis. Respir Med 1990; 84:57–59.
19. Stout JE, Yu VL. Legionellosis. New England J Med 1997; 337:682–687.
20. Schindel C, Siepmann U, Han S, Ullmann AJ, Mayer E, Fischer T, Maeurer M. Persistent *legionella* infection in a patient after bone marrow transplantation. J Clin Microbiol 2000; 38:4294–4295.
21. Kovacs JA, Gill VJ, Meshnick S, Masur H. New insights into transmission, diagnosis, and drug treatment of *Pneumocystis carinii* pneumonia. J Am Med Assoc 2001; 286:2450–2460.
22. Arend SM, Kroon FP, van't Wout JW. *Pneumocystis carinii* pneumonia in patients without AIDS, 1980 through 1993. Arch Intern Med 1995; 155:2436–2441.
23. Galgiani JN, Ampel NM, Catanzaro A, Johnson RH, Stevens DA, Williams PL. Practice guideline for the treatment of coccidioidomycosis. Clin Infect Dis 2000; 30:658–661.
24. Wheat J, Sarosi G, McKinsey D, Hamill R, Bradsher R, Johnson P, Loyd J, Kauffman C. Practice guideline for the management of patients with histoplasmosis. Clin Infect Dis 2000; 30:688–695.
25. Desachy A, Ranger-Rogez S, Francois B, Venot C, Traccard I, Gastinne H, Denis F, Vignon P. Reactivation of human herpescirus type 6 in multiple organ failure syndrome. Clin Infect Dis 2001; 32:197–203.
26. Nguyen Q, Champlin R, Giralt S, Rolston K, Raad J, Jacobson K, Ippoliti C, Hecht D, Tarrand J, Luna M, Whimbey E. Late Cytomegalovirus pneumonia in adult allogenic blood and marrow transplant recipients. Clin Infect Dis 1999; 28:618–623.
27. Chien JW, Johnson JL. Viral pneumonias, infection in the immunocompromised host. Postgrad Med 2000; 107:67–80.
28. Imbert-Marcille BM, Tang XW, Lepelletier D, Besse B, Moreau P, Billaudel S, Milpied N. Human herpesvirus 6 infection after autologous or allogenic stem cell transplantation: a single-center prospective longitudinal study of 92 patients. Clin Infect Dis 2000; 31:881–886.
29. Caserta MT, Mock DJ, Dewhurst S. Human herpesvisus 6. Clin Infect Dis 2001; 33:829–833.
30. Wendt CH, Weisdorf DJ, Jordan MC, Balfour HH Jr, Hertz MI. Para-

influenza virus respiratory infection after bone marrow transplantation. N Engl J Med 1992; 326:921–926.

31. Finegold SM. Lung abscess. In: Mandell GL, Bennett JE, Dolin R, eds. Principle and Practice of Infectious Diseases. Philadelphia: Churchill Livingstone, 2000: 751–754.

32. Marik PE. Aspiration pneumonitis and aspiration pneumonia. N Engl J Med 2001; 344:665–670.

33. Hirshberg B. Factors predicting mortality of patients with lung abscess. Chest 1999; 115:746–750.

34. Koloff MH, Schuster DP. The acute respiratory distress syndrome. N Engl J Med 1995; 332:27–37.

35. Rosenow EC III, Myers JL, Swensen SJ, Pisani RJ. Drug induced pulmonary disease: an update. Chest 1992; 102:239 250.

36. Soubani AO, Miller KB, Hassoun PM. Pulmonary complications of bone marrow transplantation. Chest 1996; 109:1066–1077.

37. Crawford SW, Hackman RC. Clinical course of idiopathic pneumonia after bone marrow transplantation. Am Rev Respir Dis 1993; 147:1393–1400.

38. Clark JG, Hansen JA, Hertz MI, Parkman R, Jensen L, Peavy HH. Idiopathic pneumonia syndrome after bone marrow transplantation. Am Rev Respir Dis 1993; 147:1601–1606.

39. Prince SE, Dominger KA, Cunha BA, Klein NC. Klebsiella pneumoniae pneumonia. Heart Lung 1997; 26:413–417.

40. Moore EH. Diffuse lung disease in the current spectrum of immunocompromised host (non-AIDS). Radiol Clin North Am 1991; 29:983–997.

41. Cailot D. Casasnovas O, Bernard A, Couaillier JF, Durand C, Cuisenier B, Solary E, Piard F, Petrella T, Bonnin A, Couillault G, Dumas M, Guy H. Improved management of invasive pulmonary aspergillosis in neutropenic patients using early thoracic computed tomographic scan and surgery. J Clin Oncol 1997; 15:139–147.

42. Berger LA. Imaging in the diagnosis of infections in immunocompromised patients. Current Opinion Infect Dis 1998; 11:431–436.

43. Wheeler JH, Fishman EK. Computed tomography in the management of chest infection: current status. Clin Infect Dis 1996; 23:232–240.

44. Stevens DA, Kan VL, Judson MA, Morrison VA, Dummer S, Denning DW, Bennett JE, Walsh TJ, Patterson TF, Pankey GA. Practice guidelines for diseases caused by *Aspergillus*. Clin Infect Dis 2000; 30:696–709.

45. Walsh FW, Rolfe MW, Rumbak MJ. The initial evaluation of the immunocompromised patient. Chest Surg Clin North Am 1999; 9:19–38.

46. Dunagan DP, Baker AM, Hurd DD, Haponik EF. Bronchoscopic evaluation of pulmonary infiltrates following bone marrow transplantation. Chest 1997; 111:135–141.

47. White P, Bonacum JT, Miller CB. Utility of fiberoptic bronchoscopy in bone marrow transplant patients. Bone Marrow Transplant 1997; 20:681–687.

48. Houston SH, Sinnott JT. Management of the transplant recipient with pulmonary infection. Infect Dis Clin North Am 1995; 9:965–983.

49. Eriksson BM, Dahl H, Wang FZ, Elvin K, Hillerdal G, Lundholm M, Linde A,

Olding-Stenkvist E. Diagnosis of pulmonary infections in immunocompromised patients by fiber-optic bronchoscopy with bronchoalveolar lavage and serology. Scan J Infect Dis 1996; 28:479–485.

50. Miller DL, Allen MS, Trastek VF, Deschamps C, Pairolero PC. Video-thoracoscopic wedge excision of the lung. Ann Thorac Surg 1992; 54:410–414.

51. Horvath JA, Dummer S. The use of respiratory-tract cultures in the diagnosis of invasive pulmonary aspergillosis. Am J Med 1996; 100:171–177.

52. Ng VL, Yajko DM, McPhaul LW, Gartner I, Byford B, Goodman CD, Nassos PS, Sanders CA, Howes EL, Leoung G, et al. Evaluation of an indirect fluorescent-antibody stain for detection of *Pneumocystis carinii* in respiratory specimens. J Clin Microbiol 1990; 28:975–979.

53. Girmenia C, Nucci M, Martino P. Clinical significance of *aspergillus fungemia* in patients with haematological malignancies and invasive aspergillosis. Br J Haematol 2001; 114:93–98.

54. Crumpacker CS. Cytomegalovirus. In: Mandell GL, Bennett JE, Dolin R. Principle and Practice of Infectious Diseases. Philadelphia: Churchill Livingstone, 1586–1594.

55. van Elden LJ, van Kraaij MG, Nijhuis M, Hendriksen KA, Dekker AW, Rozenberg-Arska M, van Loon AM. Polymerase chain reaction is more sensitive than viral culture and antigen testing for detection of respiratory viruses in adult with hematological cancer. Clin Infect Dis 2002; 34:177–183.

56. Bretagne S, Costa JM, Marmorat-Khuong A, Poron F, Cordonnier C, Vidaud M, Fleury-Feith J. Detection of *Aspergillus* species DNA in bronchoalveolar lavage sample by competitive PCR. J Clin Microbiol 1995; 33:1164–1168.

57. Buchheidt D, Baust C, Skladny H, Ritter J, Suedhoff T, Baldus M, Seifarth W, Leib-Moesch C, Hehlmann R. Detection of *Aspergillus* species in blood and bronchoalveolar lavage samples from immunocompromised patients by means of 2 step polymerase chain reaction: clinical result. Clin Infect Dis 2001; 33:428–435.

58. Ridge RJ, Finkelman MA, Rex JH. Application of a glucan-specific limulus amebocyte lysate serum assay for diagnosis of invasive fungal infection. Abstract J-842. Presented at the 41st ICAAC.

59. Herbrecht R, Letscher-Bru V, Oprea C, et al. *Aspergillus* galactomannan ELISA in onco-hematologic patients. Abstract J-842. Presented at the 42nd ICAAC.

60. Kami M, Fukui T, Ogawa S, Kazuyama Y, Machida U, Tanaka Y, Kanda Y, Kashima T, Yamazaki Y, Hamaki T, Mori S, Akiyama H, Mutou Y, Sakamaki H, Osumi K, Kimura S, Hirai H. Use of real-time PCR on blood samples for diagnosis of invasive aspergillosis. Clin Infect Dis 2001; 33:1504–1512.

61. Lin M, Lu H, Chen W. Improving efficacy of antifungal therapy by polymerase chain reaction-based strategy among febrile patients with neutropenia and cancer. Clin Infect Dis 2001; 33:1621–1627.

62. Boutboul F, Alberti C, Leblanc T, Sulahian A, Gluckman E, Derouin F, Ribaud P. Invasive aspergillosis in allogenic stem cell transplant recipients: increasing antigenemia is associated with progressive disease. Clin Infect Dis 2002; 34:939–943.

26

Cardiovascular Infections in Cancer Patients

Bernhard Unsöld
Albert-Ludwigs University of Freiburg
Freiburg, Germany

John N. Greene
University of South Florida School of Medicine
and Moffitt Cancer Center and Research Institute
Tampa, Florida, U.S.A.

ENDOCARDITIS

The annual incidence of IE is between 1.9 and 11.6 per 100,000 population. Most cases involve native heart valves. Of the patients with native valve endocarditis (NVE), 55 to 75% have predisposing conditions such as rheumatic or congenital heart disease. About one quarter of all cases represent prosthetic valve endocarditis (PVE) [1].

NVE is most often caused by oral ("viridans") streptococci which cause about 30 to 65% of all cases. The most common streptococci are those of the *sanguis* and *oralis* groups [1,2]. Enterococci, mostly *Enterococcus faecalis* are less common (5 to 15% of all cases), but their incidence is increasing [1,2]. The incidence of NVE caused by Staphylococci has increased during recent years, so that community-acquired NVE now is just as likely to be caused by

Staphylococci as by Streptococci. *S. aureus*, which causes 25 to 40% of all cases, is the most frequent Staphylococcal species, followed by coagulase negative staphylococci (3 to 8% of all cases) [1,2]. Rarer causes of NVE are gram-negative bacteria, especially those of the HACEK group (Haemophilus, Actinobacillus, Cardiobacterium, Eikenella, Kingella). PVE is more often caused by staphylococci, especially coagulase negative strains. Community-acquired PVE has a similar range of pathogens as NVE but a higher incidence of unusual organisms [2].

There is little data about the incidence of IE in patients with cancer. A postmortem study on 7,840 patients with predominantly neoplastic diseases who were autopsied between 1950 and 1971 showed IE in 0.35% of the autopsied patients. The causative organisms were *Staphylococcus aureus* (46%), streptococci (22%), half of which were Group D, gram-negative bacilli (18%) and candida (14%) [3].

STAPHYLOCOCCUS AUREUS

Several small retrospective studies of *S. aureus* bacteremia (SAB) in cancer patients found a low incidence of endocarditis in patients with SAB [4–6]. One of these studies even found a lower incidence of IE in patients with SAB and hematological malignacies and/or agranulocytosis than in other patients with SAB [6]. A more recent prospective analysis of nonneutropenic cancer patients and SAB found that of 52 patients with SAB, 15% developed IE. Patients in whom the SAB was related to an intravascular device or in whom the focus of infection was unknown had a higher risk of developing IE than patients in whom the SAB was attributed to a tissue infection [7].

VIRIDANS STREPTOCOCCI

In studies with cancer patients who had bacteremia due to viridans strepto-cocci, the incidence of IE was 6 to 8% [8,9]. The following risk factors for viridans streptococcal bacteremia were identified: profound neutropenia, bone marrow transplantation, chemotherapy-induced oral mucositis, ongo-ing therapy with histamine type 2 receptor antagonists or antacids, antibiotic prophylaxis with trimethoprim/sulfamethoxazole or a fluoroquinolone [8], colonization with viridans streptococci, the use of cytosine arabinoside, and the absence of previous therapy with parenteral antibiotics [9].

STREPTOCOCCUS BOVIS

Infections with *S. bovis*, especially *S. bovis* endocarditis, have been found to be strongly associated with colorectal cancer. *S. bovis* is a Group D nonenterococcal organism that is found significantly more often in the stool of patients with colorectal cancer than in control patients (56 vs. 10%, respectively) [10]. In patients with IE due to *S. bovis* the incidence of colonic carcinoma was found to be 18% [11]. Of 467 patients with *S. bovis* bacteremia, 62% developed endocarditis [12]. Because of the strong association, patients with *S. bovis* bacteremia or endocarditis should be screened for colorectal tumors. Endocarditis due to other gastrointestinal organisms is less often associated with colonic lesions. For example, patients with enterococcal endocarditis had an incidence of colonic carcinoma of only 2% [11]. Clostridia septicum and group B Streptococci bacteremia have been associated with colorectal cancer. However, only the latter organism is likely to cause endocarditis.

STREPTOCOCCUS AGALACTIAE

Endocarditis caused by Group B Streptococci is rare. Most cases of Group B Streptococcal IE have been reported in patients with underlying immunocompromised conditions including cancer in 25% of the cases [13,14]. One study found an association of *S. agalactiae* endocardits and villous adenomas of the colon (without foci of adenocarcinoma) in two patients [14].

IE DUE TO RARER ORGANISMS

Among the rarer causes of IE in cancer patients that have been described are four cases of chronic Q fever endocarditis (*Coxiella burnetii*). The authors suggest that suppression of cellular immunity could increase the risk of developing chronic Q fever endocarditis. Therefore Q fever should be in the differential diagnosis for patients with cancer and unexplained fever, especially if they live in areas where *C. burnetii* is endemic [15].

A study on 61 patients with Aspergillus valve endocarditis without prior cardiac surgery found that 67% of the patients had underlying immunosuppression. Forty-three percent of immunosuppressed patients had an underlying hematologic malignancy, and 7% had underlying solid tumors. The most common Aspergillus species causing endocarditis were *A. fumigatus* and *A. flavus*. Aspergillus endocarditis is characterized by bulky vegetations (average 39 mm). Peripheral signs of endocarditis are rare (only 9% of patients). Blood cultures are rarely positive, which makes diagnosis difficult. Only about one-third of aspergillus IE cases were diagnosed antemortem. The prognosis of aspergillus endocarditis is very poor with an overall mortality of 95% and a mortality of 100% in immunocompromised patients [16].

A study done on 168 cancer patients with candidiasis showed that 20% of the patients with disseminated candidiasis had cardiac involvement. None of the patients with localized candidiasis had cardiac involvement. In that study no patient with cardiac candidiasis showed involvement of the heart valve, whereas all patients had myocardial abscesses. In five patients the mural endocardium was affected from direct extension of a myocardial abscess [17]. Case reports suggest a rising incidence of *Candida parapsilosis* endocarditis in cancer patients [18,19].

In conclusion, cardiovascular infections, namely endocarditis, occur at similar rates in cancer patients as in people without cancer. However, because of the ubiquitous need of central venous access in cancer patients, catheter-associated bacteremia and endocarditis is more common, with *Staphylococcus aureus* predominating. In addition, *Streptococcus bovis* endocarditis and bacteremia is well known to be linked to colorectal cancer. Finally, because of prolonged neutropenia in patients with hematologic malignancy and the immunosuppressive effects of graft versus host disease and its treatment in patients undergoing stem cell transplantation, the incidence of candidemia and disseminated Aspergillosis is increasing. Rarely, these fungal pathogens can cause endocarditis, which is almost always fatal.

REFERENCES

1. Karchmer AW. Infective endocarditis. In: Braunwald, Zipes, Libby, eds. Heart Disease: A Textbook of Cardiovascular Medicine. 6th ed. Philadelphia: W. B. Saunders, 2001:1723–1724.
2. Eykyn SJ. Endocarditis: basics. Heart 2001; 86(4):476–480.
3. Rosen P, Armstrong D. Infective endocarditis in patients treated for malignant neoplastic diseases: a postmortem study. Am J Clin Patho 1973; 60:241–250.
4. Sotman SB, Schimpff SC, Young VM. *Staphylococcus aureus* bacteremia in patients with acute leukemia. Am J Med 1980; 69(6):814–818.
5. Carney DN, Fossieck BE, Parker RH, Minna JD. Bacteremia due to *Staphylococcus aureus* in patients with cancer: report on 45 cases in adults and review of the literature. Rev Infect Dis 1982; 4(1):1–12.
6. Espersen F, Frimodt-Moller N, Rosdahl VT, Jessen O, Faber V, Rosendal K. *Staphylococcus aureus* bacteremia in patients with hematological malignancies and/or agranulocytosis. Acta Med Scand 1987; 222(5):465–470.
7. Gopal AK, Fowler VG Jr, Shah M, Gesty-Palmer D, Marr KA, McClelland RS, Kong LK, Gottlieb GS, Lanclos K, Li J, Sexton DJ, Corey GR. Prospective analysis of *Staphylococcus aureus* bacteremia in nonneutropenic adults with malignancy. J Clin Oncol 2000; 18(5):1110–1115.
8. Elting LS, Bodey GP, Keefe BH. Septicemia and shock syndrome due to viridans streptococci: a case-control study of predisposing factors. Clin Infect Dis 1992; 14:1201–1207.
9. Bochud PY, Eggiman P, Calandra T, Van Melle G, Saghafi L, Francioli P. Bacteremia due to viridans streptococcus in neutropenic patients with cancer: clinical spectrum and risk factors. Clin Infect Dis 1994; 18:25–31.

10. Klein RS, Recco RA, Catalano MT, Edberg SC, Casey JI, Steigbigel NH. Association of streptococcus bovis with carcinoma of the colon. N Engl J Med 1977; 297:800–802.
11. Leport C, Bure A, Leport J, Vilde JL. Incidence of colonic lesions in streptococcus bovis and enterococcal endocarditis. Lancet 1987; 1(8535):748.
12. Panwalker AP. Unusual infections associated with colorectal cancer. Rev Infect Dis 1988; 10(2):347 364.
13. Akram M, Khan IA. Isolated pulmonic valve endocarditis caused by Group B Streptococcus (*Streptococcus agalactiae*)—a case report and literature review. Angiology 2001; 52:211–215.
14. Wiseman A, René P, Crelinsten GL. *Streptococcus agalactiae* endocarditis: an association with villous adenomas of the large intestine. Ann Int Med 1985; 103(6):893–894.
15. Raoult D, Brouqui P, Marchou B, Gastaut JA. Acute and chronic Q fever in patients with cancer. Clin Infect Dis 1992; 14:127–130.
16. Gumbo T, Taege AJ, Mawhorter S, McHenry MC, Lytle BH, Cosgrove DM, Gordon SM. Aspergillus valve endocarditis in patients without prior cardiac surgery. Medicine 2000; 79:261–268.
17. Ihde DC, Roberts WC, Marr KC, Brereton HD, McGuire WP, Levine AS, Young RC. Cardiac candidiasis in cancer patients. Cancer 1978; 41:2364–2371.
18. Girmenia C, Martino P, DeBernardis F, Gentile G, Boccanera M, Monaco M, Antonucci G, Cassone A. Rising incidence of *Candida parapsilosis* fungemia in patients with hematologic malignancies: clinic aspects, predisposing factors, and differential pathogenicity of the causative strains. Clin Infect Dis 1996; 23(3):506–514.
19. Inoue Y, Yozu R, Ueda T, Kawada S. A case report of *Candida parapsilosis* endocarditis. J Heart Valve Dis 1998; 7(2):240–242.

27

Gastrointestinal Infections in Cancer Patients

Todd S. Wills
University of South Florida School of Medicine
Tampa, Florida, U.S.A.

Gastrointestinal infections are common clinical entities faced in the care of patients with underlying malignant disease. Infections of the gastrointestinal tract may be related to anatomic lesions with obstructive sequelae, may result from impaired immunity or cellular function from chemotherapy, may be local manifestations of systemic infections, and even may be a complication of antibiotic therapy used in the prevention and treatment of other systemic or localized infections. Microorganisms colonizing the gastrointestinal tract frequently are pathogens leading to systemic infection in patients with hematological malignancy and neutropenia.

The goal of this chapter is to provide an overview of the diagnosis and management of the most common gastrointestinal infections in cancer patients. Abdominal infections that represent medical or surgical emergencies will be outlined. A primary focus of the chapter will be on those infectious syndromes of the gastrointestinal tract that occur in the settings of neutropenia and bone marrow transplantation.

GASTROINTESTINAL INFECTIOUS EMERGENCIES IN CANCER PATIENTS

Surgical Abdomen

The so-called acute abdomen indicative of peritonitis usually signals a need for emergent diagnosis and often exploratory surgery in the general population. The hallmarks of this presentation are pain, usually of short duration, and abdominal tenderness on examination, often with rigidity and guarding. These findings are related to acute inflammation of the peritoneum that may stem from many causes; most concerning among these is spilling of gastrointestinal contents into the peritoneum secondary to perforation of a hollow viscous. Among otherwise healthy patients, an acute abdomen may be the result of appendicitis, cholecystitis, perforated diverticulum, or perforated peptic ulcer among others. Oncology patients remain at risk for such complications even when hospitalized for other reasons or therapies. Additionally, these patients are at risk for peritonitis specifically related to underlying malignancy, such as a bulky tumor with anatomic disruption, or alteration of intestinal/gastric mucosa secondary to chemotherapy or other medications.

The management of an acute abdomen is complicated in cancer patients, where typical diagnoses must be considered equally with those unique to the oncology population. An example is the diagnostic dilemma of right lower quadrant pain in adolescents undergoing chemotherapy. Adolescent patients who may be undergoing treatment for leukemia fall into an age group with a 2 to 4% rate of appendicitis in the general population. Reviews have demonstrated a similar or even slightly higher rate of appendicitis in the adolescent population with leukemia [1]. The similar clinical presentation of neutropenic enterocolitis may lead to diagnostic difficulty. Whereas appendicitis remains a surgical disease, increasing success has been found with medical therapy in the management of neutropenic enterocolitis (see following section) [2–4].

Many factors also may mask the clinical finding of a surgical abdomen in cancer patients. Medications may affect both a patient's risk for abdominal catastrophe and hinder the evaluation of the same. Traditional exam findings of a perforated viscous may be masked by pain medications or corticosteroids in common use on an oncology ward. Additionally, corticosteroids increase the risk for stress gastric ulceration with the possibility of perforation. Neurological dysfunction from a patient's underlying malignancy, such as from spinal cord compression from tumor metastases, can also attenuate physical exam findings [5]. Further complicating evaluation of abdominal pain in the oncology population is the frequency of the complaint, with up to one-third of patients in some series experiencing acute abdominal pain during hospitalization [1]. In some cases an acute abdominal presentation may not reflect any intra-abdominal pathology. One such example is the acute neuropathic pain of herpes zoster caused by varicella-zoster virus during the prodromal period prior to the onset of a typical rash [6].

The cornerstone of therapy for an acute abdomen is surgery. In some cases, a diagnosis can be achieved prior to surgery via focal exam findings or radiological imaging, but such a diagnostic workup should not delay prompt surgical evaluation in patients where suspicion for an acute abdominal process is high. For patients who may mask the symptoms of an acute abdomen because of those factors described above, the clinician must keep a high diagnostic index of suspicion.

Patients who are clinically stable may undergo a more complete diagnostic workup prior to a final decision about exploratory surgery. Among the diagnostic tests which may be appropriate are abdominal x-ray to rule out pneumoperitoneum, abdominal computed tomography to refine a differential diagnosis, and complete blood count for marked fluctuations in leukocyte count or hemoglobin. It is appropriate to treat patients undergoing a diagnostic workup for possible peritonitis with empirical antimicrobial coverage until a diagnosis can be achieved. Antibiotic choice should be tailored to cover enteric aerobes including *Pseudomonas aeruginosa* and anaerobes including *B. fragilis*. Single-agent therapies include imipenem–cilastatin, meropenem, piperacillin–tazobactam, and ticarcillin–clavulanate [7]. Antifungal therapy should be strongly considered in the treatment of any perforated viscous, as the rate of recovery of yeast from intraoperative specimens for abdominal perforations exceeds 30% [8]. Therapy should be continued throughout the perioperative period.

Ascending and Suppurative Cholangitis in Malignancy

Cholangitis is usually the result of biliary ductal obstruction from stones in the general population. Cholangitis in cancer patients may result from cholelithiasis or more commonly from malignant lesions of the biliary tract either from primary (cholangiocarcinoma, hepatocellular carcinoma) or metastatic disease. This difference in etiology affects both the management and the prognosis of these entities in oncology patients.

The hallmark of the diagnosis of cholangitis is Charcot's triad of jaundice, fever, and abdominal pain resulting from biliary tract obstruction and infection. The differentiation between suppurative and ascending cholangitis is largely one of severity. Suppurative cholangitis is the result of complete obstruction on the biliary tract resulting in increased luminal pressure and near constant bacterial passage into the bloodstream. The result is usually progressive sepsis and death. Ascending cholangitis is the result of partial biliary ductal obstruction without increased transluminal pressure.

This results in intermittent bacterial translocation into the bloodstream with a remitting and relapsing course. Ascending cholangitis may progress to suppurative disease, making prompt therapy to prevent such progression vital.

Relief of biliary tract obstruction is the primary goal in the therapy of patients with cholangitis of either type [9]. In most cases, initial management includes endoscopic retrograde cholangiopancreatography (ERCP). Often this procedure is both diagnostic and therapeutic. In patients with known metastatic disease or with a malignancy known to be poorly responsive to treatment, an endoscopically placed biliary stent can serve as a temporizing measure to provide at least temporary relief of symptomatic biliary obstruction. Additionally, for patients in whom the underlying malignancy is not known, cytological brushings from the biliary or pancreatic ducts are sometimes diagnostic. In situations where stenting is not possible endoscopically, surgical or percutaneous relief of obstruction is warranted. Surgical intervention is preferred when cholangitis results from a tumor amenable to surgical cure or when a tumor with the potential for response to systemic chemotherapy is present. Surgery is also recommended when other diagnostic procedures have failed to arrive at a definitive etiology for biliary obstruction, so long as the patient is a reasonable surgical candidate.

Antimicrobial therapy that targets biliary tract flora is an essential component of treatment for cholangitis. Among the pathogens of concern are *Enterobacteriaceae*, *Enterococci*, *Bacteroides*, and *Clostridium* species. Initial antibiotic regimens should have activity agaisnt these organisms. After a more protracted illness, when multiple courses of antibiotics have been used, resistant bacteria and yeast predominate. These pathogens include *Pseudomonas aeruginosa* and other gram-negative bacilli and *Candida* species. The presence of chronic biliary obstruction and the continued need for an internal or external biliary stent or drainage invariably results in cholangitis. In addition, persistent biliary obstruction can result in multiple liver abscesses. Despite the most aggressive care, malignant biliary obstruction portends a poor prognosis with an estimated mortality of 67% at 2 months [10].

INFECTIONS OF THE ORAL CAVITY AND ESOPHAGUS

Oral Cavity

Infections of the oral cavity are common in cancer patients. Oropharyngeal epithelial damage is often a complication of chemotherapy. The oral cavity is the most visible area of mucosal damage from chemotherapy-induced mucositis, although any mucosal surface may be affected. Mucositis of the oral cavity is a more prominent complaint among patients because of the significant discomfort it causes associated with any oral intake. Importantly, bacterial colonization of the oral cavity can serve as a source of systemic infection in cancer patients. Mouth bacteria such as *viridans streptococci, capnocytophaga* species, and *stomatococcus* species can lead to septicemia in the setting of mucositis, especially when coupled with quantitative neutrophil deficits from chemotherapy [11]. Disseminated candidiasis may also result from oral candidiasis in the setting of mucositis [12]. A careful examination of the oral cavity for mucositis is essential in selecting empirical antibiotics in the setting of febrile neutropenia.

Herpes labialis and oropharyngeal herpes from herpes simplex virus (HSV 1) and to a lesser extent herpes simplex virus 2 (HSV 2) are common in oncology patients, especially in the setting of hematological and lymphoid malignancies, and in bone marrow transplant (BMT) patients. Reactivation of HSV 1 occurs in up to 60% of patients with hematological malignancy and in up to 80% of patients following allogeneic BMT. Lesions may be limited to isolated vesicular lesions of the vermillion border but may also manifest multiple ulcerative lesions of the oral cavity. Thrombocytopenia from marrow suppression due to chemotherapy may lead to hemorrhagic vesicles that may be confused with traumatic lesions. In the setting of neutropenia, vesicles are rarely seen. Rather a hemorrhagic ulcer or an ulcer with white base and serpengious borders is characteristic. Often herpes infections arise in areas of recent minor trauma such as sites of oral-gastric tubes and endotracheal tubes. Such atypical presentations often require diagnosis by viral culture for HSV or examination of vesicle or ulcer content for typical cellular changes via the Tzank preparation or more recently an immunoflourescent stain. In bone marrow transplant patients, pretransplant serology is helpful for planning prophylactic therapy for HSV.

One of the most common infections of the oral cavity is oral candidiasis. The most common form is the pseudomembranous form typified by white plaques, but erythematous plaques without membranes and angular chelosis are also the result of *candida* oral infection. Predisposing factors for the development of thrush in cancer patients include impaired cellular immunity secondary to primary malignancy or chemotherapy, prolonged steroid use such as that used for intracranial or spinal metastatic disease, and prolonged broad-spectrum antibiotic use [12]. In most cases, oral candidiasis is the result of *candida albicans* infection. Such infection is usually responsive to topical therapy (clotrimazole troches, nystatin suspension) or fluconazole. Lack of response to therapy may indicate a resistant *Candida albicans* strain or a nonalbicans *candida* infection (*C. glabrata, C. krusei, C. parapsilosis*) [13–15]. In such cases, systemic amphotericin has traditionally been utilized. Newer agents including caspofungin and voriconazole may offer additional choices in the treatment of such infections.

A less common but serious oral infection in patients with neutropenia is anaerobic stomatitis [16]. This primarily occurs in neutropenic patients on empirical antibiotic regimens that lack anaerobic coverage. The mucosal lesion is usually an ulcer with white base 1–4 cm in size, which may become hemorrhagic. It can easily be confused with herpes virus infection. Submandicular or cervical lymphadenopathy can frequently coexist with or without the mucosal ulcer. Culture of the ulcer is not helpful because anerobes do not grow well from a swab culturette and their presence in the mouth is normal. Only when a blood culture is positive for the organism is the entity recognized. The organisms responsible are primarily *Capnocytophaga ochracea* and *Fusobacterium* species. Clindamycin or penicillins are preferred treatment regimens. Metronidazole should also be effective.

Esophagitis

Infectious esophagitis is also frequent in the oncological population. The clinical presentation of esophagitis is typified by odynophagia with varying degrees of dysphagia. The most common etiology of esophagitis in malignancy is chemotherapy followed by candidiasis and then herpes simplex virus. Often esophagitis occurs in association with oral candidiasis, but this is not universal. In neutropenic patients, the risk of invasive esophageal candidiasis with possible systemic dissemination is increased. Additionally, thrombocytopenia predisposes these patients to greater risk of bleeding from esophagitis. Definitive diagnosis can usually be made endoscopically with primary differential diagnostic considerations including HSV and CMV esophagitis. It is important to note that candidal esophagitis may often mask endoscopic findings of an underlying coinfection with either HSV or CMV. Often esophagitis is treated empirically with systemic antifungals in oncology patients, since many patients carry increased bleeding risk secondary to pancytopenia, and an invasive endoscopic exam may carry excessive risk [12].

A less recognized clinical entity in cancer patients is bacterial esophagitis. The diagnosis of bacterial esophagitis depends on the isolations of organisms from biopsy specimens taken during endoscopy. Studies have demonstrated that bacteria isolated from biopsy specimens with tissue invasion were implicated with subsequent bacteremia. This reflects the importance of an intact epithelial lining of the GI tract in the prevention of systemic or disseminated infection [17].

DIARRHEAL INFECTIONS IN MALIGNANCY

Diagnostic Workup

Diarrhea is a common complaint in the oncological population. Although the causes of diarrhea are numerous, many of which are noninfectious, infectious etiologies are usually of primary concern. Imunnosuppression by primary malignancy, medication, chemotherapy, or recent bone marrow transplantation broadens the differential diagnosis considerably.

A detailed history and physical is important in focusing the diagnostic workup. A patient presenting from the community with new onset diarrhea raises markedly different concerns from a hospitalized patient with prolonged febrile neutropenia or a patient with recent bone marrow transplantation. The quality of diarrhea provides important clues to possible diagnoses (bloody versus watery, high volume, associated with abdominal pain, foul smelling, etc.). For patients presenting from the community, inquiries regarding dietary changes, sick contacts, recent travel, or water consumption may prove helpful.

The management of diarrheal illness for immunocompetent patients is dealt with in detail in many other texts. This discussion will focus primarily on the workup of diarrhea in patients immunosuppressed by their cancer and its treatment.

When diarrhea is a presenting complaint for admission or evaluation, community-acquired pathogens are usually of primary concern. These include enteric pathogens such as *Salmonella, Shigella, Campylobacter, Yersinia* species, and *E. coli*. For patients with exposure to unpurified water sources, parasitic infection with *Giardia intestinalis, Entamoeba histolytica*, and *Cryposporidium* is a concern [18]. Interestingly, while the diagnosis of parasitic causes for diarrhea is not uncommon within 3 days of hospitalization, it is rare for a diarrheal illness starting greater than 3 days from hospital admission to be attributable to parasitic infection [19]. An exception to this rule is reactivation of *Strongyloides stercoralis* infection with initiation of high-dose chemotherapy or immunosuppresant therapy for bone marrow transplantation, although this usually presents with disseminated disease rather than an isolated diarrheal illness [20].

Bloody diarrhea is often suggestive of enteroinvasive bacterial infection in the community population. In the oncology population, hematological and hemostatic abnormalities may increase the risk of bloody diarrhea even without mucosal invasive infection. In bone marrow transplantation, gastrointestinal infection with cytomegalovirus (CMV) may present with a diarrheal illness as a first sign. Finally, *Clostridium difficile* colitis presenting as diarrhea is common in the cancer population, especially in the setting of prolonged antibiotic therapy for febrile neutropenia.

In most cases of diarrheal illness, proper hydration is of primary concern. Empirical antimicrobial therapy is usually not recommended prior to a vigorous search for the etiology. In the oncology patient, empirical antibiotic therapy with enteric gram-negative and anerobic bacterial coverage may be indicated, especially in the setting of profound neutropenia following chemotherapy or significant immunosuppression following bone marrow transplantation. The initial workup should include a stool culture for enteric pathogens and a stool assay for *C. difficile* toxin. Although *C. difficile* infection was previously considered a risk only with a history of prolonged broad-spectrum antibiotic exposure, the incidence of community-acquired infection in patients with minimal to no antibiotic exposure also merits diagnostic consideration [21]. Examination of stool for ova and parasites is not indicated unless the patient has been in an endemic area or has persistent undiagnosed diarrhea.

In cases where stool studies have failed to arrive at a diagnosis, further diagnostic studies such as computed tomography and colonoscopy should be considered. In the BMT population, refractory diarrhea may be a harbinger of cytomegalovirus enteritis or graft-versus-host disease, which often may be distinguished only through visualization of the bowel lumen with acquisition of samples for histopathological examination. Antibiotic-associated diarrhea is a common diagnosis after other causes have been exluded. The musocal damage of the intestinal tract by chemotherapy can cause malabsorption and diarrhea from microvilli loss that can persist for weeks.

Clostridium Difficile Infections

An important cause of diarrheal illness and colitis in the oncological population is the toxin-mediated disease caused by *Clostridium difficile*. This was identified as a cause of pseudomembranous colitis associated with antibiotic use by Bartlett and associates in 1978 [22]. It is second only to *Clostridium perfringens* among anaerobes causing diarrhea, but more important to this discussion, it is the leading bacterial causative agent for nosocomial diarrhea [23].

Clostridium difficile causes disease primarily in patients whose gastrointestinal flora have been altered. The most common means of such alteration is broad-spectrum antibiotic exposure. Although agents such as 3d generation cephalosporins and clindamycin have previously been implicated as carrying increased risk of progression to *C. difficile* disease, all antimicrobial agents may be implicated in the disease. Antineoplastic therapy alone has also been linked to the development of *C. difficile* disease in the absence of antibiotic therapy [24,25].

Cancer patients, especially those undergoing therapy for hematological malignancy, carry many risks for the development of *C. difficile* disease. Common risk factors include prolonged antibiotic exposure (especially in neutropenic patients), antineoplastic therapy, and altered bowel motility through dietary and pharmacological means. Additionally, prolonged hospitalization may place patients at risk. *C. difficile* is transmissible from patient to patient either from common contact with health care workers or through environmental contact [25,26]. Thus an increased incidence of *C. difficile* in any hospital merits investigation and possible use of typing methods (serotyping, PCR fingerprinting) to rule out a common source outbreak that may mandate stricter infection control measures.

The spectrum of *C. difficile* disease extends from a mild diarrheal illness to pseudomembranous colitis (PMC). Pseudomembranous colitis is a severe illness characterized by abdominal pain and diarrhea. The hallmark of PMC is the finding of adherent raised white to yellow plaques (pseudomembranes), which may become confluent. Cytopathological damage may be so severe as to require colectomy in cases refractory to medical care. Still, the majority of *C. difficile* disease cases show a diarrheal illness of varying degrees.

The diagnosis of *C. difficile* disease is usually made through an analysis of stool for the presence of *C. difficile* toxins. Stool cultures have been used in the past with good correlation between isolation of organism and clinical disease in adults [27]. However in newborns, isolation of organism alone is not diagnostic, since as many as 70% of newborns harbor the organism for several months. For these reasons as well as the availability of rapid and reliable tests, *C. difficile* toxin assays are used most frequently. *Clostridium difficle* produces two toxins, A and B. Toxin A is an enterotoxin that produces local inflammation and is thought to be the etiology of symptomatic disease in most patients [28]. Toxin B is cytotoxic to colonic mucosal cells but is thought to be active only following tissue damage caused by toxin A. Most testing kits use enzymatic immunoassays to detect the presence of toxins A and B. Some assays detect only one of the two toxins. In most cases, both toxins are present in the setting of clinical disease; however, cases in which only a single toxin is elaborated have been described [29].

Both metronidazole and oral vancomycin are effective in the treatment of *C. difficile* disease of the GI tract. Standard initial therapy is a 10-day course of oral metronidazole, 500 mg three times a day. If patients are unable to take oral medications, intravenous metronidazole is recommended. Initial relapses are treated with a second course of metronidazole for 14 to 42 days [30].

The emergence of vancomycin-resistant enterococci as nosocomial pathogens has made oral vancomycin an alternative usually reserved for patients unresponsive to or unable to tolerate metronidazole. Enteric colonization with vancomycin-resistant enterococci is especially concerning in the neutropenic population, where gut flora are often implicated in later bacteremia and sepsis. When vancomycin is used for therapy for *C. difficile*, it is given as a 125 mg oral dose four times a day for 10 to 14 days. Intravenous vancomycin is not effective against *C. difficile*.

Cases of multiple relapses are usually due to an inability to rid the gut of *C. difficile* spores. In such cases, a long-term suppressive regimen is usually devised. Consideration of a regimen should take into account a patient's past responses. A patient who has responded to both metronidazole and vancomycin but who continues to relapse can be placed on a suppressive regimen using either agent. A patient who demonstrated no response to metronidazole but responded to vancomycin will require this as the suppressive agent. Suppressive regimens include vancomycin every other day and metronidazole at standard doses for alternating weeks. Varying degrees of success have been seen with the use of adjuvant agents such as lactobacillus and cholestyramine [30].

Diarrheal Illness Following Bone Marow Transplantation

Bone marrow transplantation (BMT) is increasingly common owing to its demonstrated success in the treatment of acute leukemias, aplastic anemia, and other hematological malignancies. This patient population is especially prone to gastrointestinal infection due to prolonged neutropenia from cytoablative chemotherapy, frequent broad-spectrum antibiotic exposure, and humoral and cellular immune deficiency until marrow engraftment is complete. Infecting agents include bacterial, fungal, and viral agents. Complicating the workup of diarrheal illness in this population are multiple noninfectious causes of diarrhea including drug toxicities and graft-versus-host disease (GVHD).

   Documented gastrointestinal infections have significant impact on survival in the bone marrow transplant population. Older studies report gastrointestinal infection rates of up to 40% with a predominance of infections caused by viral agents following bone marrow transplantation; mortality rates of 55% have been reported when any organism is isolated from the gastrointestinal tract and is implicated in clinical disease [31]. Among these common viral pathogens reported is CMV. The utility of ganciclovir as prophylaxis against CMV disease has been well documented, and its use has reduced the frequency of CMV infections following BMT [32,33]. A recent study by Cox et al. [34] at the Fred Hutchinson Cancer Research Center prospectively investigated the etiology of diarrhea in the bone marrow transplant population. This study found that most cases of diarrhea in which a cause could be found were attributable to GVHD (48%). Only 13% of diarrheal illness was associated with infection [34]. Despite such improvements, the high mortality attributed to gastrointestinal infections following BMT merits a vigorous search for infectious etiology, especially when targeted therapy offers a significant chance for recovery. Viral pathogens predominate in diarrheal infections following BMT. Among the viral pathogens implicated are astrovirus, adenovirus, rotavirus, coxsackievirus, and CMV—accounting for 65 to 80% of documented cases of infectious diarrhea following BMT. *Clostridium difficile* colitis accounts for the majority of other cases of infectious diarrhea in the BMT population, the management of which was discussed previously [31,34]. Other enteric bacterial pathogens are exceedingly rare following BMT, likely secondary to frequent exposure to broad-spectrum antibiotics.

CMV gastroenteritis remains an important diagnostic consideration in the BMT population. Although decreased in frequency secondary to the use of ganciclovir prophylaxis and now the routine use of serum CMV antigen or DNA detection systems, mortality from CMV disease may be as high as 85%, especially when CMV pneumonia is present [35]. Mortality from gastrointestinal CMV disease is approximately 40% [36]. Diagnosis and treatment of CMV disease limited to the GI tract reduces morbidity from esophagitis, gastritis, and enteritis and reduces viral excretion from systemic foci [37].

Diagnosis of CMV disease of the gastrointestinal tract usually requires multiple modalities. Clinical presentation of gastrointestinal CMV disease does not differ significantly from the presentation of noninfectious gastrointeritis, especially GVHD, in the BMT population. Primary symptoms and signs include greater than four stools/day, nausea, vomiting, and occult gastrointestinal bleeding. These symptoms are present in similar frequencies in medication-induced diarrhea and GVHD. Notably, GVHD itself is a risk factor for development of CMV disease with a relative risk of 1.8 [35]. A helpful clinical finding in GVHD is that gastrointestinal disease often parallels the presence and severity of skin and hepatic GVHD [38,39]. Gross GI bleeding is slightly more common in CMV gastroenteritis than in other causes of diarrhea in BMT patients, but it remains a rare presentation of the disease [34].

Laboratory methods for the diagnosis of CMV disease rely on the detection of virus in culture specimens, demonstration of CMV viral changes on histopathological specimens, and amplification methods such as PCR or in situ hybridization for CMV from either tissue or blood specimens [40]. Endoscopy is also important in the diagnosis of CMV disease in the BMT population. Endoscopy will usually reveal erythematous gastrointestinal mucosa in both CMV and GVHD, with mucosal ulceration possible in both diseases [41]. Biopsy of gastrointestinal mucosal is most helpful, allowing for examination for viral cytopathic effect in CMV disease and crypt cell necrosis and apoptosis in GVHD [42].

The gold standard of treatment for gastrointestinal CMV is intravenous ganciclovir. Standard dosing is 5 mg/kg every 12 hours. Although beneficial in CMV pneumonia, intravenous immunoglobulin has not been shown to improve outcomes in gastrointestinal limited CMV disease [36]. Treatment failures with ganciclovir can be managed with foscarnet, but its use is limited by significant renal toxicity. Although oral ganciclovir and valganciclovir are useful in CMV prophylaxis and for treatment of CMV infections at other sites (retinitis, viremia) in the BMT population, IV therapy should be the mainstay of therapy for gastrointestinal disease until absorption from the GI tract is judged reliable.

NEUTROPENIC ENTEROCOLITIS

Background

Neutropenic enterocolitis is a potentially life-threatening gastrointestinal infection. Although clinical definitions vary slightly, the disease is usually described as fever, diarrhea, abdominal pain, and distension in the setting of granulocytopenia [43]. Most commonly, neutropenic enterocolitis occurs in the setting of hematological malignancy and high-dose chemotherapy, but it has also been reported in patients with solid tumors receiving high-dose chemotherapy, especially in the setting of autologous stem cell transplantation [44]. Other clinical settings in which neutropenic enterocolitis has been described include solid organ transplantation, human immunodeficiency virus infection, cyclic neutropenia, and myelodysplastic syndrome [45–47].

Wagner and colleagues are usually credited with the initial definition of neutropenic enterocolitis in 1970. This initial description was of a focal necrotizing colitis of the cecum, complicating acute leukemia in children [48]. Interestingly, a similar pathological entity was described by Cooke in 1933 in her overview of the treatment of acute leukemia in children [49]. Subsequently, neutropenic enterocolitis has been described by terms including typhlitis [48], leukopenic enteropathy, and ileocecal syndrome [2]. Since its initial description, the number of reported cases has progressively increased, and cases in adults are common. Autopsy series place the incidence of neutropenic enterocolitis in leukemic patients at 12 to 46% [50].

Pathophysiology

The pathogenesis of neutropenic enterocolitis is best described for cases associated with high-dose cytotoxic chemotherapy. Agents especially associated with a clinical diagnosis of neutropenic enterocolitis include cytosine arabinoside (ARA-C), doxorubicin, and cyclophosphamide [43]. These agents contribute to neutropenic enterocolitis both through resultant mucositis and neutropenia. Mucositis, although it is usually diagnosed through visualization in the oral cavity, can affect mucosal surfaces of the entire gastrointestinal tract. Disruption of the bowel wall allows for a bacterial invasion that cannot be controlled in the setting of neutropenia. Invasive infection results in necrosis of the bowel wall to varying degrees including transmural necrosis. In

cases not associated with high-dose chemotherapy, it is presumed that local factors other than mucositis permit initial bacterial invasion.

Although this process may occur anywhere in the gastrointestinal tract, the disease most commonly affects the terminal ileum and cecum. Factors related to this predilection include relative stool stasis in the cecum, locally abundant bacteria and lymphoid associated tissue, and thin cecal mucosa [2]. Multiple bacterial species have been associated with neutropenic enterocolitis based on monobacterial blood culture isolates obtained during clinical disease. Among these, *Clostridium* species, especially *C. septicum*, are common. Gram-negative organisms including *Pseudomonas aeruginosa*, *E. coli*, *Klebsiella* sp., and *Enterobacter* sp. have been associated with neutropenic enterocolitis in multiple case series [2,51]. Gram-positive bacteria including *Staphylococcus aureus*, *Staphylococcus epidermidis*, *Enterococcus* sp., and fungal pathogens including *Candida* species and *Aspergillus* have also been implicated in neutropenic enterocolitis. Fungal pathogens likely play a greater role than would be predicted by blood culture isolates. Although one series found only 14% of neutropenic enterocolitis cases associated with a positive fungal blood culture, 53% of cases on postmortem examination demonstrated fungal invasion of the bowel wall at autopsy [51].

Diagnosis and Management

Gastrointestinal symptoms of any type in a febrile patient with neutropenia raise concern for the diagnosis of neutropenic enterocolitis. The clinical signs and symptoms of neutropenic enterocolitis include (in descending order of frequency) fever, diffuse abdominal pain, abdominal distension, diarrhea, vomiting, and nausea. Although the cecum and terminal ileum are often involved, right-sided abdominal pain is not a prerequisite for the diagnosis. Diffuse abdominal pain was up to four times more common than right lower quadrant pain in patients with a confirmed diagnosis of neutropenic enterocolitis in one case series [43].

The most important laboratory finding associated with neutropenic enterocolitis is an absolute neutrophil count <500/mL. The duration of neutropenia is also helpful. Almost three-fourths of patients in one series suffered neutropenia of greater than 1 week duration in association with neutropenic enterocolitis. The onset of gastrointestinal symptoms began on average at day 5 of neutropenia. Positive blood cultures are also strongly associated with neutropenic enterocolitis. Organisms of concern are described above. In one series, 71% of patients with neutropenic enterocolitis had positive blood cultures, 44% of these within 3 days of the onset of clinical disease [2].

Although previously considered a primarily surgical disease, medical therapy alone has been used with increased frequency in the treatment of neutropenic enterocolitis. Although traditional mortality rates for neutropenic enterocolitis were reported as high as 50 to 100%, a combined medical surgical approach to the disease has reduced overall mortality [52]. Several reviews have cited survival rates ranging from 60 to 95% with aggressive medical management of neutropenic enterocolitis [3,53]. Cornerstones of such medical therapy include aggressive hemodynamic support, fluid resuscitation, and broad-spectrum antimicrobial therapy including gram-negative and anaerobic coverage. Nadiminti et al. [2] reported a mortality rate of 15.4% for clinical neutropenic enterocolitis when anaerobic and gram-negative antibiotic coverage was present at the first sign of suspicious symptoms (abdominal pain bloating, diarrhea). In one series, aggressive medical care alone for neutropenic enterocolitis was continued unless patients developed persistent gastrointestinal bleeding, fluid retention, or vasopressor requirement; the overall mortality was 12% [52].

Abdominal plain radiographs and computed tomography scans are helpful in determining when surgical therapy may be preferred in neutropenic enterocolitis, or in confiring the diagnosis. In 85% of cases, plain radiographs will reveal only an ileus associated with the inflamed bowel [43]. The most important finding on a plain radiograph in neutropenic enterocolitis is pneumoperitoneum, a life-threatening complication usually secondary to perforation following transmural colonic necrosis [43]. Surgical therapy is urgently required. Such cases usually manifest with peritoneal signs on physical examination. In rare cases, bowel perforation is present in the absence of peritoneal signs because of medication effects or impaired neurological function due to underlying disease. Thus all abdominal pain in neutropenic patients, even in the absence of an acute abdomen, should be evaluated with abdominal radiographs.

Multiple reports have described the utility of computed tomography (CT) in the diagnosis and management on neutropenic enterocolitis [54,55]. CT scan findings in neutropenic enterocolitis include bowel wall thickening and edema, ascites, inflammatory masses, and abscesses and pneumatosis intestinalis [56,57]. CT imaging has its greatest utility in the management of indolent cases of neutropenic enterocolitis. In cases where optimal medical care, including broad-spectrum antibiotics, fails to result in clinical improvement, a CT scan may be helpful in revealing a drainable fluid collection, or it may reveal extensive bowel involvement that may best be treated with resection. Exploratory surgery should be reserved for those with marked clinical deterioration despite aggressive medical care in the absence of clear surgical indication by radiologic workup. A review of autopsy findings by Wade and colleagues finds than among 11 conservatively treated patients with clinical neutropenic enterocolitis who subsequently died, only four had pathological findings consistent with the diagnosis, and none demonstrated perforation or transmural necrosis [43]. Four of the 11 did have findings of systemic fungal infection, highlighting the multiple comorbidities found in patients with neutropenic enterocolitis, each of which must be managed optimally to improve survival.

REFERENCES

1. Skibber JM, Matter GJ, Pizzo PA, Lotze MT. Right lower quadrant pain in young patients with leukemia: a surgical perspective. Ann Surg 1987; 711–716.
2. Nadiminti U, Greene JN, Vincent AL, Sandin RL. Typhlitis in neutropenic patients: an analysis of thirty-nine patients in a cancer hospital. Infect Dis Clin Prac 2000; 9:153–158.
3. Sloas MM, Flynn PM, Kaste SC, Patrick CC. Typhlitis in children with cancer: a thirty year experience. Clin Infect Dis 1993; 17(3):484–490.
4. Starnes HF, Moore FD, Mentzer S, Osteen RT, Steele GD Jr, Wilson RE. Abdominal pain in neutropenic cancer patients. Cancer 1986; 57(3):616–621.
5. Silen W. Zachary Cope's Early Diagnosis of the Acute Abdomen. 16th ed. New York: Oxford, 1983.
6. Shiller GJ, Nimer SD, Gajewski JL, Golde DW. Abdominal presentation of varicella-zoster infection in recipients of allogeneic bone marrow transplantation. Bone Marrow Transplantation 1991; 7:489–491.
7. Nichols RL, Holmes JWC, Smith JW. Peritonitis. In: Gorbach SL, Bartlett JG, Blacklow NR, eds. Infectious Diseases. 2d ed. Philadelphia: W.B. Saunders, 1998: 800–810.
8. Sandven P, Qvist H, Skovlund E, Giercksky KE. Significance of candida recovered from intraoperative specimens with intra-abdominal perforations. Crit Care Med 2002; 30(3):541 547.
9. van den Hazel SJ, Speelman P, Tytgat GN, Dankert J, van Leeuwen DJ. Role of antibiotics in the treatment and prevention of acute and recurrent cholangitis. Clin Infect Dis 1994; 19(2):279–286.
10. Stellato TA, Shenk RR. Gastrointestinal emergencies in the oncology patient. Sem Oncology 1989; 16(6):521–531.
11. Bochud PY, Calandra T, Francioli P. Bacteremia due to viridans streptococci in neutropenic patients: a review. Am J Med 1994; 97:369.
12. Maenza JR, Merz WG. Candida albicans and related species. In: Gorbach SL, Bartlett JG, Blacklow NR, eds. Infectious Diseases. 2d ed. Philadelphia: W. B. Saunders, 1998:2313 2322.
13. Powderly WG. Mucosal candidiasis caused by non-albicans species of Candida in HIV-positive patients. AIDS 1992; 6:604.
14. Chavanet P, Lopez J, Grappin M. Cross-sectional study of the susceptibility of Candida isolates to antifungal drugs and in vitro–in vivo correlation in HIV-infected patients. AIDS 1994; 8:945.
15. Maenza JR, Keruly JC, Moore RD. Risk factors for fluconazole-resistant candidiasis in human immunodeficiency virus–infected patients. J Infect Dis 1996; 173:219.

16. Dominquez ER, Greene JN, Sandin RL. Capnocytophaga: a case series and review. Infect Med 1996; 13(3):165–166, 168, 236.

17. Walsh TJ, Belitsos NJ, Hamilton SR. Bacterial esophagitis in immunocompromised patients. Arch Intern Med 1986; 146:1345–1348.

18. Tanyuksel M, Gun H, Doganci L. Prevalence of *Cryptosporidium* sp. in patients with neoplasia and diarrhea. Scand J Infect Dis 1995; 27:69–70.

19. Siegel DL, Edelstein PH, Nachamkin I. Inappropriate testing for diarrheal diseases in the hospital. JAMA 1990; 263(7):979–982.

20. Bodey GP, Fainstein V. Infections of the gastrointestinal tract in the immunocompromised patient. Ann Rev Med 1986; 37:271–281.

21. Laing RB, Dykhuizen RS, Smith CC, Gould IW, Reid TM. Community-acquired toxigenic *Clostridium difficile* diarrhoea in the normoxaemic elderly who have received no antimicrobials: soft evidence for ischemic colitis? Scottish Med J 1996; 41(1):15–16.

22. Bartlett JG, Chang TW, Gurwith M, Gorbach SL, Onderdonk AB. Antibiotic-associated pseudomembranous colitis due to toxin-producing clostridia. N Engl J Med 1978; 298:531–534.

23. Willis AT. Historical aspects. In: Rolfe RD, Finegold SM, eds. *Clostridium difficile*: its role in intestinal disease. San Diego: University Press, 1988:15–28.

24. Anaud A, Glatt AE. *Clostridium difficile* infection associated with antineoplastic chemotherapy: a review. Clin Infect Dis 1993; 17:109–113.

25. Cudmore MA, Silva J Jr, Liepman MK, Kim KH. *Clostridium difficile* colitis associated with cancer chemotherapy. Arch Intern Med 1982; 142:333–335.

26. McFarland LV, Sramm WE. Review of *clostridium difficile*-associated diseases. Am J Infect Control 1986; 14:99–109.

27. Fekety R, Kim KH, Brown D. Epidemiology of antibiotic-associated colitis. Isolation of *Clostridium difficile* from the hospital environment. Am J Med 1981; 70:906–908.

28. Brazier JS. Role of the laboratory in investigation of *Clostridium difficile* diarrhea. Clin Infect Dis 1993; 16(suppl 4):S228–S233.

29. Markowitz JE, Brown KA, Mamula P, Drott HR, Piccoli DA, Baldassano RN. Failure of single-toxin assays to detect *clostridium difficile* infection in pediatric inflammatory bowel disease. Am J Gastroenterology 2001; 96(9):2688–2690.

30. Fekety R. Antibiotic-associated colitis. In: Mandell GL, Bennett JE, Dolin R, eds. Principles and Practice of Infectious Diseases. 4th ed. New York: Churchill Livingstone, 1995:978–986.

31. Yolken RH, Bishop CA, Townsend TR, Bolyard EA, Bartlett J, Santos SW, Saral R. Infectious gastroenteritis in bone-marrow transplant recipients. New Eng J Med 1982; 306(17):1009–1012.

32. Goodrich JM, Bowden RA, Fisher L, Keller C, Schoch G, Meyer JD. Ganciclovir prophylaxis to prevent cytomegalovirus disease after allogeneic marrow transplantation. Ann Intern Med 1993; 118:173–178.

33. Winston DJ, Chanrasekar PH, Lazarus HM, Goodman JL, Silber JL, Horowitz H, Shadduck RK, Rosenfeld CS, Ho WG, Islam MZ, Batoni K. Ganciclovir prophylaxis of cytomegalovirus infection and disease in allogeneic bone marrow

transplant recipients: results of a placebo-controlled, double blind trial. Ann Intern Med 1993; 118:179 184.

34. Cox GJ, Matsui SM, Lo RS, Hinds M, Bowden RA, Hackman RC, Meyer WG, Motomi M, Tarr PI, Oshiro LS, Ludert JE, Meyer JD, McDonald GB. Etiology and outcome of diarrhea after marrow transplantation: a prospective study. Gastroenterology 1994; 107:1398–1407.

35. Meyers JD, Flournoy N, Thomas ED. Risk factors for cytomegalovirus infection after human marrow transplantation. J Infect Dis 1986; 153(3):478–488.

36. Ljungman P, Cordonnier C, Einsele H, Bender-Gotze C, Bosi A, Dekker A, De la Camara R, Gmur J, Newland AC, Prentice HG, Robinson AJ, Rovira M, Rosler W, Veil D. Use of intravenous immunoglobulin in addition to antiviral therapy in the treatment of CMV disease in allogeneic bone marrow transplant patients. Bone Marrow Transplant 1998; 21(5):473–476.

37. Reed EC, Shepp DH, Dandliker PS, Meyers JD. Ganciclovir treatment of cytomegalovirus infection of the gastrointestinal tract after marrow transplantation. Bone Marrow Transplant 1988; 3(3):199–206.

38. McDonald GB, Shulman HM, Sullivan KM, Spencer GD. Intestinal and hepatic complications of human bone marrow transplantation. Part I. Gastroenterology 1986; 90:460–477.

39. Martin PJ, Schoch G, Fisher L, Byers V, Anasetti C, Appelbaum FR, Beatty PG, Doney K, McDonald GB, Sanders JE. A retrospective analysis of therapy for acute graft-versus-host disease: initial treatment. Blood 1990; 76:1464–1472.

40. Hackman RC, Wolford JL, Gleaves CA, Meyerson D, Beauchamp MD, Meyers JD, McDonald GB. Recognition and rapid diagnosis of upper gastrointestinal cytomegalovirus infection in marrow transplant recipients. A comparison of seven virologic methods. Transplantation 1994; 57(2):231–237.

41. Snover C, Weisdorf SA, Vercellotti GM, Rank B, Hutton S, McGlave P. A histopathologic study of gastric and small intestine graft-versus-host disease following allogeneic bone marrow transplantation. Hum Pathol 1985; 16:387–392.

42. Cox GJ, McDonald GB. Graft-versus-host disease of the intestine. Springer Semin Immunopatlol 1990; 12:283–299.

43. Wade DS, Nava HR, Douglas HO. Neutropenic enterocolitis: clinical diagnosis and treatment. Cancer 1992; 69(1):17–23.

44. Avigan D, Richardson P, Elias A, Demetri G, Shapiro M, Schnipper L, Wheeler C. Neutropenic enterocolitis as a complication of high dose chemotherapy with stem cell rescue in patients with solid tumors. Cancer 1998; 83(3):409–414.

45. Mullholland MW, Delany JP. Neutropenic enterocolitis and aplastic anemia. Ann Surg 1983; 197:84–90.

46. Sra JS, Owens MR. Typhlitis occurring in myelodysplastic syndrome. NY State J Med 1989; 2:89–90.

47. Geelhoed GW, Kane MA, Dale DC, Wells SA. Colon ulceration and perforation in cyclic neutropenia. J Pediatr Surg 1973; 8:379–382.

48. Wagner ML, Rosenberg HS, Ferbach DL, Singleton ED. Typhlitis: a complication of leukemia in childhood. AJR Am J Roetgenol 1970; 109:341.

49. Cooke JV. Acute leukemia in children. JAMA 1933; 101:432–435.
50. Steinberg D, Gold J, Brodin A. Necrotizing enterocolitis in leukemia. Arch Intern Med 1973; 131:538–544.
51. Katz JA, Wagner ML, Gresik MV, Mahoney DH Jr, Fernbach D. Typhlitis: an 18-year experience and postmortem review. Cancer 1990; 65(4):1041–1047.
52. Shamberger RC, Weinstein HJ, Delony MJ, Levy RH. The medical and surgical management of typhlitis in children with acute non-lymphocytic (myelogenous) leukemia. Cancer 1986; 57:603–609.
53. Starnes HF, Moore FD, Mentzer S, Osteen RT, Steele GD Jr, Wilson RE. Abdominal pain in neutropenic cancer patients. Cancer 1986; 57(3):616–621.
54. Keidan RD, Fanning J, Gatenby RA, Weese JL. Recurrent typhlitis, a disease resulting from aggressive chemotherapy. Dis Colon Rectum 1989; 32:206–209.
55. Vas WG, Seelig R, Mahanta B. Neutropenic colitis: evaluation with computed tomography. J Comput Tomogr 1988; 12:211–215.
56. Gootenberg JE, Abbondanzo AL. Rapid diagnosis of neutropenic enterocolitis (typhlitis) by ultrasonography. Am J Pediatr Hematol Oncol 1987; 9(3):222–227.
57. Merine D, Nussbaum AR, Fishman ED, Sanders RC. Sonographic observations in a patient with typhlitis. Clin Pediatr 1989; 28(8):377–379.

28

Genitourinary Infections in Cancer Patients

Michael J. Tan
University of South Florida School of Medicine
Tampa, Florida, U.S.A.

John N. Greene
University of South Florida School of Medicine
and Moffitt Cancer Center and Research Institute
Tampa, Florida, U.S.A.

OVERVIEW

There are numerous causes of infection of the genitourinary tract in cancer patients. Hematological abnormalities, chemotherapy, and compromise of anatomical barriers increase the susceptibility to infection. Although the pathogens are similar to those of the immunocompetent host, infections generally are more frequent and more severe. One study focusing on epidemiology of bacteremia in neutropenic patients showed a urinary tract focus in 25% of patients[1].

URINARY TRACT INFECTION

Urinary tract infections (UTI) occur when normal defence barriers are altered. These include normal perineal flora, loss of micturition ability, and the presence of indwelling devices such as Foley catheters and ureteral stents that often introduce colonizing flora [2]. The presence of an indwelling urinary catheter increases the risk of bacteriuria 5 to 10% for each day of catheterization [3]. The most common organisms responsible for these infections are *Escherichia coli, Pseudomonas aeruginosa, Serratia marcessans, Staphylococcus aureus,* and *Candida albicans* [4,5]. Systemic antibiotics that alter the normal genitourinary flora may lead to overgrowth of hospital-acquired and often resistant bacteria such as *P. aeruginosa* and *C. albicans* [6]. In most cases of bladder colonization with *C. albicans* or other yeast due to the presence of an indwelling catheter, removal of the catheter is usually sufficient to relieve colonization and symptoms. In some cases, however, fungus balls may develop in the bladder or renal pelvis leading to persistent funguria.

The presence of neoplasm within or impinging upon the GU tract may lead to urinary retention, hydronephrosis, pyelonephritis, and bacteremia. Such obstructions may cause persistent infections with the above-mentioned organisms or some less common genitourinary organisms. Clostridial infection has been documented with renal cell carcinoma [7,8]. Appell et al. in 1979 demonstrated a high incidence of bacteriuria in patients undergoing transurethral resection of bladder tumor as compared with transurethral resection of the prostate and cystoscopy [9]. They also demonstrated a correlation between the organisms recovered from the urine and the organisms recovered from the tumor tissue sample [9]. Similarly, a renal cell carcinoma has also been documented to harbor organisms as a source of recurrent UTI with *P. aeruginosa* [10]. One patient with transitional cell carcinoma presented with hemorrhagic cystitis and *N. gonorrhea* [11]. Renal abscesses associated with *Salmonella* have also been documented [12]. Urinary tract infection was also demonstrated to be more common in patients with cervical carcinoma and undergoing external pelvic radiotherapy. In this study, the most common organisms were *E. coli* and *Enterococcus* spp [13]. One patient with breast cancer metastatic to the ureter has been described with recurrent UTI with *E. coli* [14]. Treatment of UTI in cancer patients is similar to that of normal hosts, therapy being directed toward symptoms, pathogen, and pyuria. The duration of treatment may be longer since a cancer degree indicates a complicated UTI. However, antimicrobial treatment should be given to the neutropenic patient with asymptomatic bacteriuria because of the high risk of subsequent bacteremia. In addition to bladder and kidney infection, secondary bacterial prostatitis and epididymitis can occur as urethral and bladder pathogens pass through the vas deferens and prostatic ducts, and culture of the pathogens may be difficult [15,16].

URINARY STENT–RELATED INFECTIONS

Many patients with local pelvicoabdominal or metastatic cancer will develop hydronephrosis or renal failure. Placement of urinary stent frequently will relieve the obstruction and preserve renal function for a time. The presence of a urinary stent, whether internal or external, increases the risk of infection, especially pyelonephritis. Obstruction and the presence of a foreign body are key factors that lead to subsequent infectious complications. An external ureter catheter, such as a Foley urethral catheter, over time will become colonized with microorganisms. When infections occur with the former, they tend to be more complicated because the kidney is directly involved. At first the pathogens are mostly E. coli and coagulase-negative Staphylococci. Later more resistant gram-negative bacilli such as *P. aeruginosa*, *Enterococcus* species, *S. aureus*, and *Candida* species predominate [17]. Cure usually requires prolonged antimicrobials and exchange of the catheter. In fact regular changing of the external ureter catheter every 21 to 28 days may prevent the development of infection.

BLADDER CONDUIT–RELATED INFECTIONS

Bladder revisions are usually required for progressive bladder cancer or metastatic disease involving the bladder. These urinary pouches, usually fashioned from ileum, can develop chronic colonization and subsequent infection. Pyelonephritis, intra-abdominal abscess, and urosepsis are possible complications [18]. If recurrent symptomatic infections develop related to the bladder conduit, chronic suppressive antibiotics may be required. The organisms isolated include all the ones mentioned above under urinary stent-related infections.

HEMORRHAGIC CYSTITIS

Hemorrhagic cystitis (HC) is a not uncommon cause of hematuria in cancer patients. In bone marrow transplant (BMT) patients, viral etiologies have been implicated. Adenovirus type 11 hemorrhagic cystitis has been reported in healthy children [19,20]. It is a rare cause of HC in bone marrow transplant patients [21]. BK virus has been more strongly implicated as a cause of HC in the setting of bone marrow transplantation. In BMT patients treated with cyclophosphamide, Bedi et al. [22] demonstrated hemorrhagic cystitis in half of the patients who had persistent BK viral shedding. Patients that did not shed BK virus did not have hemorrhagic cystitis. Because not all patients with BK viruria have hemorrhagic cystitis, and because it tends to be a late complication, it has been postulated that healthy T lymphocytes are required for damage of the bladder epithelium [22]. At present, there is no standard medical therapy other than reducing immunosuppressive therapy, such as corticosteroids or cyclosporine A.

XANTHOGRANULOMATOUS DISEASE

Granuloma formation can occur in situations of chronic inflammation or infection. With routine imaging, granulomas can be misinterpreted as malignancy. Xanthogranulomatous pyelonephritis (XP) is frequently mistaken for renal cell carcinoma until nephrectomy reveals the true etiology. Few cases of XP associated with a malignancy are reported. Goulding and Moser reported a patient with renal cell carcinoma with concurrent xanthogranulomatous pyelonephritis and persistent *Proteus mirabilis* UTI [23].

INTRAVESICULAR BCG

The use of intravesical bacillus Calmette–Guerin (BCG) therapy for transitional cell carcinoma can lead to granuloma formation throughout the genitourinary tract and its associated structures. Extravesicular granulomas are less common. The renal parenchyma has been involved in a number of cases, and the suggested mechanism is through hematogenous spread, traumatic instillation or injection, or through vesicoureteral reflux [24,25]. Tuberculous iliac lymphadenitis has been described [26]. Truelson et al. described two cases of epididymoorchitis associated with intravesical BCG [27]. Abscesses have also been reported in the prostate and prevesical and inguinal regions [28,29]. All of the cases of granuloma and abscess secondary to BCG instillation were treated with multidrug antituberculous therapy. Fever has also been associated with BCG instillation; however, it has not necessarily been correlated with the presence of infection [30].

SUMMARY

Changes of host defense mechanisms by way of neutropenia, radiation therapy, chemotherapy, and compromise of anatomic barriers are the primary means that cancer patients develop urinary tract infections. Because of these changes, infections caused by common community-acquired and hospital-acquired organisms are most frequently encountered. Special consideration should be given to unusual presentations of common organisms when obstruction or a foreign body is present.

REFERENCES

1. Siegman-Igra T, Schwartz D, Gonen I, Konforti N. Bacteremic infections in granulopenic patients in Israel. Isr J Med Sci 1987; 23:1214–1216.
2. Korzeniowski OM. Urinary tract infection in the impaired host. Med Clin North Am 1991; 75:391–404.

3. Stamm WB. Nosocomial infections: etiologic changes, therapeutic challenges. Hosp Pract 1981; 16:75–78.
4. Fierer J. Acute pyelonephritis. Urol Clin North Am 1987; 14:251–256.
5. Armstrong D. Infectious complications of neoplastic disease: their diagnosis and management—part II. Clinical Bull 1977; 7:13–20.
6. Russo P. Urologic emergencies in the cancer patient. Seminar in Oncology 2000; 27:284–298.
7. Graham BS, Johnson AC, Sawyers JL. Clostridial infection of renal cell carcinoma. J Urol 1986; 135:354–355.
8. Bogucki MS, August DA, Andriole VT. Clostridial infection of a locally recurrent renal cell carcinoma with sepsis. Cancer 1990; 66:601–603.
9. Appell RA, Flynn JT, Paris AM, Blandy JP. Occult bacterial colonization of bladder tumors. J Urol 1980; 124:345–346.
10. Boustead GB, Beard RC, Liston TL, Wright ED. Renal cell carcinoma as a source of recurrent urinary tract infections. Br J Urol 1995; 76:670.
11. Blackwell AL, Barrow J. Carcinoma of the bladder presenting as gonococcal cystitis. Br J Vener Dis 1980; 56:105–106.
12. Olson ES, Asmussen T, Vicca AF, Osborn DE. A case report of renal abscess caused by *Salmonella virchow* phage type 1 associated with a papillary renal cell carcinoma. J Infect 1999; 38:56–57.
13. Prasad KN, Pradhan S, Datta NR. Urinary tract infection in patients of gynecological malignancies undergoing external pelvic radiotherapy. Gynecol Oncol 1995; 57:380–382.
14. Lopez-Martinez RA, Stock JA, Gump FE, Rosen JS. Carcinoma of the breast metastatic to the ureter presenting with flank pain and recurrent urinary tract infection. Am Surg 1996; 62:748–752.
15. Berger RE. Acute epididymitis: etiology and therapy. Semin Urol 1991; 9:28–31.
16. Pfau A. Prostatitis: a continuing enigma. Urol Clin North Am 1986; 13:695–715.
17. Farsi HM, Mosli HA, Al-Zemaity MF, Bahnassy AA, Alvarez M. Bacteriuria and colonization of double-pigtail ureteral stents: long-term experience with 237 patients. J Endo Urol 1995; 9:469–472.
18. Doehn C, Bohle A, Jocham D. Intra-abdominal abscess due to patient noncompliance after construction of an ileal neobladder: case report and review of the literature. Int J Urol 1999; 6:264–267.
19. Numazaki Y, Shigeta S, Kumaska T, et al. Acute hemorrhagic cystitis in children: isolation of adenovirus type 11. N Engl J Med 1968; 278:700–704.
20. Mufson MA, Belshe RB. A review of adenoviruses in the etiology of cute hemorrhagic cystitis. J Urol 1976; 115:191–194.
21. Ambinder RF, Burns W, Forman M, et al. Hemorrhagic cystitis associated with adenovirus infection in bone marrow transplantation. Arch Intern Med 1986; 146:1400–1401.
22. Bedi A, Miller CB, Hanson JL, et al. Association of BK virus with failure of prophylaxis against hemorrhagic cystitis following bone marrow transplantation. J Clin Oncol 1995; 13:1103–1109.

23. Goulding FJ, Moser A. Xanthogranulomatous pyelonephritis with associated renal cell carcinoma. Urology 1984; 23:385–386.
24. Stanisic TH, Brewer ML, Graham AR. Intravesical bacillus Calmette–Guerin therapy and associated granulomatous renal masses. J Urol 1986; 135:256–258.
25. Kondratowicz GM. BCG pyelonephritis following intravesical BCG. Br J Urol 1989; 64:649.
26. Ali-El Dein B, Nabeeh A. Tuberculous iliac lymphadenitis: a rare complication of intravesical bacillus Calmette–Guerin and cause of tumor over staging. J Urol 1996; 156:1766–1767.
27. Truelson T, Wishnow KI, Johnson DE. Epididymo-orchitis developing as a late manifestation of intravesical bacillus Calmette–Guerin therapy and masquerading as a primary testicular malignancy: a report of 2 cases. J Urol 1992; 148:1534–1535.
28. Matlaga BR, Veys JA, Thacker CC, Assimos DG. Prostate abscess following intravesical bacillus Calmette–Guerin treatment. J Urol 2002; 167:251.
29. Martinez-Caceres P, Rubio-Briones J, Palou J, Salvador J, Vicente J. Prevesical and inguinal abscess following intravesical BCG instillation. Scan J Urol Nehrol 1998; 32:409–410.
30. Schnapp DS, Weiss GH, Smith AD. Fever following intracavitary bacillus Calmette–Guerin therapy for upper tract transitional cell carcinoma. J Urol 1996; 156:386–388.

29

Bone, Joint, and Soft Tissue Infections in Cancer Patients

Lucinda M. Elko
University of South Florida School of Medicine
Tampa, Florida, U.S.A.

INTRODUCTION

Certain cancers or their treatment can predispose a patient to bone, joint, and soft tissue infections. In patients with cancer the differential diagnosis should include opportunistic pathogens. Regarding soft tissue infections, many cases of gangrene have been reported in the literature. Most reports discuss vascular insufficiency rather than an infectious process in the oncological patient. Therefore gangrene will not be discussed in this chapter.

OSTEOMYELITIS

Osteomyelitis is infection of bone. Infection can occur by hematogenous spread, direct inoculation, and spread from contiguous sites. The presentation is usually insidious. There is pain over the affected site, fever, edema, and possibly overlying cellulitis. When the infection is chronic, sinus tracts may form and drainage may occur. In reference to cancer, chronic osteomyelitis predisposes to the development of squamous cell carcinoma in the fistulous tract. The prevalence of malignant lesions arising in chronic osteomyelitis has been reported between 0.2 to 1.6% with a predilection for male patients and the lower extremities [1]. Symptoms indicating malignant transformation include increased pain, foul discharge, and hemorrhage. Other more rare cancers attributed to chronic osteomyelitis include fibrosarcoma, multiple myeloma, and lymphoma [1]. Though these cancers are usually low grade, it is important to note that aggressive therapy with limb resection/amputation is offered as the most reliable means of treating both the tumor and the chronic infection [1].

In turn, specific cancers or treatments may increase the risk of osteomyelitis. The main sites of infection include the symphysis pubis, the vertebrae, the mandible, and the sternum. The main standards of care include tissue biopsy, intravenous antibiotic therapy, and resection of necrotic bone if possible. *Mycobacterium*, especially bacillus Calmette–Guerin, can cause vertebral infections as well as infections of prior hardware in cancer patients.

There are many case reports of patients presenting with postradiotherapy osteomyelitis of the symphysis pubis. The predisposing cancers include bladder, gynecological, and prostate cancer. The onset is typically a few years after the radiotherapy has been completed. The patients presented with fistula, pain, or small bowel obstruction [2]. The organisms most commonly responsible are bowel organisms such as *Bacteroides*, *Enterococci*, and enteric gram-negative bacilli [2]. Radiographic clues to infection include a long time interval between original radiotherapy and onset of osteomyelitis, the coexistence of lytic and sclerotic bony changes, and the presence of gas within the symphysis pubis and/or an intestinal fistula [2].

Vertebral osteomyelitis can be caused by many organism classes including *Stapylococcus Streptococcus*, anaerobic bacteria, and *Mycobacteria*. Vertebral osteomyelitis can present with back pain and fever. The lumbar vertebrae are involved most frequently in hematogenous vertebral osteomyelitis, followed by the thoracic region [3]. Less commonly, patients may develop spinal cord compression, nerve root compression, or paravertebral abscesses [3]. Pockets of gas in an abscess indicate likely anaerobic growth or gas producing gram-negative aerobes such as *E. coli* or *Klebsiella* [3]. The association between *Streptococcus bovis* endocarditis and vertebral ostemyelitis is well known for its association with colon carcinoma [4]. There have also been case reports of atypical *Mycobacteria* and tuberculosis causing osteomyelitis in cancer patients.

Oral infections in cancer patients can be caused by almost any organism found in the mouth as normal oral flora. The most common are alpha hemolytic *Streptococci*, *Staphylococcus aureus*, enteric gram-negative bacilli, Prevotella, and Peptostreptococcus. In addition, several unusual organisms such as *Candida*, *Aspergillus*, *Saccharomyces*, and *Actinomyces* can cause opportunistic periodontal infections in immunosuppressed patients [5]. Patients may present with local swelling and pain in the facial region and gingivitis. Teeth may be spontaneously lost. Osteonecrosis of the mandible with subsequent mandibular osteomyelitis caused by oral flora shows the most common site for radiation-induced osteomyelitis.

Sternal osteomyelitis can also occur. One case report discusses a patient with a history of previously treated Hodgkin's disease complicated by aspergillus requiring pneumonectomy [6]. The patient presented 8 years later with night sweats, fever, general malaise, and pain in the region of the left clavicle and sternum. A technetium-99 scan had focally increased uptake in the region of the right sternoclavicular joint. Upon diagnositic biopsy, overlying necrotic bone and purulent material were removed. Cultures eventually grew *Aspergillus fumigatus* [6]. Most cases of sternal osteomyelitis are related to trauma or surgery. This case illustrates spread from a contiguous focus. Another case of sternal osteomyelitis due to *Aspergillus* developed as a primary focus with no contiguous or distant site of infection in an elderly man with chronic lymphocytic leukemia receiving chemotherapy and corticosteroids [7].

Bacillus Calmette–Guerin (BCG), an attenuated form of *Mycobacterium bovis*, is commonly used as an immunomodulator to treat transitional cell carcinoma of the bladder. One of the main side effects of BCG treatment is a reactive arthritis which occurs 1 to 5 months after therapy, especially in patients who are HLA-B27 positive [8]. The patients will suffer from a symmetrical small joint polyarthritis associated with a negative rheumatoid factor. BCG immunotherapy may also cause osteomyelitis. One case report documents spinal osteomyelitis affecting a 75-year-old man 2.5 years after intravesicular BCG administration for bladder cancer. MRI revealed destruction of the vertebral body of L3 with paraspinal soft-tissue mass extending to the left psoas muscle [9]. Biopsy of the mass proved to be *M. bovis*. The authors noted that osteoporotic compression fractures of the spine might have contributed to the development of vertebral osteomyelitis. A second case report documents a patient with remote placement of a total right hip replacement who developed osteolytic and osteoblastic radiographic changes 20 months after receiving intravesicular BCG for papillary transitional cell bladder CIS [10]. Histopathology of the right femur revealed noncaseating granulomas, and two AFB cultures yielded *M. bovis*.

SEPTIC ARTHRITIS

Septic arthritis can be a presentation of cancer as well as a complication of cancer chemotherapy. Clinical clues to the diagnosis include monoarticular joint pain, fever, joint swelling/effusions with erythema and warmth, normal to increased leukocytes, and increased sedimentation rate. Blood cultures are positive in one-third of patients. All septic arthritis cases should be treated with intravenous antibiotics as well as repeated joint aspirations and orthopedic surgery as appropriate.

Patients receiving stem cell transplantation (SCT) and those with multiple myeloma are at increased risk for septic arthritis. Recipients of SCT are susceptible to infections with encapsulated organisms commonly occurring later than 6 months after SCT. A case report documents a 15-year-old male 23 months following SCT for chronic myelogenous leukemia presented with *S. pneumoniae* pneumonia. One year later, septic arthritis of the left knee due to *S. pneumoniae* developed. Biotypes were not determined for the two organisms, but both isolates of *S. pneumoniae* had the same susceptibility pattern [11]. Bacteremia is frequent in multiple myeloma secondary to defective antibody production. Common causes of bacteremia in myeloma patients include *S. pneumoniae, S. aureus, E. coli, Klebsiella, Pseudomonas* and *H. influenzae* [12]. Strep pneumoniae and *H. influenzae* tend to occur within 8 months of myeloma diagnosis. Infections with other gram-negative bacilli typically occur in patients with refractory, advancing disease [12]. Rarely, septic arthritis can develop during the episode of bacteremia.

Rarely, fungal pathogens such as *Candida* species can cause septic arthritis in neutropenic patients. Septic arthritis caused by *Candida* species is unusual in patients who are not intravenous drug injectors. Transient candidemia in immunocompromised patients can result in seeding of a joint. One report presents an elderly woman with acute myelogenous leukemia who presented with increased sedimentation rate, fever, and knee pain at the end of a period of neutropenia. A gallium scan was positive for knee inflammation. Arthrocentesis cultures grew *Candida tropicalis* [13].

Lastly, the group G streptococci are facultative anaerobes that cause infections similar to group A streptococci and can manifest as septic arthritis. The malignancies that have been associated with group G streptococci include oropharyngeal, cervical, breast, colonic, and hematological cancers [4].

Sternoclavicular joint (SCJ) septic arthritis is a rare infection that has been described in healthy adults and immunocompromised individuals. It accounts for 1 to 9% of septic arthritis [14]. The isolated organisms are frequently related to bacteremic complications of intravenous access devices or intravenous drug abusers. The SJC is a common site for hematogenous dissemination because the subclavian vein lies just behind the SCJ. Seeding of the SCJ can readily occur if a central venous catheter or intravenous drug injection into the jugular vein produces a high concentration of bacteria in the subclavian vein. In cancer patients, *S. aureus*, Group B *Streptococcus, P. aeruginosa*, and Fusobacterium are common organisms [14].

NECROTIZING FASCIITIS

Necrotizing fasciitis can occur in normal hosts as well as oncology patients. The presentation is similar in both with severe pain, subcutaneous crepitus, fever, leukocytosis, hyperesthesia, with progression to anesthesia. Cases can be divided into two types: monomicrobial with *Streptococcus pyogenes* (group A streptococcus) as the primary pathogen or polymicrobial with mixed bacterial flora. Necrotizing fasciitis can occur after surgical procedures, and if it occurs within 48 hours postprocedure, it is more likely secondary to a single organism [15]. There is a case report in which a patient underwent resection of a superficial spreading melanoma is same-day surgery center. Two days after discharge, the patient presented with malaise, nausea, emesis, erythema, and pain at the surgical site. The excision site was leaking seropurulent fluid. A wound swab grew Group A streptococcus. Despite aggressive support, the patient expired. At autopsy there was no evidence of metastatic spread of the melanoma [15].

Necrotizing fasciitis can also be caused by bacteria other than the usual two types mentioned above in neutropenic patients such as gram negative bacilli (especially *Pseudomona aeruginosa*). It is well known that neutropenic fever is commonly related to gram-negative organisms such as *Pseudomonas*. A case report of a previously healthy young girl presented with a 2 day history of right labium edema, diffuse tenderness, and hyperesthesia. One day after admission, the patient had blood cultures positive for *Pseudomonas aeruginosa*. Incision, drainage, and fasciotomy were completed in addition to IV antibiotics. The wound cultures from surgery also grew *Pseudomonas aeruginosa*. No other organisms were identified [16]. The young girl was also diagnosed with acute lymphocytic leukemia during the hospital admission.

PYOMYOSITIS

Pyomyositis is an infection of skeletal muscle that is usually caused by *Staphylococcus aureus*. The quadriceps femoris and gluteus maximus are the muscles most commonly involved. The largest risk groups include children and young adults living n the tropics and patients with AIDS. Minor exercise or local trauma may precede the infection. Unusual organisms may cause pyomyositis in immunosuppressed cancer patients. Matsuno et al. cite the third case of pyomyositis occurring in patients with multiple myeloma [17]. *Bacteroides fragilis* pyomyositis developed in an elderly woman with multiple myeloma following chemotherapy. Successful treatment consisted of surgical incision and drainage and antibiotic therapy.

Muscle infection in patients with neutropenia can develop when bacteremia or fungemia seeds the muscle diffusely or to focal areas. The most common fungal cause of myalgia or myositis is *Candida tropicalis*. Diffuse muscle involvement occurs without the need for surgical intervention. Prolonged combination antifungal therapy and central venous catheter removal is necessary for cure. Bacterial causes of myositis include enteric gram-negative bacilli, *S. aureus*, and *Clostridia* species. If gas is present in the muscle during the period of neutropenia, *Clostridium septicum* is the most common cause. Usually, neutropenic enterocolitis (typhlitis) is the primary focus of infection. Other pathogens that can produce gas in the muscle are *Klebsiella* species and *E. coli*, usually associated with bacteremia and neutropenia. Prompt surgical incision and debridement along with appropriate antibiotics is necessary for cure.

CONCLUSION

Many infections of the bones, joints, and soft tissues can occur in cancer patients. In addition to the usual pathogens, one must consider specific infections that are unique to immunocompromised patients. These infections primarily occur during periods of neutropenia or other forms of immunodeficiency. Recognizing these vulnerable periods for infection may lead to more rapid diagnosis and intervention and possibly prevention.

REFERENCES

1. McGrory JE, Pritchard DJ, Unni KK, et al. Malignant lesions arising in chronic osteomyelitis. Clin Orthopaedics Rel Res 1999; 362:181–189.
2. Wignall TA, Carrington BM, Logue JP. Post-radiotherapy osteomyelitis of the symphysis pubis: computed tomographic features. Clin Radiol 1998; 53:126–130.
3. Bilgrami S, Pesant EL, Singh NT, et al. Spinal cord compression due to anaerobic vertebral osteomyelitis in a patient with metastatic prostate cancer. Clin Inf Dis 1995; 21:457–458.
4. Marinella MA. Streptococcus bovis endocarditis and vertebral osteomyelitis. Heart Lung 1996; 25(5):422.
5. Hovi L, Saarinen UM, Donner U, et al. Opportunistic osteomyeltitis in the jaws of children on immunosuppressive chemotherapy. J Ped Hematal Onc 1996; 18(1):90–94.
6. Allen D, Ng S, Beaton K, et al. Sternal osteomyelitis caused by Apergillus fumigatus in a patient with previously treated Hodgkin's disease. J Clin Path 2002; 55:616–618.
7. Baez-Escudero JL, Greene JN, Sandin RL. Primary sternal Aspergillus osteomyelitis. Infect Med 2000; 17:505–516.
8. Jawad ASM, Kahn L, Copland RFP, et al. Reactive arthritis associated with

Bacillus Calmette–Guerin immunotherapy for carcinoma of the bladder: a report of two cases. Brit J Rheumatol 1993; 32:1018–1020.

9. Aljada IS, Crane JK, Corriere N, et al. Mycobacterium bovis BCG causing vertebral osteomyelitis (Pott's disease) following intravesical BCG therapy. J Clin Microbiol 1999; 37(6):2106–2108.

10. Guerra CE, Betts RF, O'Keefe RG, et al. Mycobacterium bovis osteomyelitis involving a hip arthroplasty after intravesicular Bacille Calmette–Guerin for bladder cancer. Clin Infect Dis 1998; 27:639–640.

11. Schwella N, Schwerdtfeger R, Schmidt-Wolf I. Pneumococcal arthritis after allogeneic bone marrow transplantation. BMT 1993; 12:165–166.

12. Berthaud V, Milder J, El-Sadr W. Multiple myeloma presenting with Hemophilus influenzae septic arthritis: case report and review of the literature. J Nat Med Assoc 1993; 85(8):626–628.

13. Weers-Pothoff G, Havermans JF, Kamphuis J, et al. Candida tropicalis arthritis in a patient with acute myeloid leukemia successfully treated with fluconazole: case report and review of the literature. Infection 1997; 25(2):109–111.

14. Mbaga II, Greene JN, Sandin Ramon L. Sternoclavicular joint septic arthritis. Cancr Cont 1998; 5(3):260–263.

15. Gibbon KL, Bewley AP. Acquired streptococcal necrotizing fasciitis following excision of malignant melanoma. Br Assoc Dermatol 1999; 141:717–719.

16. Jaing T, Huang C, Chiu C, et al. Surgical implications of *Pseudomonas aeruginosa* necrotizing fasciitis in a child with acute lymphoblastic leukemia. J Ped Surg 2001; 36(6):948–950.

17. Matsuno O, Matsumoto T, Miyazaki E, Nakogawa H, Kumamoto T, Tsuda T. Pyomyositis associated with Bacteroides fragilis in a patient with multiple myeloma. Am J Trop Med Hyg 1998; 58:42–44.

30

Dermatological Infections in Cancer Patients

Mary Evers

UHHS-Richmond Heights Hospital
Cleveland, Ohio, U.S.A.

John N. Greene

University of South Florida School of Medicine
and Moffitt Cancer Center and Research Institute
Tampa, Florida, U.S.A.

INTRODUCTION

Cutaneous infections are not uncommon in the immunocompromised patient with cancer. The risk of infection may be due to the underlying malignancy, the therapy administered, the presence of other comorbid conditions such as diabetes, or a combination of these factors. Prolonged neutropenia and a sudden reduction in the absolute neutrophil count dramatically increases the frequency of infection. The presence of an intravascular catheter can also predispose the cancer patient to infection.

A variety of pathogens are responsible for causing cutaneous infection in patients with cancer. While our list is not all-inclusive, the more common bacterial, fungal, and viral infections seen in the immunocompromised patient will be discussed. Impaired host defenses can result in a modified clinical presentation and course. Skin lesions may result from a localized infection or be manifestations of disseminated disease. The rich blood supply of the skin provides an opportunity for metastatic spread of infection from the skin and also to the skin from other sources. Early diagnosis of disseminated cutaneous lesions may identify a silent systemic infection. Prompt recognition and treatment of cutaneous infections are crucial in reducing morbidity and mortality in cancer patients.

BACTERIA

Pseudomonas Aeruginosa

With the advent of routine prophylactic antimicrobial therapy, infections caused by *P. aeruginosa* have been declining since the 1970s in patients with cancer [1,2]. Currently, *P. aeruginosa* accounts for 5 to 10% of all bacteremia in patients with neutropenia [2]. Colonization can lead to pneumonia, typhlitis (neutropenic enterocolitis), and perineal cellulitis. Other sites of infection include the urinary tract, the skin and soft tissue, and central venous catheters [2]. Immunocompromised patients, especially neutropenics, are at greatest risk of pseudomonal infection.

Cutaneous pseudomonal infection can occur from a primary skin source or secondary to bacteremia. Manifestations of primary skin lesions include folliculitis, cellulitis, bullae, pustules, nodules, and abcesses. The pathognomonic lesion of *P. aeruginosa* septicemia is ecthyma gangrenosum (EG), seen in 30% of cases [1]. Classic EG presents as erythema, progressing to macules, nodules, and hemorrhagic bullae. Ulceration and central necrosis of the lesion follows. EG usually presents on the extremities and anogenital and axillary regions [3]. EG has also been reported in patients without clinically detectable pseudomonal bacteremia [4]. Other pathogens reported to cause EG or EG-like lesions include *Aeromonas, Serratia, Stenotrophomonas, Candida, Capnocytophaga, Aspergillus*, and *Escherichia coli* [4,5]. Conditions that mimic the other cutaneous manifestations of *P. aeurginosa* include candidiasis, aspergillosis, zygomycosis, vasculitis, and other bacterial infections [3].

Diagnosis is made by visualization of the organism in biopsy specimens or by isolation in culture. Histopathology shows necrosis and vasculitis without thrombosis [5]. Treatment consists of local incision and debridement, reversal of neutropenia, and antipseudomonal penicillins, cephalosporins, or carbapenems plus an aminoglycoside or quinolone. Resistance to all of these antibiotics may occur and result in treatment failure [2].

Aeromonas Hydrophila

Aeromonas hydrophila, a gram-negative motile rod, is found in water and soil. Tap water, hospital water sources, rivers, lakes, and swimming pools can all be reservoirs of *Aeromonas* [6]. Although stool isolates have been recovered, *Aeromonas* is not generally regarded to be part of the normal human floral [6]. Patients with hematological malignancy or bone marrow hypoplasia are at risk for *Aeromonas* bacteremia [7,8].

Ten to twenty percent of patients with *Aeromonas* bacteremia have associated skin lesions [1]. Erythematous nodules and hemorrhagic bullae with central necrosis and eschar consistent with ecthyma gangrenosum can be seen. Cellulitis, osteomyelitis, and necrotizing myositis have also been reported [6,9]. Extracutaneous manifestations of *Aeromonas* bacteremia include gastroenteritis, hepatobiliary infections, and meningitis.

Tissue biopsy and blood culture will identify the organism. Misidentification as *Enterobacteriaceae* may occur, necessitating routine testing with indophenol oxidase. *Aeromonas* is oxidase positive while *Enterobacteriaceae* are oxidase negative [10]. Other *Aeromonas* species known to cause human infection include *A. sobria*, *A. shigelloides*, and *A. punctata* [6,8]. *A. hydrophila* is susceptible to extended spectrum cephalosporins, trimethoprim-sulfamethoxazole (TMP-SMZ), and aminoglycosides [1]. Mortality from *Aeromonas* septicemia ranges from 29 to 60% [1,8].

Stenotrophomonas (Xanthomonas) Maltophilia

Stenotrophomonas maltophilia is a gram-negative bacillus that has become an important nosocomial pathogen. Sink drains and respiratory therapy equipment are known reservoirs of *S. maltophilia* in the hospital [11]. Risk factors for infection include neutropenia, hematological malignancy, prolonged hospitalization, and presence of a central venous catheter. Patients receiving broad-spectrum antibiotics, in particular imipenem-cilastatin, are at risk for superinfection with *S. maltophilia* [12].

Cutaneous manifestations include mucocutaneous ulcerations, primary cellulitis, and metastatic cellulitis. Mucocutaneous lesions commonly involve the gingival, lip, and buccal mucosa. Primary cellulitis frequently develops around catheter insertion sites. Metastatic *S. maltophilia* cellulitis can present as an erythematous tender nodule, ecthyma gangrenosum, or cellulitis with necrosis and ulceration. Vartivarian et al. reported skin, soft tissue, or mucocutaneous involvement in 15% of patients with *S. maltophilia* infection [12]. Other infections seen with this organism include pneumonia, endocarditis, mastoiditis, and meningitis [2,13].

Diagnosis can be made from a biopsy of skin lesions or a culture of skin, blood, or catheters. Removal of infected catheters, resolution of neutropenia, and administration of appropriate antibiotics are important components of treatment. TMP-SMZ with or without ticarcillin-clavulanate is the recommended antibiotic therapy for *S. maltophilia* infection.

Viridans Streptococci

Viridans streptococci, also called *alpha-hemolytic streptococci*, are major pathogens and cause bacteremia in neutropenic patients. Bochud et al. reported *S. viridans* bacteremia rates of 30% in neutropenic adults [14]. The use of cytosine arabinoside (Ara-C), prophylaxis with quinolones or TMP-SMZ, oropharyngeal mucositis, and neutropenia following chemotherapy are all risk factors for the development of *S. viridans* bacteremia [5,15]. Complications of bacteremia include endocarditis, respiratory distress syndrome, renal failure, and rash [2,5].

On examination, a maculopapular rash starting on the trunk and spreading centrifugally, desquamation of the palms and soles, petechiae, purpura, or erythema multiform–like lesions may be seen [5]. Diagnosis can be made by culture of the blood or any cutaneous source. Intravenous vancomycin can be used empirically for neutropenic fever and chemotherapy-induced mucositis, and it is generally the preferred therapy for *S. viridans* bacteremia. Penicillin resistance can occur in up to 40% of *S. viridans* isolates from neutropenic cancer patients.

Bacillus

Bacillus spp. have been reported to cause cutaneous infection in cancer patients. *B. cereus* and *B. subtilus* account for the majority of infections. Cutaneous manifestations include vesicles and pustules progressing to frank cellulitis. Gas gangrene–like infection with black necrotic lesions and ulcerations has also been reported. Approximately 50% of lesions develop at the entrance sites of indwelling intravascular catheters [5]. Extracutaneous manifestations of *B. cereus* infection include pneumonia, sepsis, and meningitis [2]. *Bacillus* spp. are notoriously resistant to *B*-lactam antibiotics. Vancomycin is the drug of choice along with removal of the vascular catheter.

Clostridium

Clostridium spp. are known pathogens in patients with hematogenous and genitourinary malignancies. Patients with occult carcinoma of the colon as well as recurrent and nonresectable gastrointestinal tumors are also at risk for infection due to *Clostridium*. One proposed mechanism of *Clostridium* bacteremia is mucosal disruption secondary to cytotoxic agents or tumor necrosis [16]. *C. perfringens* is the most common species isolated from the blood. *C. septicum* and *C. tertium* have also been isolated in severe infections [5]. *C. septicum* infection in leukemia patients is most commonly associated with typhlitis (necrotizing enterocolitis) [16].

Two types of skin lesions can occur in cancer patients with *Clostridium* bacteremia: gas gangrene (myonecrosis) and spreading cellulitis. Gas gangrene often presents with an abrupt onset of pain and swelling of an extremity. Rapid and progressive soft tissue swelling, skin discoloration, and hemorrhagic bullae follow. Confusion, malaise, or other systemic symptoms may be present. Spreading cellulitis presents as a puplish-black discoloration of the skin, often located on the flank or abdomen. Crepitation, blister formation, and appearance of new lesions are characteristic.

Tissue biopsy and blood culture can make the diagnosis. Mainstays of treatment include prompt antimicrobial therapy and surgical debridement. Metronidazole and clindamycin have both shown activity against *Clostridium*. Mortality rates are high in cancer patients with *Clostridium* septicemia with skin involvement.

Corynebacterium Jeikeium

Corynebacterium jeikeium, a gram-positive diphtheroid, is a known cutaneous commensal organism most commonly found in the rectal, inguinal, and axillary areas of hospitalized patients. Neutropenia, hematogenous malignancy, prolonged hospital stay, exposure to multiple antibiotics, and the presence of central venous catheters increases the cancer patients' risk for colonization [17]. Colonization rates of 40 to 80% have been reported in leukemic patients [5].

Skin lesions have been reported in up to 50% of patients with *C. jeikeium* bacteremia [18]. Cutaneous manifestationsof *C. jeikeium* bacteremia include pustules, nodules, ulcers, abscesses, and cellulitis. Indwelling catheters and sites of trauma such as bone marrow biopsy sites are common sources of bacteremia. Extracutaneous manifestations of infection include pneumonitis, endocarditis, peritonitis, and pyelonephritis [18,19].

In the microbiology laboratory, culture of *C. jeikeium* may be reported as normal skin flora because diphtheroids are common skin contaminants. Culturing *C. jeikeium* from the blood can make the diagnosis. Removal of central venous catheters and reversal of neutropenia are important for a favorable outcome. *C. jeikeium* is resistant to many antibiotics but is susceptible to vacomycin. Mortality rates are greater than 50% without proper treatment [2].

Mycobacterium Tuberculosis

Immunosuprressed patients, including those with malignancy and those receiving chronic immunosuppressive therapy, are at risk for active tuberculosis [5]. Cutaneous lesions may occur from exogenous or endogenous sources, or by hematogenous spread. Inoculation from an exogenous source results in a papule or granuloma in patients with no prior immunity. Regional lymphadenopathy follows, usually within 1 month. Persons with preexisting immunity develop a hyperkeratotic papule (prosector's wart). No lymphadenopathy or systemic symptoms are seen. Direct extension of an endogenous source of infection can manifest as mobile subcutaneous nodules resulting in sinus tracts that drain caseous material called scrofuloderma. Hematogenous dissemination results in three distinct patterns of cutaneous disease: lupus vulgaris, acute hematogenous dissemination, and nodules or abscesses. Lupus vulgaris is characterized by asymptomatic plaques and nodules with ulceration and scarring. Most commonly it occurs in women and is often found on the face, neck, and ear lobes. Acute hematogenous dissemination manifests as macules, papules, or purpuric truncal lesions. The nodules and abscesses of hematogenous dissemination are nontender, fluctuant, and often found on the trunk, extremities, or head [20].

Diagnosis is by tissue examination for acid-fast bacilli and culture. In pulmonic involvement, chest radiographic appearance is variable and includes nodules, infiltrates, or a diffuse reticulonodular or miliary pattern [2]. A negative tuberculin test may be seen in the immunosuppressed patient [5]. Treament consists of a four-drug regimen based on culture susceptibility results [5].

Nontuberculous Mycobacteria

Nontuberculous mycobacteria are abundant in nature and are known sources of infection in cancer patients. Runyon classified them into four groups by colony pigmentation, growth rates, and morphology:

Group I: Photochromogens
   M. marinum
   M. kansasii
Group II: Scotochromogens
   M. scrofulaceum
Group III: Nonchromogens
   M. avium-intracellulare (*MAI*)
   M. ulcerans
   M. haemophilum
Group IV: Rapid growers
   M. fortuitum
   M. chelonei
   M. abscessus
   M. vaccae

Group I are the photochromogens that produce pigment only when exposed to light. Infections with *M. marinum* usually occur through contact with contaminated water. Lesions are common on exposed areas of the skin, most commonly on the extremities. Lesions consist of papules, nodules, bullae, ulcers, and cellulitis [21,22]. Approximately 20 to 40% of patients will develop lesions in a sporotrichoid pattern [23]. *M. kansasii* has been isolated from tap water and ice machines. Although primarily a pulmonary pathogen, cutaneous lesions can develop. Common skin manifestations include papulopustules, sporotrichoid nodules, plaques, ulcers, and cellulitis. Patients with hairy cell leukemia appear to be especially susceptible to infection with *M. kansasii.*

Group II consists of mycobacteria that produce pigment in the dark and in the light called scotochromogens. *M. scrofulaceum* is most prevalent in the southeastern United States. The organism has been isolated from oysters, dairy products, water, and soil. Cutaneous involvement most commonly involves fistula formation. Nodules, ulcers, abscesses, cervical lymphadenitis, and lesions in a sporotrichoid pattern can also be seen [23].

Group III is made up of the nonchromogens that do not produce pigment. *MAI* is ubiquitous in the environment and most commonly causes pulmonary disease. Cutaneous *MAI* can occur via direct inoculation of the skin or as part of a disseminated infection. Up to 20% of patients with disseminated disease develop cutaneous lesions. Tender subcutaneous nodules or ulcerations are characteristic. *M. ulcerans* is common in warm climates that are close to bodies of water. On cutaneous exam, a nontender nodule that ulcerates and becomes necrotic known as a Buruli ulcer is seen. Rapid spread of the infection can occur with extension to the deeper tissues [23]. Lesions associated with *M. haemophilum* consist of violaceous nodules, papules, or plaques with ulceration and abscess formation. The extremities are usually involved with a diffuse distribution of lesions [5,23].

Group IV are the rapid growers, named so as a result of their fast growth characteristics. *M. fortuitum* is ubiquitous in the environment and is known to cause a wide variety of cutaneous and extracutaneous diseases. Immunocompromised patients are most likely to develop cutaneous lesions from disseminated disease. Papules, nodules, abscesses, or a generalized morbilliform rash can be seen and are usually located on the extremities. Cancer patients at risk for *M. chelonae* infection include persons on steroids and patients with long-term catheters. Cutaneous lesions usually present on an extremity and present as erythematous subcutaneous nodules with draining fistulas. *M. chelonae* infection manifesting in a sporotrichoid pattern has also been reported [24]. Cutaneous *M. abscessus* in the immunocompromised host is most likely a result of disseminated disease. Erythematous, violaceous nodules or abscesses are common and can develop at injection sites. Patients with a genetic defect in the receptor for interferon gamma are also at risk for infection with *M. abscessus* [25]. Cutaneous infections with *M. vaccae* have been reported and have a strong association with exposure to cattle. Skin lesions consist of tender erythematous nodules [26].

When a diagnosis of nontuberculous mycobacteria is suspected, adequate tissue for culture should be obtained. The microbiology laboratory should be alerted to ensure that cultures are performed in the proper media at the correct temperature. Antimicrobial therapy should be guided by antibiotic susceptibility testing of mycobacterial isolates.

Nocardia

Nocardia species are ubiquitous gram-positive, variably acid-fast aerobic bacteria that are found predominantly in the soil. Patients with leukemia and lymphoma are at high risk for nocardiosis, especially while on prolonged steroid therapy [27,28]. Cell-mediated immunodeficiency is the primary risk factor for developing *Nocardia* infection in cancer patients, whereas neutropenia is not a significant risk factor [29].

The most common cutaneous presentation of nocardiosis is a painful erythematous nodule (<2 cm diameter) located on an extremity occurring after traumatic inoculation or hematogenous dissemination from a primary lung focus. Sinus tract formation, nodular lymphangitis, and regional adenopathy may accompany the lesion. Other presentations of nocardiosis include cellulitis, abscess, ulcers, granulomas, mycetoma, and pyoderma [27,28].

The majority of infections are caused by *Nocardia asteroids* and *Nocardia brasiliensis*, with the latter responsible for the majority of the lymphangitic or sporotrichoid form of nocardiosis [27,30]. Differential diagnosis of nocardiosis includes other infectious and granulomatous diseases (including *Sporothrix schenckii*, *Mycobacterium*, and *Fusarium*) as well as a variety of tumors [31]. Gram stain, modified acid-fast stain, and culture make the diagnosis. Treatment of choice is TMP-SMZ with or without amikacin, imipenem, minocycline, or ceftriaxone [2,27]. Surgical drainage of abscesses may be required.

FUNGAL

Candida

The most common cause of invasive fungal disease in patients with hematological malignancies, and in bone marrow transplant (BMT) recipients, is *Candida* [5,32]. The incidence of disseminated candidiasis is directly related to the severity and duration of neutropenia in patients with hematologic malignancies [33]. The use of broad-spectrum antibiotics promotes *Candida* overgrowth in the oropharynx and GI tract by suppressing the normal bacterial flora [1,33]. Other risk factors for infection include hyperalimentation and central venous catheter use. Chemotherapy with resultant mucosal damage of the GI tract is also a risk factor for infection [5].

Candida can infect the lungs, liver, spleen, kidneys, eye, and skin. Oral, vaginal, and intertriginous lesions are also common. *C. albicans* is the species most commonly isolated from the blood [2]. Clinical infection can also be seen with *C. tropicalis*, *C. glabrata*, *C. parapsilosis*, *C. krusei*, *C. guilliermondii*, and *C. lusitaniae* [5,35,36]. *C. tropicalis* is more virulent, and the patient's clinical course tends to be more severe. *C. glabrata* and *C. krusei* have both been reported to be resistant to the antifungal fluconazole. The species most likely to be associated with vascular catheters and lipid formulations is *C. parapsilosis*.

Chronic disseminated candidiasis occurs primarily in leukemic patients and BMT recipients. The skin and other organs such as the liver, spleen, kidney, and lungs become seeded with *Candida* during the neutropenic period [2]. Manifestations of the disease do not usually occur until the neutrophil count returns to normal. Culture of lesions and blood are negative in half the cases.

The mucous membranes are a common site of *Candida* infection. Oral candidiasis (thrush) presents as a white curdlike plaque on the palate, buccal mucosa, tongue, or gingiva that can be partially scraped off. Erythematous mucositis without plaques can also occur. Angular chelitis due to *Candida* species may be seen and presents with ulceration and cracking of the angle of the mouth.

Cutaneous involvement with disseminated candidiasis has been reported in 10% of patients with hematological malignancy [5]. Lesions of disseminated candidiasis commonly present as multiple erythematous papules and macules with central pallor or pustulation [33,34]. Other morphological forms include purpura, necrosis with eschar, abscess, or ecthyma gangrenosum–like lesions [33].

Skin biopsies of lesions reveal budding yeast and pseudohyphae in tissue. Growth of *Candida* in culture is also diagnostic [33]. Systemic candidiasis is more difficult to diagnose, yielding positive blood cultures in only 25 to 50% of patients [33]. Treatment of *Candida* is with oral or systemic antifungal therapy. Mortality to candidemia can be as high as 60% [2].

Aspergillus

Aspergillosis is the second most common opportunistic fungal infection in cancer patients [5]. Predisposing factors include hematological malignancy, organ transplant recipients, mucous membrane disruption, long-term central venous access, chronic pulmonary disease, and the use of long-term corticosteroids, broad spectrum antibiotics, or cytotoxic agents [37–39]. Neutropenic patients may also be at risk for reactivation of a previously eradicated *Aspergillus* pulmonary infection [38].

Organ systems involved include the lungs (most common), CNS, gastrointestinal tract, and skin. Cutaneous aspergillosis is an unusual variant and may represent either a primary focus or a metastatic lesion in the immunocompromised host [37]. Primary cutaneous aspergillosis develops in areas of skin trauma, particularly intravenous catheters and dressings [40]. *Aspergillus flavus* is the pathogen responsible for most primary skin infections [5]. Metastatic lesions usually represent a pulmonary source of infection. The most common species known to cause pulmonary infection is *Aspergillus fumigatus*. Direct extension from the paranasal sinuses may also occur [37].

On cutaneous examination, primary lesions differ from metastatic lesions. Characteristics of primary lesions include erythematous to violacious papules or plaques that progress to hemorrhagic bullae and necrotic ulcers with black eschar [41].

Disseminated lesions characteristically present as a diffuse erythematous maculopapular eruption followed by pustule formation. Nonspecific chronic urticarial lesions following ingestion or inhalation of spores can also be seen [37].

Biopsy and culture will confirm the diagnosis. Other conditions that can mimic aspergillosis include echthyma gangrenosum, mucormycoses, cryptococcus, anthrax, and vasculitis [41]. Histologically *Aspergillus* demonstrates septated acute-angle branching hyphae [34]. Treatment consists of removal of any catheters, local wound care and/or surgical debridement, and systemic antifungal therapy.

Fusarium

Fusarium, a common soil saprophyte, is a known pathogen in the immunocompromised patient. Neutropenia in the setting of BMT, hematogenous malignancy, and cytoreductive chemotherapy are major risk factors for disseminated infection [42]. The most likely portals of entry for infection include the paranasal sinuses, lungs, GI tract, and skin [42,43]. Intravascular catheters can also be portals of entry for *Fusarium* spp. [44]. *F. solani* is the species most commonly isolated. *F. moniliforme*, *F. dimerum*, *F. oxysporum*, *F. chlamydosporum*, and *F. anthophilum* are also medically important species [5,42].

Fusarium skin infection can be a localized infection or a manifestation of disseminated disease. Localized skin infections include pustules, plaques, my-

cetoma, ecthyma gangrenosum–like lesions, and onychomycosis [5,44]. Periungual or interdigital cellulitis is a frequent presentation of *Fusarium* infection. Tender erythematous, purpuric, or necrotic lesions are characteristic and occur in the setting of prolonged neutropenia (greater than 1 week). Dissemination can occur and result in death. Minor trauma such as nail clipping may initiate the infection and should be discouraged during the neutropenic period. Skin lesions have been reported in 70 to 90% of immunocompromised patients with disseminated disease [5,45]. Characteristic lesions of disseminated infection are tender erythematous or purpuric macules, papules, and nodules with central necrosis. Fever, myalgia, and weakness often accompany the skin lesions.

On biopsy, *Fusarium* resembles other fungal organisms, particularly *Aspergillus*. Branching septate hyphae with a propensity for vascular wall invasion is seen. *Fusarium* may be further identified for its characteristic short-lived spores called macroconidia and microconidia and long-lived spores called chlamydospores [46]. Definitive diagnosis is made by culture. Periungual cellulitis requires removal of the nail for a diagnosis by culture and histopathology. This also improves the response to antifungal therapy by removing the nidus of infection. Rapid diagnosis and bone marrow recovery are the most important determinants for survival [44]. Treatment also consists of antifungal therapy, use of granulocyte colony-stimulating factor, removal of catheters, and surgical debridement if warranted. Mortality rates of disseminated *Fusarium* are high, reaching 80% of patients infected [44]. With the availability of Voriconazole, which has good activity against *Fusarium*, mortality rates are reduced to 40% or less.

Trichosporon

Fungi of the genus *Trichosporon*, which includes *Trichosporon beigelii* and *Trichosporon capitatum*, are known opportunistic pathogens. *T. beigelii* is found in the soil and can be part of the normal skin human flora [47]. It can be responsible for causing onychomycosis, paronychia, localized granulomas, and white piedra (a superficial infection of the hair shaft). Disseminated infection can occur and is most commonly seen in the immunocompromised host. Risk factors for disseminated infection include hematogenous malignancy, chemotherapy-induced neutropenia, corticosteroids, and hemachromatosis [47,48].

The lower respiratory and gastrointestinal tracts seem to be the portal of entry for infection [5]. The lungs, liver, kidneys, spleen, heart, and skin are the organs most frequently affected. Cutaneous involvement is seen in 30% of patients with disseminated trichosporonosis [5,47]. Purpuric papules and nodules on the trunk, arms, and face are most commonly reported [47]. Additional lesions include vesicles, necrotic ulcers, cellulitis, and desquamation of the skin [5,47].

On biopsy, the histological pattern most commonly reported is fungal dermal invasion. Microscopically, it may resemble *Candida* or *Aspergillus*. Specimens containing *T. beigelii* reveal pseudohyphae, rectangular arthroconidia, and blastoconidia [47,49]. Fungal culture is positive in greater than 90% of cutaneous lesions [47]. Susceptibility testing may help guide treatment regimens because this organism has been reported to be resistant to many antifungals including Amphotericin B [5,47].

Cryptococcus Neoformans

Cryptococcus neoformans is a ubiquitous encapsulated yeast found in soil, pigeon droppings, and fruits. Cancer patients at increased risk for cryptococcosis include those with lymphoreticular malignancy, transplant recipients, and those receiving corticosteroid therapy [5,50,51]. Inhalation is the primary mode of entry. Hematogenous dissemination to the CNS from the lungs is most common. Other organs that can become secondarily infected include the kidney, liver, spleen, prostate, and skin [5]. Skin involvement has been reported in 10 to 20% of cases of disseminated cryptococcus. Primary cutaneous cryptococcus has been reported but is rare.

Cutaneous lesions may be the sole manifestation of disseminated cryptococcus and precede systemic involvement by 1 to 13 months [51]. The most common areas involved are the head and neck. Lesions are polymorphous and can present as acneiform papules, vesicles, pustules, nodules, ulcers, palpable purpura, subcutaneous swelling, or cellulitis. Localized lymphadenopathy does not commonly occur [52]. Skin findings may resemble molloscum contagiosum, herpes simplex, vasculitis, skin cancer, syphilis, tuberculosis, sarcoidosis, or a bacterial cellulitis [53].

It is virtually impossible to make a clinical diagnosis of *Cryptococcus* on cutaneous findings alone because there is no single pathognomonic lesion. Skin scrapings and smears with India ink, Wright's stain, or Gram's stain may allow a presumptive diagnosis to be made. Confirmatory biopsy or culture is strongly recommended [52]. Two histological types are seen on biopsy: granulomatous and gelatinous. The granulomatous type is characterized by few organisms, in contrast to the gelatinous type, which shows numerous budding yeasts [50]. Tzanck smears may also be warranted in vesicular lesions to rule out herpes simplex or zoster.

A careful search for extracutaneous disease is indicated when a diagnosis of cutaneous *Cryptococcus* infection is made. A chest x-ray and lumbar puncture should be performed. In addition, culture of the blood, urine, sputum, and prostatic secretions should be obtained [54]. Left untreated, disseminated *Cryptococcus* has a mortality rate of 70 to 80% versus a mortality rate of 10 to 20% with appropriate treatment [50,54]. Intravenous Amphotericin B with flucytosine is the recommended therapy for disseminated disease [5]. Oral fluconazole remains the drug of choice for maintenance therapy [5,50].

Histoplasma Capsulatum

Histoplasma capsulatum is a dimorphic fungus that is distributed principally in the soil of the Ohio, Missouri, and Mississippi river valleys. Histoplasmosis is predominantly a disease of the lungs, but disseminated disease can occur. Immunocompromised patients, particularly those with hematological malignancy, or patients receiving corticosteroids or cytotoxic agents, are at risk for disseminated histoplasmosis [55].

Cutaneous histoplasmosis can be either a primary lesion or represent dissemination from another source. Primary cutaneous histoplasmosis is rare and the infection is usually self-limited, thus requiring no treatment. Cutaneous manifestations associated with disseminated disease have been reported in less than 10% of cases [5]. Lesions present as nontender papules, pustules, or punched-out ulcers. Ulcerative, vegetative, or nodular oropharyngeal lesions are seen more commonly and are highly characteristic for disseminated histoplasmosis. Systemic disease can also infect the lungs, bone marrow, spleen, liver, lymph nodes, genitourinary (GU) tract, adrenals, heart, and CNS [5,55].

Histopathological examination shows the presence of narrow intracellular budding yeast. Culture of the yeast will confirm the diagnosis. Immunocompromised patients with disseminated disease are treated with systemic antifungal therapy.

Blastomyces Dermatitidis

Blastomyces dermatitidis is a dimorphic fungus endemic to the Mississippi and Ohio river valleys, central and southern Canada, and parts of Africa [56]. Infection occurs by inhalation of spores from the soil into the lungs. Patients with hematological malignancy or solid tumors of the lung, and those receiving systemic corticosteroids or cytotoxic agents, are at risk for primary infection or reactivation of latent infection [57].

The skin is the most common extrapulmonary site of disseminated infection. Lesions may appear verrucous or ulcerative. The verrucous or fungating form is elevated with sharp but irregular borders [58]. Ulcers most commonly present with a heaped up border and an exudative base [58]. Subcutaneous abscesses that drain to the skin can also be seen. Oropharyngeal lesions occur less frequently than lesions due to *H. capsulatum*, with the ex-

ception of laryngeal lesions. Other common sites of disseminated blastomycosis include the bone, GU system, and CNS [5,57].

Rapid diagnosis of blastomycosis can be obtained by microscopic examination of a KOH preparation of the specimen [59]. Broad-based budding
yeast is classic for blastomycosis. Culture is confirmatory but can take 2 to 3
weeks. Skin and serological tests are unreliable for diagnosis. Immunocompromised individuals with disseminated blastomycosis should receive IV
antifungal therapy.

Coccidioides Immitis

Coccidioides immitis is a dimorphic fungus that is endemic in soil in the
southwestern United States. An estimated 100,000 infections occur each year
in the United States. Approximately 60% of these infections are asymptomatic [60]. The remainder develop manifestations of pulmonary disease.
Immunosuppressed patients are at risk for late dissemination or reactivation
of disease [5].

The cutaneous reaction patterns seen with primary pulmonary coccidiomycosis include toxic erythema, erythema nodosum, and erythema multiforme [60]. Toxic erythema is the earliest cutaneous manifestation and is
nonspecific. It can present as a pruritic erythematous maculopapular, morbilliform, or urticarial eruption. This may be accompanied by an oral exanthem and low-grade fever. Erythema nodosum, the most common reaction
pattern, is characterized by symmetric tender erythematous nodules and
plaques located predominantly on the extensor aspects of the lower extremities [34]. The presence of erythema nodosum denotes a favorable prognosis.
Erythema multiforme is more common in children and is predominantly
located on the lower extremities, particularly the inner thighs. Characteristic
target lesions are seen. Both erythema nodosum and erythema multiforme can
present with arthralgia and ocular involvement to form the "valley fever"
complex of primary pulmonary coccidiomycosis [60].

Primary cutaneous coccidiomycosis is rare. It most often presents as a
painless ulcer. Lymphangitis, regional adenopathy, and sporotrichoid nodules often accompany the lesion. Dissemination of primary cutaneous coccidiomycosis can occur.

The lesions of disseminated coccidiomycosis are morphologically indistinct. Papules, pustules, plaques, nodules, sinuses, ulcers, and abscesses
may be seen [60]. The central face, especially the nasolabial fold, is a common
site of infection. Other organs that can be involved in disseminated disease
include the lung, CNS, and bone.

Diagnosis of coccidiomycosis can be made by demonstration of pathognomonic spherules in sputum or tissue samples [2]. The organism may also be

grown in culture, but protective measures must be taken, as the filamentous form is infectious. Serological testing and skin testing for delayed hypersensitivity to coccidioidin may be negative in the immunosuppressed patient with disseminated infection. Treatment consists of antifungal therapy such as Amphotericin B, fluconazole, or itraconazole.

Mucormycosis

Mucormycosis is a term used to describe disease caused by a family of fungi in the class Zygomycetes. Within this class are the species *Rhizopus*, *Absidia*, *Cunninghamella*, and *Mucor* [61,62]. Risk factors for mucormycosis include intravenous drug abuse of amphetamines, diabetes, iron overload (with or without treatment with desferrioxamine), and the immunocompromised patient [62–64]. Myelodysplasia, myeloproliferative disorders, leukemia, and stem cell recipients are at particular risk because of iron overload from frequent transfusions. Cutaneous infection has been reported but is uncommon. More commonly the lungs, sinuses, gastrointestinal tract, kidneys, and CNS are involved [63].

In the immunocompromised patient, skin lesions commonly present as a painful purple-red plaque or nodule with areas of necrosis [34]. Biopsy and culture of the lesions are necessary to differentiate lesions of mucormycosis from other bacterial, fungal, protozoal, and viral infections; embolic or other vascular diseases; trauma; or topical or systemic cytotoxic agents. On histological examination, broad, nonseptate, right-angle branching hyphae in tissue and blood vessels are seen [63,64]. Treatment consists of surgical debridement with adjunctive medical therapy with amphotericin B or lipid formulations of amphotericin B (the latter is preferred) [63].

Malassezia

Malassezia furfur, also known as *Pityrosporum orbiculare*, is a ubiquitous fungus that colonizes normal skin. Suppression of normal bacterial skin flora by antibiotic usage may result in overgrowth of *M. furfur*. Impaired host immunity such as hematogenous malignancy, patients receiving steroids, and BMT recipients are also at risk for infection. In addition, intravascular catheter use is a risk factor for *M. furfur* infection.

In the immunocompromised host, the most common cutaneous manifestation of *M. furfur* infection is folliculitis. An erythematous maculopapular rash with a follicular and perifollicular distribution is characteristic. The development of pustules and crusts may be seen after 48 to 72 hours. Lesions are commonly located on the chest, shoulders, and upper back and may be pruritic.

Diagnosis of *M. furfur* is made by skin scraping, biopsy, and culture. Perifollicular budding yeast without hyphae or pseudohyphae that are confined to the epidermis is characteristic [65]. Growth of *M. furfur* on media requiring lipid supplementation confirms the diagnosis. Treatment consists of topical, oral, or systemic antifungal therapy. Clinical improvement in the BMT recipient may not occur until normalization of the granulocyte count [66].

VIRAL

Herpes Simplex Virus (HSV)

By age 50, more than 90% of adults have antibodies to HSV1 indicating a prior exposure to *HSV* [67]. Reactivation of latent *HSV* is the most common viral infection in neutropenic patients [68]. Patients at risk are those with hematological malignancies receiving chemotherapy, and BMT recipients. Reactivation of *HSV* is approximately 70% to 80% following induction chemotherapy for leukemia or conditioning for BMT [2].

Characteristics of recurrent *HSV* infection include tender and painful vesicles, pustules, "punched out" erosions, or ulceration. In the immunocompromised patient, the vesicular stage is often missed owing to rapid transformation of the lesion, leaving secondary hemorrhagic crusts. Numbness, itching, or burning may precede lesions. Lesions predominantly occur on the oral mucosa and nares. The danger of superinfection with bacteria or fungi may occur with prolonged ulceration. Genital and perianal *HSV* infections in the immunocompromised patient are typically more extensive. Dissemination is rare but may occur to the lung, liver, eye, and CNS [68,69]. Chronic herpes infections can develop in severely immunosuppressed patients and last for months. Confluent areas of superficial ulceration with a serpiginous border are characteristic.

Conditions that mimic recurrent *HSV* include aphthous ulcers, *Cytomegalovirus* ulcers, candida esophagitis, impetigo, and cytotoxic mucositis [69]. Finding multinucleated giant cells on Tzanck prep from an unroofed vesicle can make the diagnosis. *HSV* can also be diagnosed by culture, electron microscopy, or monoclonal antibody staining or immunoflourescent staining [68].

Patients receiving chemotherapy and transplant recipients who are neutropenic should routinely receive prophylaxis against *HSV* reactivation. Treatment of mucosal disease is with oral intravenous acyclovir 5 mg/kg every 8 hours for a minimum of 7 days [2,68]. Disseminated *HSV* disease is treated with intravenous acyclovir 10 mg/kg every 8 hours. Acyclovir-resistant strains of *HSV* have been reported and are due to a viral deficiency of thymidine kinase. The treatment of choice for resistant strains is foscarnet [68].

Cytomegalovirus (CMV)

CMV, like *HSV*, is a common viral infection with many adults testing sero-positive, indicating prior exposure [68]. *CMV* infection can occur by primary exposure, reactivation of a latent strain, or reinfection with another strain of *CMV*. Patients at risk of *CMV* disease include those receiving chemotherapy for malignant disease and BMT recipients.

CMV can affect the lungs, gastrointestinal tract, liver, pancreas, CNS, and retina [2]. Skin findings are uncommon but can occur. Haki et al. [70] reported the case of a 6-year-old boy who presented with a pruritic erythematous papular rash over the face, buttocks, arms, and legs following BMT for acute lymphocytic leukemia. A diagnosis of papular acrodermatitis of childhood (Gianotti–Crosti syndrome) associated with *CMV* antigenemia was made [70].

Histologically, *CMV* infection can be identified by finding inclusion bodies in tissue biopsy [34]. Viral culture, PCR, and antigen assay can also be used to diagnose *CMV* infection. Treatment of *CMV* infection is with ganciclovir or foscarnet; *CMV* immune globulin also may be added [34,68].

Varicella Zoster Virus (VZV)

Patients receiving long term corticosteroids and chemotheraphy or radiation therapy BMT recipients are at risk for primary and reactivated *VZV* infection [2]. Reactivation of *VZV* following BMT is typically a late complication occurring 3 or more months after transplantation. For this reason, prophylaxis of *VZV* with acyclovir is not routinely given [68]. *VZV* infection is more severe in the immunosuppressed patient and lasts longer. Complications of *VZV* infection include hemorrhagic pneumonia, encephalitis, retinal necrosis, hepatitis, thrombocytopenia, DIC, and fulminant purpura [2].

Dermatomal zoster (shingles) most commonly involves the thoracic dermatomes and is characterized by vesicles and hemorrhagic crusts. A prodrome of tingling, pain, or numbness may precede cutaneous findings. *VZV* infection may also become disseminated or present as a atypical recurrent chickenpox. Lesions may be vesicular, hyperkeratotic, verrucous, papular, or nodular. Like chronic *HSV* infection, large superficial ulcerations can occur. Patients who are thrombocytopenic may present with hemorrhagic blisters. Cutaneous exam shows the lesions to be in all stages of disease simultaneously. Secondary infection can occur and is usually due to Group A *Streptococci* or *S. aureus*.

The diagnosis of single dermatomal shingles can be made by visual inspection alone. *VZV* infection in the setting of cutaneous graft-versus-host disease can be difficult to detect and precludes a diagnostic workup. Tzanck or immunoflourescent smear, viral culture, serology, and biopsy can make the diagnosis [34]. Systemic acyclovir is the treatment of choice along with reducing immunosuppressive therapy. Oral acyclovir, famcyclovir, or valcyclovir may be used once clinical improvement has occurred.

REFERENCES

1. Bodey GP. Dermatologic manifestations of infections in neutropenic patients. In: Pankey GA, ed. Infectious Disease Clinics of North America. Philadelphia: W.B. Saunders, 1994:655–675.
2. Freeman JS Jr, Rhyner S, Snyder A, Devita VT, Hellman S, Rosenberg, SA. Cancer Principles and Practice of Oncology. 6th ed. Philadelphia: Lippincott Williams and Wilkins, 2001.
3. Kim EJ, Foad M, Travers R. Ecthyma gangrenosum in an AIDS patient with normal neutrophil count. J Am Acad Dermatol 1999; 41:840–841.
4. Baze PE, Thyss A, Vinti H, Deville A, Dellamonica P, Ortonne JP. A study of nineteen immunocompromised patients with extensive skin lesions caused by *Pseudomonas aeruginosa* with and without bacteremia. Acta Derm Venereol 1991; 71:411–415.
5. Lopez FA, Sanders CV. Dermatologic infections in the immunocompromised (non-HIV) host. In: Moellering RC Jr, ed. Infectious Disease Clinics of North America. Philadelphia: W.B. Saunders, 2001:671–702.
6. Davis WA, Kane JG, Garagusi VF. Human *Aeromonas* infections: a review of the literature and a case report of endocarditis. Medicine 1978; 57:267–277.
7. Cordingley FT, Rajanayagam A. *Aeromonas hydrophila* bacteraemia in haematological patients. Med Journ of Aust 1981; 1:364–365.
8. Funada H, Matsuda T. *Aeromonas* bacteremia in patients with hematologic diseases. Intern Med 1997; 36:171–174.
9. Moyes CD, Sykes PA, Rayner JM. *Aeromonas hydrophila* septicaemia producing ecthyma gangrenosum in a child with leukaemia. Scand J Infect Dis 1977; 9:151–153.
10. Wolff RL, Wiseman SL, Kitchens CS. *Aeromonas hydrophila* bacteremia in ambulatory immunocompromised hosts. Am J Med 1980; 68:238–242.
11. Yamadori JF, Xu G, Hojo S, Negayama K, Miyawaki H, Yamaji Y, Takahara J. Clinical features of *Stenotrophomonas maltophilia* pneumonia in immunocompromised patients. Resp Med 1996; 90:35–38.
12. Vartivarian SE, Papadakis KA, Palacios JA, Manning JT, Anaissie EJ. Mucocutaneous and soft tissue infections caused by *Xanthomonas maltophilia*. Ann Intern Med 1994; 21:969–973.
13. Burns RL, Lowe L. *Xanthomonas maltophilia* infection presenting as erythematous nodules. J Am Acad Dermatol 1997; 37:836–838.
14. Bochud PY, Eggiman P, Calandra T, Van Melle G, Saghafi L, Francioli P. Bacteremia due to *Viridans streptococcus* in neutropenic patients with cancer: clinical spectrum and risk factors. Clin Infect Dis 1994; 18:25–31.
15. Bow EJ. Infection risk and cancer chemotherapy: the impact of the chemotherapeutic regimen in patients with lymphoma and solid tissue malignancies. J Antimicrob Chemother 1998; 41:1–5.

16. Litam PP, Loughran TP Jr. *Clostridium septicum* bacteremia in a patient with large granular lymphocyte leukemia. Cancer Invest 1995; 13:492–494.

17. Van Der Lelie H, Leverstein-Van Hall M, Mertens M, Van Zaanen HCT, Van Oers RHJ, Thomas BLM, Von Dem Borne AE, Kuijperm EJ. Corynebacterium CDC Group JK (*Corynebacterium jeikeium*) sepsis in haematological patients: a report of three cases and a systematic literature review. Scand J Infect Dis 1995; 27:581–584.

18. Dan M, Somer I, Knobel B, Gutman R. Cutaneous manifestations of infection with *Corynebacterium Group JK*. Rev Infect Dis 1988; 10:1204–1207.

19. Hande KR, Witebsky FG, Brown MS, Schulman CB, Anderson SE, Levine AS, MacLowry JD, Chabner BA. Sepsis with a new species of *Corynebacterium*. Ann Intern Med 1976; 85:423–426.

20. Asnis DS, Bresciani AR. Cutaneous tuberculosis: a rare presentation of malignancy. Clin Infect Dis 1992; 15:158–160.

21. Edelstein H. *Mycobacterium marinum* skin infections. Arch Intern Med 1994; 154:1359–1364.

22. Hanau LH, Leaf A, Soeiro R, Weiss LM, Pollack SS. *Mycobacterium marinum* infection in a patient with the acquired immunodeficiency syndrome. Cutis 1994; 54:103–105.

23. Weitzul S, Eichhorn PJ, Pandya AG. Nontuberculous mycobacterial infections of the skin. Derm Clin 2000; 18:359–376.

24. Zahid MA, Klotz SA, Goldstein E, Bartholomew W. *Mycobacterium chelonae* (*M. chelonae subspecies chelonae*): report of a patient with a sporotrichoid presentation who was successfully treated with clarithromycin and ciprofloxacin. Clin Infect Dis 1994; 18:999–1001.

25. Colsky AS, Hanly A, Elgar G, Kerdel FA. Treatment of refractory disseminated *Mycobacterium abscessus* infection with interferon gamma therapy. Arch Dermatol 1999; 135:125–127.

26. Hachem R, Raad I, Rolston KVI, Whimbey E, Katz R, Tarrand J, Libshitz H. Cutaneous and pulmonary infections caused by *Mycobacterium vaccae*. Clin Infect Dis 1996; 23:173–175.

27. Odom RB, James WD, Berger TG. Andrews' Diseases of the Skin. 9th ed. Philadelphia: W. B. Saunders, 2000.

28. Berkey P, Bodey GP. Nocardial infection in patients with neoplastic disease. Rev Infect Dis 1989; 11:407–411.

29. Watkins A, Greene JN, Vincent AL, Sandin RL. Nocardial infections in cancer patients: our experience and a review of the literature. Infect Dis Clin Pract 1999; 8:294–300.

30. Nishimoto K, Ohno M. Subcutaneous abscesses caused by *Nocardia brasiliensis* complicated by malignant lymphoma. Int J Dermat 1985; 24:437–440.

31. Kostman JR, DiNubile MJ. Nodular lymphangitis: a distinctive but often unrecognized syndrome. Ann Intern Med 1993; 118:883–888.

32. Chanock SJ, Pizzo PA. Infectious complications of patients undergoing therapy for acute leukemia: current status and future prospects. Semin Oncol 1997; 24:132–139.

33. Marcus J, Grossman ME, Yunakov MJ, Rappaport F. Disseminated candid-

iasis, *Candida* arthritis, and unilateral skin lesions. J Am Acad Dermatol 1992; 26:295–297.

34. Dover JS, Jackson BA, Junkins-Hopkins JM, et al. Pocket Guide to Cutaneous Medicine and Surgery. 1st ed. Philadelphia: W. B. Saunders, 1996.

35. Spiers ASD. Primary cutaneous infections with *Candida* species associated with percutaneous intravenous catheters in patients with cancer. J Fla Med Assoc 1989; 76:386–387.

36. Booth LV, Collins AL, Lowes JA, Radford M. Skin rash associated with *Candida guilliermondii*. Med Pediatr Oncol 1988; 16:295–296.

37. Allo MD, Miller J, Townsend T, Tan C. Primary cutaneous aspergillosis associated with hickman intravenous catheters. N Engl J Med 1987; 317:1105–1108.

38. Buescher TM, Moritz DM, Killyon GW. Resection of chest wall and central veins for invasive cutaneous *Aspergillus* infection in an immunocompromised patient. Chest 1994; 105:1283–1285.

39. Carlile JR, Millet RE, Cho CT, Vats TS. Primary cutaneous aspergillosis in a leukemic child. Arch Dermatol 1978; 114:78–80.

40. Khardori N, Hayat S, Rolston K, Bodey GP. Cutaneous *Rhizopus* and *Aspergillus* infections in five patients with cancer. Arch Dermatol 1989; 125:952–956.

41. Raszka WV, Shoupe BL, Edwards EG. Isolated primary cutaneous aspergillosis of the labia. Med Pediatr Oncol 1993; 21:375–377.

42. Alvarez-Franco M, Reyes-Mugica M, Paller AS. Cutaneous *Fusarium* infection in an adolescent with acute leukemia. Pediatr Dermatol 1992; 9:62–65.

43. Anaissie E, Kantarjian H, Ro J, Hopfer R, Rolston K, Fainstein V, Bodey G. The emerging role of *Fusarium* infections in patients with cancer. Medicine 1988; 67:77–83.

44. Caux F, Aractingi S, Baurmann H, Reygagne P, Dombret H, Romand S, Dubertret L. *Fusarium solani* cutaneous infection in a neutropenic patient. Dermatol 1993; 186:232–235.

45. Poblete SJP, Greene JN, Sandin RL. Disseminated *Fusarium* in the immunocompromised host. Infect Dis Clin Pract 1998; 7:339–344.

46. Mowbray DN, Paller AS, Nelson PE, Kaplan RL. Disseminated *Fusarium solani* infection with cutaneous nodules in a bone marrow transplant patient. Int J Dermatol 1988; 27:698–701.

47. Nahass GT, Rosenberg SP, Leonardi CL, Penneys NS. Disseminated infection with *Trichosporon beigelii*. Arch Dermatol 1993; 129:1020–1023.

48. Pierard GE, Read D, Pierard-Franchimont C, Lother Y, Rurangirwa A, Estrada JA. Cutaneous manifestations in systemic trichosporonosis. Clin Exp Dermatol 1992; 17:79–82.

49. Haupt HM, Merz WG, Beschorner WE, Vaughn WP, Saral R. Colonization and infection with *Trichosporon* species in the immunosuppressed host. J Infect Dis 1983; 147:199–203.

50. Durden FM, Elewski B. Cutaneous involvement with *Cryptococcus neoformans* in AIDS. J Am Acad Dermatol 1994; 30:844–848.

51. Kim JH, Shin DH, Oh MD, Park S, Kim BK, Choe KW. A case of disseminated cryptococcosis with skin eruption in a patient with acute leukemia. Scand J Infect Dis 2001; 33:234–235.

52. Hernandez AD. Cutaneous cryptococcosis. Dermatol Clin 1989; 7:269–274.
53. Haight DO, Esperanza LE, Greene JN, Sandin RL, DeGregorio R, Spiers ASD. Case report: cutaneous manifestations of cryptococcosis. Am J Med Sci 1994; 308:192–195.
54. Anderson DJ, Schmidt C, Goodman J, Pomeroy C. Cryptococcal disease presenting as cellulitis. Clin Infect Dis 1992; 14:666–672.
55. Kauffman CA, Israel KS, Smith JW, White AC, Schwarz J, Brooks GF. *Histoplasmosis* in immunosuppressed patients. Am J Med 1978; 64:923–932.
56. Pappas PG, Threlkeld MG, Bedsole GD, Cleveland KO, Gelfand MS, Dismukes WE. *Blastomycosis* in immunocompromised patients. Medicine 1993; 72:311–325.
57. Winquist EW, Walmsley SL, Berinstein NL. Reactivation and dissemination of *Blastomycosis* complicating Hodgkin's disease: a case report and review of the literature. Am J Hematol 1993; 43:129–132.
58. Bradsher RW. *Histoplasmosis* and *Blastomycosis*. Clin Infect Dis 1996; 22:S102–S111.
59. Recht LD, Daview SF, Eckman MR, Sarosi GA. *Blastomycosis* in immunosuppressed patients. Am Rev Respir Dis 1982; 125:359–362.
60. Hobbs ER. *Coccidioidomycosis*. Dermatol Clin 1989; 7:227–239.
61. Trigg ME, Comito MA, Rumelhart SL. Cutaneous *Mucor* infection treated with wide excision in two children who underwent marrow transplantation. J Pediatr Surg 1996; 31:976–977.
62. Ringeroth JD, Roth RS, Talcott JA, Rinaldi MG. *Zygomycosis* due to *Mucor circinelloides* in a neutropenic patient receiving chemotherapy for acute myelogenous leukemia. Clin Infect Dis 1994; 19:135–137.
63. Nomura J, Ruskin J, Sahebi F, Kogut N, Falk PM. *Mucormycosis* of the vulva following bone marrow transplantation. Bone Marrow Transplant 1997; 19:859–860.
64. MacDonald ML, Weiss PJ, Deloach-Banta LJ, Comer SW. Primary cutaneous *Mucormycosis* with a *Mucor* species: is iron overload a factor? Cutis 1994; 54:275–278.
65. Klotz SA, Drutz DJ, Huppert M, Johnson JE. *Pityrosporum* folliculitis. Arch Intern Med 1982; 142:2126–2129.
66. Bufill JA, Lum LG, Caya JG, Chitambar CR, Ritch PS, Anderson T, Ash RC. *Pityrosporum* folliculitis after bone marrow transplantation. Ann Intern Med 1988; 108:560–563.
67. Mandell GL, Bennett JE, Dolin R. Principles and Practice of Infectious Diseases. 5th ed. Philadelphia: Churchill Livingstone, 2000.
68. Wood MJ. Viral infections in neutropenia-current problems and chemotherapeutic control. J Antimicrob Chemother 1998; 41:81–93.
69. Fitzpatrick TB, Johnson RA, Wolff K. Color Atlas and Synopsis of Clinical Dermatology. 3d ed. New York: McGraw-Hill, 1997.
70. Haki M, Tsuchida M, Kotsuji M, Iijima S, Tamura K, Koike K, Izumi I, Tanaka M, Hirano T. Gianotti–Crosti syndrome associated with *Cytomegalovirus* antigenemia after bone marrow transplantation. Bone Marrow Transplant 1997; 20:691–693.

31

Infections Associated with Radiation Therapy

Brent W. Laartz and John N. Greene
University of South Florida, School of Medicine
and Moffitt Cancer Center and Research Institute
Tampa, Florida, U.S.A.

OVERVIEW

Radiation therapy has been utilized effectively in the last 30 years as an adjunct and sometimes as primary therapy for controlling malignant tumor growth. It has been refined significantly in recent years to narrow the focus of the beam and lower the levels of radiation required for tumor control. However, the effect of the irradiation on the host immune cells, endothelial cells, and fibroblasts can create problems with healing and soft tissue infections. The combination of radiation with surgery necessarily creates problems with healing that can manifest as wound infections and abscess formation.

EFFECTS OF RADIATION ON IMMUNITY AND HEALING

Radiation inflicts its damage on rapidly dividing cells, by damaging DNA. Cells have differing susceptibilities to the damage from radiation. There are two types of radiation damage: early phase and late phase. Early phase

367

damage occurs to rapidly proliferating cells such as epithelial cells, causing mucositis, xerostomia, proctitis, and skin damage. Late phase damage occurs 6 or more months later with depletion of fibroblasts and stem cells, thus impairing the capacity for subsequent wound healing; this can lead to fistula formation and fibrosis [1,2]. Another late effect is decreased vascularity, which likewise could affect the ability of tissues to heal and also affects the ability to fight infections in the irradiated field [1].

There is a modest short-lived effect of radiation on host immunity. The migratory function of neutrophils in tissue is diminished by irradiation [3,4]. Additionally, the function of neutrophils in releasing reactive oxygen species in response to phorbol myristate was inhibited by irradiation; however, upon stimulation with tumor cells, their capacity for increased reactive oxygen species release was preserved [4]. Neutrophils are locally replaced every three days, so this effect may only be observed immediately postirradiation.

ENT INFECTIONS

The extensive use of adjunctive radiation in head and neck cancers and the close relation of epithelial layers with visceral structures have resulted in many reports of associated infections. Xerostomia, resulting from temporary destruction of salivary gland epithelial cells, decreases the amount of secretory enzymes and IgA in the oral cavity. The mucositis related to radiation allows local invasion of oral microbial flora into the submucosal region. Possible organisms causing these local infections include *Candida* species, gram-negative bacilli, *Staphylococcus aureus*, anaerobic streptococcus, and herpes simplex virus [5].

In one study, oral *Candida* colonization occurred in 73% of patients receiving radiation for head and neck cancer, and infection occurred in 27%. Fifty-nine percent of the isolates were nonalbicans *Candida* species. However, 100% of the infections responded to appropriate therapy [6]. In addition, one must be wary of invasive mold infections, especially in those receiving concomitant chemotherapy or in those who have functionally suppressed immune systems as in diabetes, leukemia, or lymphoma. One case report of laryngeal aspergillosis following radiation therapy was found in a diabetic patient which was cauterized by laser with no evidence of recurrence [7].

SKIN AND SOFT TISSUE INFECTIONS

Following radiation, especially to lymphatic beds such as the abdomen, pelvis, neck, axillary, and inguinal regions, lymphatic drainage is compromised. This is compounded by the often accompanying surgical resection of lymph nodes. The resulting lymphedema can predispose to cellulitis and fasciitis of the area drained by the irradiated lymph nodes. Common organisms are group A *Streptococcus*, *Staphylococcus aureus* and gram-negative organisms. Synergistic gangrene can occur with mixed aerobic and anaerobic organisms.

Postoperative wound infections commonly occur when the incision is made in an area previously or subsequently exposed to radiation. Waiting 3 weeks after radiation to perform surgery or waiting 3 weeks after surgery to perform radiation have been found to help prevent wound breakdown [1,2].

OSTEORADIONECROSIS AND OSTEOMYELITIS

Osteoradionecrosis is a well-documented complication of radiation to the head and neck region, to long bones and to the spine [8–13]. The necrotic region is predisposed to developing osteomyelitis and overlying cellulitis. Whenever cellulitis is present in an irradiated area in close proximity to bone, one must rule out underlying osteonecrosis and osteomyelitis. Organisms causing infection include those that frequently inhabit the area in question, such as *Staphylococcus epidermidis*, *Staphylococcus aureus*, *Candida* species, and gram-negative bacilli.

CHEST INFECTIONS

Chest irradiation for a variety of tumors including lung cancer and breast cancer can cause pleuritis, mediastinitis, pneumonitis, and bronchiolitis obliterans, which may mimic infection. Radiation pneumonitis refers to a syndrome of dyspnea, nonproductive cough, and fever with pulmonary infiltrates [14]. Bronchiolitis obliterans and organizing pneumonia (BOOP) has a similar presenation with effective response to steroid therapy. CT and histological findings usually assist in diagnosis [15,16]. However, it is often difficult to discern whether an infiltrate is caused by one of these noninfectious causes or by a bacterial or fungal pneumonia. Antibiotics are commonly given in addition to steroids. See Chapter 15 for a more detailed discussion on radiation pneumonitis and BOOP.

Infectious pneumonia can also occur after radiation secondary to decreased ability to regenerate normal alveolar architecture. Organisms involved are similar to those of community-acquired and nosocomial pneumonia, depending on the patient's exposure to hospital-acquired organisms. Pneumococcal and gram negative organisms are frequent. *Aspergillus* and other molds can infect an irradiated lung and should be considered, especially if the infiltrate looks nodular or cavitary. Recurrent pneumonia after irradiation must alert clinicians to the possibility of tracheoesophageal fistula formation.

Chest irradiation also may predispose to radiation-induced esophagitis or infectious esophagitis. Endoscopy is necessary to distinguish these two entities. Infectious causes of esophagitis include *Candida* species, herpes simplex virus, and cytomegalovirus. Of 16 patients with esophagitis following radiation who underwent endoscopy, 5 patients had documented *Candida* esophagitis and 1 patient had herpes simplex virus [17].

GI AND GU INFECTIONS

Radiation for prostate and rectal carcinomas often results in proctitis, a syndrome of diarrhea, rectal pain, and bleeding. The syndrome can be acute or chronic, and complications include ulceraton, fistulation, abscess formation, and perforation [18]. Infections such as abscess formation are commonly caused by bowel microbial flora such as gram-negative bacteria, *Enterococcus*, anaerobes, and *Candida* species. Herpes simplex virus infection can also complicate proctitis associated with radiation.

Colovesicle fistulae and anovaginal fistulae formation can lead to frequent urinary tract infections or perineal abscess formation [19]. Fournier's gangrene has also been reported following radiation therapy [20,21]. Organisms involved in these infections are commonly mixed aerobic and anaerobic bacteria.

PREVENTION AND NEW MODALITIES

Prevention of infection following radiation involves treatment of the mucositis aggressively with therapies such as peridex mouthwashes and fluoride treatments for oral mucositis and metronidazole and sucralfate for radiation proctitis [22–24]. Hyperbaric oxygen treatment represents an exciting new modality to treat proctitis [25], cystitis [26], lymphedema [27], neurosurgical infections [28], and postoperative wound infections in irradiated fields. Hyperbaric oxygen is also indicated for treatment of osteoradionecrosis [29,30]. Vacuum-assisted drainage dressings also have been employed to promote wound healing.

REFERENCES

1. Hom DB, Adams GL, Monyak D. Irradiated soft tissue and its management. Otolaryngol Clin North Am 1995; 28(5):1003–1019.
2. Moore MJ. The effect of radiation on connective tissue. Otolaryngol Clin North Am 1984; 17:389–399.

3. Frumento G, Bonvini E, Minervini F, Dallegri F, Patrone F, Sacchetti C. Defective neutrophil mobilization to skin chambers in cancer patients. J Cancer Res Clin Oncol 1984; 107:53–56.
4. De Vries A, Holzberger P, Kunc M, Hengster P. Influence of irradiation on neutrophilic granulocyte function. Cancer 2001; 92(9):2444–2450.
5. Nikoskelainen J. Oral infections related to radiation and immunosuppressive therapy. J Clin Periodontal 1990; 17:504–507.
6. Redding SW, Zellars RC, Kirkpatrick WR, McAfee RK, Caceres MA, Fothergill AW, Lopez-Ribot JL, Bailey CW, Rinaldi MG, Patterson TF. Epidemiology of oropharyngeal Candida colonization and infection in patients receiving radiation for head and neck cancer. J Clin Micriobiol 1999; 37:3896–3900.
7. Ogawa Y, Nishiyama N, Hagiwara A, Ami T, Fujita H, Yoshida T, Suzuki M. A case of laryngeal aspergillosis following radiation therapy. Auris Nasus Larynx 2002; 29:73–76.
8. Warscotte L, Duprez T, Lonneux M, Michaux L, Renard L, Sindic CJ, Lecouvet FE. Concurrent spinal cord and vertebral bone marrow radionecrosis 8 years after therapeutic irradiation. Neuroradiology 2002; 44(3):245–248.
9. Jereczek-Fossa BA, Orecchia R. Radiotherapy-induced mandibular bone complications. Cancer Treatment Reviews 2002; 28(1):65–74.
10. Celik N, Wei FC, Chen HC, Cheng MH, Huang WC, Tsai FC, Chen YC. Osteoradionecrosis of the mandible after oromandibular cancer surgery. Plastic and Reconstructive Surgery 2002; 109(6):1875–1881.
11. Schwartz HC, Kagan AR. Osteoradionecrosis of the mandible: scientific basis for clinical staging. American Journal of Clinical Oncology 2002; 25(2):168–171.
12. Lieblich SE, Piecuch JF. Infections of the jaws, including infected fractures, osteomyelitis, and osteoradionecrosis. Atlas of the Oral & Maxillofacial Surgery Clinics of North America 2000; 8(1):121–132.
13. Vanderpuye V, Goldson A. Osteoradionecrosis of the mandible. Journal of the National Medical Association 2000; 92(12):579–584.
14. Salinas FV, Winterbauer RH. Radiation pneumonitis: a mimic of infectious pneumonitis. Semin Respir Infect 1995; 10(3):143–153.
15. Epler GR. Bronchiolitis obliterans organizing pneumonia. Semin Respir Infect 1995; 10(2):65–77.
16. Stover DE, Milite F, Zakowski M. A newly recognized syndrome—radiation-related bronchiolitis and organizing pneumonia. Respiration 2001; 68:540–544.
17. Perez RA, Early DS. Endoscopy in patients receiving radiation therapy to the thorax. Dig Dis Sci 2002; 47(1):79–83.
18. Ramirez PT. Sigmoid perforation following radiation therapy in patients with cervical cancer. Gynecol Oncol 2001; 82(1):150–155.
19. Senatore PJ. Anovaginal fistulae. Surg Clin North Am 1994; 74(6):1361–1375.
20. Laucks SS. Fournier's gangrene. Surg Clin North Am 1994; 74(6):1339–1352.
21. Khan S, Smith NL, Gonder M, Ravo B, Siddharth P. Gangrene of male external genitalia in a patient with colorectal disease. Dis Colon Rectum 1985; 28:519.

22. Epstein JB. Infection prevention in bone marrow transplantation in bone marrow transplantation and radiation patients. NCI Monogr 1990; 9:73–85.
23. Fleming TJ. Oral tissue changes of radiation oncology and their management. Dent Clin North Am 1990; 34(2):223–237.
24. Denton A, Forbes A, Andreyev J, Maher EJ. Non-surgical interventions for late radiation proctitis in patients who have received radical radiotherapy to the pelvis. The Cochrane Library 2. Oxford: Update Software, 2002.
25. Kitta T, Shinohara N, Shirato H, Otsuka H, Koyanagi T. The treatment of chronic radiation proctitis with hyperbaric oxygen in patients with prostate cancer. BJU International 2000; 85:372–374.
26. Mayer R, Klemen H, Quehenberger F, Sankin O, Mayer E, Hackl A, Smolle-Juettner FM. Hyperbaric oxygen—an effective tool to treat radiation morbidity in prostate cancer. Radiotherapy and Oncology 2001; 61:151–156.
27. Carl UM, Feldmeier JJ, Schmitt G, Hartmann KA. Hyperbaric oxygen therapy for late sequelae in women receiving radiation after breast-conserving surgery. Int J Radiat Biol Oncol Phys 2001; 49(4):1029–1031.
28. Larsson A, Engstrom M, Uusijarvi J, Kihlstrom L, Lind F, Mathiesen T. Hyperbaric oxygen treatment of postoperative neurosurgical infections. Neurosurg 2002; 50:287–296.
29. Porter BR, Brian JE Jr. Hyperbaric oxygen therapy and osteoradionecrosis. Iowa Dental Journal 1999; 85(3):23–27.
30. Maier A, Gaggl A, Klemen H, Santler G, Anegg U, Fell B, Karcher H, Smolle-Juttner FM, Friehs GB. Review of severe osteoradionecrosis treated by surgery alone or surgery with postoperative hyperbaric oxygen. Br J Oral Maxillofac Surg 2000; 38:167–246.

32

Complications of Surgery in Cancer Patients

John N. Greene

University of South Florida, School of Medicine
and Moffitt Cancer Center and Research Institute
Tampa, Florida, U.S.A.

Nick Nicoonahad

Shriner's Hospital
Tampa, Florida, U.S.A.

Cancer patients are at increased risk for surgical site infections (SSI) due to malnutrition, and immunosuppression from their malignancy or its therapy. They have a higher incidence of colonization of the skin with *Staphylococcus aureus*, including methicillin-resistant *S. aureus* (MRSA). Chronic skin colonization with *Staphylococcus aureus* frequently precedes an SSI. In addition, corticosteroid therapy, chemotherapy, and radiotherapy delay wound healing and closure which can lead to an SSI. Another risk factor for poor wound healing and SSI is cigarette smoking. A history of a prior SSI increases the risk of subsequent wound infection. A review of SSI unique to cancer patients based on the type of malignancy is presented.

BRAIN CANCER

Infection following brain cancer resection includes superficial wound infections, subgaleal fluid collection infection, meningitis, and brain abscess. The risk of SSI following neurosurgery in cancer patients is increased in patients with prior neurosurgery, chemotherapy, radiotherapy, prolonged use of corticosteroids, a history of prior wound infection, prolonged intraoperative time, and the placement of a gliadel (BCNU) chemotherapy wafer into the brain tumor cavity. A cerebral spinal fluid (CSF) leak is a significant risk factor for meningitis. When a CSF leak is present, prophylactic antibiotics are warranted. The most common causes of superficial and deep-seated post-neurosurgical infections are *Staphylococcus aureus* and enteric gram-negative bacilli (GNB), especially *P. aeruginosa* and *Enterobacter* species. Propionobacter acnes is a rare but life-threatening cause of brain abscess or meningitis following neurosurgery. If a foreign body is in place such as a bone plate or a ventriculoperitoneal shunt, then coagulase-negative *Staphylococci* are the most common cause of neurosurgical infections. Rarely, anaerobes such as anaerobic Streptococci and Peptostreptococcus can cause a deep-seated infection if the sinuses are entered during surgery.

The drugs of choice for deep-seated brain infections include intravenous Vancomycin and Meropenem or Cefepime for 3 to 6 weeks to treat the aforementioned pathogens. Osteomyelitis of the skull plate may rarely develop and require removal of the bone plate followed by placement of a titanium plate. Radionecrosis of surrounding bone may lead to recurrent infection and chronic osteomyelitis despite the best of resection procedures.

HEAD AND NECK CANCER

Patients requiring major oncological head and neck surgery are at high risk for postoperative wound infection when the surgical site is contaminated with oropharyngeal secretions (i.e., saliva) [1]. The bacterial load in saliva is several orders of magnitude greater than that used to define soft tissue infection (10^8 cells/mL versus 10^5 cells/g tissue, respectively) [2]. With this in mind, prophylaxis antibiotics commonly used for head and neck surgery in cancer patients include clindamycin or ampicillin/sulbactam [1]. These agents are very effective at reducing the common flora found in the mouth, pharynx, and sinuses as well as the skin, namely *S. aureus*, *Streptococci* and anaerobic bacteria. However, when infections do occur while receiving these agents, resistant pathogens tend to predominate. These organisms include enteric gram-negative bacilli, MRSA, and *Candida* species [2,3]. MRSA is a significant cause of SSI in patients with head and neck cancer. Parton et al. report four cases of serious MRSA SSI following head and neck surgery with one death attributed to local spread of the infection [4].

Even in the presence of appropriate antibiotic prophylaxis, infections can occur in 10 to 20% of surgical procedures for head and neck cancer [5]. A study that evaluated complications in head and neck surgical procedures found several risk factors [6]. Prior radiotherapy, prolonged operative time, perioperative transfusion, and flap reconstruction were all associated with a significantly higher overall complication rate. Only prior radiotherapy correlated with an increase in SSI in this study. In another report, bilateral neck dissections, advanced disease, type of laryngectomy, and history of prior tracheostomy increased the risk of SSI following head and neck surgery [7]. Radionecrosis of the mandible may result in osteomyelitis that is polymicrobial and is mentioned in detail in the chapter "Bone, Joint, and Soft Tissue Infections."

BREAST CANCER

Infections following surgery for breast cancer include SSI from lumpectomy, mastectomy, and axillary lymph node dissection. Breast expanders or implants can likewise become infected with pathogens common with a foreign device. Myocutaneous flaps can develop necrosis, failure to engraft, and infection. As with other types of surgery, smoking is a risk factor for postmastectomy wound infection and skin flap necrosis [8]. The risk factors for SSI following breast cancer surgery is the same for other locations of the body, namely, hematoma or seroma formation, prolonged surgical drains, lymphedema, prior chemotherapy or radiation therapy, and a history of a prior SSI. *S. aureus* (including MRSA) is the most common pathogen followed by beta-hemolytic *Streptococci*, enteric gram-negative bacilli, and occasionally rapidly growing *Mycobacterium*. Rarely, chest wall infection (ribs and cartilage) can develop, especially if a mesh is present. *S. aureus* and *Pseudomonas aeruginosa* predominate, the latter especially when cartilage of the costochondral junction is involved.

LUNG CANCER AND ESOPHAGEAL CANCER

Surgical-related infections following lung cancer resection includes pneumonia, empyema, SSI, and bronchopleural fistula (BPF) formation. Empyema due to chest tube placement usually is due to *S. aureus* (including MRSA) originating from skin colonization. Occasionally enteric GNB, and alpha-hemolytic *Streptococci* and *Candida* species, can cause empyema, especially if a BPF or esophageal anastomosis leak is present. The mainstay of treatment is surgical drainage of pockets of fluid collection and appropriate antimicrobial therapy for 3 to 6 weeks. BPF may close spontaneously in time, but subsequent reoperation is frequently required. Chronic drainage of pleural fluid collections is necessary to prevent recurrent empyema and pneumonia.

COLORECTAL AND GYNECOLOGICAL CANCER

The primary infections following colorectal surgery besides SSI are peritonitis, bowel perforation, intra-abdominal abscess and sepsis. Abdominal wall mesh infections may develop in patients requiring hernia repair following abdominal surgery for colorectal cancer. Enterocutaneous fistula may develop and require prolonged bowel rest, and frequently future surgical repair. Perineum infections can occur after abdominal perineal resection, as well as a presacral abscess, and rarely sacral osteomyelitis [9]. The predominant pathogens include *S. aureus* (including MRSA), enteric GNB, enteric anaerobes, *Enterococci*, and *Candida* species, usually in combination as a polymicrobial infection. Broad-spectrum antibiotics, and antifungals for prolonged periods of time, along with surgical debridement and drainage, are necessary for successful management.

When the cancer is progressive, especially with a necrotic center, secondary fistula and abscess formation that is polymicrobial may develop. Lifelong antimicrobial therapy may be needed to prevent further spread of infection. Aggressive radiation therapy may result in radiation colits with perforation and fistula formation, which may require resection and a colostomy. When the patient is not a surgical candidate, prolonged antibiotics may prevent further spread of infection. In summary, surgery in cancer patients is known to carry a higher risk for an SSI. However, with a better understanding of risk factors for infections, preventive measures can be taken to reduce the risk of and complications from a SSI.

REFERENCES

1. Johnson JT, Kachman K, Wagner RL, Myers EN. Comparison of ampicillin/sulbactam versus clindamycin in the prevention of infection in patients undergoing head and neck surgery. Head Neck 1997; 19:367–371.
2. Barry B. Pharyngeal flora in patients undergoing head and neck oncologic surgery. Acta Otorhinolaryngol Belg 1999; 53:237–240.
3. Callender DL. Antibiotic prophylaxis in head and neck oncologic surgery: the role of gram-negative coverage. Int J Antimicrob Agents 1999; 12(suppl 1):S21-S27.
4. Parton M, Beasley NJ, Harvey G, Houghton D, Jones AS. Four cases of aggressive MRSA wound infection following head and neck surgery. J Laryngol Otol 1997; 111:874–876.
5. Simons JP, Johnson JT, Yu VL, Vickers RM, Gooding WE, Myers EN, Pou

AM, Wagner RL, Grandis JR. The role of topical antibiotic prophylaxis in patients undergoing contaminated head and neck surgery with flap reconstruction. Laryngoscope 2001; 111:329–335.

6. Penel N, Lefebvre D, Fournier C, Sarini J, Kara A, Lefevbre JL. Risk factors for wound infection in head and neck cancer surgery: a prospective study. Head Neck 2001; 23:447–455.

7. Barry B, Lucet JC, Kosmann MJ, Gehanno P. Risk factors for surgical wound infections in patients undergoing head and neck oncologic surgery. Acta Otorhinolaryngol Belg 1999; 53:241–244.

8. Sorensen LT, Horby J, Friis E, Pilsgraad B, Jorgensen T. Smoking as a risk factor for wound healing and infection in breast cancer surgery. Eur Jour Surg Oncol 2002; 28:815–820.

9. Poulin EC, Schlachta CM, Seshadri PA, Cadeddu MO, Gregoire R, Mamazza J. Septic complications of elective laparascopic colorectal resection. Surg Endosc 2001; 15:203–208.

33

Catheter-Related Infections

Ioannis Chatzinikolaou and Issam I. Raad
The University of Texas, M. D. Anderson Cancer Center
Houston, Texas, U.S.A.

INTRODUCTION

Significance of Central Venous Catheters and the Cost of Related Infections

The use of catheters has revolutionized the way cancer patients are treated, and the advent of catheter technology is closely related to the improvement of the quality of cancer care and of the life of cancer patients. Effective cancer care can be considered only if there is a safe and reliable intravascular access in order to administer chemotherapy, blood products, antibiotics, fluids, electrolytes, and nutritional support.

The most common and life-threatening complication of catheters is infection. Catheter-related bloodstream infection (CRBSI) is the most common type of nosocomial infection, and it is associated with significant morbidity and mortality [1–6]. Additionally they contribute to the majority of nosocomial cases of septicemia caused by *Staphylococcus epidermidis*, *Staphylococcus aureus*, and *Candida* spp. [6–8]. In cancer patients the risk of CRBSI is even higher than in other patients owing to a multitude of host factors (compromised skin due to radiation therapy or bioimmunotherapy such as interleukin-2, increased use of intensive chemotherapeutic regimens leading to profound and prolonged neutropenia, and aggressive surgery).

Approximately 5 million central venous catheters (CVC) are inserted annually in the United States, and 1 out of 20 of them is anticipated to be associated with at least one episode of bacteremia despite the use of antiseptic technique during catheter insertion and maintenance [9]. The attributable mortality of such infections is calculated to be 12 to 25%. In critically ill patients, CRBSI result in an additional 6.5 days stay in the ICU with extra attributable costs per survivor averaging in excess of $28,000 [2]. It is estimated that approximately 80,000 episodes of CRBSI occur annually in U.S. intensive care units alone, thus raising the cost of medical care an additional $296 million to $2.3 billion [10,11].

Types of Catheters

There is no standard agreed-upon definition of the types of catheters based on the duration of dwell time. For the purposes of this chapter we are going to define long-term catheters as the ones that stay in place for >30 days [12]. Consequently, short-term catheters are devices that remain in place for < 30 days. Although both types of catheters are extensively used in cancer patients, it is the long-term central venous catheters that are predominantly used in this type of patient population. Additionally, central venous catheters are associated with more serious infections, and their relative risk for a CRBSI is 2 to 855 times higher than that of peripheral venous catheters [13–15]. For the reasons mentioned above, our chapter will focus on long-term central venous catheters (CVC).

Currently there are four types of long-term CVC (Table 1): tunneled catheters (Broviac, Hickman, Groshong), nontunneled CVC (e.g., Hohn), peripherally inserted central catheters (PICCs), and implantable ports (ports).

Tunneled Catheters

The catheter tips of the tunneled silicone catheters end in the superior vena cava. Their exit is tunneled under the skin on the chest. In 1973, Broviac and his colleagues described the first tunneled catheter to be used in pediatric patients in need of total parenteral nutrition [16]. In 1979, a different type of tunneled catheter for cancer patients undergoing bone marrow transplantation was introduced by Hickman et al. [17]. The Hickman catheter has a wider lumen and thicker wall. About 1 inch before the exit site there is a small Dacron cuff that serves as both an anchor and a barrier to infection. Hickman catheters are the more widely used tunneled catheters. The Groshong catheter is a newer version of the Hickman, with thinner walls and a narrower lumen. It has a rounded, closed tip and the Groshong valve.

TABLE 1 Characteristics of Different Types of Long-Term Central Venous Catheters (CVC)

Type of catheter	Advantages	Disadvantages
Tunneled catheter (TC)	—Low risk of infection	—Surgical procedure —High cost
Nontunneled catheters (NTC)	—Lower cost than tunneled —Comparable infection rate to TC during first 6 months of placement	—Lower durability than TC and IP
Peripherally inserted CVCs (PICC)	—Inserter can be a trained healthcare worker other than physician —Low cost —No risk of pneumothorax —Comparable infection rate to TC during first 3 months after placement	—High incidence of mechanical irritation (phlebitis) —Limited durability
Implantable ports (IP)	—Lowest infection rate —Minimally interfering with regular activities —Minimal maintenance required	—Most expensive —Most extensive surgical procedure

The valve remains closed when the catheter is not in use, sealing the fluid inside the catheter and thus preventing contact with the blood. During an infusion, the pressure of the incoming fluid opens the valve, letting the fluid enter the bloodstream. When suction is applied, i.e., through a syringe, the negative pressure causes the valve to open inwards, letting blood flow through the catheter into the syringe. The valve eliminates the need for routine clamping of the catheter. A Groshong catheter does not need heparin flushes; weekly flushing with saline is all that is required to ensure the patency of the catheter. Tunneled catheters are available in single, double, and triple lumen.

Nontunneled Long-Term Catheters

Nontunneled silicone catheters can remain in place for a period up to 400 days without complication [18], making them a possible alternative to tunneled catheters, when long catheterization is needed. Since they are inserted percutaneously, their insertion/removal or exchange can take place in an outpatient setting, associating them with lower cost than tunneled catheters. Additionally, they can be exchanged over a guide wire, increasing patients' comfort.

There are two types of nontunneled silicone catheters: nontunneled subclavian catheters and peripherally inserted central catheters (PICC). The nontunneled subclavian catheters (e.g., Hohn catheters) are inserted percutaneously in the subclavian vein. They are available in single, double, and triple lumen. A PICC is inserted in the antecubital space (cephalic or basilic veins). Trained nurses, members of an infusion therapy team, can insert these single-lumen catheters, so PICC are highly cost-effective [18]. Their main disadvantage is that they are associated with high rates of mechanical irritation (aseptic phlebitis). This type of catheter can stay in place for an average of 3 months and is associated with low infection rates [18].

Implantable Ports

These single or double-lumen silicone catheters consist of a reservoir that is surgically implanted in a subcutaneous pocket usually on the upper chest (central ports) [19]. A small catheter is tunneled through the subcutaneous tissue and it terminates in the superior vena cava. The reservoir can be accessed through the skin, using a needle, whenever a medication infusion or blood draw is necessary. Since these devices are completely covered by skin they do not interfere with the patient's body image or lifestyle. Maintenance is minimal, rendering them suitable for pediatric patients or others with active lifestyles [20]. Ports are, though, the most expensive long-term intravascular devices.

PATHOGENESIS AND MICROBIOLOGY

The pathogenesis of bloodstream catheter infections is a complex and dynamic interplay between four protagonists: the catheter material/surface, the microbes, the human factor, and the iatrogenic factor. The first scene of the play is the colonization of the catheter by microorganisms. For short-term nontunneled catheters, the external surface of the catheter is more likely the source of CRBSI. The breach of a naturally occurring barrier, the skin, by the inserted catheter, permits the migration of members of the skin flora, such as *Staphylococcus aureus* and coagulase-negative staphylococci. Microorganisms migrate from the skin insertion site, through the cutaneous catheter tract, to the catheter, colonizing the external catheter surface and eventually the catheter tip [9,21–23] (Fig. 1). Another albeit less frequent way of colonization of the external surface of the catheter is through hematogenous seeding from a distant site [24–27]. With long-term catheters, the contamination of the catheter hub, leading to intraluminal microbial colonization, becomes a more important source of CRBSI [28–33]. Additional supportive evidence is provided by electron microscopy studies [12] suggesting that hub/lumen contamination is the most likely mechanism of CRBSI for long-term

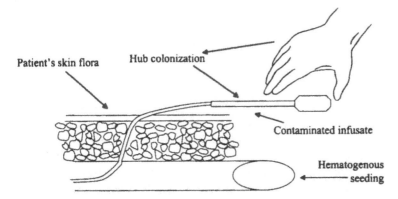

FIGURE 1   Potential sources of contamination of intravascular catheters. Catheter-related infection develops most commonly from microorganisms colonizing the skin surface, followed by the hub and much less frequently from infusion fluid or hematogenous seeding.

catheters (>30 days dwell time), whereas for short-term catheters the skin is more likely to be the source of infection [9,21,28,31,34]. A much less commonly reported source of CRBSI is through contaminated intravenous fluids [1,35].

Vascular catheters within a short time after insertion become uniformly colonized with biofilm, an architecturally complex structure that is rich in exopolysaccharides. Following their attachment on the catheter surface, microorganisms, such as *S. aureus*, coagulase-negative *Staphylococci*, and *Candida parapsilosis*, undergo phenotypic and enzymatic changes resulting in the production of exopolysaccharide, a major component of the biofilm [36–46]. Recent studies on *S. epidermidis* have described a polysaccharide adhesin (PS/A) that is crucial to the pathogenesis of CRBSI [47]. Similar work on *Saccharomyces cerevisiae* and a genomic library from *C. albicans* lead to the identification of the ALA gene, whose product seems to play a crucial role in adherence to fibronectin, laminin, type IV collagen, and epithelial cells [48]. Recently, the genetic control of biofilm production has begun to be elucidated in *S. epidermidis*, *S. aureus*, and *C. albicans* [43,44,49,50]. Synthesis of the capsular polysaccharide in *Staphylococcus* spp. is mediated by the *ica* operon. The key event in biofilm formation is a phenomenon called quorum sensing [51]. Quorum sensing is an intermicrobial communication system vital for the regulation of a diverse array of processes, such as plasmid transfer, the activation of virulence factors, and biofilm formation. This communication is accomplished via chemical messengers like acyl-homoserine-lactone [52] and other peptides. Quorum sensing has been reported in all the major pathogens involved in CRBSI (*S. aureus, Staphylococcus epidermidis*, and *Candida* spp.) [53–55]. The microorganisms that are embedded in the biofilm layer become more resistant to different antibiotics [37,56,57], especially the glycopeptides [58], since they live in a microenvironment that acts as a barrier to circulating antibiotics.

Various host-derived proteins enhance the process of adherence and colonization. Soon after insertion a thrombin sheath is formed around the internal and external surface of the catheter. This sheath is rich in host-derived proteins, such as laminin, fibrin, fibronectin, thrombospondin [59,60]. These proteins become the receptors to which various organisms, like *S. aureus, S. epidermidis*, and *C. albicans* attach themselves [61–67].

An additional factor that determines the pathogenesis of CRBSI is the material forming the catheters. Physical properties of the material, such as hydrophobicity, surface charges, irregularities, and defects as well as the thrombogenicity of the catheter surface, contribute to the process of microbial attachment [60,68]. Staphylococci preferentially adhere to silicone [61,69–71]. This is because silicone has a qualitative and quantitative negative effect on neutrophils, altering their chemotactic abilities [72–74]. Additionally, excessive complement activation by silicone surfaces, leading to local complement depletion, may interfere with neutrophil chemotaxis toward bacteria [74]. Recent attempts aim to develop materials resistant to microorganism adherence. Coating polyurethane with polyvinyl pyrrolidone led to decreased adhesion by both *S. aureus* and *S. epidermidis* [75].

Various iatrogenic factors are involved in the pathogenesis of CRBSI. Total parenteral nutrition (TPN) has been associated with increased risk for vascular catheter–related infection [76]. TPN solutions being nutritiously rich are more likely than conventional intravenous fluids to grow microbes, once contaminated [77–81]. Additionally the use of interleukin-2 (IL-2) has been associated with an increase in CRBSI, particularly with staphylococci [82–84].

The microorganisms most commonly implicated in CRBSI are predominantly skin organisms: *S. aureus* and coagulase-negative staphylococci [85] (Table 1). *Staphylococcus aureus* and coagulase-negative Staphylococci are considered to be introduced through the skin and contaminated hubs, whereas *C. albicans* and *C. parapsilosis* are thought to seed in the bloodstream from the gastrointestinal system [86], especially in cancer patients who receive cytotoxic immunosuppressive therapy. Other skin organisms such as *Bacillus* spp. and *Corynebacterium* spp. (especially the JK strains) have been reported frequently as the cause of CRBSI [87–89]. Gram-negative microorganisms such as *Pseudomonas aeruginosa, Stenotrophomonas maltophilia*, and *Acinetobacter* spp. are frequent causes of CRBSI, since they can contaminate the hands of medical personnel, IV fluids, and other fomites of the hospital environment [90,91]. Microorganisms emerging as CRBSI pathogens are

Micrococcus spp. [92], *Achromobacter* spp. [93], *Rhodococcus* spp. [94], *Mycobacterium chelonei* [95], *Mycobacterium fortuitum* [96], and fungi such as *Rhodotorula* spp. [97], *Fusarium* ssp. [98–100], and *Hansenula anomala* [101,102].

EPIDEMIOLOGY

More than 150 million intravascular devices are purchased annually by clinics and hospitals in the USA [85]. The majority of these devices are peripheral venous catheters, but more than five million CVCs are inserted each year. More than 200,000 nosocomial bloodstream infections occur annually in the United States [1]. Most of these infections are related to different types of intravascular devices, especially the nontunneled CVC [5,103]. The rates of device-related bloodstream infections vary by hospital size, hospital unit, and type of device. According to a report from the National Nosocomial Infection Surveillance (NNIS) System, the rates of central CRBSI range from 2.1 (respiratory ICU) to 30.2 (burn ICU) per 1,000 central catheter days. The rates of noncentral CRBSI were lower, ranging from 0 (medical, medical-surgical, and coronary ICU) to 2.0 (trauma ICU) per 1,000 noncentral catheter-days [5].

The incidence of CRBSI with long-term silicone catheters ranges from 1.4 to 1.9 episodes per 1,000 catheter-days [104–107]. Tunneled catheters have been shown to predispose less to CRBSI than nontunneled catheters [28,107–114]. However, two studies, one randomized, failed to demonstrate any difference in the infection rates among tunneled and nontunneled catheters [18,115]. Additional data, from a center that maintains an infusion therapy team, showed that tunneled catheters have comparable rates of infectious complications when compared to nontunneled catheters or PICC [116,117]. Totally implantable intravascular devices (ports), being totally covered by the skin, have been associated with the lowest rate of infection when compared to other long-term catheters [118–128].

Multilumen catheters have been associated with a higher risk of infection than single lumen catheters [129–133], although in more than 50% of the triple lumen catheters only a single port is being used [134]. This significant difference in infection rates is independent to underlying disease severity [129]. However, a prospective randomized study failed to demonstrate any difference in the CRBSI rate in triple lumen catheters when compared to single lumen ones [135].

The catheter insertion site is another factor influencing the rate of CRBSI. In general, the internal jugular vein is related to higher risk for infections than the subclavian vein [136–140].

The role of neutropenia as an independent risk factor for CRBSI is controversial. In a study in cancer patients with long-term tunneled CVCs [106], neutropenia (< 500 neutrophils/mm^3) was proven to be an independent risk factor for CRBSI, whereas a similar study conducted in M. D. Anderson Cancer Center [18], failed to show such an association. In the latter study [18] the only statistically significant risk factor for CRBSI was hematological malignancy, something that is supported by the study of Groeger et al. [118].

A postmortem study has demonstrated that 38% of the catheterized veins with long-term catheters had evidence of mural thrombosis and that vascular mural thrombosis of the catheterized vessels was independently associated with catheter-related septicemia [59]. Two other studies evaluating a related question failed to document an association between clotting of the catheter and risk of infection [106,118]. An analysis of data from a prospective randomized study showed that the administration of blood products through central venous catheters was a risk factor for CRBSI, whereas thrombocytopenia during catheterization may have a protective role against CRBSI [141].

CLINICAL MANIFESTATIONS

The clinical manifestations of CRBSI can be specific and nonspecific. Particularly in immunocompromised cancer patients, whose inability to launch an immune response to infectious stimuli obscures the signs and symptoms of any infectious process, the diagnosis of CRBSI can be a significant diagnostic challenge.

Nonspecific manifestations of CRBSI include fever, chills, and occasionally hypotension. Hypotension is often associated with CRBSIs caused by gram-negative bacilli or *Candida* spp.

More specific signs, like inflammation and/or purulence from the catheter site, palpable vessel cord, and occasionally purulent secretions at the skin insertion site, indicate catheter exit site infection. A quantitative culture of the affected skin or of the excretions from the insertion site can help in distinguishing sterile inflammation from an exit site infection [142]. This is particularly helpful in peripherally inserted central catheters (PICC), where local exit site inflammation can be the aftermath of mechanical irritation of the proportionately small basilic and cephalic veins and not true infection.

In tunneled catheters a greater than 2 cm inflammation extending proximally from the catheter exit site is an indication of tunnel infection.

Pocket space abscess formation should be suspected in case of inflammation or cellulitis overlying the catheter hub.

Although the majority of CRBSIs are uncomplicated, occasionally septic thrombophlebitis or deep-seated infections can occur [143]. This is particularly true with virulent microorganisms like *S. aureus*, *C. albicans*, and *Pseudomonas aeruginosa*. Septic thrombosis is suspected in the presence of swelling above the site of the thrombotic catheterized vein (swelling in the neck, shoulder or arm ipsilateral to the catheter insertion site). Imaging proof of the presence of thrombus (venography, or Doppler ultrasonography) in the vein with an indwelling catheter and positive blood cultures with clinical manifestations of sepsis establish the diagnosis. Infrequently, deep-seated infections like endocarditis, osteomyelitis, septic pulmonary emboli, and retinitis (in case of candidemia) can complicate a CRBSI [143,144].

DIAGNOSIS

Catheter-related bloodstream infection is to be suspected if a patient has (1) clinical signs and symptoms of bloodstream infection (i.e., fever, chills, hypotension), (2) blood culture(s) positive for an organism often associated with CRBSIs, such as *S. epidermidis, S. aureus, Bacillus* spp., or *C. parapsilosis*, (3) the absence of any other source for the bloodstream infection except the catheter, and (4) local catheter infection, such as exit site inflammation, tunnel tract inflammation, a port pocket abscess formation associated with bloodstream infection (Table 2).

Culture of the catheter was considered to be the gold standard for the diagnosis of catheter infection, especially in the absence of local catheter site infection. Usually the distal tip of the catheter (3–5 cm) is cultured. Culturing the subcutaneous catheter segment does not add to the diagnostic yield of the currently used methods of catheter culture [145]. A number of different methods are available for culturing vascular catheters [24,27,137,146]. The roll plate semiquantitative culture method is the most widely used [27]. This involves aseptic removal of the catheter, rolling it across an agar plate several times and counting the number of colonies of microorganisms after overnight incubation. The limiting factor of this method is that it cultures only the external surface of the catheters and does not retrieve organisms that are well embedded in the biofilm layer that covers the internal lumen of the catheter. Consequently the roll-plate semiquantitative technique is of limited usefulness in long-term catheters, in which the internal surface of the catheter is the predominant source of bloodstream infection [12].

Some laboratories use quantitative methods that are more labor intensive and more expensive. Such methods are (1) sonication [146], or (2) vortexing a catheter segment [137], or (3) infusing the catheter lumen with a known volume of broth [24]. The cutoff point differs between the various methods. It is greater than 15 colony-forming units (CFUs) for the semiquantitative [27] or at least 100 CFUs for the quantitative methods [147]. Quantitative methods have been proven to be of higher sensitivity than semiquantitative methods [147,148]. The limitation of the semiquantitative and quantitative catheter culture methods is that they require removal of the catheter [149], often resulting in wasteful removal of noncolonized catheters, in increased medical costs, and in patient inconvenience.

TABLE 2   Diagnosis of Long-Term Catheter-Related Infections

I. Criteria to suspect catheter-related infection
   1. Clinical manifestations of infection (i.e., fever, chills)
   2. Blood culture positive for likely organism (coagulase negative staphylococci, *S. aureus*, *Bacillus* spp., *Corynebacterium* spp., *Candida* spp.)
   3. No apparent source of bacteremia other than the catheter
II. Criteria to confirm the diagnosis of catheter-related infection
   1. Clinical evidence of catheter site and/or tunnel infection/inflammation (purulent discharge, erythema, tenderness, warmth)
   2. Response to antibiotic therapy within 48 hours after catheter removal; after 48 hours without response
   3. 5:1 CFU ratio of the same organism from CVC-blood culture compared to simultaneously collected peripheral blood culture
   4. ≥15 CFU (roll plate) or ≥1000 CFU (sonication) from CVC tip of the same organism as the one growing from peripheral blood culture
   5. CVC collected blood culture is positive <2 hours prior to simultaneous peripheral blood culture

CFU: colony forming units.

Catheter-related bloodstream infections can be diagnosed using simultaneous quantitative blood cultures without removing the catheter [150]. This involves drawing one set of blood cultures through the catheter and one from a percutaneous site. If both blood cultures are positive for the same microorganism and the number of CFUs in the catheter-drawn specimen is at least 5 times (≥5:1 ratio) higher than the number of CFUs from the peripheral venipuncture blood, this strongly suggests catheter-related bloodstream infection. The sensitivity of this method is higher in long-term catheters, where intraluminal transmission of microbes to the bloodstream is more common [12]. The limitation of the method is that it is costly and labor intensive, so not many hospitals use quantitative cultures in their microbiology laboratory.

A way to bypass the above-mentioned restriction and preserve the catheter in place is to use the differential time to positivity method. This requires simultaneous collection of blood through the catheter and through a peripheral venipuncture. If growth is detected in the catheter-drawn blood at least 2 hours earlier than in the simultaneously collected peripheral blood, this suggests CRBSI [151,152]. This is a simple technique and can be practiced worldwide, since many laboratories have adopted the use of automated continuously monitored blood systems. The value of this approach has been challenged by a recent study involving a small number of patients in medical/surgical ICUs [153]. However, a large prospective clinical study at M. D. Anderson Cancer Center verified the value of this method in diagnosing CRBSI [154].

Catheter related bloodstream infections can also be diagnosed using an endoluminal brush technique that involves brushing the lumen of the catheter and performing an acridine orange leukocyte cytospin (AOLC) test on blood drawn through colonized catheters [155]. Although this approach has 95% specificity and 84% sensitivity, it has been associated with induction of transient bacteremia in 6% of the study patients. Staining catheter-drawn blood with AOLC was shown to be 96% specific and 92% sensitive when diagnosing CRBSI [156]. Further larger studies are required to support such a finding.

MANAGEMENT

The optimal management of catheter related infections requires taking many parameters into account, such as the condition of the host, the type of the infecting organism, and the site and severity of infection. Especially in cancer patients, a crucial question is added: Should we remove the catheter or not? (Table 3). The rationale for removing the catheter is to eliminate the nidus of infection that continuously sheds microorganisms in the bloodstream, possibly seeding other target organs. This action, however, may lead to increased morbidity and mortality, not to mention increased cost. Since the catheter is literally the lifeline of a cancer patient, removal of a long-term catheter usually necessitates an insertion of a similar catheter at least at a different site, preferably after the infection is treated. In Hickman/Broviac or port-type catheters, this translates to another surgical procedure, which may be particularly hazardous in a patient who has thrombocytopenia or some other coagulopathy. An additional complication of insertion of new catheters is the possibility of pneumothorax.

Antibiotic lock therapy (ALT) is a new concept developed to reduce the need of catheter removal, when long-term catheters are infected. As stated earlier, the majority of these infections originate from microbes colonizing the internal lumen of the catheters. Recent studies have shown that many antibiotics are unable to kill microorganisms growing in biofilm, when used in therapeutic concentrations. Concentrations 100 to 1000 times greater are required in order to kill bacteria embedded in biofilm (sessile) than to kill planktonic (in solution) bacteria [157–160]. ALT consists of installation and holding for hours or days pharmacological concentrations of antibiotics into the catheter lumen of the infected catheter. Antibiotic solutions that contain the desired antimicrobial agent are mixed with heparin or normal saline, in sufficient volume to fill the catheter lumen (usually 2–5 mL) and are "locked" (installed) into the catheter lumen during periods when the catheter is not being used (e.g., during nighttime) [161,162]. The volume of locked antibiotic is removed before infusion of the next dose of intravenous medication or fluids through the catheter. Although the duration of ALT varies, in the

TABLE 3   Factors That May Influence the
Decision of Catheter Removal in Patients
with Catheter Infection

Factors[a]	Need for CVC removal
Type of organism	
S. epidermidis	Low
S. aureus	High
Candida spp.	High
Gram-negative	High
Type of CVC	
Tunneled	Low
Nontunneled	High
PICC	High
Port	Low
Patient's condition	
Thrombocytopenia	Low
Compromised vascular access	Low
Hypotensive shock	High
Deep seated infection	High
Tunnel infection	High

[a] None of these factors will determine removal by itself, but a combination thereof will.

majority of clinical studies [162–169] it is most often done for 2 weeks. Antibiotics that are usually used in these solutions are vancomycin at a concentration of 1 to 5 mg/mL, gentamycin and amikacin (1 to 2 mg/mL), and ciprofloxacin (1 to 2 mg/mL) [170]. Several trials of ALT on tunneled CRBSI, with or without concomitant intravenous antibiotic therapy, have reported response and catheter salvage rate in 82% of the episodes of CRBSI [170]. Since the rationale behind ALT is to sterilize the lumen of the catheter, it should be used in cancer patients with long-term catheters, whose signs of catheter-related infection indicate an intraluminal source of infection.

Exit site infections can be cured by antibiotics locally and systemically, usually without removal of the catheter [107,171]. If the infection persists for more than 48 hours, or if Pseudomonas spp. are cultured from the exit site, the removal of the catheter may be required for the eradication of the infection [107].

Tunnel infections and port pocket infections (abscesses) can sometimes be associated with significant local morbidity and even mortality. Catheter removal and 10 to 14 days of antibiotic therapy are required in order to cure the infection [170]. In the treatment of *Mycobacterium fortuitum* and *Mycobacterium chelonei* tunnel infections, surgical excision of the infected tunnel may be required [172] in addition to CVC removal.

Managing catheter-related bloodstream infections means their categorization into three groups: low, moderate, and high risk. The risk stratification depends on the virulence of the organism involved and whether the CRBSI is complicated or uncomplicated. A CRBSI is characterized as complicated if (1) the accompanying fever and/or positive blood culture(s) persist more than 48 hours despite appropriate antimicrobial therapy, (2) it is associated with hypotension, organ hypoperfusion, septic thrombosis, septic emboli, or deep-seated infections such as endocarditis [143,144] and (3) there is concurrent tunnel or port pocket infection.

A CRBSI is considered to be of low risk if it is uncomplicated and caused by a low-virulence microorganism, such as coagulase-negative staphylococci [173], the most frequent cause of bacteremia in neutropenic patients [174]. These microorganisms are not usually associated with deep-seated infections, and their dramatic increase as pathogens parallels the use of long-term catheters, accounting for the majority of CRBSI occurring annually [174–179]. From the family of coagulase-negative staphylococci, *S. epidermidis* is most commonly isolated in bloodstream infections [174]. In the case of a single positive blood culture for coagulase-negative staphylococci, the question arises if this represents a true bacteremia or just a catheter colonization or specimen contamination. Multiple positive blood cultures, isolation of the same microorganism from catheter and percutaneous blood cultures, as well as quantitative blood cultures collected through CVC, growing more than 100 cfu/mL, indicate true bloodstream infection [180]. A low-risk CRBSI can be treated without removal of the long-term catheter [173,181], with systemic administration of appropriate antibiotics for usually 10 days [170]. If the CVC is removed, appropriate systemic antibiotic therapy is recommended for 5 to 7 days [170]. If the CVC is retained and there is a high suspicion for intraluminal infection, patients should be treated with systemic antibiotics and antibiotic lock therapy for 10 to 14 days [170]. Treatment failure manifesting as persistent fever, persistently positive blood cultures, or relapse of the infection after the antibiotic therapy has been completed is a clear indication for catheter removal [170]. Vancomycin is the drug of choice in the case of methicillin-resistant *S. epidermidis*. In patients who are either allergic to vancomycin or colonized with vancomycin-resistant enterococci, novel agents such as quinopristin-dalfopristin or linezolid can be used [182–186]. In the absence of methicillin-resistant microorganisms, penicillinase-resistant penicillins (nafcillin, oxacillin) or a first-generation cephalosporin may be used if the patient is not allergic to β-lactam antibiotics. *Staphylococcus haemolyticus* is less frequently isolated from clinical specimens [175]. Its resistance pattern to multiple antibiotics, including vancomycin [175], may impose catheter removal whenever *S. haemolyticus* is implicated in CRBSI.

A moderate-risk CRBSI is an uncomplicated CRBSI caused by moderate- to high-virulence microorganisms such as *S. aureus* and *Candida* spp. These microorganisms can be associated with serious complications such as deep-seated infection or fatal septic shock [143,187]. In such cases the CRBSI is considered to be a high-risk one, especially if it occurs in an immunocompromised patient [188,189].

Owing to its high virulence and high rates of complications, *S. aureus* CRBSI requires prompt antibiotic therapy and in most cases catheter removal [143,190]. Serious complications such as deep-seated infections (endocarditis, septic thrombophlebitis, and osteomyelitis) or fatal septic shock occur at a frequency of 20 to 30% following CRBSI caused by *S. aureus* [190]. In the case of uncomplicated CRBSI a 10 to 14 day course of antibiotic therapy is sufficient to treat the infection after the catheter is removed [170,190,191]. Removal of nontunneled catheters that are infected with *S. aureus* has been associated with more rapid response to therapy and higher cure rate [143,188,191,192]. If a new catheter has to be inserted, a different site has to be chosen. Tunneled CVCs or ports should definitely be removed if there is evidence of tunnel, pocket, or exit-site infection [170]. However, in the case of patients with long-term tunneled catheters or implantable ports, in the absence of tunnel, pocket, or exit-site infection, owing to the difficulty and expenses involved with the removal of such catheters, they may be preserved, and antibiotic lock therapy may be considered in addition to 14 days of systemic antibiotic therapy [170]. The clinician is to err on the side of caution and remove the catheter. If the CVC cannot be removed, then systemic and antibiotic lock therapy are to be considered. For patients who remain febrile and/ or have positive blood cultures >3 days after appropriate antibiotic therapy has been instituted and/or the catheter has been removed, the possibility of a deep-seated infection, especially endocarditis, should be investigated [193,194]. In this case, transesophageal echocardiography (TEE) may help in the decision to remove the catheter and to guide therapy [195]. Provided that TEE is available, the use of transthoracic echocardiography for excluding a diagnosis of catheter-related endocarditis is not recommended [170] because of its low sensitivity [196]. For patients with TEE: negative results, and from whom the catheter has been removed, a 14-day systemic antibiotic therapy is recommended [170]. *Staphylococcus aureus* CRBSI complicated by a deep-seated infection, such as septic thrombosis, endocarditis, osteomyelitis, septic emboli abscesses, and septic arthritis, should be treated for 4 to 6 weeks [143,170]. Determining the duration of therapy based on findings provided by TEE is a cost-effective alternative to the administration of therapy for 1 month to all patients with *S. aureus* bacteremia [195]. The first choice for antibiotic therapy, of CRBSI caused by methicillin-susceptible *S. aureus*, should be intravenously administered β-lactam antibiotics (penicillinase-resistant penicillins, i.e., nafcillin or oxacillin [170]. In case of penicillin allergy without anaphylaxis or angioedema, first- or second-generation cephalosporins such as cefazolin or cefuroxime can be used [170]. The addition of aminoglycosides (gentamycin) for the first 5 to 7 days of therapy may improve eradication of the *S. aureus* infection [6]. For patients who are allergic to β-lactam antibiotics, and for those with methicillin-resistant *S.aureus*, vancomycin is the drug of choice [170]. In case of *S. aureus* isolates with reduced susceptibility to vancomycin, the use of linezolid or quinopristin/dalfopristin is a therapeutic alternative.

All patients with candidemia should be treated [170]. Candidemia is the third or fourth most common cause of nosocomial bloodstream infections. It occurs usually in seriously ill patients with multiple catheters and is associated with high attributable mortality rate, as high as 38% [197]. Hemodynamically stable patients with CRBSI caused by *C. albicans* or *C. parapsilosis* can be treated with fluconazole provided that it has not been recently used either prophylactically or therapeutically [198,199]. A 14-day regimen of fluconazole (400 mg/day) has been proven as effective as and less toxic than amphotericin B (0.5 mg/kg/day) given for the same length of time [198]. Amphotericin B is recommended in patients with catheter-related candidemia who are hemodynamically unstable. Additionally, infections caused by fluconazole-resistant *Candida* spp. such as *C. krusei* should be treated with high-dose amphotericin B (1.0 mg/kg/day) [200–202]. Treatment should be provided for 14 days after the last positive culture result and when signs and symptoms of infection have resolved [170]. Since *C. albicans* and other candida species adhere avidly to materials used in vascular catheters [203], the removal of all central catheters from all patients with candidemia is considered to be standard practice and reinforced by recent consensus guidelines [170,200]. In neutropenic cancer patients, however, who have mucositis (ex. acute leukemia, bone marrow transplantation), independent of the vascular catheter, the gastrointestinal system is an important source of *C. albicans* [204–207]. Vascular catheters may, however, be the primary source of fungemia [208–210]. Predictors of catheter-related candidemia include quantitative blood cultures suggestive of CRBSI (≥5:1 CFU ratio from blood collected through the catheter, compared to blood collected from a peripheral vein); indicative differential time to positivity (>2 hours for blood collected from a percutaneous venipuncture, compared with the one drawn through the CVC); isolation of *C. parapsilosis* from blood samples; candidemia in a non-neutropenic patient who has a CVC in place and no other apparent source of bloodstream infection; candidemia in a patient who is receiving TPN through the catheter; and persistent fungemia in a patient with a CVC, who is not responding to systemic antifungal therapy [170]. Several studies have evaluated the impact of CVC removal on the outcome of candidemia [189,211–223]. In the majority of these studies, catheter removal was associated with decreased duration of fungemia, recurrence of infection, and improved survival [189,211–222]. In a prospective observational study, in 145 cases of candidemia in patients with different underlying conditions, catheter retention was the only variable associated with increased risk of death on multivariate analysis [212]. However, when the same scientific team looked into the risk factors for death in cancer patients with fungemia, the variables associated with an increased risk for death in multivariate analysis were older age, persistent neutropenia, and low performance status [215]. In a large multicenter prospective observational study of 427 consecutive patients with candidemia, CVC retention was an independent risk factor for persistence of candidemia after 72 hours of antifungal therapy and was associated with higher mortality [211]. In a review of the existing literature, with the notable absence of a prospective randomized study whose primary endpoint is the evaluation of the effect of vascular catheter removal in patients with candidemia, the consensus of catheter removal in all patients with candidemia was not substantiated [224]. Given the limitations of the studies published today, and based on our experience, we believe that early therapy with a parenteral agent is important, since sustained fungemia is associated with poor outcome [189]. An organism as adherent as *Candida* spp. to catheter surface can be more predictive of catheter-related candidemia [225], even in the setting of neutropenic cancer patients. Removal of the catheter is a common-sense therapeutic approach, especially if there is evidence implicating the catheter as the possible source of fungemia. Such predictors are (1) no prior chemotherapy for the last month, indicating the possible absence of gastrointestinal mucositis that enhances the risk of gut originating candidemia [206], (2) no prior steroid therapy, which has been associated with breakthrough candidemia [226,227], and (3) no other apparent source of the candidemia. Additionally, evidence of septic thrombophlebitis (ex. through angiography) and invasion of the vascular wall [228] is another indication for catheter removal, since it may further increase the difficulty of eradicating the infection with medical therapy only. If the catheter is retained, the parenteral antifungal agents should be administered through all the lumens of the catheter, and the patient should be very closely monitored. If the patient is severely ill or has 72 hours of fungemia or persistent fever while on appropriate antifungal therapy, then removal of all CVCs is advised. Fungemia with *C. parapsilosis* is strongly associated with direct catheter infection [229] and would indicate catheter removal.

Malassezia furfur is a lipophilic yeast that requires an exogenous lipid source to grow. Infection with this organism generally occurs in premature infants, but it has also been described in older children and adults, especially in critically ill patients hospitalized in ICU. Risk factors include the presence of a venous catheter and the administration of a lipid-enriched solution, like total parenteral nutrition. The basis of treatment is systemic administration of amphotericin B, discontinuation of the parenteral lipid supplements, and removal of the catheter, especially with nontunneled catheter infections [170,230,231].

Although staphylococci and *Candida* spp. are the most frequent pathogens implicated in CRBSI, a number of other microorganisms have been reported as causing catheter-related bacteremia [232]. The incidence of CRBSI due to gram-negative rods, including *Pseudomonas* spp., *Acinetobacter* spp., and *Stenotrophomonas maltophilia* is increasing, especially in cancer patients and immunocompromised hosts [233,234]. These microorganisms are occasionally associated with contaminated infusate [1], and they can cause infections associated with a high rate of failure when the catheter remains in place [90]. There are no controlled trials evaluating the optimal antibiotics or the optimal duration of therapy for CRBSI caused by gram-negatives. In addition, there is a similar lack of controlled trials encompassing the management of the catheter implicated in such infections. Catheter removal within 48 to 72 hours of the onset of the CRBSI has been proven to prevent relapse of the infection [235]. A course of 10 to 14 days of therapy with appropriate antibiotics is sufficient in the majority of cases [170]. If the catheter cannot be removed and there is no evidence of tissue hypoperfusion, a combination of 14 days systemic therapy and antibiotic lock therapy is advised [170]. In any case of persistence of fever and/or of positive blood cultures despite appropriate systemic antibiotic therapy, removal of the implicated catheter(s) should be seriously considered [170]. Empirical antibiotic therapy, in cancer patients with gram-negative infections, should always cover *P. aeruginosa* [236].

Treatment of CRBSI caused by mycobacteria, notably *M. fortuitum* and *M. chelonae*, requires, in addition to systemic therapy with appropriate antibiotics, removal of the catheter [170,237].

PREVENTION

Most CVC infections are preventable. Several protective measures have been suggested to guard against long-term catheter CRBSI.

Precautions During Catheter Insertion

Careful handwashing and attention to aseptic technique during insertion is paramount for the prevention of infections in any type of catheter. For long-term central venous catheters, though, the level of precaution should be greater than just handwashing, wearing gloves, and using a small drape. The use of maximal sterile barriers (sterile gloves, mask, gown, cap, and a large drape) has been linked to a four-fold decrease in the rate of bacteremia related to pulmonary-artery catheters [21] and to a more than sixfold decrease in the rate of bacteremia related to CVCs [238]. The presence of an experienced infusion therapy team that inserts and maintains catheters has been proven to decrease the rate of CRBSI by up to eight times [239,240]. Thus such a team is cost-effective in large centers with a high number of central vascular catheter insertions.

Catheter-Site Care

The use of skin antiseptics at the insertion site is a very important measure for preventing CRBSI. In a trial of cutaneous antiseptics, 2% chlorhexidine gluconate was shown to be superior to both 10% povidone–iodine and 70% alcohol in preventing CRBSI [241]. The application of antimicrobial ointments to the catheter site at the time of catheter insertion or during routine dressing changes has been done to reduce the microbial burden at the skin insertion site. The use of a topical polyantibiotic regimen (polymyxin β, neomycin, bacitracin) is associated with a significantly lower rate of CRBSI [242]; but the overall protective effect of the topical antibiotic regimen is offset by a higher risk of catheter colonization and infection with *Candida* spp. [242,243]. The use of mupirocin, a nonsystemic antistaphylococcal agent with proven efficacy in reducing staphylococcal spp. nasal carriage, has been proven to reduce fivefold the colonization of internal jugular catheters in cardiac surgery patients [244].

Transparent dressings have become popular for dressing catheter-insertion sites, since they reliably secure the device, permit patients to bathe without saturating the dressing, permit continuous visual inspection of the catheter site, and require less frequent changes. In a meta-analysis the risk for CRBSI did not differ for the group using transparent dressings compared with gauze dressings, to cover CVC insertion sites, despite a significantly higher incidence of catheter-tip colonization in the transparent dressing group [245]. A study reported an increased risk of CRBSI among CVCs with a transparent dressing compared with those covered with gauze [246]. However, in another study no significant difference in the incidence of CRBSI was observed between patients with gauze and those with transparent dressings [247].

Tunneled Catheters

Tunneling of short-term polyurethane internal jugular catheters reduces significantly the risk for CRBSI compared to nontunneled catheters [248]. However, a prospective randomized study investigating the effect of tunneling of long-term CVCs, in immunocompromised patients failed to show a significant benefit in reducing the rate of CRBSI [115]. The risk of CRBSI was 2% with tunneled and 5% with nontunneled catheters. The difference was not significant, probably because of the small power of the study (107 tunneled and 105 nontunneled patients). In the study that showed the greatest benefit from tunneling [248], the potential colonization of the catheter hubs was minimized because the catheters were not used for drawing blood. More studies are required, especially in long-term silicone catheters, in order to investigate the impact of tunneling in reducing CRBSI.

Intraluminal Antibiotic Locks

The intraluminal antibiotic lock consists of flushing and filling the lumen of the CVC with a combination of anticoagulant and antimicrobial agents. This flushing solution is then locked into the catheter for the time period that the catheter is not being used. This procedure is particularly useful for long-term catheters where hub contamination leads to lumen colonization and ultimately to bloodstream infection [29,31,249]. Vancomycin in combination with heparin has been used as a daily flush solution for tunneled CVCs in five prospective randomized studies [250–254]. Four of them have demonstrated the benefit of heparin-vancomycin lock solution in preventing CRBSI caused by vancomycin-susceptible microorganisms [250–253]. A smaller prospective randomized controlled trial in pediatric patients, the majority of whom had cancer, failed to show any benefit of heparin-vancomycin lock solution over heparin alone in preventing CRBSI caused by vancomycin-susceptible microorganism [254]. The major drawback of this lock solution is that the use of vancomycin, even in minute quantities, could lead to the emergence of vancomycin-resistant gram-positive organisms.

A different antimicrobial/anticoagulant combination as a lock solution is the combination of minocycline with edetic-acid (EDTA). EDTA is a potent calcium and iron chelator with antistaphylococcal and anti-*Candida* activity, in addition to its anticoagulant properties [255,256]. Minocycline has broad antistaphylococcal activity. The combination of minocycline/ EDTA in animal studies has been proven to be superior to heparin–vancomycin and heparin alone in preventing catheter colonization, catheter-related bacteremia, and phlebitis [257]. Additional evidence from clinical studies has demonstrated the ability of minocycline/EDTA to provide anti-infective and anticoagulant protection to CVCs [258,259].

Antimicrobial Coating of Catheters

Microorganisms can be prevented from colonizing catheter surfaces by coating the external and/or internal surfaces of the catheter with antimicrobial agents.

Catheters coated with chlorhexidine and silver sulfadiazine (CHSS) were two times less likely to become colonized and were at least four times less likely to cause bacteremia than noncoated catheters [260]. The catheters used in this study were coated only in the external surface (first-generation CHSS catheters) and thus do not provide the luminal protection that is needed in long-term catheters (> 2 weeks) [261,262]. Additionally, these catheters have a short antimicrobial durability [262]. Several clinical studies reflect these weaknesses of the first-generation CHSS catheters, especially when used for longer than 2 weeks [261,263–265]. A meta-analysis of 12 studies did show a benefit in using the first-generation CHSS catheters as short-term catheters [266], as these catheters are associated with a decrease in CRBSI [10]. A second generation CHSS polyurethane catheter has been tested in an animal model [267]. The second-generation CHSS catheter (CS2) has both the external and internal surfaces coated and may retain antimicrobial activity longer than the first-generation CHSS catheters [267]. Clinical trials of this catheter are pending. Given that only short-term polyurethane CVCs are coated with CHSS, these catheters may not be useful in cancer patients requiring long-term catheterization.

Catheters impregnated with minocycline and rifampin (MR) have both their external and internal surfaces coated. The MR catheters have broad-spectrum activity against the most common microorganisms implicated in CRBSI, including *C. albicans*. In addition, these catheters demonstrated superior inhibitory activity against these microorganisms over the CHSS catheters [268,269]. Both an animal model and a large-multicenter prospective randomized clinical trial demonstrated that the MR catheters are safe and efficacious in preventing CRBSI [269,270]. A prospective randomized multicenter trial comparing the MR and the CHSS catheters concluded that the MR catheters were 12 times less likely to be associated with CRBSI and three times less likely to be colonized than those coated only externally with CHSS [271]. The MR catheters are coated both on the external surface and on their lumen, and the antimicrobial durability of these catheters extends to more than 4 weeks [271,272]. No resistance thus far has been detected in the hundreds of MR catheters that have been studied. However the risk for development of such resistance still exists. Although an in vitro study suggests that the susceptibility of *S. epidermidis* to rifampin may decrease after repeated exposure of the organism to MR catheters [273], a surveillance study demonstrated that susceptibility patterns for minocycline and rifampin, among staphylococcal isolates from clinical service that uses the MR catheters, are comparable to those in patients not using antibiotic-coated catheters, in spite of a longer use of tetracyclines in the former group [274]. The use of the MR catheters in the ICU of a cancer hospital resulted in a significant decrease in the frequency of nosocomial vancomycin-resistant enterococci-related bacteremia [275].

Antimicrobially coated catheters should be used when the following are fulfilled [276]: (1) femoral or internal jugular vein insertion (greater risk of infection than subclavian vein catheterization [21]), (2) catheterization expected to last longer than 4 days, (3) units with risk of CRBSI greater than 3% or 3.3/1000 catheter days, (4) patient with neutropenia or undergoing transplantation, (5) patients receiving TPN, (6) patients with burns, (7) patients undergoing hemodialysis, (8) patients with short-bowel syndrome, (9) patients colonized with methicillin-resistant *S aureus*, (10) insertion or exchange in a patient with known infection or bacteremia.

REFERENCES

1. Maki DG. Infections due to infusion therapy. In: Bennett JV, Brachman PS, eds. Hospital Infections. Boston: Little, Brown, 1992:849–898.
2. Pittet D, Tarara D, Wenzel RP. Nosocomial bloodstream infection in critically ill patients. Excess length of stay, extra costs, and attributable mortality. JAMA 1994; 271:1598–1601. See comments.
3. Richards MJ, Edwards JR, Culver DH, Gaynes RP. Nosocomial infections in combined medical-surgical intensive care units in the United States. Infect Control Hosp Epidemiol 2000; 21:510–515.
4. Soufir L, Timsit JF, Mahe C, Carlet J, Regnier B, Chevret S. Attributable morbidity and mortality of catheter-related septicemia in critically ill patients: a matched, risk-adjusted, cohort study. Infect Control Hosp Epidemiol 1999; 20: 396–401.
5. Jarvis WR, Edwards JR, Culver DH, Hughes JM, Horan T, Emori TG, Banerjee S, Tolson J, Henderson T, Gaynes RP. Nosocomial infection rates in adult and pediatric intensive care units in the United States. National Nosocomial Infections Surveillance System. American Journal of Medicine 1991; 91:185S–191S.
6. Raad II, Bodey GP. Infectious complications of indwelling vascular catheters. Clin Infect Dis 1992; 15:197–208.
7. Bross J, Talbot GH, Maislin G, Hurwitz S, Strom BL. Risk factors for nosocomial candidemia: a case-control study in adults without leukemia. Am J Med 1989; 87:614–620.
8. Fraser VJ, Jones M, Dunkel J, Storfer S, Medoff G, Dunagan WC. Candidemia in a tertiary care hospital: epidemiology, risk factors, and predictors of mortality. Clin Infect Dis 1992; 15:414–421.
9. Maki DG, Cobb L, Garman JK, Shapiro JM, Ringer M, Helgerson RB. An attachable silver-impregnated cuff for prevention of infection with central venous catheters: a prospective randomized multicenter trial. Am J Med 1988; 85:307–314.
10. Mermel LA. Prevention of intravascular catheter-related infections. Ann Intern Med 2000; 132:391–402.
11. Mermel LA. Preventing intravascular catheter-related infections [letter]. Ann Intern Med 2000; 133:395.

12. Raad I, Costerton W, Sabharwal U, Sacilowski M, Anaissie E, Bodey GP. Ultrastructural analysis of indwelling vascular catheters: a quantitative relationship between luminal colonization and duration of placement. J Infect Dis 1993; 168:400–407.

13. Maki DG. Skin as a source of nosocomial infection: directions for future research. Infect Control 1986; 7:113–117.

14. Richet H, Hubert B, Nitemberg G, Andremont A, Buu-Hoi A, Ourbak P, Galicier C, Veron M, Boisivon A, Bouvier AM, et al. Prospective multicenter study of vascular-catheter-related complications and risk factors for positive central-catheter cultures in intensive care unit patients. J Clin Microbiol 1990; 28:2520–2525.

15. Collignon PJ. Intravascular catheter associated sepsis: a common problem. Australian Study on Intravascular Catheter Associated Sepsis. Med J Aust 1994; 161:374–378.

16. Broviac JW, Cole JJ, Scribner BH. A silicone rubber atrial catheter for prolonged parenteral alimentation. Surg Gynecol Obstet 1973; 136:602–606.

17. Hickman RO, Buckner CD, Clift RA, Sanders JE, Stewart P, Thomas ED. A modified right atrial catheter for access to the venous system in marrow transplant recipients. Surg Gynecol Obstet 1979; 148:871–875.

18. Raad I, Davis S, Becker M, Hohn D, Houston D, Umphrey J, Bodey GP. Low infection rate and long durability of nontunneled silastic catheters. A safe and cost-effective alternative for long-term venous access. Arch Intern Med 1993; 153:1791–1796.

19. Goodman MS, Wickham R. Venous access devices: an overview. Oncol Nurs Forum 1984; 11:16–23.

20. Bagnall H, Ruccione K. Experience with a totally implanted venous access device in children with malignant disease. Oncol Nurs Forum 1987; 14:51–56.

21. Mermel LA, McCormick RD, Springman SR, Maki DG. The pathogenesis and epidemiology of catheter-related infection with pulmonary artery Swan–Ganz catheters: a prospective study utilizing molecular subtyping. Am J Med 1991; 91:197S–205S.

22. Bjornson HS, Colley R, Bower RH, Duty VP, Schwartz-Fulton JT, Fischer JE. Association between microorganism growth at the catheter insertion site and colonization of the catheter in patients receiving total parenteral nutrition. Surgery 1982; 92:720–727.

23. Cooper GL, Hopkins CC. Rapid diagnosis of intravascular catheter-associated infection by direct Gram staining of catheter segments. N Engl J Med 1985; 312:1142–1147.

24. Cleri DJ, Corrado ML, Seligman SJ. Quantitative culture of intravenous catheters and other intravascular inserts. J Infect Dis 1980; 141:781–786.

25. Band JD, Maki DG. Infections caused by aterial catheters used for hemodynamic monitoring. Am J Med 1979; 67:735–741.

26. Maki DG, Hassemer CA. Endemic rate of fluid contamination and related septicemia in arterial pressure monitoring. Am J Med 1981; 70:733–738.

27. Maki DG, Weise CE, Sarafin HW. A semiquantitative culture method for

identifying intravenous-catheter-related infection. N Engl J Med 1977; 296: 1305–1309.

28. Weightman NC, Simpson EM, Speller DC, Mott MG, Oakhill A. Bacteraemia related to indwelling central venous catheters: prevention, diagnosis and treatment. Eur J Clin Microbiol Infect Dis 1988; 7:125–129.

29. Salzman MB, Isenberg HD, Shapiro JF, Lipsitz PJ, Rubin LG. A prospective study of the catheter hub as the portal of entry for microorganisms causing catheter-related sepsis in neonates. J Infect Dis 1993; 167:487–490.

30. Peters G, Locci R, Pulverer G. Adherence and growth of coagulase-negative staphylococci on surfaces of intravenous catheters. J Infect Dis 1982; 146:479–482.

31. Linares J, Sitges-Serra A, Garau J, Perez JL, Martin R. Pathogenesis of catheter sepsis: a prospective study with quantitative and semiquantitative cultures of catheter hub and segments. J Clin Microbiol 1985; 21:357–360.

32. de Cicco M, Panarello G, Chiaradia V, Fracasso A, Veronesi A, Testa V, Santini G, Tesio F. Source and route of microbial colonisation of parenteral nutrition catheters. Lancet 1989; 2:1258–1261.

33. Capell S, Linares J, Sitges-Serra A. Catheter sepsis due to coagulase-negative staphylococci in patients on total parenteral nutrition. Eur J Clin Microbiol 1986; 5:40–42.

34. Flowers RH III, Schwenzer KJ, Kopel RF, Fisch MJ, Tucker SI, Farr BM. Efficacy of an attachable subcutaneous cuff for the prevention of intravascular catheter-related infection. A randomized, controlled trial. JAMA 1989; 261: 878–883.

35. Sherertz RJ. Pathogenesis of vascular catheter-related infections. In: Seifert H, Jansen B, Farr BM, eds. Catheter-Related Infections. New York: Marcel Dekker, 1997:1–30.

36. Tojo M, Yamashita N, Goldmann DA, Pier GB. Isolation and characterization of a capsular polysaccharide adhesin from *Staphylococcus epidermidis*. J Infect Dis 1988; 157:713–722.

37. Sheth NK, Franson TR, Sohnle PG. Influence of bacterial adherence to intravascular catheters on in-vitro antibiotic susceptibility. Lancet 1985; 2:1266–1268.

38. Falcieri E, Vaudaux P, Huggler E, Lew D, Waldvogel F. Role of bacterial exopolymers and host factors on adherence and phagocytosis of *Staphylococcus aureus* in foreign body infection. J Infect Dis 1987; 155:524–531.

39. Costerton JW, Irvin RT, Cheng KJ. The bacterial glycocalyx in nature and disease. Annu Rev Microbiol 1981; 35:299–324.

40. Christensen GD, Simpson WA, Bisno AL, Beachey EH. Adherence of slime-producing strains of *Staphylococcus epidermidis* to smooth surfaces. Infect Immun 1982; 37:318–326.

41. Christensen GD, Simpson WA, Younger JJ, Baddour LM, Barrett FF, Melton DM, Beachey EH. Adherence of coagulase-negative staphylococci to plastic tissue culture plates: a quantitative model for the adherence of staphylococci to medical devices. J Clin Microbiol 1985; 22:996–1006.

42. Montanaro L, Arciola CR, Borsetti E, Brigotti M, Baldassarri L. A polymerase chain reaction (PCR) method for the identification of collagen adhesin gene (CNA) in Staphylococcus-induced prosthesis infections. New Microbiol 1998; 21:359–363.

43. McKenney D, Pouliot KL, Wang Y, Murthy V, Ulrich M, Doring G, Lee JC, Goldmann DA, Pier GB. Broadly protective vaccine for *Staphylococcus aureus* based on an in vivo–expressed antigen. Science 1999; 284:1523–1527.

44. Cramton SE, Gerke C, Schnell NF, Nichols WW, Gotz F. The intercellular adhesion (ica) locus is present in *Staphylococcus aureus* and is required for biofilm formation. Infect Immun 1999; 67:5427–5433.

45. Arciola CR, Montanaro L, Baldassarri L, Borsetti E, Cavedagna D, Donati E. Slime production by Staphylococci isolated from prosthesis-associated infections. New Microbiol 1999; 22:337–341.

46. Ammendolia MG, Di Rosa R, Montanaro L, Arciola CR, Baldassarri L. Slime production and expression of the slime-associated antigen by staphylococcal clinical isolates. J Clin Microbiol 1999; 37:3235–3238.

47. McKenney D, Hubner J, Muller E, Wang Y, Goldmann DA, Pier GB. The ica locus of *Staphylococcus epidermidis* encodes production of the capsular polysaccharide/adhesin. Infect Immun 1998; 66:4711–4720.

48. Gaur NK, Klotz SA. Expression, cloning, and characterization of a *Candida albicans* gene, ALA1, that confers adherence properties upon *Saccharomyces cerevisiae* for extracellular matrix proteins. Infect Immun 1997; 65:5289–5294.

49. Gerke C, Kraft A, Sussmuth R, Schweitzer O, Gotz F. Characterization of the *N*-acetylglucosaminyltransferase activity involved in the biosynthesis of the *Staphylococcus epidermidis* polysaccharide intercellular adhesin. J Biol Chem 1998; 273:18586–18593.

50. Lewis RE, Lo HJ, Raad II, Kontoyiannis DP. Lack of catheter infection by the efg1/efg1cph1/cph1 double-null mutant, a *Candida albicans* strain that is defective in filamentous growth. Antimicrob Agents Chemother 2002; 46:1153–1155.

51. Hardman AM, Stewart GS, Williams P. Quorum sensing and the cell–cell communication dependent regulation of gene expression in pathogenic and nonpathogenic bacteria. Antonie Van Leeuwenhoek 1998; 74:199–210.

52. Parsek MR, Val DL, Hanzelka BL, Cronan JE Jr, Greenberg EP. Acyl homoserine–lactone quorum-sensing signal generation. Proc Natl Acad Sci USA 1999; 96:4360–4365.

53. Wesson CA, Liou LE, Todd KM, Bohach GA, Trumble WR, Bayles KW. *Staphylococcus aureus* Agr and Sar global regulators influence internalization and induction of apoptosis. Infect Immun 1998; 66:5238–5243.

54. Otto M, Sussmuth R, Jung G, Gotz F. Structure of the pheromone peptide of the *Staphylococcus epidermidis* agr system. FEBS Lett 1998; 424:89–94.

55. Hornby JM, Jensen EC, Lisec AD, Tasto JJ, Jahnke B, Shoemaker R, Dussault P, Nickerson KW. Quorum sensing in the dimorphic fungus *Candida albicans* is mediated by farnesol. Appl Environ Microbiol 2001; 67:2982–2992.

56. Stewart PS, Costerton JW. Antibiotic resistance of bacteria in biofilms. Lancet 2001; 358:135–138.
57. Pfaller MA, Messer SA, Hollis RJ. Variations in DNA subtype, antifungal susceptibility, and slime production among clinical isolates of *Candida parapsilosis*. Diagn Microbiol Infect Dis 1995; 21:9–14.
58. Farber BF, Kaplan MH, Clogston AG. Staphylococcus epidermidis extracted slime inhibits the antimicrobial action of glycopeptide antibiotics. J Infect Dis 1990; 161:37–40.
59. Raad II, Luna M, Khalil SA, Costerton JW, Lam C, Bodey GP. The relationship between the thrombotic and infectious complications of central venous catheters. Jama 1994; 271:1014–1016.
60. Raad II, Safar H. Long-term central venous catheters. Infectious complications and cost. In: Seifert H, Jansen B, Farr BM, eds. Catheter-Related Infections. New York: Marcel Dekker, 1997:307–324.
61. Vaudaux P, Pittet D, Haeberli A, Lerch PG, Morgenthaler JJ, Proctor RA, Waldvogel FA, Lew DP. Fibronectin is more active than fibrin or fibrinogen in promoting *Staphylococcus aureus* adherence to inserted intravascular catheters. J Infect Dis 1993; 167:633–641.
62. Herrmann M, Vaudaux PE, Pittet D, Auckenthaler R, Lew PD, Schumacher-Perdreau F, Peters G, Waldvogel FA. Fibronectin, fibrinogen, and laminin act as mediators of adherence of clinical staphylococcal isolates to foreign material. J Infect Dis 1988; 158:693–701.
63. Herrmann M, Suchard SJ, Boxer LA, Waldvogel FA, Lew PD. Thrombospondin binds to *Staphylococcus aureus* and promotes staphylococcal adherence to surfaces. Infect Immun 1991; 59:279–288.
64. Lopes JD, dos Reis M, Brentani RR. Presence of laminin receptors in *Staphylococcus aureus*. Science 1985; 229:275–277.
65. Hawiger J, Timmons S, Strong DD, Cottrell BA, Riley M, Doolittle RF. Identification of a region of human fibrinogen interacting with staphylococcal clumping factor. Biochemistry 1982; 21:1407–1413.
66. Vaudaux P, Pittet D, Haeberli A, Huggler E, Nydegger UE, Lew DP, Waldvogel FA. Host factors selectively increase staphylococcal adherence on inserted catheters: a role for fibronectin and fibrinogen or fibrin. J Infect Dis 1989; 160:865–875.
67. Bouali A, Robert R, Tronchin G, Senet JM. Characterization of binding of human fibrinogen to the surface of germ-tubes and mycelium of *Candida albicans*. J Gen Microbiol 1987; 133:545–551.
68. Bailly AL, Laurent A, Lu H, Elalami I, Jacob P, Mundler O, Merland JJ, Lautier A, Soria J, Soria C. Fibrinogen binding and platelet retention: relationship with the thrombogenicity of catheters. J Biomed Mater Res 1996; 30:101–108.
69. Kreft B, Ilic S, Ziebuhr W, Kahl A, Frei U, Sack K, Trautmann M. Adherence of *Staphylococcus aureus* isolated in peritoneal dialysis-related exit-site infections to HEp-2 cells and silicone peritoneal catheter materials. Nephrol Dial Transplant 1998; 13:3160–3164.

70. Galliani S, Cremieux A, van der Auwera P, Viot M. Influence of strain, biomaterial, proteins, and oncostatic chemotherapy on *Staphylococcus epidermidis* adhesion to intravascular catheters in vitro. J Lab Clin Med 1996; 127:71 80.

71. Sherertz RJ, Carruth WA, Marosok RD, Espeland MA, Johnson RA, Solomon DD. Contribution of vascular catheter material to the pathogenesis of infection: the enhanced risk of silicone in vivo. J Biomed Mater Res 1995; 29:635–645.

72. Lopez-Lopez G, Pascual A, Martinez-Martinez L, Perea EJ. Effect of a siliconized latex urinary catheter on bacterial adherence and human neutrophil activity. Diagn Microbiol Infect Dis 1991; 14:1–6.

73. Lopez-Lopez G, Pascual A, Perea EJ. Effect of plastic catheters on the phagocytic activity of human polymorphonuclear leukocytes. Eur J Clin Microbiol Infect Dis 1990; 9:324–328.

74. Marosok R, Washburn R, Indorf A, Solomon D, Sherertz R. Contribution of vascular catheter material to the pathogenesis of infection: depletion of complement by silicone elastomer in vitro. J Biomed Mater Res 1996; 30:245–250.

75. Francois P, Vaudaux P, Nurdin N, Mathieu HJ, Descouts P, Lew DP. Physical and biological effects of a surface coating procedure on polyurethane catheters. Biomaterials 1996; 17:667–678.

76. Fuchs PC, Gustafson ME, King JT, Goodall PT. Assessment of catheter-associated infection risk with the Hickman right atrial catheter. Infect Control 1984; 5:226–230.

77. Goldmann DA, Martin WT, Worthington JW. Growth of bacteria and fungi in total parenteral nutrition solutions. Am J Surg 1973; 126:314–318.

78. Gelbart SM, Reinhardt GF, Greenlee HB. Multiplication of nosocomial pathogens in intravenous feeding solutions. Appl Microbiol 1973; 26:874–879.

79. Dugleux G, Le Coutour X, Hecquard C, Oblin I. Septicemia caused by contaminated parenteral nutrition pouches: the refrigerator as an unusual cause. J Parenter Enteral Nutr 1991; 15:474–475.

80. Llop JM, Mangues I, Perez JL, Lopez P, Tubau M. Staphylococcus saprophyticus sepsis related to total parenteral nutrition admixtures contamination. J Parenter Enteral Nutr 1993; 17:575–577.

81. Scheckelhoff DJ, Mirtallo JM, Ayers LW, Visconti JA. Growth of bacteria and fungi in total nutrient admixtures. Am J Hosp Pharm 1986; 43:73–77.

82. Murphy PM, Lane HC, Gallin JI, Fauci AS. Marked disparity in incidence of bacterial infections in patients with the acquired immunodeficiency syndrome receiving interleukin-2 or interferon-gamma. Ann Intern Med 1988; 108:36–41.

83. Bock SN, Lee RE, Fisher B, Rubin JT, Schwartzentruber DJ, Wei JP, Callender DP, Yang JC, Lotze MT, Pizzo PA, et al. A prospective randomized trial evaluating prophylactic antibiotics to prevent triple-lumen catheter-related sepsis in patients treated with immunotherapy. J Clin Oncol 1990; 8:161–169.

84. Siegel JP, Puri RK. Interleukin-2 toxicity. J Clin Oncol 1991; 9:694–704.

85. Maki DG. Infection caused by intravascular devices: pathogenesis, strategies for prevention. London: Royal Society of Medicine Services, 1991.

86. Maki DG. Pathogenesis, prevention and management of infections due to intravascular devices used for infusion therapy. In: Bisno AL, Waldvogel FA,

eds. Infections Associated with Indwelling Medical Devices. Washington: Americal Society for Microbiology, 1989:161–177.

87. Cotton DJ, Gill VJ, Marshall DJ, Gress J, Thaler M, Pizzo PA. Clinical features and therapeutic interventions in 17 cases of Bacillus bacteremia in an immunosuppressed patient population. J Clin Microbiol 1987; 25:672–674.

88. Riebel W, Frantz N, Adelstein D, Spagnuolo PJ. Corynebacterium JK: a cause of nosocomial device-related infection. Rev Infect Dis 1986; 8:42–49.

89. Saleh RA, Schorin MA. *Bacillus* sp. sepsis associated with Hickman catheters in patients with neoplastic disease. Pediatr Infect Dis J 1987; 6:851–856.

90. Elting LS, Bodey GP. Septicemia due to *Xanthomonas* species and non-aeruginosa *Pseudomonas* species: increasing incidence of catheter-related infections. Medicine (Baltimore) 1990; 69:296–306.

91. Seifert H, Strate A, Schulze A, Pulverer G. Vascular catheter–related bloodstream infection due to *Acinetobacter johnsonii* (formerly *Acinetobacter calcoaceticus* var. lwoffi): report of 13 cases. Clin Infect Dis 1993; 17:632–636.

92. Ambler MW, Homans AC, O'Shea PA. An unusual central nervous system infection in a young immunocompromised host. Arch Pathol Lab Med 1986; 110:497–501.

93. Hernandez JA, Martino R, Pericas R, Sureda A, Brunet S, Domingo-Albos A. *Achromobacter xylosoxidans* bacteremia in patients with hematologic malignancies. Haematologica 1998; 83:284–285.

94. Chatzinikolaou I, Rolston K, Raad I. Central venous catheter–related *Rhodococcus* spp. bacteremia in cancer patients. Fourth Decennial International Conference on Nosocomial and Healthcare–Associated Infections in Conjuction with the 10th Annual Meeting of SHEA, Atlanta, Georgia 2000.

95. Engler HD, Hass A, Hodes DS, Bottone EJ. *Mycobacterium chelonei* infection of a Broviac catheter insertion site. Eur J Clin Microbiol Infect Dis 1989; 8:521–523.

96. Swanson DS. Central venous catheter-related infections due to nontuberculous *Mycobacterium* species. Pediatr Infect Dis J 1998; 17:1163–1164.

97. Chung JW, Kim BN, Kim YS. Central venous catheter–related *Rhodotorula rubra*. fungemia. J Infect Chemother 2002; 8:109–110.

98. Ammari LK, Puck JM, McGowan KL. Catheter-related *Fusarium solani* fungemia and pulmonary infection in a patient with leukemia in remission. Clin Infect Dis 1993; 16:148–150.

99. Kiehn TE, Nelson PE, Bernard EM, Edwards FF, Koziner B, Armstrong D. Catheter-associated fungemia caused by *Fusarium chlamydosporum* in a patient with lymphocytic lymphoma. J Clin Microbiol 1985; 21:501–504.

100. Raad I, Hachem R. Treatment of central venous catheter–related fungemia due to *Fusarium oxysporum*. Clin Infect Dis 1995; 20:709–711.

101. Klein AS, Tortora GT, Malowitz R, Greene WH. Hansenula anomala: a new fungal pathogen. Two case reports and a review of the literature. Arch Intern Med 1988; 148:1210–1213.

102. Haron E, Anaissie E, Dumphy F, McCredie K, Fainstein V. Hansenula anomala fungemia. Rev Infect Dis 1988; 10:1182–1186.

103. Pearson ML. Guideline for prevention of intravascular device–related infections. Hospital Infection Control Practices Advisory Committee. Infect Control Hosp Epidemiol 1996; 17:438–473. See comments.
104. Clarke DE, Raffin TA. Infectious complications of indwelling long-term central venous catheters. Chest 1990; 97:966–972.
105. Decker MD, Edwards KM. Central venous catheter infections. Pediatr Clin North Am 1988; 35:579–612.
106. Howell PB, Walters PE, Donowitz GR, Farr BM. Risk factors for infection of adult patients with cancer who have tunnelled central venous catheters. Cancer 1995; 75:1367–1375.
107. Press OW, Ramsey PG, Larson EB, Fefer A, Hickman RO. Hickman catheter infections in patients with malignancies. Medicine (Baltimore) 1984; 63:189–200.
108. Abrahm JL, Mullen JL. A prospective study of prolonged central venous access in leukemia. JAMA 1982; 248:2868–2873.
109. Darbyshire PJ, Weightman NC, Speller DC. Problems associated with indwelling central venous catheters. Arch Dis Child 1985; 60:129–134.
110. Pessa ME, Howard RJ. Complications of Hickman-Broviac catheters. Surg Gynecol Obstet 1985; 161:257–260.
111. Schuman ES, Winters V, Gross GF, Hayes JF. Management of Hickman catheter sepsis. Am J Surg 1985; 149:627–628.
112. Shapiro ED, Wald ER, Nelson KA, Spiegelman KN. Broviac catheter-related bacteremia in oncology patients. Am J Dis Child 1982; 136:679–681.
113. Shulman RJ, Smith EO, Rahman S, Gardner P, Reed T, Mahoney D. Single- vs. double-lumen central venous catheters in pediatric oncology patients. Am J Dis Child 1988; 142:893–895.
114. Rannem T, Ladefoged K, Tvede M, Lorentzen JE, Jarnum S. Catheter-related septicaemia in patients receiving home parenteral nutrition. Scand J Gastroenterol 1986; 21:455–460.
115. Andrivet P, Bacquer A, Ngoc CV, Ferme C, Letinier JY, Gautier H, Gallet CB, Brun-Buisson C. Lack of clinical benefit from subcutaneous tunnel insertion of central venous catheters in immunocompromised patients. Clin Infect Dis 1994; 18:199–206.
116. Raad I, Hanna H, McFadyen S, Marts K, Richardson D, Mansfield P. Non-tunneled subclavian central venous catheters (NTSC) vs. tunneled central venous catheters (CVCs) and ports in cancer patients. Forty-first Annual Interscience Conference on Antimicrobial Agents and Chemotherapy (ICAAC), Chicago, IL, USA, 2001.
117. Hanna H, McFadyen S, Marts K, Richardson D, Hachem R, Raad I. Prospective evaluation of 1.67 million catheter-days of peripherally inserted central catheters (PICCs) in cancer patients: long durability and low infection rate. Forty-first Annual Interscience Conference on Antimicrobial Agents and Chemotherapy (ICAAC), Chicago, IL, USA, 2001.
118. Groeger JS, Lucas AB, Thaler HT, Friedlander-Klar H, Brown AE, Kiehn TE, Armstrong D. Infectious morbidity associated with long-term use of venous access devices in patients with cancer. Ann Intern Med 1993; 119:1168–1174.

119. van der Pijl H, Frissen PH. Experience with a totally implantable venous access device (Port-A-Cath) in patients with AIDS. AIDS 1992; 6:709–713.

120. Khoury MD, Lloyd LR, Burrows J, Berg R, Yap J. A totally implanted venous access system for the delivery of chemotherapy. Cancer 1985; 56:1231–1234.

121. Kappers-Klunne MC, Degener JE, Stijnen T, Abels J. Complications from long-term indwelling central venous catheters in hematologic patients with special reference to infection. Cancer 1989; 64:1747–1752.

122. Carde P, Cosset-Delaigue MF, Laplanche A, Chareau I. Classical external indwelling central venous catheter versus totally implanted venous access systems for chemotherapy administration: a randomized trial in 100 patients with solid tumors. Eur J Cancer Clin Oncol 1989; 25:939–944.

123. Brincker H, Saeter G. Fifty-five patient years' experience with a totally implanted system for intravenous chemotherapy. Cancer 1986; 57:1124–1129.

124. Gyves JW, Ensminger WD, Niederhuber JE, Dent T, Walker S, Gilbertson S, Cozzi E, Saran P. A totally implanted injection port system for blood sampling and chemotherapy administration. JAMA 1984; 251:2538–2541.

125. Lokich JJ, Bothe A Jr, Benotti P, Moore C. Complications and management of implanted venous access catheters. J Clin Oncol 1985; 3:710–717.

126. Pegues D, Axelrod P, McClarren C, Eisenberg BL, Hoffman JP, Ottery FD, Keidan RD, Boraas M, Weese J. Comparison of infections in Hickman and implanted port catheters in adult solid tumor patients. J Surg Oncol 1992; 49: 156–162.

127. McDowell HP, Hart CA, Martin J. Implantable subcutaneous venous catheters. Arch Dis Child 1986; 61:1037 1038.

128. Wurzel CL, Halom K, Feldman JG, Rubin LG. Infection rates of Broviac-Hickman catheters and implantable venous devices. Am J Dis Child 1988; 142: 536–540.

129. Clark-Christoff N, Watters VA, Sparks W, Snyder P, Grant JP. Use of triple-lumen subclavian catheters for administration of total parenteral nutrition. J Parenter Enteral Nutr 1992; 16:403–407.

130. Hilton E, Haslett TM, Borenstein MT, Tucci V, Isenberg HD, Singer C. Central catheter infections: single- versus triple-lumen catheters. Influence of guide wires on infection rates when used for replacement of catheters. Am J Med 1988; 84:667–672.

131. McCarthy MC, Shives JK, Robison RJ, Broadie TA. Prospective evaluation of single and triple lumen catheters in total parenteral nutrition. J Parenter Enteral Nutr 1987; 11:259–262.

132. Pemberton LB, Lyman B, Lander V, Covinsky J. Sepsis from triple- vs. single-lumen catheters during total parenteral nutrition in surgical or critically ill patients. Arch Surg 1986; 121:591–594.

133. Yeung C, May J, Hughes R. Infection rate for single lumen v. triple lumen subclavian catheters. Infect Control Hosp Epidemiol 1988; 9:154–158.

134. Lee RB, Buckner M, Sharp KW. Do multi-lumen catheters increase central venous catheter sepsis compared to single-lumen catheters? J Trauma 1988; 28:1472–1475.

135. Farkas JC, Liu N, Bleriot JP, Chevret S, Goldstein FW, Carlet J. Single- versus

triple-lumen central catheter-related sepsis: a prospective randomized study in a critically ill population. Am J Med 1992; 93:277–282.

136. Collignon PJ, Soni N, Pearson IY, Woods WP, Munro R, Sorrell TC. Is semiquantitative culture of central vein catheter tips useful in the diagnosis of catheter-associated bacteremia? J Clin Microbiol 1986; 24:532–535.

137. Brun-Buisson C, Abrouk F, Legrand P, Huet Y, Larabi S, Rapin M. Diagnosis of central venous catheter-related sepsis. Critical level of quantitative tip cultures. Arch Intern Med 1987; 147:873–877.

138. Prager RL, Silva J Jr. Colonization of central venous catheters. South Med J 1984; 77:458–461.

139. Richet H, Hubert B, Nitemberg G, Andremont A, Buu-Hoi A, Ourbak P, Galicier C, Veron M, Boisivon A, Bouvier AM, et al. Prospective multicenter study of vascular-catheter-related complications and risk factors for positive central-catheter cultures in intensive care unit patients. J Clin Microbiol 1990; 28:2520–2525.

140. Snydman DR, Gorbea HF, Pober BR, Majka JA, Murray SA, Perry LK. Predictive value of surveillance skin cultures in total-parenteral-nutrition-related infection. Lancet 1982; 2:1385–1388.

141. Hanna HA, Raad I. Blood products: a significant risk factor for long-term catheter-related bloodstream infections in cancer patients. Infect Control Hosp Epidemiol 2001; 22:165–166.

142. Raad II, Baba M, Bodey GP. Diagnosis of catheter-related infections: the role of surveillance and targeted quantitative skin cultures. Clin Infect Dis 1995; 20:593–597.

143. Raad I, Narro J, Khan A, Tarrand J, Vartivarian S, Bodey GP. Serious complications of vascular catheter-related *Staphylococcus aureus* bacteremia in cancer patients. Eur J Clin Microbiol Infect Dis 1992; 11:675–682.

144. Strinden WD, Helgerson RB, Maki DG. Candida septic thrombosis of the great central veins associated with central catheters. Clinical features and management. Ann Surg 1985; 202:653–658.

145. Raad II, Hanna HA, Darouiche RO. Diagnosis of catheter-related bloodstream infections: is it necessary to culture the subcutaneous catheter segment? Eur J Clin Microbiol Infect Dis 2001; 20:566–568.

146. Sherertz RJ, Raad II, Belani A, Koo LC, Rand KH, Pickett DL, Straub SA, Fauerbach LL. Three-year experience with sonicated vascular catheter cultures in a clinical microbiology laboratory. J Clin Microbiol 1990; 28:76–82.

147. Sherertz RJ, Heard SO, Raad II. Diagnosis of triple-lumen catheter infection: comparison of roll plate, sonication, and flushing methodologies. J Clin Microbiol 1997; 35:641–646.

148. Siegman-Igra Y, Anglim AM, Shapiro DE, Adal KA, Strain BA, Farr BM. Diagnosis of vascular catheter-related bloodstream infection: a meta-analysis. J Clin Microbiol 1997; 35:928–936.

149. Widmer AF, Nettleman M, Flint K, Wenzel RP. The clinical impact of culturing central venous catheters. A prospective study. Arch Intern Med 1992; 152:1299–1302.

150. Capdevila JA, Planes AM, Palomar M, Gasser I, Almirante B, Pahissa A,

Crespo E, Martinez-Vazquez JM. Value of differential quantitative blood cultures in the diagnosis of catheter-related sepsis. Eur J Clin Microbiol Infect Dis 1992; 11:403–407.

151. Blot F, Schmidt E, Nitenberg G, Tancrede C, Leclercq B, Laplanche A, Andremont A. Earlier positivity of central-venous-versus peripheral-blood cultures is highly predictive of catheter-related sepsis. J Clin Microbiol 1998; 36:105–109.

152. Blot F, Nitenberg G, Chachaty E, Raynard B, Germann N, Antoun S, Laplanche A, Brun-Buisson C, Tancrede C. Diagnosis of catheter-related bacteraemia: a prospective comparison of the time to positivity of hub-blood versus peripheral-blood cultures. Lancet 1999; 354:1071–1077.

153. Rijnders BJ, Verwaest C, Peetermans WE, Wilmer A, Vandecasteele S, Van Eldere J, Van Wijngaerden E. Difference in time to positivity of hub-blood versus nonhub-blood cultures is not useful for the diagnosis of catheter-related bloodstream infection in critically ill patients. Crit Care Med 2001; 29:1399–1403.

154. Raad I, Hanna H, Alakech B, Chatzinikolaou I, Whimbey E, Rolston KV, Tarrand J. Diagnosis of catheter-related bloodstream infections (CRBSI): correlation of differential time to positivity (DTP) with quantitative blood cultures (QBC) for short- and long-term central venous catheters (CVC). Fortieth Interscience Conference on Antimicrobial Agents and Chemotherapy (ICAAC), Toronto, Ontario, Canada, 2000.

155. Kite P, Dobbins BM, Wilcox MH, Fawley WN, Kindon AJ, Thomas D, Tighe MJ, McMahon MJ. Evaluation of a novel endoluminal brush method for in situ diagnosis of catheter related sepsis. J Clin Pathol 1997; 50:278–282.

156. Kite P, Dobbins BM, Wilcox MH, McMahon MJ. Rapid diagnosis of central-venous-catheter-related bloodstream infection without catheter removal. Lancet 1999; 354:1504–1507.

157. Pascual A, Ramirez de Arellano E, Martinez Martinez L, Perea EJ. Effect of polyurethane catheters and bacterial biofilms on the in-vitro activity of antimicrobials against Staphylococcus epidermidis. J Hosp Infect 1993; 24:211–218.

158. Guggenbichler JP, Berchtold D, Allerberger F, Bonatti H, Hager J, Pfaller W, Dierich MP. In vitro and in vivo effect of antibiotics on catheters colonized by staphylococci. Eur J Clin Microbiol Infect Dis 1992; 11:408–415.

159. Ramirez de Arellano E, Pascual A, Martinez-Martinez L, Perea EJ. Activity of eight antibacterial agents on Staphylococcus epidermidis attached to Teflon catheters. J Med Microbiol 1994; 40:43–47.

160. Gaillard JL, Merlino R, Pajot N, Goulet O, Fauchere JL, Ricour C, Veron M. Conventional and nonconventional modes of vancomycin administration to decontaminate the internal surface of catheters colonized with coagulase-negative staphylococci. J Parenter Enteral Nutr 1990; 14:593–597.

161. Cowan CE. Antibiotic lock technique. J Intraven Nurs 1992; 15:283–287.

162. Messing B, Peitra-Cohen S, Debure A, Beliah M, Bernier JJ. Antibiotic-lock technique: a new approach to optimal therapy for catheter-related sepsis in home-parenteral nutrition patients. J Parenter Enteral Nutr 1988; 12:185–189.

163. Douard MC, Arlet G, Leverger G, Paulien R, Waintrop C, Clementi E, Eurin B,

Schaison G. Quantitative blood cultures for diagnosis and management of catheter-related sepsis in pediatric hematology and oncology patients. Intensive Care Med 1991; 17:30–35.

164. Johnson DC, Johnson FL, Goldman S. Preliminary results treating persistent central venous catheter infections with the antibiotic lock technique in pediatric patients. Pediatr Infect Dis J 1994; 13:930–931.

165. Williams N, Carlson GL, Scott NA, Irving MH. Incidence and management of catheter-related sepsis in patients receiving home parenteral nutrition. Br J Surg 1994; 81:392–394.

166. Benoit JL, Carandang G, Sitrin M, Arnow PM. Intraluminal antibiotic treatment of central venous catheter infections in patients receiving parenteral nutrition at home. Clin Infect Dis 1995; 21:1286–1288.

167. Krzywda EA, Andris DA, Edmiston CE Jr, Quebbeman EJ. Treatment of Hickman catheter sepsis using antibiotic lock technique. Infect Control Hosp Epidemiol 1995; 16:596–598.

168. Capdevila JA, Segarra A, Planes AM, Ramirez-Arellano M, Pahissa A, Piera L, Martinez-Vazquez JM. Successful treatment of haemodialysis catheter-related sepsis without catheter removal. Nephrol Dial Transplant 1993; 8:231–234.

169. Rao JS, O'Meara A, Harvey T, Breatnach F. A new approach to the management of Broviac catheter infection. J Hosp Infect 1992; 22:109–116.

170. Mermel LA, Farr BM, Sherertz RJ, Raad II, O'Grady N, Harris JS, Craven DE. Guidelines for the management of intravascular catheter-related infections. Clin Infect Dis 2001; 32:1249–1272.

171. Raad I, Davis S, Khan A, Tarrand J, Elting L, Bodey GP. Impact of central venous catheter removal on the recurrence of catheter-related coagulase-negative staphylococcal bacteremia. Infect Control Hosp Epidemiol 1992; 13:215–221.

172. Raad II, Vartivarian S, Khan A, Bodey GP. Catheter-related infections caused by the Mycobacterium fortuitum complex: 15 cases and review. Rev Infect Dis 1991; 13:1120–1125.

173. Fidalgo S, Vazquez F, Mendoza MC, Perez F, Mendez FJ. Bacteremia due to Staphylococcus epidermidis: microbiologic, epidemiologic, clinical, and prognostic features. Rev Infect Dis 1990; 12:520–528.

174. Rupp ME, Archer GL. Coagulase-negative staphylococci: pathogens associated with medical progress. Clin Infect Dis 1994; 19:231–243; quiz 244–235.

175. Froggatt JW, Johnston JL, Galetto DW, Archer GL. Antimicrobial resistance in nosocomial isolates of Staphylococcus haemolyticus. Antimicrob Agents Chemother 1989; 33:460–466.

176. Christensen GD, Bisno AL, Parisi JT, McLaughlin B, Hester MG, Luther RW. Nosocomial septicemia due to multiply antibiotic-resistant Staphylococcus epidermidis. Ann Intern Med 1982; 96:1–10.

177. Winston DJ, Dudnick DV, Chapin M, Ho WG, Gale RP, Martin WJ. Coagulase-negative staphylococcal bacteremia in patients receiving immunosuppressive therapy. Arch Intern Med 1983; 143:32–36.

178. Sattler FR, Foderaro JB, Aber RC. Staphylococcus epidermidis bacteremia

associated with vascular catheters: an important cause of febrile morbidity in hospitalized patients. Infect Control 1984; 5:279–283.

179. Sherertz RJ, Falk RJ, Huffman KA, Thomann CA, Mattern WD. Infections associated with subclavian Uldall catheters. Arch Intern Med 1983; 143:52–56.

180. Herwaldt LA, Geiss M, Kao C, Pfaller MA. The positive predictive value of isolating coagulase-negative staphylococci from blood cultures. Clin Infect Dis 1996; 22:14–20. See comments.

181. Raad I, Davis S, Khan A, Tarrand J, Elting L, Bodey GP. Impact of central venous catheter removal on the recurrence of catheter-related coagulase-negative staphylococcal bacteremia. Infect Control Hosp Epidemiol 1992; 13:215–221.

182. Raad I, Bompart F, Hachem R. Prospective, randomized dose-ranging open phase II pilot study of quinupristin/dalfopristin versus vancomycin in the treatment of catheter-related staphylococcal bacteremia. Eur J Clin Microbiol Infect Dis 1999; 18:199–202.

183. Garcia R, Raad I. In vitro study of the potential role of quinupristin/dalfopristin in the treatment of catheter-related staphylococcal infections. Eur J Clin Microbiol Infect Dis 1996; 15:933–936.

184. Jones RN, Johnson DM, Erwin ME. In vitro antimicrobial activities and spectra of U-100592 and U-100766, two novel fluorinated oxazolidinones. Antimicrob Agents Chemother 1996; 40:720–726.

185. Kaatz GW, Seo SM. In vitro activities of oxazolidinone compounds U100592 and U100766 against *Staphylococcus aureus* and *Staphylococcus epidermidis*. Antimicrob Agents Chemother 1996; 40:799–801.

186. Moellering RC Jr. A novel antimicrobial agent joins the battle against resistant bacteria. Ann Intern Med 1999; 130:155–157.

187. Rose HD. Venous catheter-associated candidemia. Am J Med Sci 1978; 275:265–269.

188. Dugdale DC, Ramsey PG. *Staphylococcus aureus* bacteremia in patients with Hickman catheters. Am J Med 1990; 89:137–141.

189. Lecciones JA, Lee JW, Navarro EE, Witebsky FG, Marshall D, Steinberg SM, Pizzo PA, Walsh TJ. Vascular catheter-associated fungemia in patients with cancer: analysis of 155 episodes. Clin Infect Dis 1992; 14:875–883.

190. Raad II, Sabbagh MF. Optimal duration of therapy for catheter-related *Staphylococcus aureus* bacteremia: a study of 55 cases and review. Clin Infect Dis 1992; 14:75–82. See comments.

191. Malanoski GJ, Samore MH, Pefanis A, Karchmer AW. *Staphylococcus aureus* catheter-associated bacteremia. Minimal effective therapy and unusual infectious complications associated with arterial sheath catheters. Arch Intern Med 1995; 155:1161–1166. See comments.

192. Fowler VG Jr, Sanders LL, Sexton DJ, Kong L, Marr KA, Gopal AK, Gottlieb G, McClelland RS, Corey GR. Outcome of *Staphylococcus aureus* bacteremia according to compliance with recommendations of infectious diseases specialists: experience with 244 patients. Clin Infect Dis 1998; 27:478–486.

193. Libman H, Arbeit RD. Complications associated with *Staphylococcus aureus* bacteremia. Arch Intern Med 1984; 144:541–545.

194. Maki DG, McCormick RD, Uman SJ, Wirtanen GW. Septic endarteritis due to intra-arterial catheters for cancer chemotherapy. I. Evaluation of an outbreak. II. Risk factors, clinical features and management. III. Guidelines for prevention. Cancer 1979; 44:1228–1240.

195. Rosen AB, Fowler VG Jr, Corey GR, Downs SM, Biddle AK, Li J, Jollis JG. Cost-effectiveness of transesophageal echocardiography to determine the duration of therapy for intravascular catheter-associated *Staphylococcus aureus* bacteremia. Ann Intern Med 1999; 130:810–820.

196. Fowler VG Jr, Li J, Corey GR, Boley J, Marr KA, Gopal AK, Kong LK, Gottlieb G, Donovan CL, Sexton DJ, Ryan T. Role of echocardiography in evaluation of patients with *Staphylococcus aureus* bacteremia: experience in 103 patients. J Am Coll Cardiol 1997; 30:1072–1078.

197. Wey SB, Mori M, Pfaller MA, Woolson RF, Wenzel RP. Hospital-acquired candidemia. The attributable mortality and excess length of stay. Arch Intern Med 1988; 148:2642–2645.

198. Rex JH, Bennett JE, Sugar AM, Pappas PG, van der Horst CM, Edwards JE, Washburn RG, Scheld WM, Karchmer AW, Dine AP, et al. A randomized trial comparing fluconazole with amphotericin B for the treatment of candidemia in patients without neutropenia. Candidemia Study Group and the National Institute. N Engl J Med 1994; 331:1325–1330.

199. Anaissie EJ, Vartivarian SE, Abi-Said D, Uzun O, Pinczowski H, Kontoyiannis DP, Khoury P, Papadakis K, Gardner A, Raad II, Gilbreath J, Bodey GP. Fluconazole versus amphotericin B in the treatment of hematogenous candidiasis: a matched cohort study. Am J Med 1996; 101:170–176.

200. Rex JH, Walsh TJ, Sobel JD, Filler SG, Pappas PG, Dismukes WE, Edwards JE. Practice guidelines for the treatment of candidiasis. Infectious Diseases Society of America. Clin Infect Dis 2000; 30:662–678.

201. Berrouane YF, Hollis RJ, Pfaller MA. Strain variation among and antifungal susceptibilities of isolates of *Candida krusei*. J Clin Microbiol 1996; 34:1856–1858.

202. Pfaller MA, Barry AL. In vitro susceptibilities of clinical yeast isolates to three antifungal agents determined by the microdilution method. Mycopathologia 1995; 130:3–9.

203. Chandra J, Kuhn DM, Mukherjee PK, Hoyer LL, McCormick T, Ghannoum MA. Biofilm formation by the fungal pathogen *Candida albicans*: development, architecture, and drug resistance. Journal of Bacteriology 2001; 183:5385–5394.

204. Cole GT, Halawa AA, Anaissie EJ. The role of the gastrointestinal tract in hematogenous candidiasis: from the laboratory to the bedside. Clin Infect Dis 1996; 22(suppl 2):S73–S88.

205. Pittet D, Monod M, Suter PM, Frenk E, Auckenthaler R. Candida colonization and subsequent infections in critically ill surgical patients. Annals of Surgery 1994; 220:751–758.

206. Reagan DR, Pfaller MA, Hollis RJ, Wenzel RP. Characterization of the sequence of colonization and nosocomial candidemia using DNA fingerprinting and a DNA probe. Journal of Clinical Microbiology 1990; 28:2733-2738.
207. Walsh TJ, Merz WG. Pathologic features in the human alimentary tract associated with invasiveness of *Candida tropicalis*. American Journal of Clinical Pathology 1986; 85:498-502.
208. McNeil MM, Lasker BA, Lott TJ, Jarvis WR. Postsurgical *Candida albicans* infections associated with an extrinsically contaminated intravenous anesthetic agent. Journal of Clinical Microbiology 1999; 37:1398-1403.
209. Solomon SL, Alexander H, Eley JW, Anderson RL, Goodpasture HC, Smart S, Furman RM, Martone WJ. Nosocomial fungemia in neonates associated with intravascular pressure-monitoring devices. Pediatric Infectious Disease 1986; 5:680-685.
210. Solomon SL, Khabbaz RF, Parker RH, Anderson RL, Geraghty MA, Furman RM, Martone WJ. An outbreak of Candida parapsilosis bloodstream infections in patients receiving parenteral nutrition. Journal of Infectious Diseases 1984; 149:98-102.
211. Nguyen MH, Peacock JE Jr, Tanner DC, Morris AJ, Nguyen ML, Snydman DR, Wagener MM, Yu VL. Therapeutic approaches in patients with candidemia. Evaluation in a multicenter, prospective, observational study. Arch Intern Med 1995; 155:2429 2435.
212. Nucci M, Colombo AL, Silveira F, Richtmann R, Salomao R, Branchini ML, Spector N. Risk factors for death in patients with candidemia. Infect Control Hosp Epidemiol 1998; 19:846-850.
213. Hung CC, Chen YC, Chang SC, Luh KT, Hsieh WC. Nosocomial candidemia in a university hospital in Taiwan. J Formos Med Assoc 1996; 95:19-28.
214. Rex JH, Bennett JE, Sugar AM, Pappas PG, Serody J, Edwards JE, Washburn RG. Intravascular catheter exchange and duration of candidemia. NIAID Mycoses Study Group and the Candidemia Study Group. Clin Infect Dis 1995; 21:994-996.
215. Nucci M, Silveira MI, Spector N, Silveira F, Velasco E, Akiti T, Barreiros G, Derossi A, Colombo AL, Pulcheri W. Risk factors for death among cancer patients with fungemia. Clin Infect Dis 1998; 27:107-111.
216. Karlowicz MG, Hashimoto LN, Kelly RE Jr, Buescher ES. Should central venous catheters be removed as soon as candidemia is detected in neonates? Pediatrics 2000; 106:E63.
217. Anaissie EJ, Rex JH, Uzun O, Vartivarian S. Predictors of adverse outcome in cancer patients with candidemia. Am J Med 1998; 104:238-245.
218. Luzzati R, Amalfitano G, Lazzarini L, Soldani F, Bellino S, Solbiati M, Danzi MC, Vento S, Todeschini G, Vivenza C, Concia E. Nosocomial candidemia in nonneutropenic patients at an Italian tertiary care hospital. Eur J Clin Microbiol Infect Dis 2000; 19:602-607.
219. Girmenia C, Martino P, De Bernardis F, Gentile G, Boccanera M, Monaco M, Antonucci G, Cassone A. Rising incidence of *Candida parapsilosis* fungemia in patients with hematologic malignancies: clinical aspects, predisposing factors,

and differential pathogenicity of the causative strains. Clin Infect Dis 1996; 23: 506–514.

220. Stamos JK, Rowley AH. Candidemia in a pediatric population. Clin Infect Dis 1995; 20:571–575.

221. Dato VM, Dajani AS. Candidemia in children with central venous catheters: role of catheter removal and amphotericin B therapy. Pediatr Infect Dis J 1990; 9:309–314.

222. Eppes SC, Troutman JL, Gutman LT. Outcome of treatment of candidemia in children whose central catheters were removed or retained. Pediatr Infect Dis J 1989; 8:99–104.

223. Goodrich JM, Reed EC, Mori M, Fisher LD, Skerrett S, Dandliker PS, Klis B, Counts GW, Meyers JD. Clinical features and analysis of risk factors for invasive candidal infection after marrow transplantation. J Infect Dis 1991; 164:731–740.

224. Nucci M, Anaissie E. Should vascular catheters be removed from all patients with candidemia? An evidence-based review. Clin Infect Dis 2002; 34:591–599.

225. Telenti A, Steckelberg JM, Stockman L, Edson RS, Roberts GD. Quantitative blood cultures in candidemia. Mayo Clin Proc 1991; 66:1120–1123.

226. Uzun O, Ascioglu S, Anaissie EJ, Rex JH. Risk factors and predictors of outcome in patients with cancer and breakthrough candidemia. Clin Infect Dis 2001; 32:1713–1717.

227. Nucci M, Colombo AL. Risk factors for breakthrough candidemia. Eur J Clin Microbiol Infect Dis 2002; 21:209–211.

228. Anaissie E. Opportunistic mycoses in the immunocompromised host: experience at a cancer center and review. Clin Infect Dis 1992; 14(suppl 1):S43–S53.

229. Abi-Said D, Anaissie E, Uzun O, Raad I, Pinzcowski H, Vartivarian S. The epidemiology of hematogenous candidiasis caused by different *Candida* species. Clin Infect Dis 1997; 24:1122–1128.

230. Barber GR, Brown AE, Kiehn TE, Edwards FF, Armstrong D. Catheter-related *Malassezia furfur* fungemia in immunocompromised patients. Am J Med 1993; 95:365–370.

231. Marcon MJ, Powell DA. Human infections due to *Malassezia* spp. Clin Microbiol Rev 1992; 5:101–119.

232. Kiehn TE, Armstrong D. Changes in the spectrum of organisms causing bacteremia and fungemia in immunocompromised patients due to venous access devices. Eur J Clin Microbiol Infect Dis 1990; 9:869–872.

233. Seifert H. Catheter-related infections due to gram-negative bacilli. In: Seifert H, Jansen B, Farr BM, eds. Catheter-Related Infections. New York: Marcel Dekker, 1997:111–138.

234. Maki DG, Mermel LA. Infections due to infusion therapy. In: Bennett JV, Brachman PS, eds. Hospital Infections. Philadelphia: Lippincott-Raven, 1998: 689–724.

235. Afif C, Hanna H, Alakech B, Boktour M, Tarrand J, Hachem R, Raad I.

Central venous catheter-related gram negative bacteremia (CRGNB): significance of catheter removal in preventing relapse. Thirty-ninth Annual Meeting of the Infectious Diseases Society of America (IDSA), San Francisco, California, USA, 2001.

236. Chatzinikolaou I, Abi-Said D, Bodey GP, Rolston KV, Tarrand JJ, Samonis G. Recent experience with *Pseudomonas aeruginosa* bacteremia in patients with cancer: retrospective analysis of 245 episodes. Arch Intern Med 2000; 160:501–509.

237. Voss A. Miscellaneous organisms. In: Seifert H, Jansen B, Farr BM, eds. Catheter-Related Infections. New York: Marcel Dekker, 1997:157–182.

238. Raad II, Hohn DC, Gilbreath BJ, Suleiman N, Hill LA, Bruso PA, Marts K, Mansfield PF, Bodey GP. Prevention of central venous catheter-related infections by using maximal sterile barrier precautions during insertion. Infect Control Hosp Epidemiol 1994; 15:231–238. See comments.

239. Maki DG. Yes, Virginia, aseptic technique is very important: maximal barrier precautions during insertion reduce the risk of central venous catheter-related bacteremia. Infect Control Hosp Epidemiol 1994; 15:227–230.

240. Faubion WC, Wesley JR, Khalidi N, Silva J. Total parenteral nutrition catheter sepsis: impact of the team approach. J Parenter Enteral Nutr 1986; 10:642–645.

241. Maki DG, Ringer M, Alvarado CJ. Prospective randomised trial of povidone-iodine, alcohol, and chlorhexidine for prevention of infection associated with central venous and arterial catheters. Lancet 1991; 338:339 343. See comments.

242. Maki DG, Band JD. A comparative study of polyantibiotic and iodophor ointments in prevention of vascular catheter-related infection. Am J Med 1981; 70:739–744.

243. Zinner SH, Denny-Brown BC, Braun P, Burke JP, Toala P, Kass EH. Risk of infection with intravenous indwelling catheters: effect of application of antibiotic ointment. J Infect Dis 1969; 120:616–619.

244. Hill RL, Fisher AP, Ware RJ, Wilson S, Casewell MW. Mupirocin for the reduction of colonization of internal jugular cannulae—a randomized controlled trial. J Hosp Infect 1990; 15:311–321.

245. Hoffmann KK, Weber DJ, Samsa GP, Rutala WA. Transparent polyurethane film as an intravenous catheter dressing. A meta-analysis of the infection risks. JAMA 1992; 267:2072–2076.

246. Conly JM, Grieves K, Peters B. A prospective, randomized study comparing transparent and dry gauze dressings for central venous catheters. J Infect Dis 1989; 159:310–319.

247. Maki DG, Stolz SS, Wheeler S, Mermel LA. A prospective, randomized trial of gauze and two polyurethane dressings for site care of pulmonary artery catheters: implications for catheter management. Crit Care Med 1994; 22:1729–1737.

248. Timsit JF, Sebille V, Farkas JC, Misset B, Martin JB, Chevret S, Carlet J. Effect of subcutaneous tunneling on internal jugular catheter-related sepsis in critically ill patients: a prospective randomized multicenter study. JAMA 1996; 276: 1416–1420.

249. Sitges-Serra A, Puig P, Linares J, Perez JL, Farrero N, Jaurrieta E, Garau J. Hub colonization as the initial step in an outbreak of catheter-related sepsis due to coagulase negative staphylococci during parenteral nutrition. J Parenter Enteral Nutr 1984; 8:668–672.

250. Schwartz C, Henrickson KJ, Roghmann K, Powell K. Prevention of bacteremia attributed to luminal colonization of tunneled central venous catheters with vancomycin-susceptible organisms. J Clin Oncol 1990; 8:1591–1597.

251. Henrickson KJ, Axtell RA, Hoover SM, Kuhn SM, Pritchett J, Kehl SC, Klein JP. Prevention of central venous catheter-related infections and thrombotic events in immunocompromised children by the use of vancomycin/ciprofloxacin/heparin flush solution: a randomized, multicenter, double-blind trial. J Clin Oncol 2000; 18:1269–1278.

252. Carratala J, Niubo J, Fernandez-Sevilla A, Juve E, Castellsague X, Berlanga J, Linares J, Gudiol F. Randomized, double-blind trial of an antibiotic-lock technique for prevention of gram-positive central venous catheter-related infection in neutropenic patients with cancer. Antimicrob Agents Chemother 1999; 43:2200–2204.

253. Maki D, Garland J, Alex C, Henrickson K. A randomized trial of a vancomycin-heparin lock solution (VHLS) for prevention of catheter-related bloodstream infection (CRBSI) in a NNICU. Twelfth Annual Scientific Meeting of the Society for Healthcare Epidemiology of America (SHEA), Salt Lake City, Utah, USA, Apr 6–9, 2002.

254. Rackoff WR, Weiman M, Jakobowski D, Hirschl R, Stallings V, Bilodeau J, Danz P, Bell L, Lange B. A randomized, controlled trial of the efficacy of a heparin and vancomycin solution in preventing central venous catheter infections in children. J Pediatr 1995; 127:147–151. See comments.

255. Gil ML, Casanova M, Martinez JP. Changes in the cell wall glycoprotein composition of *Candida albicans* associated to the inhibition of germ tube formation by EDTA. Arch Microbiol 1994; 161:489–494.

256. Root JL, McIntyre OR, Jacobs NJ, Daghlian CP. Inhibitory effect of disodium EDTA upon the growth of *Staphylococcus epidermidis* in vitro: relation to infection prophylaxis of Hickman catheters. Antimicrob Agents Chemother 1988; 32:1627–1631.

257. Raad I, Hachem R, Tcholakian RK, Sherertz R. Efficacy of minocycline and EDTA lock solution in preventing catheter-related bacteremia, septic phlebitis, and endocarditis in rabbits. Antimicrob Agents Chemother 2002; 46:327–332.

258. Raad I, Buzaid A, Rhyne J, Hachem R, Darouiche R, Safar H, Albitar M, Sherertz RJ. Minocycline and ethylenediaminetetraacetate for the prevention of recurrent vascular catheter infections. Clin Infect Dis 1997; 25:149–151.

259. Bleyer A, Mason L, Raad I, Sherertz R. A randomized, double-blind trial comparing minocycline/EDTA vs heparin as flush solutions for hemodialysis catheters. Fourth Decennial International Conference on Nosocomial and Healthcare-Associated Infections, in conjunction with the 10th Annual Meeting of the Society for Healthcare Epidemiology of America (SHEA), Atlanta, Georgia, USA, 2000:91. Abstract No. P-S1-31.

260. Maki DG, Stolz SM, Wheeler S, Mermel LA. Prevention of central venous catheter-related bloodstream infection by use of an antiseptic-impregnated catheter. A randomized, controlled trial. Ann Intern Med 1997; 127:257–266. See comments.

261. Logghe C, Van Ossel C, D'Hoore W, Ezzedine H, Wauters G, Haxhe JJ. Evaluation of chlorhexidine and silver-sulfadiazine impregnated central venous catheters for the prevention of bloodstream infection in leukaemic patients: a randomized controlled trial. J Hosp Infect 1997; 37:145–156. See comments.

262. Bach A, Schmidt H, Bottiger B, Schreiber B, Bohrer H, Motsch J, Martin E, Sonntag HG. Retention of antibacterial activity and bacterial colonization of antiseptic-bonded central venous catheters. J Antimicrob Chemother 1996; 37: 315–322.

263. Ciresi DL, Albrecht RM, Volkers PA, Scholten DJ. Failure of antiseptic bonding to prevent central venous catheter-related infection and sepsis. Am Surg 1996; 62:641–646.

264. Heard SO, Wagle M, Vijayakumar E, McLean S, Brueggemann A, Napolitano LM, Edwards LP, O'Connell FM, Puyana JC, Doern GV. Influence of triple-lumen central venous catheters coated with chlorhexidine and silver sulfadiazine on the incidence of catheter-related bacteremia. Arch Intern Med 1998; 158:81–87.

265. Pemberton LB, Ross V, Cuddy P, Kremer H, Fessler T, McGurk E. No difference in catheter sepsis between standard and antiseptic central venous catheters. A prospective randomized trial. Arch Surg 1996; 131:986–989.

266. Veenstra DL, Saint S, Saha S, Lumley T, Sullivan SD. Efficacy of antiseptic-impregnated central venous catheters in preventing catheter-related bloodstream infection: a meta-analysis. JAMA 1999; 281:261–267. See comments.

267. Bassetti S, Hu J, D'Agostino RB Jr, Sherertz RJ. Prolonged antimicrobial activity of a catheter containing chlorhexidine-silver sulfadiazine extends protection against catheter infections in vivo. Antimicrob Agents Chemother 2001; 45:1535–1538.

268. Raad I, Darouiche R, Hachem R, Sacilowski M, Bodey GP. Antibiotics and prevention of microbial colonization of catheters. Antimicrob Agents Chemother 1995; 39:2397–2400.

269. Raad I, Darouiche R, Hachem R, Mansouri M, Bodey GP. The broad-spectrum activity and efficacy of catheters coated with minocycline and rifampin. J Infect Dis 1996; 173:418–424.

270. Raad I, Darouiche R, Dupuis J, Abi-Said D, Gabrielli A, Hachem R, Wall M, Harris R, Jones J, Buzaid A, Robertson C, Shenaq S, Curling P, Burke T, Ericsson C. Central venous catheters coated with minocycline and rifampin for the prevention of catheter-related colonization and bloodstream infections. A randomized, double-blind trial. Texas Medical Center Catheter Study Group. Ann Intern Med 1997; 127:267–274. See comments.

271. Darouiche RO, Raad II, Heard SO, Thornby JI, Wenker OC, Gabrielli A, Berg J, Khardori N, Hanna H, Hachem R, Harris RL, Mayhall G. A comparison

of two antimicrobial-impregnated central venous catheters. Catheter Study Group. N Engl J Med 1999; 340:1–8. See comments.

272.   Raad II, Darouiche RO, Hachem R, Abi-Said D, Safar H, Darnule T, Mansouri M, Morck D. Antimicrobial durability and rare ultrastructural colonization of indwelling central catheters coated with minocycline and rifampin. Crit Care Med 1998; 26:219–224. See comments.

273.   Tambe SM, Sampath L, Modak SM. In vitro evaluation of the risk of developing bacterial resistance to antiseptics and antibiotics used in medical devices. J Antimicrob Chemother 2001; 47:589–598.

274.   Hanna H, Graviss L, Chaiban G, Dvorak T, Arbuckle R, Estey E, Munsell M, Hachem R, Champlin R. Susceptibility patterns of *Staphylococcus* organisms in leukemia and bone marrow transplant (BMT) services after the use of minocycline/rifampin-impregnated central venous catheters (MR-CVCs) in a cancer hospital. Forty-Second Annual Conference of the Interscience Conference on Antimicrobial Agents and Chemotherapy (ICAAC), San Diego, CA, USA, 2002.

275.   Raad II, Hackett B, Hanna HA, Graviss L, Botz R. Use of antibiotic impregnated catheters associated with significant decrease in nosocomial bloodstream infections in critically ill cancer patients [abstr]. Programs and Abstracts of the 4th Decennial Conference on Nososcomial and Healthcare-Associated Infections, in conjuction with the 10th Annual Meeting of the Society for Healthcare Epidemiology of America, Atlanta, Georgia, 2000.

276.   Raad II, Hanna HA. Intravascular catheter-related infections: new horizons and recent advances. Arch Intern Med 2002; 162:871–878.

34

Fungal Infections in Cancer Patients

Magnus Gottfredsson
Landspitali University Hospital
Reykjavik, Iceland

John R. Perfect
Duke University Medical Center
Durham, North Carolina, U.S.A.

INTRODUCTION

Fungal pathogens have emerged during the past two decades as important causes of morbidity and mortality in immunocompromised patients, particularly in patients with malignancies and during their treatment. According to the National Nosocomial Infections Surveillance (NNIS) system, *Candida* species constitute the fourth most common causes of nosocomial bloodstream infections in the U.S. Moreover, *Aspergillus* species have become the most common infectious cause of death due to pneumonia in bone marrow/stem cell transplant (BMT) recipients. Other emerging mold infections have caused very high morbidity and mortality in BMT patients [1]. An international autopsy survey of patients with cancer identified fungal infections in 25% of leukemic patients and transplant recipients [2]. The development of drug resistance to antifungal agents and the emergence of new pathogenic fungi is a mounting problem in immunosuppressed patients with cancer. In this chapter we will focus on important clinical aspects of the increasing problem of serious fungal infections among oncological patients.

EPIDEMIOLOGY

In general, the incidence of invasive fungal infections is highly correlated with the number of immunosuppressed patients in the population. For instance, a recent prospective surveillance study for candidemia in Iowa showed that the annual incidence of candidemia in the state is 6.0 infections per 100,000 of the population [3]. A similar figure has been found in a nationwide study in Iceland where the incidence has increased more than fourfold in the past 20 years [4]. In addition to bloodstream yeast infections, chronic disseminated candidiasis such as hepatosplenic candidiasis is a major problem in patients with prolonged neutropenia. A study from Finland on patients with acute leukemia and hepatosplenic candidiasis during 1980 to 1993 reported a fivefold increase in the incidence of this infection during the study period. Interestingly, the incidence was higher among patients with acute lymphatic leukemia (11.3%) than among those with acute myeloid leukemia (5.1%) [5].

During the 1990s, molds have emerged as a major cause of mortality related to infection in patients with hematological malignancies and in BMT patients. In particular, aspergillosis seems to be increasing in incidence in this high-risk population. According to one study among patients with acute leukemia the incidence of proven or probable invasive aspergillosis (IA) was 7.1%, with a vast majority of the patients (92%) being neutropenic at the time of diagnosis [6]. In a cohort of marrow transplant patients, the incidence of IA increased from 5.7% to 11.2% during 1987 to 1993 at the Fred Hutchinson Cancer Research Center [7]. In the allogeneic BMT population, aspergillosis peaks occur during neutropenia, during graft vs. host disease and its management, and possibly a third peak during the latter part of the first posttransplant year. The emergence of infections caused by other molds, such as *Fusarium* species, zygomycetes, and dematiaceous fungi, has been described by several investigators in the high-risk population of BMT recipients [1,8–11].

MICROBIOLOGY

The most common fungal pathogens causing serious infections in immunocompromised patients are listed in Table 1. According to the NNIS data, *Candida* species are the most common nosocomial fungal pathogens, accounting for 72.1% of isolates in the study [12]. Although *Candida albicans* is still the most common *Candida* species causing infections in patients with solid tumors, non*albicans Candida* species have become common causes of infection in patients with hematological malignancies and BMT recipients

[13]. For instance, *Candida glabrata* and *Candida krusei* seem to be causing an increasing number of infections in cancer patients, and especially among patients who have received fluconazole prophylaxis [13,14]. Furthermore, *C. glabrata* fungemia has been shown to be associated with higher mortality than infections caused by other species of *Candida* [15]. This finding likely reflects the severity of the underlying disease rather than the intrinsic virulence of this yeast species, since higher mortality was associated with older age and more advanced malignancies. Other non*albicans Candida* species, such as *C. tropicalis*, with its ability to transmigrate through the gastrointestinal tract, and *C. parapsilosis*, with its ability to contaminate fluids and catheters, are also frequently found to produce infection in cancer patients and can even cause outbreaks [15a]. Fungemias caused by other yeast species are less common, but they are increasingly reported in patients with malignancies [16]. These yeasts or yeastlike structures in tissue include *Malassezia furfur*, *Rhodotorula rubra*, *Saccharomyces cerevisiae*, *Candida lusitaniae*, *Cryptococcus laurentii*, and *Hansenula anomala* [16–18].

Aspergillus fumigatus represents the most common *Aspergillus* species to produce a mold infection in patients with malignancies. Other *Aspergillus* species can also cause serious infections, including *A. flavus*, *A. terreus*, and *A. niger*. In comparison to other *Aspergillus* species, isolation of both *A. terreus* and *A. flavus* has been found to be more commonly associated with invasive disease than with colonization [19].

Hyaline septate filamentous fungi, such as *Trichosporon beigelii*, *Fusarium* species, *Acremonium* species, Paecilomyces species, and *Trichoderma* species, can cause invasive mycoses in severely immunosuppressed patients, and these infections are often refractory to conventional therapy. *Trichosporon beigelii*, in particular, has emerged as a life-threatening opportunist in granulocytopenic and immunocompromised hosts. This pathogen is a yeast in tissue but can produce hyphae in culture, and it can produce a false-positive cryptococcal antigen test in patients with disseminated trichosporonosis. *Fusarium* species can start infection from onychomycosis or contaminate a catheter. In a neutropenic patient, disseminated disease can develop rapidly with positive blood cultures [60–70% of cases]. *Blastoschizomyces capitatus*, another filamentous fungus, is also an important emerging opportunist in the compromised host, and most frequently infects patients with acute leukaemia, after chemotherapy treatment [20].

Dematiaceous septate filamentous fungi, such as *Alternaria* species, *Pseudallescheria boydii*, *Bipolaris* species, and *Cladophialophora bantiana* can cause severe pneumonia, sinusitis, and infections of the central nervous system, which may respond poorly to antifungal drug therapy in cancer patients (Table 1) [10,21].

Several zygomycetes, such as *Rhizopus* sp. or *Cunninghamella* sp., can cause lethal infections in cancer patients, despite aggressive medical and

TABLE 1 Common Pathogenic Yeast and Molds Which Cause Infections in Patients with Malignancies

Class	Genus, species	Common sites of infection	Unique characteristics
Yeasts	Candida albicans	Oropharyngeal, esophageal, gastrointestinal, catheter-associated bloodstream infections, candiduria, endocarditis, acute disseminated candidiasis, chronic disseminated candidiasis	Most virulent and most common of the Candida species
	Candida glabrata	Bloodstream, candiduria, intra-abdominal	Associated with fluconazole use
	Candida tropicalis	Bloodstream, intra-abdominal, skin	Pustular skin lesions and dissemination
	Candida parapsilosis	Bloodstream, catheter-associated bloodsteam infections, candiduria	Catheter-associated
	Candida krusei	Bloodstream, candiduria	Fluconazole-resistant, but not resistant to all azoles
	Candida guillermondii	Bloodstream	Frequently resistant to amphotericin B and nystatin
	Candida lusitaniae	Bloodstream	Frequently resistant to amphotericin B and nystatin
	Malassezia furfur	Bloodstream, contaminated i.v. lipids	Requires special lipid-supplemented medium for culture

Trichosporon beigelii	Bloodstream, cutaneous lesions, pulmonary infiltrates, and azotemia	Biopsy of skin lesions, blood cultures positive late in course. Causes false-positive cryptococcal antigen test
Cryptococcus neoformans	Lung, central nervous system	Associated with defects in cell-mediated immunity, steroids, and fludarabine use
Molds		
Aspergillus fumigatus, A. flavus, A. terreus, A. niger	Acute invasive pulmonary aspergillosis, chronic necrotizing aspergillosis, involving lungs and sinuses	Angioinvasive properties. May disseminate to central nervous system, skin, and other organs
Zygomycetes: *Mucor* sp., *Rhizopus* sp., *Cunninghamella* sp.	Sinuses, central nervous system, skin, lung	Direct tissue invasion, may disseminate
Fusarium sp.	Bloodstream, skin, sinus, lung, toes, and toenails	Frequently positive blood cultures and skin lesions
Scedosporium sp.	Bloodstream, skin, lung, central nervous system	Frequently positive blood cultures and skin lesions
Alternaria sp.	Sinuses, skin	Biopsy and culture of sinus mucosa
Bipolaris sp.	Sinuses	Biopsy and culture of sinus mucosa
Curvularia sp.	Sinuses	Biopsy and culture of sinus mucosa
Cladophialophora bantiana	Sinus, central nervous system, lung	Neurotropic

surgical interventions; and in most series of zygomycoses, outcome in cancer patients is worse than for those with diabetes.

In regions of the world where specific mycoses are endemic, such as penicilliosis, coccidioidomycosis, and histoplasmosis, the growing number of susceptible hosts has resulted in increased numbers of patients who either develop or reactivate these infections during cancer or its treatment. Therefore a thorough history of residence in an endemic area in the past should be undertaken [22].

RISK FACTORS

Candidiasis

Over the past three decades, risk factors for candidemia in cancer patients have been studied extensively. Well-established risk factors include the immunosuppression of malignancies and their treatments (e.g., neutropenia), administration of broad-spectrum antibacterial agents, and the use of indwelling central venous catheters [23]. In addition it has been shown that during chemotherapy, a characteristic profile of cytotoxic therapy–related damage is produced to the functional integrity of the intestinal epithelium, dependent on the chemotherapeutic regimen used. This damage is independent of the myelosuppression and is predictive for invasive infectious complications such as candidemia and hepatosplenic candidiasis [24]. The depth and duration of neutropenia has frequently been found to be the one of the most important risk factors for invasive candidiasis because it is easily measured. However it is more likely that a break in the integrity of the mucosa represents the single biggest risk to development of invasive candidiasis.

Aspergillosis

In a large hospital-based survey of aspergillosis the strongest risk factors for invasive infection were allogeneic BMT, neutropenia, and hematologic malignancies (Table 2). For instance, in patients with a positive culture for *Aspergillus* sp. from nonsterile body sites, these three clinical entities had a risk of IA that ranges from 50 to 64% [19]. Among BMT patients, the onset of IA is bimodal, peaking at 16 and 96 days after transplant [7], and there is concern that a third peak may occur later in the first year posttransplant. In BMT patients, underlying disease, donor type, season, and transplant outside of laminar airflow rooms are associated with a significant risk for IA within 40 days from the transplant. For patients presenting with IA > 40 days after transplant, age, underlying disease, donor type, graft-versus-host disease (GVHD), neutropenia, and corticosteroids were associated with increased risk. Interestingly, in this patient population with later onset of disease, only 31% of infected patients were neutropenic at the time of diagnosis [7].

TABLE 2   Risk Factors for IA Among Patients Who Have a
Positive Culture for *Aspergillus* sp. from Clinical Primarily
Nonsterile Specimens

Risk category, feature	Risk of IA (no. of cases, %)[a]
High	
Allogeneic BMT	25/39 (64)
Neutropenia	39/61 (64)
Hematologic cancer	53/106 (50)
Intermediate	
Autologous BMT	4/14 (28)
Malnutrition	27/99 (27)
Corticosteroids	78/381 (20)
HIV	26/138 (19)
Solid-organ transplant	21/124 (17)
Diabetes	17/151 (11)
Underlying pulmonary disease	45/477 (9)
Solid-organ cancer	10/126 (8)
Low	
Cystic fibrosis	1/127 (0.7)
Connective tissue disease	0/28 (0)

A case can be included in disease classification.
[a] Numerator, no. of cases of IA; denominator, no. of cases in which an *Aspergillus*
species was isolated.
Source: Ref. 19.

Corticosteroid prophylaxis and moderate-to-severe GVHD and its management posttransplant play major roles in the development of IA [25]. The
impact of hospital construction and the value of high-efficiency particulate air
filtration (HEPA) has been clearly demonstrated on cases of IA. For instance,
Oren and colleagues observed a nosocomial IA infection rate of 50% among
patients with acute leukemia during extensive hospital construction and
indoor renovation [26]. Then a new hematology ward was opened with HEPA
filters, and none of the acute leukemia or BMT patients who were hospitalized
exclusively on this hematology ward developed IA over a 3-year period [26].
In addition to the air quality as a source for IA in high-risk cancer patients,
recent studies suggest that the hospital water systems may also be a source of
nosocomial aspergillosis [27], and this concern about a water source for
infection has been extended to the other waterborne fungi such as *Fusarium*
sp. [28].

CLINICAL SYNDROMES

Candidiasis

Mucosal candidiasis (thrush) is a common entity among patients who receive cytotoxic therapy and antibacterial therapy. Thrush is particularly common in the treatment of head and neck cancers and probably reflects the impact of local irradiation, systemic chemotherapy, and possibly the use of antibacterials. These infections frequently produce dysphagia, odynophagia, and even abdominal pain. The absence of oral thrush does not exclude mucosal candidiasis elsewhere in the gastrointestinal tract. Mucosal candida infections are associated with substantial morbidity but do not directly increase patient mortality. However, heavy colonization of the skin or luminal surfaces with *Candida* is a risk factor for invasive, systemic spread of the infection, especially in the presence of severe mucositis and long-lasting neutropenia. Disseminated candidasis carries a substantial mortality in this patient population.

Candidemia is a common nosocomial infection, especially among patients with central venous catheters. Patients frequently present with fever and hypotension. In addition, tachypnea, evidence of infection at catheter insertion sites, and a pustular or papular rash are possible findings in patients with candidemia and cancer.

Molecular-relatedness studies strongly suggested that the gut is a primary source for the development of this infection [29]. In patients with cancer and candidemia a mortality rate of 33–75% has been reported. Host factors and the extent of infection (rather than infecting *Candida* species) are the main predictors of mortality [30]. Early diagnosis and treatment is therefore of paramount importance to prevent dissemination, which is the most severe complication of candidemia. In the syndrome of acute disseminated candidiasis during cancer with neutropenia, the infection frequently spreads to many organs including the liver, spleen, and kidneys. In addition, meningitis, endophthalmitis, endocarditis, and myositis are occasionally seen. Mortality in the acute disseminated candidiasis syndrome is as high as 50% [31].

Chronic disseminated candidiasis (CDC) is a potentially life-threatening complication of cytotoxic therapy for malignant diseases, particularly acute leukemia. As reflected by the older but more restrictive terminology, hepatosplenic candidiasis, this infection most commonly affects the liver (96%) and spleen (38%), with lungs and kidneys being less frequently involved [32]. In most instances, dissemination takes place during neutropenia, but diagnosis is usually made after recovery of the neutrophils. Symptoms are relatively nonspecific, fever and abdominal pain being most common. Elevation of alkaline phosphatase (3–5-fold the upper normal limit) is seen in most patients [32]. It is important to note that less than one third of the patients have history of documented candidemia [32]. In patients with acute leukemia, younger age, neutropenia of 15 days or longer, and the use of prophylactic quinolone antibiotics have been shown to be independent risk factors related to the development of CDC [33]. Diagnosis is made by abdominal ultrasonography or computed tomography (CT) scanning of the abdomen. However, hepatic or splenic lesions may transiently disappear during neutropenia, and antifungal therapy should therefore not be discontinued on the basis of radiologic findings alone [34].

Primary pneumonia caused by *Candida* sp. is uncommon, and the diagnosis can be difficult owing to the high prevalence of positive cultures for *Candida* from respiratory secretions in hospitalized patients receiving antibiotics. In one large series, less than one-third of the patients had severe neutropenia [35]. Most infections seem to be limited to the upper gastrointestinal tract and lung, suggesting aspiration as the main mechanism of entry to the lungs. The major clinical manifestations of primary *Candida* pneumonia are fever and tachypnea. Patchy infiltrates can be seen on chest radiographs, but the findings are nonspecific. Primary *Candida* pneumonia can be life-threatening in patients with cancer, since it has been shown to directly contribute to the death of 84% of the patients [35]. The diagnosis can be difficult owing to low specificity of sputum and bronchoalveolar lavage cultures, even among patients at highest risk [36]. Tissue biopsy is therefore needed to establish the diagnosis.

Candiduria is a common problem in hospitalised patients. In cancer patients with fungal urinary tract infections, the etiological agent is most commonly *C. albicans* (72%), but other yeasts may be found in urine [37]. Risk factors for funguria are frequently multiple, such as prior antibiotic therapy, other concomitant fungal infections, skin colonization with the same species, and urinary catheterization. Risk factors unique to cancer patients include corticosteriod use and neutropenia. Response to systemic antifungal therapy for this localized infection/colonization is generally good [37].

Aspergillosis

Aspergillus species can produce a broad spectrum of infections. These are categorized as invasive aspergillosis (IA), chronic necrotizing aspergillosis, aspergilloma, ("fungus ball"), and allergic bronchopulmonary aspergillosis. In patients with invasive pulmonary Aspergillosis (IPA), 56 to 90% present with respiratory symptoms and abnormal pulmonary chest radiograph [6,38,39]. The diagnosis of IA can be elusive and it may not be suspected before the diagnosis is made. In addition, most patients have concominant infections, which may lead the clinician astray [38]. In patients with acute leukemia and IPA, the infection disseminates to extrapulmonary sites in up to one-third of the patients [6]. The diagnosis of IPA should be entertained in patients with fever not responding to antibiotics, and/or typical findings ("halo sign," "air-cresecent sign") on a CT scan of the chest. A CT scan of the chest is relatively sensitive in suggesting aspergillosis in high-risk patients such as those with acute leukemia or BMT. Other common sites of infection with aspergillus include the paranasal sinuses, central nervous system, and skin.

Trichosporonosis

Disseminated trichosporonosis is increasingly reported, especially among patients with granulocytopenia. It often presents as fungemia, cutaneous lesions, pulmonary infiltrates, and azotemia [39a]. Trichosporonosis is associated with a high mortality [18,40]. A good response to azole therapy has occasionally been reported in a limited number of patients [41], but rapid immunological recovery is the single most important factor for a favorable outcome [17].

Fusariosis

This ubiquitous mold has become difficult to treat; it causes life-threatening disseminated infections in cancer patients with neutropenia. With disseminated infection, >60% of patients will have positive blood cultures, which is dramatically higher than other mold infections like *Aspergillus* and the zygomycetes [8,42,43]. This finding is likely due to the ability of this fungus to produce adventitial yeastlike propagules in tissue [44]. The most common portals of entry are the skin (33%) and the sinopulmonary tract (30%) [8]. Clinically, disseminated fusariosis can mimic aspergillosis with fever and severe myalgias during neutropenia, and disseminated ecthyma gangrenosumlike lesions may appear on the skin [42]. From a treatment standpoint, *Fusarium* infections respond inconsistently to amphotericin B and thus microbiological distinction from aspergillosis is of paramount importance. Voriconazole, a new extended-spectrum triazole, can successfully manage approximately 50% of cases of invasive disease. Immunological recovery is again the single most important predictor for survival.

Scedosporiosis

The emergence of both *Scedosporium prolificans* and *S. apiospermum* in cancer patients and particularly during neutropenia has become problematic. Both pathogens respond poorly to amphotericin B, and while *S. apiospermum* may respond to voriconazole, *S. prolificans* is frequently resistant to all presently used antifungal agents. It also has a propensity for being found in blood cultures in cases of disseminated disease.

Cryptococcosis

Because of the pandemic of HIV infection, cryptococcosis has probably become the most common invasive mycosis in the world. In cancer patients, it has always been observed at a measurable level and particularly in those with lymphomas and chronic leukemias. It is likely that the cell-mediated immune defects associated with these neoplasms combined with the frequent use of corticosteroids made these patient groups susceptible to infection. If medications for cancer therapies impact chronically on cellular immunity like fludarabine, cryptococcosis will become a more frequent opportunistic infection in this patient population. On the other hand, patients with solid tumor malignancies or BMT recipients without other risk factors appear to be unlikely to develop cryptococcosis. The primary sites for infection are the lung and the central nervous system.

DIAGNOSIS OF FUNGAL INFECTIONS

Candidiasis

Traditional culture-based methods remain the most clinically valuable diagnostic tools in patients with candidiasis. The sensitivity of blood cultures in patients with disseminated candidiasis ranges between 43 and 73% [45,46]. It is also important to note that fluconazole and other antifungals are increasingly being used prophylactically in patients with cancer and impaired immune function, and recent data show that this practice may further decrease the sensitivity of traditional blood cultures [47]. In order to improve the sensitivity of blood cultures it has therefore been proposed that the bottles should contain chemicals that inactivate fluconazole, but currently no such systems are commercially available [47]. Unfortunately, at the present time, blood cultures clearly lack the sensitivity needed consistently to rule out invasive *Candida* infections in high-risk patients. Therefore, clinicians need to have a low threshold for performing biopsies of skin lesions and other potentially infectious foci, followed by histopathological analysis.

Given the limitations of traditional cultures, several molecular methods, such as the polymerase chain reaction (PCR), have been developed to facilitate the diagnosis of fungal infections but remain to be critically tested in the clinical arena [48]. Similarly, other tests, such as antigen tests (enolase, β-glucan) and measurements of fungal metabolites such as D-arabinitol have been tested but are not currently being used in routine clinical practice.

Aspergillosis

The diagnosis of IA is difficult owing to lack of sensitivity of diagnostic procedures and the high incidence of concomitant infections. According to one study of 35 patients with IA, *Aspergillus* spp. were recovered from sputum in 75% of patients and from bronchoalveolar lavage in only 52% [38]. In many clinical cases with low or moderate risk for infection, a positive *Aspergillus* culture from a nonsterile body site did not represent disease [19]. However, in high-risk populations, such as allogeneic BMT recipients, persons with hematological malignancies, and those with neutropenia or malnutrition, a positive culture is frequently associated with invasive disease (Table 2) [19]. If aspergillosis is being considered, diagnosis should be sought by biopsy of the affected organ with histopathological examination. Several investigators have used PCR to facilitate diagnosis, but this techique is currently not standardized for clinical use and is unavailable outside research laboratories. In neutropenic patients, thoracic CT exam with halo and/or air-crescent signs in or around a lesion is recognized as highly suggestive of IPA and may occur early in infection. For instance, by sequential CT scanning of patients with histologically-proven IPA it has been demonstrated that these two characteristics are highly dependent on the timing of the scans [49]. In a recent study by Caillot and colleagues the halo sign was present in 68, 22, and 19% of IPA cases on days 3, 7, and 14, respectively. In contrast, the air-crescent sign was seen in 8, 28, and 63% of cases on the same days. These researchers also showed that the median volume of the necrotic pulmonary lesions increased fourfold during the first week, despite antifungal treatment, whereas it remained stable during the second week. In clinical practice it is therefore important to note the value of early CT scans in the diagnosis of IPA. On the other hand, an increase in the size of an *Aspergillus* lesion is not necessarily correlated with a poor immediate outcome when a combined medical-surgical approach is used for treatment [49].

In addition to clinical symptoms and imaging studies in high-risk patients, the *Aspergillus* galactomannan antigen by enzyme-linked immuno-sorbent assay (ELISA) has been advocated as a marker for IA. A recent clinical study involving cancer patients addressed the sensitivity and the specificity of this test [50]. Four patient groups were studied: those with fever of unknown origin during neutropenia, patients with suspected pulmonary infection, or nonpulmonary aspergillosis, and those undergoing surveillance after hematopoietic stem-cell transplantation. Sensitivity of the ELISA was 64.5% in definite IA, but only 16.4%, and 25.5% in probable and possible cases of IA, respectively, casting some doubts on the clinical usefulness of this test [50]. On the other hand, another prospective study designed to monitor BMT recipients serially showed a very respectable performance (sensitivity 90%, specificity 98%) over half the cases diagnosed prior to clinical suspicion of an infection [51]. It is likely that this test will need to be further evaluated as it is placed in a management algorithm in very high risk patients such as BMT recipients and those with hematological malignancies receiving aggressive chemotherapy. Its accuracy along with its success in early diagnosis compared to other modalities such as radiographs and PCR need to be further defined, but it remains promising. In addition, serial measurements of the galactomannan antigen may have a role for monitoring response to antifungal therapy for aspergillosis [52]. Since diagnostic tests from cultures to serologies still have some need for improvement in certain cancer patients with high risk for fungal infections, we need to emphasize prophylactic and empirical strategies for management. The concept is that prevention or early treatment of fungal infections may lead to better patient outcomes.

ANTIFUNGAL PROPHYLAXIS FOR AFEBRILE NEUTROPENIC PATIENTS

Antifungal prophylaxis with fluconazole has been shown to reduce the frequency of both superficial and systemic infections in patients who undergo BMT. Importantly, one study reported improved long-term survival for patients receiving fluconazole prophylaxis [53–57]. These findings have been incorporated into the most recent guidelines from the Centers for Disease Control and Prevention (CDC), Infectious Diseases Society of America (IDSA), and American Society of Blood and Bone Marrow Transplantation, which recommend the administration of fluconazole prophylaxis (400 mg/ day) from the day of hematopoietic stem cell transplantation until engraftment for the prevention of candidiasis [58].

   Antifungal prophylaxis with itraconazole has been studied in two large randomized double-blind trials for neutropenic patients with hematological malignancies. In one of the studies, itraconazole was associated with a significant reduction in the frequency of systemic fungal infection due to *Candida* species, and mortality related to candidemia was reduced (0/201 of patients receiving itraconazole vs. 4/204 patients receiving placebo, $p = 0.06$) [59,60]. However, both studies included a large number of patients in whom antifungal prophylaxis with fluconazole would now be considered, based on the IDSA guidelines. No studies have been conducted where fluconazole and itraconazole are compared in neutropenic patients with hematological malignancies and those who undergo BMT.

   Furthermore, for patients with malignancies and neutropenia who do not require BMT, inconsistent results have been found with fluconazole prophylaxis. A recent meta-analysis was conducted to evaluate the efficacy of fluconazole prophylaxis in this patient group. This analysis of 3,734 patients with neutropenia receiving fluconazole prophylaxis did not show an impact on mortality, although a significant reduction in superficial fungal infections was noted [61]. These results likely show that patients with low-risk neutropenia (i.e., of short duration and not associated with severe mucositis or transplantation) benefit little from azole prophylaxis. A consensus at present is that the routine use of fluconazole or itraconazole for all patients with neutropenia is not recommended by the IDSA guidelines [62].

EMPIRICAL ANTIFUNGAL THERAPY AND PROPHYLAXIS IN PATIENTS WITH FEVER AND NEUTROPENIA

At least one-half of neutropenic patients who become febrile have an established or occult infection, and at least one-fifth of febrile patients with neutrophil counts of <100 cells/mm^3 have bacteremia [62]. Gram-positive bacteria account for 70% of microbiologically documented infections, although the rate of gram-negative infections may be higher in some centers. After initiation of empirical antibacterial therapy, the clinician may wait 5 days to make any changes in the antimicrobial regimen, even though the patient remains febrile, unless a change is mandated by clinical deterioration or the results of a new culture. If the fever persists after 5 days of antibiotic therapy and reassessment does not yield a cause, the clinician has three choices: to continue treatment with the initial antibiotic(s), to change or add antibiotic(s), or to add an antifungal drug (amphotericin B) to the regimen, with or without changing the antibiotics. Two studies from the 1980s suggest that up to one-third of patients with fever and neutropenia who do not respond to a 7-day course of antibacterial therapy have systemic fungal infections [63,64]. Therefore, empirical antifungal therapy has become the standard of care in many patients who remain febrile and neutropenic for ≥5 days, despite the administration of adequate empirical antibacterial therapy [62]. According to a recent meta-analysis, intravenous amphotericin B is the only antifungal agent which has a documented effect on mortality, in cancer patients with neutropenia, and has been the preferred empirical antifungal therapy [65]. In this meta-analysis 29 randomized trials were evaluated, comparing various antifungals with placebo or no treatment in a total of 3,875 patients. Based on 8 trials, intravenous amphotericin B reduced total mortality (relative risk 0.72, 95% confidence interval 0.51 to 1.02, $P = 0.06$) [65]. For these reasons amphotericin B remains the most commonly chosen agent in patients with neutropenia where empirical antifungal therapy is indicated. Due to the poor tolerability of amphotericin B, however, alternative lipid formulations of amphotericin B and new antifungal agents have been sought for this indication. Table 3 summarizes a series of large comparative studies of empirical antifungal therapy during febrile neutropenia. The efficacy of the new lipid formulations, liposomal amphotericin B (L-AmB, AmBisome), amphotericin B lipid-complex (ABLC, Abelcet), and amphotericin B colloidal dispersion (ABCD, Amphotec , Amphocil) seems to be comparable to amphotericin B deoxycholate (AmB, Fungizone®). Importantly, however, the lipid products have a better safety profile (Table 3)

TABLE 3 Summary of Studies on Empirical Antifungal Therapy During Febrile Neutropenia

Regimen	Number of patients	Success	Toxicity	Final outcome	Ref.
L-AmB vs AmB	687	L-Amb (50%) AmB (49%)	AmB > L-AmB	AmB = L-AmB	Walsh et al. (67)
AmB vs FLU	317	AmB (67%) FLU (68%)	AmB > FLU	AmB = FLU	Winston et al. (71)
L-AmB vs ABLC	244	L-AmB (42%) ABLC (33%)	ABLC > L-AmB	L-AmB = ABLC	Wingard et al. (68)
AmB vs ITZ	360	AmB (38%) ITZ (47%)	AmB > ITZ	AmB = ITZ	Boogaerts et al. (72)
L-AmB vs vori	837	L-AmB (31%) vori (26%)	L-Amb > vori	L-Amb = vori (?)	Walsh et al. (73)

AmB: Amphotericin B deoxycholate ("regular amphotericin B", Fungizone).
L-AmB: Liposomal amphotericin B (AmBisome).
ABLC: Amphotericin B lipid complex (Abelcet).
FLU: Fluconazole.
ITZ: Itraconazole.
vori: Voriconazole.
(?) = Noninferiority of voriconazole was not proven but outcomes were similar.

[66–68]. However, all lipid products are not created equal. For example, the safety profiles of the two most commonly-used products, ABLC with L-AmB, are different. Wingard and colleagues have shown that L-AmB has superior safety to ABLC and a similar therapeutic success rate [68]. In another study comparing ABLC and L-AmB, these agents were again found to be equally effective for the treatment of suspected and documented fungal infections in patients with leukaemia, with similar frequency of severe adverse effects on the kidneys or liver. However, infusion-related toxic reactions and nephrotoxicity were more commonly seen with ABLC, and more liver function test abnormalities were associated with L-AmB [66]. In many hospitals, the high costs of the lipid formulations of amphotericin B have resulted in restrictions on their use, and hospital-based policies have been developed to ensure optimization of resources [69]. Regardless of the formulation being used, clinicians using amphotericin B need to perform regular monitoring of creatinine and electrolyte levels in their patients.

Fluconazole is not considered the "gold standard" in empirical antifungal therapy for patients with febrile neutropenia, in part because this agent lacks activity against molds and certain species of yeasts. However, it has been suggested that this agent could be used in institutions where mold infections (most commonly *Aspergillus* sp.) and azole-resistant yeasts are uncommon. Before initiation of empiric fluconazole in this setting, patients at risk should be evaluated by chest radiograph, CT scanning, and appropriate cultures [70,71].

Itraconazole has also been studied for empiric use in patients with neutropenia and persistent fever who are receiving broad-spectrum antibacterial therapy. In a recent randomized study of patients with febrile neutropenia, itraconazole and amphotericin B were shown to have similar efficacy to empirical antifungal therapy, but itraconazole was less toxic (Table 3) [72].

Voriconazole, a novel extended-spectrum triazole, has recently been compared to L-AmB for empirical therapy of patients with neutropenia and persistent fever despite antibacterial therapy (Table 3) [73]. Patients receiving voriconazole were found to have fewer breakthrough fungal infections than those receiving L-AmB. The safety profile of voriconazole was also favorable, with a lower risk of infusion-related symptoms and nephrotoxicity, but with higher risk of transient visual changes and hallucinations compared to L-AmB. The final outcome of patients was similar for both patient groups [73]. However, the study did not prove that voriconazole was superior to L-AmB which was a primary endpoint of the study [74].

The optimum duration of empirical antifungal therapy in the setting of febrile neutropenia is unknown, but many clinicians continue therapy until the ANC $> 500/mm^3$. After the resolution of neutropenia, and if the patient is clinically well, amphotericin B may be discontinued if imaging studies of the chest and abdomen reveal no suspicious lesions [75,76]. For patients with prolonged neutropenia who are doing well clinically, the drug may be stopped after 2 weeks of therapy if no discernible lesions can be found by clinical evaluation and appropriate imaging studies [77,78]. However, there is a consensus that therapy with antibiotics and amphotericin B should be continued throughout the neutropenic episode in patients who appear ill or are at very high risk for fungal infection [62].

EMPIRICAL USE OF HEMATOPOIETIC GROWTH FACTORS IN FEBRILE NEUTROPENIA

Use of colony-stimulating factors such as G-CSF (filgrastim) and GM-CSF (sargramostim) as adjunctive therapy to antimicrobial therapy for febrile neutropenic patients has been studied in several clinical trials. Although these growth factors can consistently shorten the duration of neutropenia, they do not consistently and significantly reduce other measures of febrile morbidity, such as duration of fever, use of anti-infectives, or costs of management. In addition, no study has shown a significant reduction in infection-related mortality. Routine use of hematopoietic growth factor in uncomplicated cases of fever and neutropenia is therefore not recommended by the American Society of Clinical Oncology guidelines [79]. However, under certain conditions such as systemic fungal infections, multiorgan dysfunction secondary to sepsis, and documented infections that do not respond to appropriate antimicrobial therapy, the use of these agents may improve the response to antibiotic and antifungal treatment [80,81]. However, it is important to emphasize that at times a too rapid return of granulocytes during a fungal pneumonia may induce cellular damage at the site of infection and particularly in the lung, which may even result in acute respiratory distress syndrome. Use of other cytokines such as interferon-γ, interleukin-1, and tumor necrosis factor α for immune reconstitution in patients with systemic fungal infections remains investigational, and these agents are used on an individual basis [82].

TREATMENT FOR DOCUMENTED FUNGAL INFECTIONS

Candidiasis

Therapy for candidiasis is summarized in Table 4. Although topical agents such as nystatin suspension or clotrimazole troches may be helpful for mucosal infections, fluconazole has become more commonly used among patients with suppressed immune function. Alternatively, caspofungin has recently been shown to be equally effective to fluconazole in the management of esophageal candidiasis [82a]. Treatment of candidemia needs to be individualized in patients with suppressed immune function. These patients are at increased risk of developing acute disseminated candidiasis, which in most instances is treated with amphotericin B initially, but once the patient has stabilized a switch can be made to fluconazole for susceptible yeast species. However, recent data from a large randomized study suggest that caspofungin may be at least equally effective or even superior to conventional amphotericin B in the management of invasive candidiasis, including candidemia [82b]. Fluconazole therapy has yielded a clinical response of 67% and 86% in cases of acute and chronic disseminated candidiasis, respectively [31]. In patients with CDC who have failed polyene therapy, fluconazole has successfully managed cases [83]. However, some cases of chronic disseminated infection can be difficult to treat, and they may actually require combination antifungal therapy. In cases of chronic disseminated candidiasis, antifungal therapy is commonly administered for 6 to 12 months. β-glucan synthase inhibitors such as caspofungin and related compounds will likely gain more widespread use in the future in the treatment of invasive candidiasis, including patients with neutropenia. Regardless of the antifungal agent being used, it is important to emphasize that catheter-associated candidemia

TABLE 4 Suggested Treatment Guidelines for Patients with Candidiasis

Site of Candida infection	Treatment	Dose/day	Duration	Alternatives
Oropharyngeal	Fluconazole, Clotrimazole troches	100 mg 10 mg × 5	5 days[a] 5 days	Nystatin suspension
Esophageal	Fluconazole	200 mg	14–21 days	Itraconazole oral solution, ≥200 mg/day, amphotericin B i.v. 0.3–0.7 mg/kg/day caspofungin 50 mg i.v./day
Urinary bladder	Fluconazole, removal of catheter	200 mg	7–14 days	amphotericin B 50 mg/d, "bladder wash" × 5 d, amphotericin B 0.5 mg/kg i.v. 7–10 days
Bloodstream[b]	AmB, removal of vascular catheters	0.5–1[c] mg/kg/day	14 days[d] after last pos. blood culture	L-AMB 3 mg/kg/day ABLC 5 mg/kg/day ABCD 2–6 mg/kg/day[e]
	Fluconazole[f], removal of vascular catheters	400 mg	14 days after last pos. blood culture	"High-dose" fluconazole, up to 800 mg/day for less susceptible strains
	Caspofungin, removal of vascular catheters	70 mg i.v./day (loading), followed by 50 mg i.v./day	14 days after last pos. blood culture	

Endocarditis[g]	AmB with 5-FC, consider surgery	AmB: 0.6–1.0 mg/kg/day 5-FC: 100 mg/kg/day[h] in four divided doses	Individualized	L-AmB 5 mg/kg/day[e], Voriconazole 4 mg/kg/d bid, Caspofungin 50 mg/day
Hepatosplenic candidiasis	Fluconazole Lipid AmB, Caspofungin	400–800 mg 3.0–5.0 mg/kg/d 50 mg/d	Individualized	Single agent vs. combination
Meningitis	AmB with 5-FC, removal of prosthetic devices	AmB: 0.7–1.0 mg/kg/day 5-FC: 100 mg/kg/day [h,i] in four divided doses	Individualized, 4–6 weeks	L-AmB 4-5 mg/kg/day[e], Fluconazole 400–800 mg/day

[a] Optimal duration of antifungal therapy for oropharyngeal candidiasis is poorly studied; favorable results with a single 100 mg dose have been published. Duration depends on immune function of the host and susceptibility of the offending pathogen.

[b] Amphotericin B has been the agent of choice in neutropenic patients, although clinical data indicate similar success rates for fluconazole and amphotericin B in the nonneutropenic population. Caspofungin may become a treatment choice in candidiasis. Candida glabrata, Candida krusei, and Candida norvegensis are frequently resistant to fluconazole.

[c] Usual dose is 0.5–0.7 mg/kg/day, but higher doses may be needed in cases of failure to respond.

[d] Duration of therapy is calculated from last positive blood culture.

[e] In patients with impaired renal function or on nephrotoxic drugs, lipid preparations of amphotericin B are preferred over amphotericin B deoxycholate.

[f] Therapy can be switched to fluconazole in cases of candidemia by fluconazole-susceptible strains.

[g] Therapy needs to be individualized. Patients with prosthetic-valve candida endocarditis need valve replacement and many patients with native-valve infection may need surgery.

[h] Dose needs adjustment based on serum levels. Aim for peak of <100 mg/L to avoid bone marrow complications.

[i] Therapy should de initiated with amphotericin B and 5-FC (flucytosine), but therapy can be switched to fluconazole after 2 weeks [102].

often responds poorly to antifungal treatment alone, and prompt removal of
the catheter is recommended, if possible [84,85].

Aspergillosis

Therapy for aspergillosis is summarized in Table 5. Until recently, amphotericin B had been considered the gold-standard for the treatment of severe
Aspergillus infections, and a higher dose is used than for candidiasis (1.0 to 1.5
mg/kg/day). As a testament to the difficulty of treatment of these infections, a
poor response rate is usually seen (average, 37%) [86]. In addition, nephrotoxicity during amphotericin B therapy is common, and elevated creatinine
levels during treatment are associated with a substantial risk for hemodialysis
and a higher mortality rate [87]. Voriconazole has recently been compared to
AmB in a large randomized multicenter study of acute IA [88]. In this
landmark trial, patients received either voriconazole (two doses of 6 mg/kg
on day 1, then 4 mg/kg daily for at least seven days, followed by 200 mg orally
twice daily) or intravenous amphotericin B deoxycholate (at 1.0–1.5 mg/kg/
day). In most patients, the underlying condition was allogeneic hematopoietic
cell transplantation, acute leukemia, or other hematologic disease. A complete or partial response was seen in 52.8% in the voriconazole group,
compared to 31.6% of patients receiving amphotericin B [88]. The survival
rate at 12 weeks was 70.8% among patients treated with voriconazole,
compared to 57.9% in the amphotericin B group. In addition, fewer severe
drug-related adverse events were noted in the voriconazole group [88]. As a
result of these findings, it is likely that voriconazole will replace amphotericin
B as a first-line agent in the primary treatment of IA, and these findings have
been incorporated in the treatment recommendations given in Table 5.

Itraconazole, which has in vitro activity against *Aspergillus* sp. has been
the most commonly used alternative to amphotericin B, and the oral use of
this agent has reported complete or partial response rates of 39–63% [89,90].
Itraconazole is now available for intravenous use, and a recent study has
shown a complete or partial response rate of 48% in immunosuppressed
patients with IPA who receive intravenous treatment for 2 weeks, followed by
oral treatment for 12 weeks [91]. Owing to the erratic absorption of itraconazole, serum levels of this agent need to be monitored regularly during
treatment. No clinical trials have compared itraconazole to voriconazole in
the management of IA.

Caspofungin is a novel antifungal agent of the echinocandin class; it
inhibits synthesis of the fungal cell wall and specifically hyphal tip growth of
aspergillus. This drug has been approved by the FDA for the treatment of
invasive aspergillosis refractory to amphotericin B and itraconazole [92]. In
this report, clinical improvement or complete response occurred in 41% of

TABLE 5 Suggested Therapy for Aspergillosis

Diagnosis	Treatment	Dose/day	Duration	Alternatives
Allergic bronchopulmonary aspergillosis	Itraconazole	200–400 mg/day	Individualized, tapered treatment with steroids	Prednisone
Aspergilloma	Surgical resection, perioperative amphotericin B[a]	1 mg/kg/day	perioperative	Observation
Chronic necrotizing	Itraconazole. Resection or debridement of the affected tissue	200–400 mg/day[b]	3–6 months	Voriconazole, 200 mg/po bid
Acute invasive	*Induction:* Voriconazole Resection or debridement of the affected tissue	Two doses of 6 mg/kg on day 1, then 4 mg/kg bid	At least 7 days	L-AmB > 3 mg/kg/day, ABLC ≥ 5 mg/kg/day, Itraconazole 400–800 mg/day[b], Caspofungin 50 mg/day
	Maintenance: Voriconazole	200 mg bid	12 weeks—needs to be individualized	Itraconazole, 400–600 mg/day

[a] During the operation, intracavitary instillation of amphotericin B (10–20 mg) is sometimes used.
[b] Itraconazole oral solution (elixir) is preferred over the capsules, since the absorbtion is better, but diarrhea may become a problem.

caspofungin-treated patients. In addition, reports have been published describing its successful use in combination with Itraconazole or L-AmB for IA [93,93a].

Despite some improvement in outcome with present antifungals, aspergillosis is still difficult to manage. Thus it is likely that future studies will attempt to determine if combination regimens might be more successful.

Cryptococcosis

Cryptococcal meningitis is generally treated with induction therapy of AmB (0.7 mg/kg/d) and flucytosine (100 mg/kg/d in four divided doses) for 2 weeks, then a switch is made to fluconazole (400 to 800 mg/d) for 8 weeks. Subsequently, the dose is reduced to 200 mg/d and therapy continued for 6 to 12 months [94]. In patients with AIDS, therapy is continued indefinitely but this may be reevaluated in the era of highly active antiretroviral therapy. An alternative to combination therapy for induction is liposomal AmB at 4 mg/kg/day. There may be circumstances where fluconazole is used initially, but in our opinion this is not optimal therapy. In patients with cancer, the above recommendations are probably reasonable but may need to be adjusted on an individual basis. Both symtomatic and asymptomatic pulmonary cryptococcosis in patients with cancer should be treated. Fluconazole (200 to 400 mg/day) is a reasonable first choice antifungal agent and should be administered for 3 to 6 months [94].

OUTCOME

Candidiasis

The mortality directly attributable to candidemia is 38% according to a widely quoted study by Wey and colleagues [95]. Other authors, however, have reported lower mortality rates [15a,56,96], but neutropenia does increase mortality in candidemic patients [96]. It is conceivable that in addition to host factors, treatment-related factors such as retention of central venous lines, and pathogen-related factors such as virulence and antifungal drug resistance, may influence the eventual outcome of patients with candidemia. For example, it has been shown that cancer patients who develop candidemia while receiving systemic antifungal therapy have a mortality of 76%, whereas other candidemic patients had a mortality of 50% [97].

The median survival of patients with acute leukemia and hepatosplenic candidiasis has been reported as 9.5 months and is related to the stage of leukemia [5]. It has been debated whether hepatosplenic candidiasis should be considered to be a contraindication to BMT. At present, this infection should not be considered to be an absolute contraindication to BMT when patients receive amphotericin B therapy before transplant and continue some type of antifungal therapy until engraftment is established. This recommendation is in part based on a study by Bjerke and colleagues, who administered AmB (0.5 mg/kg/day) to BMT patients with a prior history of hepatosplenic candidiasis from conditioning through marrow engraftment [98]. The drug was discontinued if CT evidence of disease was stable or improved. After transplant, 3 of 15 patients died (20%) with evidence of fungal disease, compared with a historical mortality rate of 90% for this patient group [98].

Invasive Aspergillosis

Patients with cancer and IA have traditionally been considered to have poor prognosis, with a mortality of 65 to 90% [38,39]. However, this grim prognosis can be improved if the diagnosis is made early and appropriate antifungal therapy administered, including surgery when necessary. For instance, in one series of patients with acute leukemia, 27% failed to respond to early antifungal therapy and died whereas 73% were cured [6]. Surgery is always an individual decision, but large necrotic lung lesions that are amenable to surgical extirpation should be considered for removal even when smaller lesions are left in other areas of the lung for medical treatment.

Among patients with prior IA who undergo BMT, 33% suffer from relapse of the infection, with a mortality of 88% [99]. However, patients who receive secondary prophylaxis are at a lower risk for relapsing IA [99]. L-AmB or itraconazole have both been administered in this setting, with favorable results [6]. It is likely that similar or even better results will be seen with voriconazole under such circumstances.

Cryptococcosis

There have been several reviews of outcomes regarding cryptococcosis and neoplasms. In a review by Kaplan et al., there were no patients with an underlying malignancy and cryptococcosis that survived longer than 2 yr after the fungal infection diagnosis [100]. In many cases this infection was a marker for progression of the underlying neoplasm. White et al. compared cryptococcosis in patients with AIDS vs. malignancy. The median overall survival for AIDS patients was 9 months, compared to 2 months in those with neoplastic disease. This survival rate correlated with the finding that 78% of AIDS patients and 43% of patients with neoplastic disease had their infection controlled initially with treatment [101]. Furthermore, cancer patients were older and in many respects were more immunosuppressed, as suggested by longer duration of underlying illness, extensive prior chemotherapy, and advanced stage of illness. Cryptococcosis dramatically illustrates an important concept in the management of fungal infections in cancer patients, which is that the underlying disease controls the outcome of the infection to a large extent.

Mold Infections

The prognosis of immunosuppressed patients with mold infections remains dismal. According to Marr and colleagues the overall 1-year survival rate of hematopoietic stem cell transplant recipients with mold infections is only 20% [1]. Similarly, in a recent study on cancer patients with zygomycosis, two-thirds of the patients died. Favorable outcome was associated with lack of pulmonary involvement [9].

Ultimately, progress in the treatment of malignancies involves improvements in control of the underlying diseases as well as more potent anti-infectives. With several important advances in antifungal therapy in the past decade, the future holds promise for better management of fungal infections in cancer patients.

ACKNOWLEDGMENT

This work was supported in part by a grant from Landspitali University Hospital science fund.

REFERENCES

1. Marr KA, Carter RA, Crippa F, Wald A, Corey L. Epidemiology and outcome of mould infections in hematopoietic stem cell transplant recipients. Clin Infect Dis 2002; 34:909–917.
2. Bodey G, Bueltmann B, Duguid W, Gibbs D, Hanak H, Hotchi M, Mall G, Martino P, Meunier F, Milliken S, et al. Fungal infections in cancer patients: an international autopsy survey. Eur J Clin Microbiol Infect Dis 1992; 11:99–109.
3. Diekema DJ, Messer SA, Brueggemann AB, Coffman SL, Doern GV, Herwaldt LA, Pfaller MA. Epidemiology of candidemia: 3-year results from the emerging infections and the epidemiology of Iowa organisms study. J Clin Microbiol 2002; 40:1298–1302.
4. Asmundsdóttir LR, Erlendsdóttir H, Gottfredsson M. Increasing incidence of Candidemia: results from a 20-year nationwide study in Iceland. J Clin Microbiol 2002; 40:3489–3492.
5. Anttila VJ, Elonen E, Nordling S, Sivonen A, Ruutu T, Ruutu P. Hepatosplenic candidiasis in patients with acute leukemia: incidence and prognostic implications. Clin Infect Dis 1997; 24:375–380.
6. Nosari A, Oreste P, Cairoli R, Montillo M, Carrafiello G, Astolfi A, Muti G, Marbello L, Tedeschi A, Magliano E, Morra E. Invasive aspergillosis in haematological malignancies: clinical findings and management for intensive chemotherapy completion. Am J Hematol 2001; 68:231–236.
7. Wald A, Leisenring W, van Burik JA, Bowden RA. Epidemiology of Aspergillus infections in a large cohort of patients undergoing bone marrow transplantation. J Infect Dis 1997; 175:1459–1466.

8. Boutati EI, Anaissie EJ. Fusarium, a significant emerging pathogen in patients with hematologic malignancy: ten years' experience at a cancer center and implications for management. Blood 1997; 90:999–1008.

9. Kontoyiannis D, Wessel V, Bodey G, Rolston K. Zygomycosis in the 1990s in a tertiary-care cancer center. Clin Infect Dis 2000; 30:851–856.

10. Morrison V, Haake R, Weisdorf D. Non-*Candida* fungal infections after bone marrow transplantation: risk factors and outcome. Am J Med 1994; 96:497–503.

11. Rossmann S, Cernoch P, Davis J. Dematiaceous fungi are an increasing cause of human disease. Clin Infect Dis 1996; 22:73–80.

12. Jarvis WR. Epidemiology of nosocomial fungal infections, with emphasis on *Candida* species. Clin Infect Dis 1995; 20:1526–1530.

13. Abi-Said D, Anaissie E, Uzun O, Raad I, Pinzcowski H, Vartivarian S. The epidemiology of hematogenous candidiasis caused by different *Candida* species. Clin Infect Dis 1997; 24:1122–1128. Erratum in: Clin Infect Dis 1997; 25:352.

14. Bodey GP, Mardani M, Hanna HA, Boktour M, Abbas J, Girgawy E, Hachem RY, Kontoyiannis DP, Raad II. The epidemiology of *Candida glabrata* and *Candida albicans* fungemia in immunocompromised patients with cancer. Am J Med 2002; 112:380–385.

15. Viscoli C, Girmenia C, Marinus A, Collette L, Martino P, Vandercam B, Doyen C, Lebeau B, Spence D, Krcmery V, De Pauw B, Meunier F. Candidemia in cancer patients: a prospective, multicenter surveillance study by the Invasive Fungal Infection Group (IFIG) of the European Organization for Research and Treatment of Cancer (EORTC). Clin Infect Dis 1999; 28:1071–1079.

15a. Gottfredsson M, Vredenburgh JJ, Xu J, Schell WA, Perfect JR. Candidemia in women with breast carcinoma treated with high-dose chemotherapy and autologous bone marrow transplantation. Cancer 2003; 89:24–30.

16. Krcmery V, Krupova I, Denning DW. Invasive yeast infections other than *Candida* spp. in acute leukaemia. J Hosp Infect 1999; 41:181–194.

17. Erer B, Galimberti M, Lucarelli G, Giardini C, Polchi P, Baronciani D, Gaziev D, Angelucci E, Izzi G. Trichosporon beigelii: a life-threatening pathogen in immunocompromised hosts. Bone Marrow Transplant 2000; 25:745–749.

18. Krcmery V Jr, Mateicka F, Kunova A, Spanik S, Gyarfas J, Sycova Z, Trupl J. Hematogenous trichosporonosis in cancer patients: report of 12 cases including 5 during prophylaxis with itraconazol. Support Care Cancer 1999; 7:39–43.

19. Perfect JR, Cox GM, Lee JY, Kauffman CA, de Repentigny L, Chapman SW, Morrison VA, Pappas P, Hiemenz JW, Stevens DA, Mycoses Study Group. The impact of culture isolation of *Aspergillus* species: a hospital-based survey of aspergillosis. Clin Infect Dis 2001; 33:1824–1833.

20. Perez-Sanchez I, Anguita J, Martin-Rabadan P, Munoz P, Serrano D, Escudero A, Pintado T. Blastoschizomyces capitatus infection in acute leukemia patients. Leuk Lymphoma 2000; 39:209–212.

21. Jahagirdar BN, Morrison VA. Emerging fungal pathogens in patients with hematologic malignancies and marrow/stem-cell transplant recipients. Semin Respir Infect 2002; 17:113–120.

22. Kauffman CA. Endemic mycoses in patients with hematologic malignancies. Semin Respir Infect 2002; 17:106–112.

23. Wright WL, Wenzel RP. Nosocomial *Candida*. Epidemiology, transmission, and prevention. Infect Dis Clin North Am 1997; 11:411–425.

24. Bow EJ, Loewen R, Cheang MS, Shore TB, Rubinger M, Schacter B. Cytotoxic therapy-induced D-xylose malabsorption and invasive infection during remission-induction therapy for acute myeloid leukemia in adults. J Clin Oncol 1997; 15:2254–2261.

25. Martino R, Subira M, Rovira M, Solano C, Vazquez L, Sanz GF, Urbano-Ispizua A, Brunet S, De la Camara R, alloPBSCT Infectious/Non-infectious Complications Subcommittees of the Grupo Espanol de Trasplante Hematopoyetico (GETH). Invasive fungal infections after allogeneic peripheral blood stem cell transplantation: incidence and risk factors in 395 patients. Br J Haematol 2002; 116:475–482.

26. Oren I, Haddad N, Finkelstein R, Rowe JM. Invasive pulmonary aspergillosis in neutropenic patients during hospital construction: before and after chemoprophylaxis and institution of HEPA filters. Am J Hematol 2001; 66:257–262.

27. Anaissie EJ, Stratton SL, Dignani MC, Summerbell RC, Rex JH, Monson TP, Spencer T, Kasai M, Francesconi A, Walsh TJ. Pathogenic Aspergillus species recovered from a hospital water system: a 3-year prospective study. Clin Infect Dis 2002; 34:780–789.

28. Anaissie EJ, Kuchar RT, Rex JH, Francesconi A, Kasai M, Muller FM, Lozano-Chiu M, Summerbell RC, Dignani MC, Chanock SJ, Walsh TJ. Fusariosis associated with pathogenic *Fusarium* species colonization of a hospital water system: a new paradigm for the epidemiology of opportunistic mold infections. Clin Infect Dis 2001; 33:1871–1878.

29. Nucci M, Anaissie E. Revisiting the source of candidemia: skin or gut? Clin Infect Dis 2001; 33:1959–1967.

30. Uzun O, Anaissie EJ. Predictors of outcome in cancer patients with candidemia. Ann Oncol 2000; 11:1517–1521.

31. de Pauw BE, Raemaekers JM, Donnelly JP, Kullberg BJ, Meis JF. An open study on the safety and efficacy of fluconazole in the treatment of disseminated *Candida* infections in patients treated for hematological malignancy. Ann Hematol 1995; 70:83–87.

32. Pagano L, Mele L, Fianchi L, Melillo L, Martino B, D'Antonio D, Tosti ME, Posteraro B, Sanguinetti M, Trape G, Equitani F, Carotenuto M, Leone G. Chronic disseminated candidiasis in patients with hematologic malignancies. Clinical features and outcome of 29 episodes. Haematologica 2002; 87:535–541.

33. Sallah S, Wan JY, Nguyen NP, Vos P, Sigounas G. Analysis of factors related to the occurrence of chronic disseminated candidiasis in patients with acute leukemia in a non–bone marrow transplant setting: a follow-up study. Cancer 2001; 92:1349–1353.

34. Pestalozzi BC, Krestin GP, Schanz U, Jacky E, Gmur J. Hepatic lesions of chronic disseminated candidiasis may become invisible during neutropenia. Blood 1997; 90:3858–3864.

35. Haron E, Vartivarian S, Anaissie E, Dekmezian R, Bodey GP. Primary *Candida*

pneumonia. Experience at a large cancer center and review of the literature. Medicine (Baltimore) 1993; 72:137–142.

36. Kontoyiannis DP, Reddy BT, Torres HA, Luna M, Lewis RE, Tarrand J, Bodey GP, Raad II. Pulmonary candidiasis in patients with cancer: an autopsy study. Clin Infect Dis 2002; 34:400–403.

37. Oravcova E, Lacka J, Drgona L, Studena M, Sevcikova L, Spanik S, Svec J, Kukuckova E, Grey E, Silva J, Krcmery V. Funguria in cancer patients: analysis of risk factors, clinical presentation and outcome in 50 patients. Infection 1996; 24:319–323.

38. Kaiser L, Huguenin T, Lew PD, Chapuis B, Pittet D. Invasive aspergillosis. Clinical features of 35 proven cases at a single institution. Medicine (Baltimore) 1998; 77:188–194.

39. Patterson TF, Kirkpatrick WR, White M, Hiemenz JW, Wingard JR, Dupont B, Rinaldi MG, Stevens DA, Graybill JR, I3 Aspergillus Study Group. Invasive aspergillosis. Disease spectrum, treatment practices, and outcomes. Medicine (Baltimore) 2000; 79:250–260.

39a. Walsh TJ, Newman KR, Moody M, Wharton RC, Wade JC. Trichosporonosis in patients with neoplastic disease. Medicine (Baltimore) 1986; 65:268–279.

40. Walsh TJ, Melcher GP, Rinaldi MG, Lecciones J, McGough DA, Kelly P, Lee J, Callender D, Rubin M, Pizzo PA. Trichosporon beigelii, an emerging pathogen resistant to amphotericin B. J Clin Microbiol 1990; 28:1616–1622.

41. Anaissie E, Gokaslan A, Hachem R, Rubin R, Griffin G, Robinson R, Sobel J, Bodey G. Azole therapy for trichosporonosis: clinical evaluation of eight patients, experimental therapy for murine infection, and review. Clin Infect Dis 1992; 15:781–787.

42. Martino P, Gastaldi R, Raccah R, Girmenia C. Clinical patterns of *Fusarium* infections in immunocompromised patients. J Infect 1994; 28(suppl 1):7–15.

43. Nelson PE, Dignani MC, Anaissie EJ. Taxonomy, biology, and clinical aspects of *Fusarium* species. Clin Microbiol Rev 1994; 7:479–504.

44. Liu K, Howell DN, Perfect JR, Schell WA. Morphologic criteria for the preliminary identification of *Fusarium, Paecilomyces,* and *Acremonium* species by histopathology. Am J Clin Pathol 1998; 109:45–54.

45. Berenguer J, Buck M, Witebsky F, Stock F, Pizzo PA, Walsh TJ. Lysis-centrifugation blood cultures in the detection of tissue-proven invasive candidiasis. Disseminated versus single-organ infection. Diagn Microbiol Infect Dis 1993; 17:103–109.

46. Telenti A, Roberts GD. Fungal blood cultures. Eur J Clin Microbiol Infect Dis 1989; 8:825–831.

47. Kami M, Machida U, Okuzumi K, Matsumura T, Mori Si S, Hori A, Kashima T, Kanda Y, Takaue Y, Sakamaki H, Hirai H, Yoneyama A, Mutou Y. Effect of fluconazole prophylaxis on fungal blood cultures: an autopsy-based study involving 720 patients with haematological malignancy. Br J Haematol 2002; 117:40–46.

48. Gottfredsson M, Cox GM, Perfect JR. Molecular methods for epidemiological and diagnostic studies of fungal infections. Pathology 1998; 30:405–418.

49. Caillot D, Couaillier JF, Bernard A, Casasnovas O, Denning DW, Mannone L, Lopez J, Couillault G, Piard F, Vagner O, Guy H. Increasing volume and changing characteristics of invasive pulmonary aspergillosis on sequential thoracic computed tomography scans in patients with neutropenia. J Clin Oncol 2001; 19:253–259.

50. Herbrecht R, Letscher-Bru V, Oprea C, Lioure B, Waller J, Campos F, Villard O, Liu KL, Natarajan-Ame S, Lutz P, Dufour P, Bergerat JP, Candolfi E. Aspergillus galactomannan detection in the diagnosis of invasive aspergillosis in cancer patients. J Clin Oncol 2002; 20:1898–1906.

51. Maertens J, Verhaegen J, Lagrou K, Van Eldere J, Boogaerts M. Screening for circulating galactomannan as a noninvasive diagnostic tool for invasive aspergillosis in prolonged neutropenic patients and stem cell transplantation recipients: a prospective validation. Blood 2001; 97:1604–1610.

52. Boutboul F, Alberti C, Leblanc T, Sulahian A, Gluckman E, Derouin F, Ribaud P. Invasive aspergillosis in allogeneic stem cell transplant recipients: increasing antigenemia is associated with progressive disease. Clin Infect Dis 2002; 34:939–943.

53. Ellis ME, Clink H, Ernst P, Halim MA, Padmos A, Spence D, Kalin M, Hussain Qadri SM, Burnie J, Greer W. Controlled study of fluconazole in the prevention of fungal infections in neutropenic patients with haematological malignancies and bone marrow transplant recipients. Eur J Clin Microbiol Infect Dis 1994; 13:3–11.

54. Goodman JL, Winston DJ, Greenfield RA, Chandrasekar PH, Fox B, Kaizer H, Shadduck RK, Shea TC, Stiff P, Friedman DJ, et al. A controlled trial of fluconazole to prevent fungal infections in patients undergoing bone marrow transplantation. N Engl J Med 1992; 326:845–851.

55. Marr KA, Seidel K, Slavin MA, Bowden RA, Schoch HG, Flowers ME, Corey L, Boeckh M. Prolonged fluconazole prophylaxis is associated with persistent protection against candidiasis-related death in allogeneic marrow transplant recipients: long-term follow-up of a randomized, placebo-controlled trial. Blood 2000; 96:2055–2061.

56. Marr KA, Seidel K, White TC, Bowden RA. Candidemia in allogeneic blood and marrow transplant recipients: evolution of risk factors after the adoption of prophylactic fluconazole. J Infect Dis 2000; 181:309–316.

57. Rotstein C, Bow EJ, Laverdiere M, Ioannou S, Carr D, Moghaddam N, the Canadian Fluconazole Prophylaxis Study Group. Randomized placebo-controlled trial of fluconazole prophylaxis for neutropenic cancer patients: benefit based on purpose and intensity of cytotoxic therapy. Clin Infect Dis 1999; 28:331–340.

58. Centers for Disease Control and Prevention. Guidelines for preventing opportunistic infections among hematopoietic stem cell transplant recipients—recommendations of CDC, the Infectious Diseases Society of America, and the American Society of Blood and Transplantation. MMWR Morb Mortal Wkly Rep 2000; 49(RR-10):1–125.

59. Menichetti F, Del Favero A, Martino P, Bucaneve G, Micozzi A, Girmenia C,

Barbabietola G, Pagano L, Leoni P, Specchia G, Caiozzo A, Raimondi R, Mandelli F. Itraconazole oral solution as prophylaxis for fungal infections inneutropenic patients with hematologic malignancies: a randomized, placebo-controlled, double-blind, multicenter trial. GIMEMA Infection Program. Gruppo Italiano Malattie Ematologiche dell' Adulto. Clin Infect Dis 1999; 28:250–255.

60. Nucci M, Biasoli I, Akiti T, Silveira F, Solza C, Barreiros G, Spector N, Derossi A, Pulcheri W. A double-blind, randomized, placebo-controlled trial of itraconazole capsules as antifungal prophylaxis for neutropenic patients. Clin Infect Dis 2000; 30:300–305.

61. Kanda Y, Yamamoto R, Chizuka A, Hamaki T, Suguro M, Arai C, Matsuyama T, Takezako N, Miwa A, Kern W, Kami M, Akiyama H, Hirai H, Togawa A. Prophylactic action of oral fluconazole against fungal infection in neutropenic patients. A meta-analysis of 16 randomized, controlled trials. Cancer 2000; 89:1611–1625.

62. Hughes WT, Armstrong D, Bodey GP, Bow EJ, Brown AE, Calandra T, Feld R, Pizzo PA, Rolston KV, Shenep JL, Young LS. 2002 guidelines for the use of antimicrobial agents in neutropenic patients with cancer. Clin Infect Dis 2002; 34:730–751.

63. EORTC International Antimicrobial Therapy Cooperative Project Group. Empiric antifungal therapy in febrile granulocytopenic patients. Am J Med 1989; 86:668–672.

64. Pizzo PA, Robichaud KJ, Gill FA, Witebsky FG. Empiric antibiotic and antifungal therapy for cancer patients with prolonged fever and granulocytopenia. Am J Med 1982; 72:101–111.

65. Gotzsche PC, Johansen HK. Routine versus selective antifungal administration for control of fungal infections in patients with cancer. Cochrane Database Syst Rev 2000; (4):CD000026.

66. Fleming RV, Kantarjian HM, Husni R, Rolston K, Lim J, Raad I, Pierce S, Cortes J, Estey E. Comparison of amphotericin B lipid complex (ABLC) vs. ambisome in the treatment of suspected or documented fungal infections in patients with leukemia. Leuk Lymphoma 2001; 40:511–520.

67. Walsh TJ, Finberg RW, Arndt C, Hiemenz J, Schwartz C, Bodensteiner D, Pappas P, Seibel N, Greenberg RN, Dummer S, Schuster M, Holcenberg JS, National Institute of Allergy and Infectious Diseases Mycoses Study Group. Liposomal amphotericin B for empirical therapy in patients with persistent fever and neutropenia. N Engl J Med 1999; 340:764–771.

68. Wingard JR, White MH, Anaissie E, Raffalli J, Goodman J, Arrieta A, L Amph/ABLC Collaborative Study Group. A randomized, double-blind comparative trial evaluating the safety of liposomal amphotericin B versus amphotericin lipid complex in the empirical treatment of febrile neutropenia. Clin Infect Dis 2000; 31:1155–1163.

69. Bennett J. Editorial response: choosing amphotericin B formulation—between a rock and a hard place. Clin Infect Dis 2000; 31:1164–1165.

70. Viscoli C, Castagnola E, Van Lint MT, Moroni C, Garaventa A, Rossi MR,

Fanci R, Menichetti F, Caselli D, Giacchino M, Congiu M. Fluconazole versus amphotericin B as empirical antifungal therapy of unexplained fever in granulocytopenic cancer patients. Eur J Cancer 1996; 32A:814–820.

71. Winston DJ, Hathorn JW, Schuster MG, Schiller GJ, Territo MC. A multi-center randomized trial of fluconazole versus amphotericin B for empiric antifungal therapy of febrile neutropenic patients with cancer. Am J Med 2000; 108:282–289.

72. Boogaerts M, Winston DJ, Bow EJ, Garber G, Reboli AC, Schwarer AP, Novitzky N, Boehme A, Chwetzoff E, De Beule K, Itraconazole Neutropenia Study Group. Intravenous and oral itraconazole versus intravenous amphotericin B deoxycholate as empirical antifungal therapy for persistent fever in neutropenic patients with cancer who are receiving broad-spectrum antibacterial therapy. A randomized, controlled trial. Ann Intern Med 2001; 135:412–422.

73. Walsh TJ, Pappas P, Winston DJ, Lazarus HM, Petersen F, Raffalli J, Yanovich S, Stiff P, Greenberg R, Donowitz G, Schuster M, Reboli A, Wingard J, Arndt C, Reinhardt J, Hadley S, Finberg R, Laverdiere M, Perfect J, Garber G, Fioritoni G, Anaissie E, Lee J, National Institute of Allergy and Infectious Diseases Mycoses Study Group. Voriconazole compared with liposomal amphotericin B for empirical antifungal therapy in patients with neutropenia and persistent fever. N Engl J Med 2002; 346:225–234.

74. Marr KA. Empirical antifungal therapy—new options, new tradeoffs. N Engl J Med 2002; 346:278–280.

75. Heussel CP, Kauczor HU, Heussel G, Fischer B, Mildenberger P, Thelen M. Early detection of pneumonia in febrile neutropenic patients: use of thin-section CT. AJR Am J Roentgenol 1997; 169:1347–1353.

76. Santhosh-Kumar CR, Ajarim DS, Harakati MS, al Momen AK, al Mohareb F, Zeitany RG. Ceftazidime and amikacin as empiric treatment of febrile episodes in neutropenic patients in Saudi Arabia. J Infect 1992; 25:11–19.

77. Bartley DL, Hughes WT, Parvey LS, Parham D. Computed tomography of hepatic and splenic fungal abscesses in leukemic children. Pediatr Infect Dis 1982; 1:317–321.

78. Flynn PM, Shenep JL, Crawford R, Hughes WT. Use of abdominal computed tomography for identifying disseminated fungal infection in pediatric cancer patients. Clin Infect Dis 1995; 20:964–970.

79. Ozer H, Armitage JO, Bennett CL, Crawford J, Demetri GD, Pizzo PA, Schiffer CA, Smith TJ, Somlo G, Wade JC, Wade JL 3d, Winn RJ, Wozniak AJ, Somerfield MR. American Society of Clinical Oncology. 2000 update of recommendations for the use of hematopoietic colony-stimulating factors: evidence-based, clinical practice guidelines. American Society of Clinical Oncology Growth Factors Expert Panel. J Clin Oncol 2000; 18:3558–3585.

80. Bodey GP, Anaissie E, Gutterman J, Vadhan-Raj S. Role of granulocyte-macrophage colony-stimulating factor as adjuvant therapy for fungal infection in patients with cancer. Clin Infect Dis 1993; 17:705–707.

81. Bodey GP, Anaissie E, Gutterman J, Vadhan-Raj S. Role of granulocyte-macrophage colony-stimulating factor as adjuvant treatment in neutropenic

patients with bacterial and fungal infection. Eur J Clin Microbiol Infect Dis 1994; 13(suppl 2):S18–S22.

82. Roilides E, Dignani MC, Anaissie EJ, Rex JH. The role of immunoreconstitution in the management of refractory opportunistic fungal infections. Med Mycol 1998; 36(suppl 1):12–25.

82a. Villanueva A, Gotuzzo E, Arathoon EG, Noriega LM, Kartsonis NA, Lipinacci RJ, Smietana JM, DiNubile MJ, Sable CA. A randomized double-blind study of caspofungin versus fluconazole for the treatment of esophageal candidiasis. Am J Med 2002; 113:294–299.

82b. Mora-Duarte J, Betts R, Rotstein C, Colombo AL, Thompson-Moya L, Smietana J, Lupinacci R, Sable C, Kartsonis N, Perfect J. Caspofungin invasive candidiasis study group. Comparison of caspofungin and amphotericin B for invasive candidiasis. New Engl J Med 2002; 347:2020–2029.

83. Anaissie E, Bodey GP, Kantarjian H, David C, Barnett K, Bow E, Defelice R, Downs N, File T, Karam G, et al. Fluconazole therapy for chronic disseminated candidiasis in patients with leukemia and prior amphotericin B therapy. Am J Med 1991; 91:142–150.

84. Mermel LA, Farr BM, Sherertz RJ, Raad II, O'Grady N, Harris JS, Craven DE. Infectious Diseases Society of America; American College of Critical Care Medicine; Society for Healthcare Epidemiology of America. Guidelines for the management of intravascular catheter—related infection. Clin Infect Dis 2001; 32:1249–1272.

85. Nucci M, Anaissie E. Should vascular catheters be removed from all patients with candidemia? An evidence-based review. Clin Infect Dis 2002; 34:591–599.

86. Perea S, Patterson TF. Invasive Aspergillus infections in hematologic malignancy patients. Semin Respir Infect 2002; 17:99–105.

87. Wingard JR, Kubilis P, Lee L, Yee G, White M, Walshe L, Bowden R, Anaissie E, Hiemenz J, Lister J. Clinical significance of nephrotoxicity in patients treated with amphotericin B for suspected or proven aspergillosis. Clin Infect Dis 1999; 29:1402–1407.

88. Herbrecht R, Denning DW, Patterson TF, Bennett JE, Greene RE, Oestmann JW, Kern WV, Marr KA, Ribaud P, Lortholary O, Sylvester R, Rubin RH, Wingard JR, Stark P, Durand C, Caillot D, Thiel E, Chandrasekar PH, Hodges MR, Schlamm HT, Troke PF, de Pauw B, Invasive Fungal Infections Group of the European Organisation for Research and Treatment of Cancer and the Global Aspergillus Study Group. Voriconazole versus amphotericin B for primary therapy of invasive aspergillosis. N Engl J Med 2002; 347:408–415.

89. Denning DW, Lee JY, Hostetler JS, Pappas P, Kauffman CA, Dewsnup DH, Galgiani JN, Graybill JR, Sugar AM, Catanzaro A, et al. NIAID Mycoses Study Group Multicenter Trial of Oral Itraconazole Therapy for Invasive Aspergillosis. Am J Med 1994; 97:135–144. Erratum in: Am J Med 1994;97:497.

90. van't Wout JW, Novakova I, Verhagen CA, Fibbe WE, de Pauw BE, van der Meer JW. The efficacy of itraconazole against systemic fungal infections in neutropenic patients: a randomised comparative study with amphotericin B. J Infect 1991; 22:45–52.

91. Caillot D, Bassaris H, McGeer A, Arthur C, Prentice HG, Seifert W, De Beule K. Intravenous itraconazole followed by oral itraconazole in the treatment of invasive pulmonary aspergillosis in patients with hematologic malignancies, chronic granulomatous disease, or AIDS. Clin Infect Dis 2001; 33:e83–e90.

92. Maertens J, Raad I, Sable CA, et al. Multicenter, noncomparative study to evaluate safety and efficacy of caspofungin (CAS) in adults with invasive aspergillosis (IA) refractory or intolerant to amphotericin B (AMB), AMB lipid formulations (lipid AMB), or azoles [abstr 1103]. In: Programs and abstracts of the 40th Interscience Conference on Antimicrobial Agents and Chemotherapy (Toronto). Washington, DC: American Society for Microbiology, 2000:371.

93. Rubin MA, Carroll KC, Cahill BC. Caspofungin in combination with itraconazole for the treatment of invasive aspergillosis in humans. Clin Infect Dis 2002; 34:1160–1161.

93a. Kontoyiannis DP, Hachem R, Lewis RE, Rivero GA, Torres HA, Thornby J, Champlin R, Kantarjian H, Bodey GP, Raad II. Efficacy and toxicity of caspofungin in combination with liposomal amphotericin B as primary or salvage treatment of invasive aspergillosis in patients with hematologic malignancies. Cancer 2003; 98:292–299.

94. Casadevall A, Perfect JR. Therapy of cryptococcosis. In: *Cryptococcus neoformans*. American Society for Microbiology, 1999:457–518.

95. Wey SB, Mori M, Pfaller MA, Woolson RF, Wenzel RP. Hospital-acquired candidemia. The attributable mortality and excess length of stay. Arch Intern Med 1988; 148:2642–2645.

96. Pagano L, Antinori A, Ammassari A, Mele L, Nosari A, Melillo L, Martino B, Sanguinetti M, Equitani F, Nobile F, Carotenuto M, Morra E, Morace G, Leone G. Retrospective study of candidemia in patients with hematological malignancies. Clinical features, risk factors and outcome of 76 episodes. Eur J Haematol 1999; 63:77–85.

97. Uzun O, Ascioglu S, Anaissie EJ, Rex JH. Risk factors and predictors of outcome in patients with cancer and breakthrough candidemia. Clin Infect Dis 2001; 32:1713–1717. Erratum in: Clin Infect Dis 2001; 33:749.

98. Bjerke JW, Meyers JD, Bowden RA. Hepatosplenic candidiasis—a contraindication to marrow transplantation? Blood 1994; 84:2811–2814.

99. Offner F, Cordonnier C, Ljungman P, Prentice HG, Engelhard D, De Bacquer D, Meunier F, De Pauw B. Impact of previous aspergillosis on the outcome of bone marrow transplantation. Clin Infect Dis 1998; 26:1098–1103.

100. Kaplan MH, Rosen PP, Armstrong D. Cryptococcosis in a cancer hospital: clinical and pathological correlates in forty-six patients. Cancer 1977; 39:2265–2274.

101. White M, Cirrincione C, Blevens A, Armstrong D. Cryptococcal meningitis with AIDS and patients with neoplastic disease. J Infect Dis 1992; 165:960–966.

102. Gottfredsson M, Perfect JR. Fungal meningitis. Semin Neurol 2000; 20:307–322.

35

Parasitic Diseases as Complications of Cancer

Albert L. Vincent
University of South Florida College of Medicine
and Moffitt Cancer Center and Research Institute
Tampa, Florida, U.S.A.

INTRODUCTION

Parasitic diseases remain a concern as the new millennium dawns. Even as new diseases emerge in the developed world, hopes for control of some long-established tropical diseases have faded over the past few decades. Exotic organisms are constantly introduced by international air travel, immigration, and military deployment. Other cosmopolitan agents are increasingly encountered in the course of aggressive cancer treatments, solid organ transplants, and HIV infections.

Reviews of infectious complications of cancer have now become somewhat dated, dealing with infectious diseases generally [1], infections in bone marrow transplant (BMT) recipients [2], and with nonbacterial complications of neoplastic disease [3]. From a less clinical perspective, recent reviews have dealt with some of the more common parasites in various immunodeficiency states [4–6]. Recent clinical overviews of infectious diseases among immunocompromised patients have also been oriented by organ system, including the lungs [7–10], CNS [11,12], and bowel [13–16]. Here we present a comprehensive review of parasitic diseases specifically in cancer patients, emphasizing their recognition and sources, behavior in the cancer patient, clinical experiences from illustrative cases, and the basis of successful therapy.

GIARDIA

The duodenal flagellate *Giardia intestinalis* (*G. lamblia*) is a common intestinal protozoon in the U.S. and is one of the most frequent causes of parasitic diarrhea globally. The pear-shaped binucleated trophozoite may proliferate in great numbers and, adhering to the mucosa by its sucking disc, injure the brush border [17]. Clinical presentation, if any, varies from an acute watery diarrhea to a severe, recurrent bloating and steatorrhea with characteristic foul-smelling stools. Chronic disease with malabsorbtion syndrome has long been linked to hypogammaglobulinemia but apparently not with AIDS. Bromiker et al. [18] reported the first two cases of severe giardiasis in two young males undergoing BMT. One, in his peritransplant period, developed marked weight loss, chronic diarrhea, abdominal distension, and an intestinal biopsy histologically consistent with giardiasis. The other, following documented graft-versus-host disease, presented with diarrhea and hypoalbuminemia several months into the posttransplant period and responded to a course of metronidazole. Another case was a 12-year-old girl with Ewing's sarcoma of the sacrum 10 months into a combination radiotherapy and chemotherapy protocol, who developed severe diarrhea, with ten or more stools per day, colicky central abdominal pain, anorexia, and a weight loss of 6 kg. After interruption of the protocol and detection of *Giardia* in a repeated stool exam, she promptly responded to a 10-day course of metronidazole, 250 mg daily [19]. *Giardia* diarrhea has also been seen in pediatric patients undergoing bone marrow transplant for Cooley's disease [20]. Because asymptomatic carriage is not uncommon in the general population of developed countries, patients undergoing BMT might benefit from a routine stool examination for trophzoites or cysts.

A cure rate of about 90% can be expected from a 5 to 7 day course of metronidazole (Flagyl) or a single dose of tinidazole. Immunocompromised patients may require prolonged treatment with a combination of two drugs such as a nitroimidazole with quinacrine [21]. Cysts and trophozoites are often shed intermittently, requiring at least three stool examinations on nonconsecutive days to rule out infection. The Entero-Test string capsule, duodenal biopsy, or aspirate may also be used to pursue the diagnosis. Antigen detection by commercially available enzyme immunoassay is highly sensitive and specific but overlooks other pathogens detectible by light microcroscopy [22].

ENTAMOEBA

Although usually an asymptomatic lumen-dweller, *Entamoeba histolytica* may ulcerate the colon, cause hepatic abscesses, and disseminate widely in some persons not known to be immunodeficient [5]. Metronidazole-resistant amoebic colitis and dysentery without systemic invasion have been reported in three male patients with acute nonlymphoblastic leukemia. During GVHD, which followed allogeneic BMT [20,23], a direct stool smear revealed the hematophagous trophozoites of *E. histolytica* [23], and rectosigmoido-scopy showed the characteristic flask-shaped ulcers upon edematous mucosa. Steroid treatment may worsen the disease and enhance resistance to standard chemotherapy.

BLASTOCYSTIS

Blastocystis and *Dientamoeba* are other bowel protozoa that, although not invasive, are suspected by some as occasional causes of diarrhea. Large numbers of *Blastocystis* were encountered in a 21-year-old female who developed acute GVHD diarrhea following allogeneic BMT for CML [24]. Metronidazole is the treatment of choice when indicated.

CRYTOSPORIDIA AND MICROSPORIDIA

The coccidia of man include three species of food-borne or water-borne minimally invasive protozoa that replicate in the epithelium of the small bowel and pass oocysts in the feces, namely *Crytosporidium*, *Isospora*, and *Cyclospora*. The watery diarrhea is usually self-limiting and not life-threatening except in immunocompromised patients infected with *Cryptosporidium* [25,26]. *C. parvum* is a zoonotic, ubiquitous coccidian passing small (4–6 μm) unsporulated (preinfective) oocysts that are easily overlooked in a routine ova and parasite exam. In the immunocompetent host, the organism is asymptomatic or may cause a watery diarrhea of 30 days duration or less. In immunocompromised individuals, those with AIDS or undergoing cancer chemotherapy, prolonged diarrhea can lead to severe dehydration, biliary obstruction, pancreatitis, and death [27]. Case reports indicate that children with leukemia or other hematological malignancies are at risk for severe or recurrent infection [28–30]. Of six patients reported by Foot et al. [30], the pathogen was eradicated after modification of the chemotherapy regimen, while two died with evidence of persistent infection. Withdrawal of immunosuppressive treatment also led to resolution of infection in a patient with ALL [29]. Stein et al. [28] reported spontaneous remission of cryptosporidiosis in another case of ALL. Pulmonary involvement from *Cryptosporidium* accompanied by *Cryptococcus albidus* fungemia was reported by Wells et al. [31] in a child with ALL. Gentile et al. [32] suggested that infection may remain asymptomatic or self-limited in some leukemia patients but become more severe in malignancies that carry a less favorable outcome. Nosocomial outbreaks have been described [33] and bone marrow transplant units may be involved [34,35].

Paromomycin or azithromycin may be beneficial, but no clear guidelines for treatment have been developed. A newly approved oral regimen of nitazoxanide is a promising treatment for *Cryptosporidium* and also effectively kills *Giardia*. In symptomatic cases rehydration and redress of electrolyte imbalances is indicated. Clinicians suspecting *Cryptosporidium* should specify the formalin-ethyl acetate method or sucrose flotation to concentrate oocysts, followed by the Kinyoun acid-fast stain. Immunoassay procedures for examination of stools are more sensitive and avoid confusion with *Isospora* [5].

ISOSPORA

Isospora belli, like *Cryptosporidium*, is a widespread coccidian that is transmitted by a fecal–oral route and may cause weight loss and watery diarrhea. Symptomatic cases have been reported from patients with acute T-cell leukemia (ATL) in Japan [36,37] and in an ALL case in India [38]. The oocysts are large (30 µm) and ellipsoidal; clinical disease responds well to trimethoprim-sulfamethoxazole or pyrimethamine sulfadoxine.

CYCLOSPORA

The oocysts of *Cyclospora cayetanensis* are smaller (8–10 µm) and spherical, but they take on a variable red after Ziehl–Neelson acid fast staining. A 35-year-old male in India developed a one-day course of loose stools without blood, 18 days after his last chemotherapy for AML. Although TMP-SMX is the treatment of choice, his *Cyclospora* infection apparently responded well to empirical metronidazole treatment [39].

MICROSPORIDIA

An undetermined species of Microsporidia was found to cause endophthalmitis and intracerebral lesions in a 22-month-old neutropenic boy with AML. The diagnostic polar filament was recognized by the "gold standard" of transmission electron microscopy. Manifestations resolved after treatment with albendazole [40]. *Enterocytozoon bieneusi*, well known as a cause of diarrhea in organ transplant or HIV-positive patients, has apparently not yet been documented in cancer or BMT patients [41].

TRICHOMONAS

A flagellate protozoon, *Trichomonas tenax* is a bacteria-feeding commensal of the oral cavity, especially in patients with pyorrhea. Beyond its usual site, large numbers of organisms have been encountered among bacterial exudates in preexisting lung disease, including bronchiogenic carcinoma [42], and from the empyemic pleural space in an advanced rectal carcinoma [43].

ACANTHAMOEBA

A free-living opportunist in soil or water, *Acanthamoeba* is best known as a cause of dentritic keratosis in contact lens users and granulomatous amebic encephalitis (GAE) in debilitated or immunocompromised hosts [44–45]. Anderlini et al. [46] presented two cases of GAE in steroid-treated leukemia patients, six and nine months post-BMT. Both gave a history of sinusitis. As is usually the case, diagnosis was made only at autopsy, by recognizing the large karyosome ("owl eye" nucleolus) and surrounding halo characteristic of both the trophozoites and the cysts. Dissemination to the lungs, skin, and adrenal gland were also noted. Another fatal case of *Acanthamoeba* meningo-encephalitis was reported by Feingold et al. [47] after autologous stem cell transplantation for non-Hodgkin's lymphoma. Therapeutic success in disseminated disease has recently been reported using a combination of pentamidine, 5-fluorcytosine, itraconazole, and a topical chlorhexidine gluconate/ketoconazole cream [48].

TOXOPLASMA

Toxoplasma gondii is a cosmopolitan protozoon that causes a zoonosis among many mammalian and avian hosts. The principal definitive host of this coccidian is the domestic cat, which passes small (10–12 μm) unsporulated oocysts in the feces. Ingested by pet owners with normal T cell responses [49], bradyzoites develop within tissue cysts, usually without significant clinical events beyond cervical adenopathy and a few other nonspecific symptoms. In undercooked meat, these tissue cysts are infective to man. Cysts in the human choroid, retina, CNS, and elsewhere probably remain viable for life, making toxoplasmosis one of the most prevalent of all latent infectious diseases and the most significant parasite in oncology. Serological surveys indicate that up to 70% of the general population has been exposed, either by oocysts in cat feces or tissue cysts in meat [50].

Among cancer patients, fulminant or disseminated toxoplasmosis has been most often encountered in Hodgkin's lymphoma, followed at some distance by non-Hodgkin's lymphoma, acute and chronic leukemia, multiple myeloma, myeloid metaplasia, and less frequently by other hematological or lymphoroliferative disorders [51,52]. The infection rate in Hodgkin's disease has been estimated at 3%. The T cell dysfunction associated with lymphomas seems to predispose to toxoplasmosis even in the absence of cytotoxic agents. Breast or lung carcinomas being treated with antineoplastic agents may also awaken dormant toxoplasmosis.

Toxoplasmosis and non-Hodgkin's lymphoma may be difficult to distinguish, since both may produce adenopathy [53]. The brain, lungs, and heart are most often involved. Brain involvement may be diffuse, multicentric, or focal, and most patients show encephalitis and altered mental states. Definitive diagnosis can be made by visualization of organisms in the CSF, electron microscopy, or immunoperoxidase staining. Decreased visual acuity, exudative retinal lesions, and vitrial haziness may be the first manifestations of life-threatening toxoplasmosis in patients with malignancies. ALL is most often incriminated in toxoplasmal congestive heart failure, pericarditis, and arrhythmia. Unexplained adenopathy [54] or a culture-negative sepsis syndrome [55] should arouse suspicion of toxoplasmosis. Pulmonary involvement is clinically nonspecific but may be established by Giema-stained BAL fluid or transbronchial biopsy material. IgG antibodies, usually detected by IFA or enzyme immunoassay, peak about 6 weeks after infection and remain positive indefinitely. The treatment of choice is a combination of pyrimethamine and sulfadiazine [56].

Among BMT patients, toxoplasmosis is an infrequent but usually fatal complication if left untreated. Most cases occur in seropositive allograft recipients [57]. In about 60 cases of post-BMT disseminated toxoplasmosis, diagnosis was usually made at autopsy [58]. Specific odds ratios for mortality vs. various clinical parameters have been calculated by Mele et al. [59].

PLASMODIUM

In terms of global morbidity and mortality, malaria is the most significant of all parasitic diseases, each year killing one to two million persons globally [60]. As an intracellular parasite of erythrocytes, the protozoon *Plasmodium* induces its classic symptoms, paroxysms of chills, fever, and sweating. The *Anopheles* mosquito is the natural vector, but congenital, transfusion, and transplantation infections are also well documented. There have been at least four reported cases of *P. falciparum* caused by contaminated allogeneic marrow transplants [61]. Falciparum malaria infection, although often fatal in children and the elderly, does not persist as a latent infection once the parasitemia has been cleared. Untreated *P. vivax* by contrast, persists indefinitely in hepatic schizonts, which may trigger a relapse of clinical disease when the immune system is later weakened. On day 8 after autologous BMT, a 20-year-old female from Bangladesh developed a febrile neutropenia which was unresponsive to broad spectrum antibiotics and amphotericin B. Fever persisted despite resolution of neutropenia. On day 14, Giemsa-stained thin films revealed the trophozoites of *P. vivax* in 4% of erythrocytes. Fever responded within 48 h to oral chloroquine (1 mg/kg/day) followed by primaquine (15.3 mg/day for 2 weeks) to eliminate hepatic schizonts [62]. As a source of anemia and thrombocytopenia, vivax malaria may misleadingly suggest the acceleration of a CML process [63]. Among patients treated for cancer, it may relapse even two decades after leaving the endemic area [64].

TRYPANOSOMA CRUZI

Chagas' disease or South American trypanosomiasis is a zoonosis that infects 18 million Latin Americans. Peridomestic triatomid or "kissing bugs" are the natural vectors, but contaminated transfusions remain a threat to local blood supplies. The acute phase often occurs in rural children, accompanied by the characteristic Romana's sign and C-shaped trypomastigotes of *Trypanosoma cruzi* in the peripheral blood. As adults, most infected persons enter an indeterminate phase, without overt progression of disease. In others, slow replication of the intracellular amastigotes may lead to megaesophagus, megacolon, or in many cases, destruction of myocardium and fatal heart disease [65].

Of five infected Argentinian patients undergoing BMT for leukemia or lymphoma, one showed signs or symptoms of reactivation. This 31-year-old male, unaware of his chronic infection, developed parasitemia during neutropenia secondary to treatment for non-Hodgkin's' lymphoma [66]. Reactivated Chagas' disease was also reported in a 27-year-old man undergoing allogeneic BMT for CML. The patient remained free of parasitemia for 2 years after a 7 week course of benznidazole [67]. Chemotherapy for Hodgkin's disease exacerbated a myocardial focus of amastigotes, leading to a fatal cardiac arrest in a 46-year-old man [68].

An uncommon form of localized encephalitis may appear in HIV or ALL patients in whom myriads of amastigotes may be seen within glial cells. Imaging studies show an intracerebral mass lesion suggesting toxoplasmosis in immunocompromised patients [69]. A 73-year-old Brazilian male presented with lymphocytic leukemia, intracranial hypertension, and a tumorlike brain mass. Flagellate forms of *T. cruzi* were encountered in the CSF, prompting a successful course of benznidazole treatment [70]. Chemotherapy has recently been reviewed by Coural and de Castro [71].

LEISHMANIA

Leishmaniasis is a zoonosis transmitted by sandflies in both the New and Old Worlds. As obligate intracellular parasites of macrophages and monocytes, the small (1–3 μm) amastigotes of *Leishmania* species produce one of three major clinical syndromes: (1) cutaneous disease (e.g., oriental sore), with one or more ulcers that typically resolve spontaneously, (2) mucocutaneous involvement (espundia), with metastasis to the oropharyngeal mucosa and progressive tissue destruction, and (3) visceral leishmaniasis (kala-azar), with systemic dissemination of infected cells, marked by fever, wasting disease, hepatosplenomegaley, and pancytopenia [72–74].

Di Cataldo et al. [75] describe three cases of visceral leishmaniasis diagnosed in Sicily. All were children in complete remission after treatment for ALL (two cases) or AML (one case). Fever, hepatosplenomegaly, and pancytopenia were first interpreted as either a relapse of ALL or a bone marrow hypoplasia secondary to chemotherapy. These symptoms proved unresponsive to antibiotics, and interruption of chemotherapy and bone marrow smears revealed the amastigotes of an unspecified *Leishmania* species. Although immune suppression was likely, IFA titers were high and confirmatory. The infection responded well to megluamine antimonate and allopurinol. Encountering fever and a progressively enlarging spleen, others have mistaken childhood visceral leishmaniasis for active leukemia but were likewise alerted by the appearance of amastigotes in the bone marrow [76].

Visceral infection is typically quiescent, characterized by low antibody titers and skin test reactivity. Latency depends on normal T cell populations and cellular responsiveness. Forty years after leaving his native Sicily, a 75 year-old CLL patient developed progressive cutaneous lesions of the normally viscerotrophic *L. infantum* that responded well to sodium stibogluconate [77]. In southern Europe, immunosuppressive treatment for organ transplants or malignancies often lead to reactivation of asymptomatic visceral leishmaniasis or facilitation of new infections [78]. Cutaneous ulceration may become quite extensive in leukemia patients yet respond well to conservative treatment and resolve without contracture or scarring [79]. Resistance to pentavalent antimony injections can be overcome by amphoterecin B, aminosidine, or miltefosine [80].

CESTODES

Although unusual in cancer patients, the tissue stages of various species of tapeworms may enlarge, become invasive, or assume atypical forms, behavior reminiscent of cancer itself. The cosmopolitan dwarf tapeworm *Hymenolepis nana* produces small cysticercoids in the duodenal epithelium, enabling a cycle of internal autoinfection. Atypical cystic structures, presumably aberrant growths of *H. nana*, appeared in the blood vessels and all deep organs of a patient with Hodgkin's disease [81]. Massive cardiopulmonary cysticercosis (presumably *Taenia solium*) caused acute heart failure and death in a 53-year-old woman treated for AML [82]. An odd, aberrant sparganum proliferated and disseminated throughout the body of a man who died of Hodgkin's disease [83]. Presenting usually as cystic masses in soft tissue, however, the immature phases of tapeworms are primarily of differential diagnostic interest. Cysticercosis may mimic various tumors [84], while the hydatid cyst of echinoccosis has been both mistaken for a tumor [85] and simulated by a cystic lymphangioma [86]. Among other flatworms, the flukes and schistosomes are of major interest primarily as causes of cancers, especially of the liver and urinary bladder [87].

NEMATODES

Strongyloides stercoralis, the threadworm, is one of the few helminths capable of replication entirely within a single individual host, making it the most significant nematode in clinical oncology. Unsuspected subclinical infections, sometimes marked only by an unexplained eosinophilia, may persist as long as 65 years after leaving the endemic area [88,89]. Parthenogenetic female adult worms, up to 2.7 mm in length, inhabit the mucosa of the duodenum and upper jejunum. Thin-shelled ovoid eggs quickly hatch into rhabditoid larvae (380 μm) that are irregularly shed in the feces and feed on organic detritus in the soil. Molting leads to slender infective or filariform larvae (up to 630 μm) capable of penetrating unprotected skin and initiating infection within the new host. Under poorly understood conditions, however, the filariform stage is attained before passage in the stool, opening the door to internal autoinfection and, in immunosuppressed patients, disseminated, overwhelming hyperinfection [90]. Predisposing factors include steroid treatment, organ transplantations, therapy for nephrotic syndrome [5], Hodgkin's lymphoma, lymphocytic and lymphoblastic leukemia, HTLV-1, and various solid tumors [91–93]. The clinical manifestations of hyperinfection are highly variable, reflecting the predisposing cause, the level of infection, and the target organs: usually the bowel, lungs, and central nervous system. Intestinal symptoms may include a spruelike syndrome, weight loss, puffiness of the face and ankles, flatulence, abdominal distention, and, in some cases, evidence of intestinal obstruction. A wheezing dyspnea and productive cough may lead to recovery of the filariform larvae in sputum [88]. Recurrent sepsis with bowel flora, meningitis, and brain abscess are important clues.

    Early detection and treatment of smoldering *Strongyloides* infections would undoubtedly reduce the 85% fatality rate of disseminated disease.

Distribution of the parasite is cosmopolitan, but a residential history is somewhat helpful. Special consideration should be given to gay men, institutionalized persons, those having lived at any time in the past in the U. S. Appalachian mountain region, especially Tennessee, or in developing countries, particularly those of Latin America and Southeast Asia [89]. A pathognomonic sign, a larva current is a linear urticarial tract migrating from the perianal area at the rate of several centimeters per hour [89]. As with giardiasis, at least three stools must be collected on nonconsecutive days to rule out infection. Other methods, including sputum examination, duodenal aspiration or biopsy, and the "string test" may be useful in particular settings [88].

Traditionally used for strongyloidiasis, thiabendazole is unreliable, toxic, and not available for intravenous administration. Given over a period of several weeks, mebendazole appears to be active against adult worms in the bowel and against larvae returning from tissue during the course of treatment. The newer albendazole appears to have greater larvacidal activity. Ivermectin, a macrolide antibiotic, seems to be more effective than either of its predecessors, but multiple doses are still indicated to assure complete elimination rather than mere suppression of infection to undetectable levels. Steroids should be decreased.

Nematodes other than *Strongyloides* may be encountered in cancer patients. A 55-year-old man was treated with steroids for mycosis fungoides and aggressive cytotoxic therapy for lymphoma. After he developed fever, myalgia, and pneumonia unresponsive to antibiotics, biopsies of skin and liver showed the larvae of *Toxocara canis*, a dog ascarid. In spite of mebendazole therapy, the patient died from complications of severe, disseminated visceral larva migrans [94]. *Ascaris lumbricoides*, the giant intestinal roundworm (20 cm) affects one fifth or more of the world's population. Of diagnostic interest, this formidable-looking nematode is apparently killed by total body irradiation and may be passed harmlessly in the emesis [95] or undoubtedly in the feces. Movement of live worms, however, occasionally leads to dangerous abdominal complications [5].

ECTOPARASITES

Demodex folliculorum is a small mite (300 μm) that normally lives as a commensal in the facial hair follicles of nearly all senior adults. Infestations are less common in healthy children, presumably because their sebum production is low. Nevertheless, during maintenance chemotherapy for ALL, mites may proliferate, leading to erythematous, papular, and pustular eruptions [96–98]. Large numbers of the stubby legged, cigar-shaped organisms appear in 10% KOH preparations. Perioral dermatitis seems to be highly suggestive [96], but dermatophyte infections, candidiasis, drug eruptions, impetigo, folliculitis, and acneiform reactions must also be considered [98]. The lesions respond well to a single overnight application of 5% permethrin cream [97,98] or 1% lindane cream in a single overnight application per week for two successive weeks [96].

Sarcoptes scabei, the human mange mite, is a microscopic (330–450 μm) ovoid arthropod that burrows in the stratum corneum of the skin, creating serpiginous trails several millimeters to a few centimeters in length. The female deposits thin-shelled, ovoid eggs as well as minute fecal pellets believed to cause the intense pruritus and excoriation that are the hallmarks of infestation in the immunocompetent host. The moist, warm intertrigenous areas of the skin are favored: the interdigital folds, flexor aspects of the wrists, extensor surfaces of the elbows, and similar sites on the trunk, including the genitalia. Transmission is by close physical contact, including sexual intercourse.

Norwegian or crusted scabies appears in some debilitated, senile, or immunocompromised individuals, including those with AIDS. Mites proliferate in enormous numbers, provoking widespread hyperkeratosis and scaling of highly infectious crusts. The characteristic pruritus may be absent, and superinfection by β-hemolytic streptococci carries the added risk of acute glomerulonephritis. On day 5 of induction chemotherapy for AML, disseminated scabies appeared on a 34-year-old male. Treated with oral ivermectin and topical lindane, the infestation resolved completely, in spite of ongoing neutropenia and other significant infectious complications [99]. Scabies has been recognized in HTLV-1 infection with associated myelopathy [100] and with herpes simplex in CLL and hypogammaglobulinemia [101,102]. Of five infested Australian aboriginal patients [103] and six native Guyanese of low socioeconomic backgrounds [104], all tested positive for HTLV-1.

Massive scabies infection should be considered when confronted with a generalized cutaneous involvement in any HTLV-1 patient [99,105]. Topical steroid use and irradiation may also predispose to heavy infestation [102,106].

Diagnosis is established by microscopic examination of skin scrapings collected in mineral oil from burrows that are not heavily excoriated. Even minimal contact with an encrusted patient may result in transmission, and institutional outbreaks are common [107]. Because the potential for fomite transmission is high, hot water laundering of the patient's underwear, clothing, and bedsheets should be used to kill mites and eggs 48 hours prior to treatment. Oral ivermectin is indicated for infections refractory to synthetic pyrethroid, lindane, or crotamiton, or where these topical medications are contraindicated.

CONCLUSIONS

Parasitic organisms that complicate neoplasms are for the most part those protozoa that replicate within cells or tissues, helminths that are capable of internal autoinfection, or small mites whose entire life cycle is passed within the skin. The neoplasms involved are overwhelmingly the leukemias and lymphomas, often treated with BMT. As examples of incidental findings, histological examination of oropharyngeal carcinomas may uncover asymptomatic parasites of skeletal muscle, *Sarcocystis* [108], or *Trichinella* [109]. Parasitic diseases, which complicate neoplasia or their therapy also complicate solid organ transplants or AIDS, but many authors whom we reviewed did not report the HIV status of their cases. Many case reports have appeared within the past decade, often from nations adjacent to the developing world, including those of the Mediterranean Sea and temperate South America. New examples will undoubtedly continue to emerge. In countries between Japan and Egypt, the small jejunal nematode *Capillaria philippinensis* is acquired by eating raw fish. Reminiscent of *Strongyloides*, it is capable of internal autoinfection and severe bowel disease [110]. Although we have seen no published reports, *C. philippensis* infections might also be exacerbated in leukemias or lymphomas or other immunodeficiency states.

Among the parasites discussed, two species of tissue protozoa enter structurally based indefinite latent periods after the mobile, disease-producing forms have been cleared away in the course of a healthy immune response. The bradyzoites of *Toxoplasma* become protected within the tissue cyst, as are the exoerythrocytic forms of vivax malaria within hepatic schizonts. Subsequent weakening of immune protection may trigger a clinical relapse with renewal of erythrocytic schizogony by merozoites (malaria) or further dissemination of tachyzoites (toxoplasmosis). In visceral leishmaniasis and Chagas' disease, accelerated replication of intracellular amastigotes leads to recrudesence of clinical disease.

High rates of asymptomatic carriage are characteristic of the lumen-dwelling protozoa (*Entamoeba*, *Giardia*, *Blastocystis*) in normal hosts; the fecal–oral life cycle is common to this group of protozoa. Diarrheal pathogens may be acquired before onset of cancer or after discharge while on maintenance chemotherapy.

In some parasitic diseases, infection is clearly acquired before treatment of the neoplasm. Vivax malaria [64], Chagas' disease [66–68], leishmaniasis [77], and toxoplasmosis may lie dormant for years or even decades. The bone marrow transplant itself may be a source of falciparum malaria [61] or visceral leishmaniasis [75] and probably for toxoplasmosis. *Cryptosporidium* [33–35] and *Sarcoptes* [107] may be transmitted within the hospital. Therapeutic immunosuppression may facilitate the acquisition of acanthamoebiasis or leishmaniasis [78].

Complications from parasitic diseases pose special diagnostic challenges to the oncologist. Clinical manifestations of some organisms are highly variable, depending on the organs involved in disseminated disease (toxoplasmosis, strongyloidiasis). Parasitic diseases may be misleading in a mindset of leukemias, lymphomas, and complications of their therapy, presenting fever and hepatosplenomegaly (visceral leishmaniasis), anemia with thrombocytopenia or pancytopenia (vivax malaria), lymphadenopathy (toxoplasmosis), or diarrhea (amebiasis). On the other hand, eosinophilia, a useful indication of tissue helminths, is usually absent in lymphoma patients with *Strongyloides*. Even the most common single manifestation, diarrhea, is more likely to be caused by viruses, bacteria, GVH disease, or chemotherapy [15]. While a history of travel or residence in a developing country is important for some of the more unusual parasites, dangerous pathogens (*Toxoplasma*, *Strongyloides*) are endemic to the U.S., and some are zoonoses. Strongyloidiasis has been recognized in the setting of cancer for several decades, whereas coccidial and microsporidial diseases are themselves considered to be still emerging diseases [4]. Screening and prophylaxis, although often advocated by authors in retrospect, are probably not justifiable in most cases, and in practice the clinician and the laboratory technician must rely on their awareness of these organisms. The correct diagnosis may come unexpectedly, as with *Strongyloides* larvae in a bronchoalveolar lavage. Even in immunosuppressed patients, parasites may be difficult to demonstrate. Laboratory diagnosis may be confounded where organisms are not regularly shed in the feces (*Giardia*, *Strongyloides*) or are inconspicuous and require special methods (*Cryptosporidium*) that must be requested by the clinician. Definitive diagnosis of parasitic diseases still relies heavily on recovery and morphological study of the organism [111]. Recognition of confusing artifacts or odd "pseudoparasites" sometimes requires a practiced eye [111,112]. Infection may still lack clear treatment guidelines (cryptosporidiosis), become severe and refractory during GVHD (amebiasis), or disseminate quickly, and be unable to halt a downward course of disease (acanthamoebiasis).

REFERENCES

1. Polsky B, Armstrong D. Infectious complications of neoplastic disease. Am J Infect Control 1985; 13(5):199–209.
2. Engelhard D. Bacterial and fungal infections in children undergoing bone marrow transplantation. Bone Marrow Transplant 1998; 21(suppl 2):S78–S80.
3. Armstrong D, Chmel H, Singer C, Tapper M, Rosen PP. Non-bacterial infections associated with neoplastic disease. Eur J Cancer 1975; 11(suppl):79–94.
4. Ambroise-Thomas P. Parasitic diseases and immunodeficiencies. Parasitology 2001; 122(suppl):S65 S71.
5. Garcia LS. Diagnostic Medical Parasitiology. ASM Press, 2001.
6. Ferreira MS, Borges AS. Some aspects of protozoan infections in immunocompromised patients: a review. Mem Inst Oswaldo Cruz 2002; 97(4):443–457.

7. Rolston KV. The spectrum of pulmonary infections in cancer patients. Curr Opin Oncol 2001; 13(4):218–223.
8. Aronchick JM. Pulmonary infections in cancer and bone marrow transplant patients. Semin Roentgenol 2000; 35(2):140–151.
9. Oh YW, Effmann EL, Godwin JD. Pulmonary infections in immunocompromised hosts: the importance of correlating the conventional radiologic appearance with the clinical setting. Radiology 2000; 217(3):647–656.
10. Rosen MJ. Respiratory infections in patients with HIV. Curr Opin Pulm Med 1995; 1(3):216–222.
11. Cunha BA. Central nervous system infections in the compromised host: diagnostic approach. Infect Dis Clin North Am 2001; 5(2):567–590.
12. Bia FJ, Barry M. Parasitic infections of the central nervous system. Neurol Clin 1986; 4(1):171–206.
13. Cohen J, West AB, Bini EJ. Infectious diarrhea in human immunodeficiency virus. Gastroenterol Clin North Am 2001; 30(3):637–664.
14. Khan SA, Wingard JR. Infection and mucosal injury in cancer treatment. J Natl Cancer Inst Monogr 2001; 29:31–36.
15. Rotterdam H, Tsang P. Gastrointestinal disease in the immunocompromised patient. Hum Pathol 1994; 25(11):1123–1140.
16. Smith PD. Infectious diarrheas in patients with AIDS. Gastroenterol Clin North Am 1993; 22(3):535–548.
17. Thompson RC, Reynoldson JA, Mendis AH. Giardia and giardiasis. Adv Parasitol 1993; 32:71–160.
18. Bromiker R, Korman SH, Or R, Hardan I, Naparstek E, Cohen P, Ben-Shahar M, Engelhard D. Severe giardiasis in two patients undergoing bone marrow transplantation. Bone Marrow Transplantation 1989; 4(6):701–703.
19. Korman SH, Granot E, Ramu N. Severe giardiasis in a child during cancer therapy. Am J Gastroenterol 84(4):450–451.
20. Bavaro P, Di Girolamo G, Di Bartolomeo P, Angrilli F, Olioso P, Papalinetti G, Del Vecchio A, Torlontano G. Amebiasis after bone marrow transplantation. Bone Marrow Transplantation 1994; 13(2):213–214.
21. Gardner TB, Hill DR. Treatment of giardiasis. Clin Microbiol Rev 2001; 4(1):114–128.
22. Schunk M, Jelinek T, Wetzel K, Nothdurft HD. Detection of Giardia lamblia and Entamoeba histolytica in stool samples by two enzyme immunoassays. Eur J Clin Microbiol Infect Dis 2001; 20(6):389–391.
23. Perret C, Harris PR, Rivera M, Vial P, Duarte I, Barriga F. Refractory enteric amebiasis in pediatric patients with acute graft-versus-host disease after allogeneic bone marrow transplantation. J Pediatr Gastroenterol Nutr 2000; 31(1):86–90.
24. Ghosh K, Ayyaril M, Nirmala V. Acute GVHD involving the gastrointestinal tract and infestation with Blastocystis hominis in a patient with chronic myeloid leukemia following allogeneic bone marrow transplantation. Bone Marrow Transplant 1998; 22(11):1115–1117.
25. Collins R. Protozoan parasites of the intestinal tract: a review of Coccidia and Microsporida. J Am Osteopath Assoc 1997; 97(10):593–598.

26. Weiss LM, Keohane EM. The uncommon gastrointestinal Protozoa: Microsporidia, Blastocystis, Isospora, Dientamoeba and Balantidium. Curr Clin Top Infect Dis 1997; 17:147–187.
27. Laurent F, McCole D, Eckmann L, Kagnoff MF. Pathogenesis of Cryptosporidium parvum infection. Microbes and Infection 1999; 1(2):141–148.
28. Stine KC, Harris JS, Lindsey NJ, Cho CT. Spontaneous remission of cryptosporidiosis in a child with acute lymphocytic leukemia. Clinical Pediatrics 1985; 24(12):722–724.
29. Lewis IJ, Hart CA, Baxby D. Diarrhoea due to Cryptosporidium in acute lymphoblastic leukemia. Archives of Disease in Childhood 1985; 60(1):60–62.
30. Foot AB, Oakhill A, Mott MG. Cryptosporidiosis and acute leukemia. Archives of Disease in Childhood 1990; 65(2):236–237.
31. Wells GM, Gajjar A, Pearson TA, Hale KL, Shenep JL. Pulmonary Cryptosporidiosis and Cryptococcus albidus fungemia in a child with acute lymphocytic leukemia. Medical and Pediatric Oncology 1998; 31(6):544–546.
32. Gentile G, Venditii M, Micozzi A, Caprioli A, Donelli G, Tirindelli C, Meloni G, Arcese W, Martino P. Cryptosporidiosis in patients with hematologic malignancies. Rev Infec Dis 1991; 13(5):842–846.
33. Hunter PR, Nichols G. Epidemiology and clinical features of Cryptosporidium infection in immunocompromised patients. Clin Microbiol Rev 2002; 15(1): 145–154.
34. Martino P, Gentile G, Caprioli A, Baldassarri L, Donelli G, Arcese W, Fenu S, Micozzi A, Venditti M, Mandelli F. Hospital-acquired cryptosporidiosis in a bone marrow transplantation unit. J Inf Dis 1988; 158(3):647–648.
35. Travis WD, Schmidt K, MacLowry JD, Masur H, Condron KS, Fojo AT. Respiratory cryptosporidiosis in a patient with malignant lymphoma. Report of a case and review of the literature. Arch Path Lab Med 1990; 114(5):519–522.
36. Kawano F, Nishida K, Kurisaki H, Tsukamoto A, Satoh M, Sanada I, Shido T, Obata S, Kimura K, Sasaki Y. Isospora belli infection in a patient with adult T-cell leukemia. Rinsho Ketsuek—Japanese Journal of Clinical Hematology 1992; 33(5):683–687.
37. Yamane T, Takekawa K, Tanaka K, Hasuike T, Hirai M, Misu K, Ota K, Ohira H, Nakao Y, Yasui Y. Isospora belli infection in a patient with adult T-cell leukemia. Risho Byori—Japanese Journal of Clinical Pathology 1993; 41(3):303–306.
38. Jayshree RS, Acharya RS, Sridhar H. Isospora belli infection in a patient with acute lymphoblastic leukemia in India. Journal of Diarrhoeal Diseases Research 1996; 14(1):44–45.
39. Jayshree RS, Acharya RS, Sridhar H. Cyclospora cayetanensis-associated diarrhoea in a patient with acute myeloid leukemia. J Diarrhoeal Dis Res 1998; 16(4):254–255.
40. Yoken J, Forbes B, Maguire AM, Prenner JL, Carpentieri D. Microsporidial endophthalmitis in a patient with acute myelogenous leukemia. Retina 2002; 22(1):123–125.
41. Kotler DP, Orenstein JM. Clinical syndromes associated with microsporidiosis. Adv Parasitol 1998; 40:321–349.

42. Stratakis DF, Lang SM, Eichenlaub S, Loscher T, Stein R, Huber RM. Pulmonary trichomoniasis diagnosis based on identification of irritation in bronchoalveolar lavage. Pneumologie 1999; 53(12):617–619.
43. Shiota T, Arizono N, Morimoto T, Shimatsu A, Nakao K. Trichomonas tenax empyema in an immunocompromised patient with advanced cancer. Parasite 1998; 5(4):375–377.
44. Marciano-Cabral F, Puffenbarger R, Cabral GA. The increasing importance of Acanthamoeba infections. Journal of Eukaryotic Microbiology 2000; 47(1):29–36.
45. Illingworth CD, Cook SD. Acanthamoeba keratitis. Survey of Ophthalmology 1998; 42(6):493–508.
46. Anderlini P, Przepiorka D, Luna M, Langford L, Andreeff M, Claxton D, Deisseroth AB. Acanthamoeba meningoencephalitis after bone marrow transplantation. Bone Marrow Transplantation 1994; 14(3):459–461.
47. Feingold JM, Abraham J, Bilgrami S, Ngo N, Visvesara GS, Edwards RL, Tutschka PJ. Acanthamoeba meningoencephalitis following autologous peripheral stem cell transplantation. Bone Marrow Transplantation 1998; 22(3): 297–300.
48. Oliva S, Jantz M, Tiernan R, Cook DL, Judson MA. Successful treatment of widely disseminated acanthamoebiasis. Southern Medical Journal 1999; 92(1): 55–57.
49. Subauste CS, Remington JS. Immunity to Toxoplasma gondii. Curr Opin Immunol 1993; 5(4):532–537.
50. Dubey JP. Advances in the life cycle of toxoplasma gondii. Int J Parasitol 1998; 28(7):1019–1024.
51. Israelski DM, Remington JS. Toxoplasmosis in patients with cancer. Clin Inf Dis 1993; 17(suppl 2):S423–S435.
52. Sing A, Leitritz L, Roggenkamp A, Kolb HJ, Szabados A, Fingerle V, Autenrieth IB, Heesemann J. Pulmonary toxoplasmosis in bone marrow transplant recipients: report of two cases and review. Clin Inf Dis 1999; 29(2):429–433.
53. Mighell A, Carton A, Carey P, High A. Toxoplasmosis masking non-Hodgkin's lymphoma: a case report. Br J Oral Maxillofac Surg 1995; 33(6):388–390.
54. McCabe RE. Current diagnosis and management of toxoplasmosis in cancer patients. Oncology (Huntington) 1990; 4(10):81–90; discussion 93–94.
55. Arnold SJ, Kinney MC, McCormick MS, Dummer S, Scott MA. Disseminated toxoplasmosis. Unusual presentations in the immunocompromised host. Arch Pathol Lab Med 1997; 121(8):869–873.
56. Israelski DM, Remington JS. Toxoplasmosis in patients with cancer. Clin Inf Dis 1993; 17(suppl 2):S423–S435.
57. Chandrasekar PH, Momin F. Disseminated toxoplasmosis in marrow recipients: a report of three cases and a review of the literature. Bone Marrow Transplantion 1997; 19(7):685–689.
58. de Medeiros BC, de Medeiros CR, Werner B, Neto JZ, Loddo G, Pasquini R, Bleggi-Torres LF. Central nervous system infections following bone marrow transplantation: an autopsy report of 27 cases. Journal of Hematology and Stem Cell Research 2000; 9(4):535–540.

59. Mele A, Paterson PJ, Prentice HG, Leoni P, Kibbler CC. Toxoplasmosis in bone marrow transplantation: a report of two cases and systemic review of the literature. Bone Marrow Transplant 2002; 29(8):691–698.
60. English M, Newton CR. Malaria: pathogenicity and disease. Chem Immunol 2002; 80:50–69.
61. Villeneuve L, Cassaing S, Magnaval JF, Boisseau M, Huynh A, Demur C, Calot JP. Plasmodium falciparium infection following allogeneic bone-marrow transplantation. Ann Trop Med Parasitol 1999; 93(5):533–535.
62. Salutari P, Sica S, Chiusolo P, Micciulli G, Plaisant P, Nacci A, Antinori A, Leone G. Plasmodium vivax malaria after autologous bone marrow transplantation: an unusual complication. Bone Marrow Transplant 1996; 18(4): 805–806.
63. Jain P, Kumar R, Kumar L, Gujral S, Singh HP, Gupta S, Goel S. Chronic myeloid leukemia complicated by megaloblastic anemia and malaria: an unusual association confounding the assessment of the phase of CML. Med Pediatr Oncol 1999; 33(4):403–404.
64. Maslin J, Cuguillere A, Bonnet D, Martet G. Malaria attack: a very late relapse due to Plasmodium vivax. Bull Soc Exot 1997; 90(1):25–26.
65. Rassi A Jr, Rassi A, Little WC. Chagas' heart disease. Clin Cardiolo 2000; 23(12):883–889.
66. Dictar M, Sinagra A, Veron MT, Luna C, Dengra C, DeRissio A, Bayo R, Ceraso D, Segura E, Koziner B, Riarte A. Recipients and donors of bone marrow transplants suffering from Chagas' disease: management and preemptive therapy of parasitemia. Bone Marrow Transplantation 1998; 21(4): 391–393.
67. Altclas J, Sinagra A, Jaimovich G, Salgueira C, Luna C, Requejo A, Milovic V, De Rissio A, Feldman L, Riarte A. Reactivation of chronic Chagas' disease following allogeneic bone marrow transplantation and successful preemptive therapy with benznidazole.
68. Metze K, Lorand-Metze I, De Almeida EA, De Moraes SL. Reactivation of Chagas' myocarditis during therapy of Hodgkin's disease. Trop Geoge Med 1991; 43(1–2):228–230.
69. Di Lorenzo GA, Pagano MA, Taratuto AL, Garau ML, Meli FJ, Pomsztein MD. Chagasic granulomatous encephalitis in immunosuppressed patients. Computed tomography and magnetic resonance imaging findings. J Neuroimaging 6(2):94–97.
70. Salgado PR, Gorski AG, Aleixo AR, de Barros EO. Tumor-like lesion due to Chagas' disease in a patient with lymphocytic leukemia. Rev Inst Med Trop Sao Paulo; 1996; 38(4):285–288.
71. Coural JR, de Castro SL. A critical review on Chagas' disease chemotherapy. Mem Inst Oswaldo Cruz, Rio de Janeiro 2002; 97.
72. Guerin PJ, Olliaro P, Sundar S, Boelaert M, Croft SL, Desjeux P, Wasunna MK, Bryceson AD. Visceral leishmaniasis: current status of control, diagnosis, and treatment and a proposed research and development agenda. Lancet Infect Dis 2002; 2(8):494–501.
73. Herwaldt BL. Leishmaniasis. Lancet 1999; 354(9185):1191–1199.

74. Solbach W, Laskay T. The host response to Leishmania infection. Advances in Immunology 2000; 74:275–317.

75. Di Cataldo A, Lo Nigro L, Marino S, Schiliro G. Visceral leishmaniasis in three children with leukemia. Pediatr Infect Dis J 1996; 15(10):916–918.

76. Aguado JM, Gomez Berne J, Figuera A, de Villalobos E, Fernandez-Guerrero ML, Sanchez Fayos J. Visceral leishmaniasis (kala-azar) complicating acute leukaemia. J Infect 1983; 7(3):272–274.

77. Jewell AP, Giles FJ. Cutaneous manifestation of leishmaniasis 40 years after exposure in a patient with chronic lymphocytic leukaemia. Leuk Lymphoma 1996; 21(3–4):347–349.

78. Dedet JP, Pratlong F. Leishmania, Trypanosoma and monoxenous trypanosomatids as emerging opportunistic agents. J Eukaryot Microbiol 2000; 47(1):37–39.

79. Al-Qattan MM. Extensive cutaneous leishmaniasis of the upper limb in a patient with leukemia. Ann Plast Surg 2002; 48(6):670–671.

80. Murray HW. Treatment of visceral leishmaniasis (kala-azar): a decade of progress and future approaches. Int J Infect Dis 2000; 4(3):158–177.

81. Lucas SB, Hassounah OA, Doenhoff M, Muller R. Aberrant form of Hymenolepis nana: possible opportunistic infection in immunosuppressed patients. Lancet 1979; 2(8156–8157):1372–1373.

82. Mauad T, Battlehner CN, Bedrikow CL, Capelozzi VL, Saldiva PH. Case report: massive cardiopulmonary cysticercosis in a leukemic patient. Pathol Res Pract 1997; 193(7):527–529.

83. Connor DH, Sparks AK, Strano AJ, Neafie RC, Juvelier B. Disseminated parasitosis in an immunosuppressed patient. Possibly a mutated sparganum. Arch Pathol Lab Med 1976; 100(2):65–68.

84. Ogilvie CM, Kasten P, Rovinsky D, Workman KL, Johnston JO. Cysticercosis of the triceps—an unusual pseudotumor: case report and review. Clin Orthop 2001; (382):217–221.

85. Nanassis K, Alexiadou-Rudolf C, Tsitsopoulos P, Tzioufa V, Petsas G, Grigoriou K. Solid cerebral echinococcosis mimicking a primary brain tumor. Neurosurg Rev 1999; 22(1):58–61.

86. Anadol AZ, Oguz M, Bayramoglu H, Edali MN. Cystic lymphangioma of the spleen mimicking hydatid disease. J Clin Gastroenterol 1998; 26(4):309–311.

87. IARC Monographs on the Evaluation of Carcinogenic Risks to Humans 61. World Health Organization, 1994.

88. Grove DI. Human strongyloidiasis. Advanced in Parasitology 1996; 38:251–309.

89. Genta RM. Global prevalence of strongyloidiasis: critical review with epidemiologic insights into the prevention of disseminated disease. Rev Infect Dis 1989; 11(5):755–767.

90. Jamil SA, Hilton E. The strongyloides hyperinfection syndrome. New York State Journal of Medicine 1992; 92(2):67–68.

91. Adedayo O, Grell G, Bellot P. Hyperinfective strongyloidiasis in the medical ward: review of 27 cases in 5 years.

92. Aydin H, Doppl W, Battmann A, Bohle RM, Klor HU. Opportunistic strongyloides stercoralis hyperinfection in lymphoma patients undergoing chemotherapy and/or radiotherapy—report of a case and review of the literature. Acta Oncologica 1994; 33(1):78–80.

93. Purvis RS, Beightler EL, Diven DG, Sanchez RL, Tyring SK. *Strongyloides stercoralis* hyperinfection. International Journal of Dermatology 1992; 31(3): 160–164.

94. Kremery V Jr, Gould I, Sobota K, Spanik S. Two cases of disseminated toxocariasis in compromised hosts successfully treated with mebendazole. Chemotherapy 1992; 38(5):367–368.

95. Jurcic JG, Koll B, Brown AE, Crown JP, Yahalom J, Gulati SC. Excretion of Ascaris lumbricoides during total body irradiation. Bone Marrow Transplantation 1994; 13(4):491–493.

96. Castanet J, Monpoux F, Mariana R, Ortonne JP, Lacour JP. Demodicidosis in an immunodeficient child. Pediatric Dermatology 1997; 14(3):219–220.

97. Ivy SP, Mackall CL, Gore L, Gress RE, Hartley AH. Demodicidosis in childhood acute lymphoblastic leukemia; an opportunistic infection occurring with immunosuppression. Journal of Pediatrics 1995; 127(5):751–754.

98. Sahn EE, Sheridan DM. Demodicidosis in a child with leukemia. Journal of the American Academy of Dermatology 1992; 27(5 pt 2):799–801.

99. Trendelenburg M, Buchner S, Passweg J, Ratz Bravo AR, Gratwohl A. Disseminated scabies evolving in a patient undergoing induction chemotherapy for acute myeloblastic leukaemia. Ann Hematol 2001; 80(2):116–118.

100. Bergman JN, Dodd WA, Trotter MJ, Oger JJ, Dutz JP. Crusted scabies in association with human T-cell lymphotropic virus 1. Journal of Cutaneous Medicine and Surgery 1999; 3(3):148–152.

101. Tibbs CJ, Wilson DJ. Norwegian scabies and herpes simplex in a patient with chronic lymphatic leukemia and hypogammaglobulinemia. British Journal of Dermatology 1992; 126(5):523–524.

102. McGregor DH, Yang Q, Fan F, Talley RL, Topalovski M. Scabies associated with radiation therapy for cutaneous T-cell lymphoma. Ann Clin Lab Sci 2001; 31(1):103–107.

103. Mollison LC, Lo ST, Marning G. HTLV-I and scabies in Australian aborigines. Lancet 1993; 341(8855):1281–1282.

104. Del Giudice P, Sainte Marie D, Gerard Y, Couppie P, Pradinaud R. Is crusted (Norwegian) scabies a marker of adult T cell leukemia/lymphoma in human T lymphotropic virus type 1-seropositive patients? Journal of Infectious Diseases 1997; 176(4):1090–1092.

105. Takeshita T, Takeshita H. Crusted (Norwegian) scabies in a patient with smoldering adult T-cell leukemia. J Dermatol 2000; 27(10):677–679.

106. Belsito DV, Flotte TJ, Lim HW, Baer RL, Thorbecke GJ, Gigli I. Effect of glucocorticosteroids on epidermal Langerhans cells. J Exp Med 155(1):291–302.

107. Obasanjo OO, Wu P, Conlon M, Karanfil LV, Pryor P, Moler G, Anhalt G, Chaisson RE, Perl TM. An outbreak of scabies in a teaching hospital: lessons learned. Infect Control Hosp Epidemiol, 2001; (1):13–18.

108. Pathmanathan R, Kan SP. Three cases of human sarcocystis infection with a review of human muscular sarcocystosis in Malaysia. Tropical and Geographical Medicine 1992; 44:102–108.
109. Simaskos N, Palaiologos Y, Eliopoulos PN. Trichinosis and cancer of the larynx. J Laryngol Otol 1992; 106(2):171–172.
110. Cross JH. Intestinal capillariasis. Clin Microbiol Rev 1992; 5(2):120–129.
111. Ash LW, Orihel TC. Atlas of Human Parasitology. 4th ed. Chicago: American Society of Clinical Pathologists Press, 1997.
112. Burgers JA, Sluitlers JF, de Jong DW, Cornelissen JJ, van Meerbeeck JP. Pseudoparasitic pneumonia after bone marrow transplantation. Neth J Med 2001; 59(4):170–176.

36

HIV-Related Malignancies

Kadry Allaboun
University of South Florida College of Medicine
Tampa, Florida, U.S.A.

John N. Greene
University of South Florida College of Medicine
and Moffitt Cancer Center and Research Institute
Tampa, Florida, U.S.A.

AIDS-DEFINING MALIGNANCIES

HIV-infected patients are at an increased risk for developing cancer. According to the CDC staging criteria classification, three types of cancer are considered to be AIDS-defining illnesses: Kaposi's sarcoma (KS), B-cell non-Hodgkin's lymphoma (NHL) and invasive carcinoma of the cervix. Their incidence has increased in conjunction with the epidemic of human immunodeficiency virus (HIV) disease [1].

An increased incidence of malignant tumors has recently become a major concern in patients with acquired immunodeficiency, which can be induced by chemotherapy or radiotherapy for cancer, immunosuppression following organ transplantation, and HIV infection. Approximately 40% of all patients with AIDS have developed cancer during the course of HIV infection [2,3].

Immunodeficiency alters the risk of cancer. Every specific state of immunodeficiency is associated with an increased incidence of certain types of cancer. Most of the immunodeficiency-associated tumors are virus induced, and they are accompanied by a persistent viral infection, including human herpes virus 8 (HHV-8) in Kaposi's sarcoma, Epstein–Barr virus (EBV) in non-Hodgkin's lymphoma (NHL), and human papillomavirus (HPV) in cervical cancer. HIV itself rarely causes cancer; rather, it helps oncogenic viruses to escape the immune system and induce cancer [4,5].

Patients infected with HIV are living longer owing to advances in antiretroviral therapy and prophylaxis against opportunistic infections. The risk of developing cancer increases as the period of cell-mediated immune impairment increases. The most common malignancies are Kaposi's sarcoma and non-Hodgkin's lymphoma.

NON-HODGKIN'S LYMPHOMA

Non-Hodgkin's lymphoma (NHL) is a frequent complication of human immunodeficiency virus (HIV) infection. NHL has been recognized as an AIDS-defining diagnosis since 1985. The vast majority of NHL in patients with HIV are of B-cell origin. It commonly presents with constitutional symptoms and involvement of extranodal sites (central nervous system, bone marrow, gastrointestinal tract, and liver). HIV-associated NHL affects all HIV-infected groups, regardless of mode of transmission. The risk of developing NHL increases with duration of HIV infection and age. Epstein–Barr virus has been implicated in the pathogenesis of NHL [6].

High-grade histologies represent the most common presentations of HIV-associated NHL. The incidence has declined only slightly with highly active antiretroviral therapy (HAART). After an initial rapid increase, the proportion of AIDS patients with KS steadily declined in the USA and in Europe, while the proportion of AIDS-related NHL has been stable during the last decade in the USA and Europe [7,8].

The most common oral cancers in HIV infected patients are Kaposi's sarcoma and non-Hodgkin's lymphoma. NHL can frequently involve the head and neck. Either nodal (cervical nodes) or extranodal locations such as the oral cavity and the maxillary sinus are the most common sites. Patients with AIDS-associated sinonasal NHL more frequently develop bony erosion and present with signs and symptoms referable to adjacent structures, such as the orbit, than do HIV-infected patients with sinusitis. However, the clinical manifestations of these conditions overlap; thus a high index of suspicion for NHL is imperative for prompt diagnosis. Extranodal NHL requires testing for HIV infection. These lymphomas typically are of high grade and disseminate early with a poor prognosis [9].

The overall outcome of patients with HIV-related NHL is generally poor because of the high-grade morphology and the frequent presence of opportunistic infections. Long-term survival and possibly a cure can be obtained in some patients with HIV-associated NHL. These in particular have a better performance status and less advanced immune dysfunction [10,11].

KAPOSI'S SARCOMA

Kaposi's sarcoma has been associated with AIDS since the onset of the epidemic in 1981. Its incidence has declined during the late 1990s with use of HAART. The tumor itself has various clinical manifestations, ranging from indolent cutaneous tumors to rapidly growing tumors involving skin, lung and the gastrointestinal tract. Clinical manifestations include nodules, plaques, lymph node enlargement, and signs and symptoms of visceral involvement [12].

Kaposi's sarcoma is the most common neoplastic disease in patients with AIDS. KS is closely linked to immunodeficiency and preferentially affects homosexual men. It arises from mesenchymal cells owing to uncontrolled expression of latency genes of human herpes virus-8 (HHV-8), influenced by cytokines or growth factors and environmental factors. HHV-8 has been identified in over 90% of KS lesions from patients with and without AIDS, suggesting its etiological importance in the development of KS. Treatment options include local therapy (radiotherapy, intralesional chemotherapy, cryotherapy) and systemic therapy (chemotherapy, interferon-alpha).

AIDS-RELATED MALIGNANCIES

Persons infected with HIV appear to be at increased risk for developing non-AIDS-defining malignancies. The natural history of cancers in patients with HIV infection differs from that of the general population. Tumors in patients with HIV infection have unusual aspects of tumor localization, growth behavior, and therapeutical response, which distinguish them from tumors that occur in patients without HIV infection. In general, HIV-related malignancies are more aggressive, respond poorly to treatment, and are associated with an extremely high rate of mortality.

The incidence of HIV-related malignancies is expected to increase as more effective therapies for HIV and associated opportunistic infections allow patients to live longer in an advanced state of immunodeficiency. A number of other malignancies may occur at an increased incidence in persons with HIV infection, including cancer of the conjunctiva (in HIV-infected individuals in sub-Saharan Africa, which is uncommon in Western countries), oral cancer, squamous-cell carcinoma of the head and neck, thyroid carcinoma, cancer of the larynx, leukemias, multiple myeloma, Hodgkin's disease, skin cancer, prostate cancer, bladder cancer, carcinoma of the penis, gastric carcinoid, colon cancer, and adenocarcinoma of the rectum. HIV-induced immunosuppression has been linked to an acceleration of cervical and anal neoplasia. Patients with and without HIV infection who develop germ-cell malignancies are similar in presentation and tumor histology [13–15].

Lung cancer is also seen with a higher frequency in AIDS patients. Lung cancer in HIV-infected patients presents at a younger age, with more advanced disease, and more commonly with adenocarcinoma. Malignant tumors are more aggressive in this group of patients as compared with the general population. Prognosis is poor. Mean overall survival is 6 months [16,17].

Leiomyosarcoma and benign leiomyomas have increased in incidence in HIV-infected children but are unusual in HIV-infected adults, perhaps because of hormonal or growth-promoting factors. Other rare tumors related to HIV infection in childhood, such as cervical, thyroid, and pulmonary carcinoma, have been reported. In contrast to HIV-infected adults, Kaposi's sarcoma is rare in children in industrialized countries, but not in children living in sub-Saharan Africa. HIV-infected children who develop cancer are likely to benefit from aggressive treatment combined with adequate supportive care. Prevention and management of HIV-associated cancers are becoming increasingly important as the HIV epidemic continues to expand [18,19].

REFERENCES

1. Spano JP, Atlan D, Breau JL, Farge D. AIDS and non-AIDS-related malignancies: a new vexing challenge in HIV-positive patients. Part I: Kaposi's sarcoma, non-Hodgkin's lymphoma, and Hodgkin's lymphoma. Eur J Intern Med 2002; 13(3):170–179.
2. Levine AM. AIDS-related malignancies: the emerging epidemic. J Natl Cancer Inst 1993; 85(17):1382–1397.
3. Hiddemann W. What's new in malignant tumors in acquired immunodeficiency disorders? Pathol Res Pract 1989; 185(6):930–934.
4. Scadden DT. AIDS-related malignancies. Annu Rev Med 2003; 54:285–303.
5. Brockmeyer N, Barthel B. Clinical manifestations and therapies of AIDS associated tumors. Eur J Med Res 1998; 3(3):127–147.
6. Rabkin CS. Epidemiology of AIDS-related malignancies. Curr Opin Oncol 1994; 6(5):492–496.
7. Nasti G, Vaccher E, Errante D, Tirelli U. Malignant tumors and AIDS. Biomed Pharmacother 1997; 51(6-7):243–251.
8. Goeder JJ. The epidemiology of acquired immunodeficiency syndrome malignancies. Semin Oncol 2000; 27(4):390–401.
9. Zapater E, Bagan JV, Campos A, Armengot M, Abril V, Basterra J. Non-

Hodgkin's lymphoma of the head and neck in association with HIV infection. Ann Otolaryngol Chir Cervicofac 1996; 113(2):69–72.

10. Pomilla PV, Morris AB, Jaworek A. Sinonasal non-Hodgkin's lymphoma in patients infected with human immunodeficiency virus: report of three cases and review. Clin Infect Dis 1995; 21(1):137–149.

11. Tirelli U, Errante D, Spina M, Vaccher E, Serraino D, Boiocchi M, Gloghini A, Carbone A. Long-term survival of patients with HIV-related systemic non-Hodgkin's lymphomas. Hematol Oncol 1996; 14(1):7–15.

12. Mitsuyasu RT. Clinical aspects of AIDS-related Kaposi's sarcoma. Curr Opin Oncol 1993; 5(5):835–844.

13. Santos J, Palacios R, Ruiz J, Gonzalez M, Marquez M. Unusual malignant tumors in patients with HIV infection. Int J STD AIDS 2002; 13(10):674–676.

14. Rabkin CS, Blattner WA. HIV infection and cancers other than non-Hodgkin lymphoma and Kaposi's sarcoma. Cancer Surv 1991; 10:151–160.

15. Cooksley CD, Hwang LY, Waller DK, Ford CE. HIV-related malignancies: community-based study using linkage of cancer registry and HIV registry data. Int J STD AIDS 1999; 10(12):795–802.

16. Katariya K, Thurer RJ. Thoracic malignancies associated with AIDS. Semin Thorac Cardiovasc Surg 2000; 12(2):148–153.

17. Gunthel CJ, Northfelt DW. Cancers not associated with immunodeficiency in HIV infected persons. Oncology (Huntingt) 1994; 8(7):59–64; discussion 64, 67–68, 70.

18. Mueller BU. Cancers in human immunodeficiency virus-infected children. J Natl Cancer Inst Monogr 1998; 23:31–35.

19. Rabkin CS. Association of non-acquired immunodeficiency syndrome—defining cancers with human immunodeficiency virus infection. J Natl Cancer Inst Monogr 1998; 23:23–25.

37

Prevention of Infection in Cancer Patients

Patrick Roth
Freiburg University
Freiburg, Germany

Despite improved measures of therapy and supportive care, infections remain a major cause of morbidity and mortality in cancer patients. Furthermore, infections represent physical and emotional stress, prolong the duration of hospitalization, and raise the cost of therapy. Prophylactic strategies have therefore been the goal of many studies that have been performed during the last 30 years. Many of the evaluated strategies have been dropped for several reasons such as a lack of proven effectiveness, patient unacceptability and consequent problems with compliance, and extreme expense.

There are numerous reasons that cancer patients are at high risk for infectious complications. Briefly, it can be said that the cancer itself can lead to an abnormality in immune function, especially in hematological malignancies. Moreover, solid tumors can cause obstruction of hollow organs and thereby alter the normal mechanisms of defense. Additional risk factors among cancer patients are malnutrition, common use of intravenous access devices and disruption of the integument by venipuncture or procedures, and chemotherapy induced mucositis. By far the most common reason for an increased risk of infection is leukopenia, especially neutropenia, which can often be found in patients with hematological malignancies. Additionally, the number of patients undergoing neutropenia has markedly increased because of the expanding use of dose-intensive chemotherapy in patients with solid tumors. It has been recognized for a long time that there exists a relationship between the degree and the duration of neutropenia, and the risk for serious infectious complications [1–3]. Because of its importance and commonness, the majority of investigations concerning prophylactic strategies have focused on neutropenic patients.

Although many clinical trials investigated the efficacy of various measures to prevent or reduce the occurrence of infection, the most effective and reproducible ways of infection prevention have been the simplest. Especially strict hand washing by physicians, nurses, and others in close contact with patients has to be emphasized. A cooked food diet that excludes fresh fruits and vegetables during periods of neutropenia is generally recommended, because these foods are often contaminated with gram-negative bacteria (especially *Klebsiella peumoniae*, *Escherichia coli*, and *Pseudomonas aeruginosa*) and fungal spores. To decrease excessive microbial colonization, invasive procedures should be minimized.

To reduce the acquisition of potential pathogens, isolation of neutropenic cancer patients has been investigated extensively. The technique of reverse isolation has not been shown to be superior to an environment where strict hand washing was performed [4]. On top of that, the totally protected environment was developed. It consists of rooms with constant laminar airflow, high-efficiency particle air filters, and aggressive measures of surface decontamination: sterilization of all objects that enter the room, topical antiseptics, and oral nonabsorbable antibiotics. The maintenance of the totally protected environment is very expensive and extremely time-consuming, so the failure of some studies to demonstrate a clear survival advantage has led to its reduced use. In addition, the total protected environment was made dispensable by the introduction of new measures, such as the use of colony-stimulating factors, which reduce the duration of neutropenia. Airflow rooms and particle air filters remain important for certain high-risk patients with profound neutropenia, such as those undergoing bone marrow transplantation [5].

ANTIBACTERIAL PROPHYLAXIS

Bacterial pathogens are by far the most common cause of an infection in neutropenic patients. For this reason, a large number of clinical trials, focused on the utility of prophylactic antibiotic regimes, have been conducted. Regrettably, many of the early studies included a very small number of patients, failed to document compliance with the prophylactic drug regimen, and utilized different endpoints, which makes it difficult to compare and interpret them. In addition, the type of pathogens underlying bacterial infections has changed during the last decades. When antibiotic prophylaxis was introduced about 30 years ago, the majority of bacterial pathogens found in neutropenic patients were gram-negative rods. However, during the last decade, gram-positive cocci have replaced the gram-negative rods as the leading cause of microbiologically documented infections in febrile neutropenia [6]. Nonetheless, the use of antibacterial agents remains a viable way to prevent bacterial infection in neutropenic patients.

ORAL NONABSORBABLE ANTIBIOTICS

The source of many infections in neutropenic patients may be the microflora that colonize the skin, the alimentary tract, and other mucosal surfaces [7]. Fifty years ago, oral antibiotics were used to diminish the frequency of postoperative infections subsequent to surgery of the colon [8]. Following this concept, several investigators treated cancer patients with a regimen of oral nonabsorbable antibiotics to decrease the endogenous gastrointestinal flora. Unfortunately, the available data confirming a beneficial effect of these measures is limited. Two studies showed a statistically significant reduction in infections and bacteremias in patients with good compliance [9]. Additional studies that used framycetin, colistin, and nystatin, or gentamicin, vancomycin, and nystatin, respectively, showed a reduced number of febrile episodes and fewer clinically and bacteriologically documented infections [10,11]. However, other studies did not prove beneficial for oral nonabsorbable antibiotics when compared to a control group [12]. Furthermore, it was found that an abrupt discontinuation of the oral antibiotics causes severe and life-threatening infections [13]. These controversial findings, and the poor tolerance of the administered drugs, which leads to difficulties in maintaining compliance, may explain why oral nonabsorbable antibiotic regimens cannot be established as a standard treatment. Finally, several studies showed the emergence of infections with organisms resistant to the regimens instituted, making their use even more questionable [14,15].

SELECTIVE GASTROINTESTINAL DECONTAMINATION

For a better understanding of selective decontamination of the gastrointestinal flora, the relationship between microbial colonization and pathogenicity has to be mentioned. Experiments in mice showed that normal anaerobic gut flora offer a certain level of protection against colonization and infection when challenged by exogenous gram-negative aerobic bacteria [16]. This concept of colonization resistance was developed about 30 years ago. It represents the basis for the use of antibiotic regimens that reduce the number of enteric aerobes while leaving anaerobic gut flora intact [17]. First studies in humans were performed with nonabsorbable antibiotics, often combined with a polyene antifungal (e.g., colistin, neomycin, nystatin). They showed a clearly reduced occurrence of gram-negative infections and bacteremia in the treatment group compared to placebo [18,19]. These studies on selective gastrointestinal decontamination used antibiotic regimens similar to those employed in the early trials with nonabsorbable antibiotics. Consequently, they suffered from comparable problems. Side effects like nausea and diarrhea combined with a poor compliance and the development of drug-resistant pathogens did not allow a broad use of these regimens. Crucial progress was only made with the introduction of trimethoprim-sulfamethoxazole (TMP-SMZ) and the fluoroquinolones.

PROPHYLAXIS WITH TRIMETHOPRIM-SULFAMETHOXAZOLE

Unlike the classic nonabsorbable antibiotics, TMP-SMZ reaches therapeutic levels in the blood, leading both to systemic and gut decontamination. The first study that showed a beneficial effect of TMP-SMZ was performed in 1977. Although it was originally planned to investigate the prevention of *Pneumocystis carinii* pneumonia with TMP-SMZ in children with leukaemia, this study demonstrated that children given placebo not only developed more often pneumonia due to PCP but also were found to have bacterial sepsis, acute otitis media, and cellulitis more frequently [20]. The meaningfulness of these findings was somewhat limited because the majority of patients included in this study were not suffering from profound neutropenia. However, numerous further studies with patients undergoing high-dose chemoterapy, thus being severely neutropenic, confirmed these findings. A precise comparison of these studies is not possible because of differences in degree and duration of neutropenia, inclusion and exclusion criteria, and definitions of infection and endpoint. Numerous studies demonstrated a decrease in the total number of acquired infections and febrile days in patients receiving TMP-SMZ prophylaxis compared to placebo [21,22]. Side effects were remarkably rare when compared to patients getting prophylaxis with oral nonabsorbable antibiotics, leading to a much better compliance.

Although many studies demonstrated benefits from TMP-SMZ prophylaxis, a number of additional trials failed to confirm a decrease in the incidence of febrile episodes or bacterial sepsis and showed no influence on infection-related mortality [23–25]. Several studies documented a reduction in episodes of bacteremia but no difference in the mean number of febrile days.

Therefore it was assumed that TMP-SMZ simply masks the feasibility to detect infections [26,27]. Besides these controversial findings, the problem of resistance to TMP-SMZ and an increased colonization with fungi became more and more important [28]. A large trial conducted by the International Antimicrobial Therapy Project Group (EORTC) reported a significantly higher number of resistant organisms in the blood of patients receiving TMP-SMZ prophylaxis in comparison with placebo recipients [29]. In addition, the spectrum of TMP-SMZ does not include *Pseudomonas aeruginosa*, a major pathogen causing fever and bacteremia in neutropenic patients. The addition of colistin to TMP-SMZ led to a reduction of isolated resistant strains and a better effectiveness against *P. aeruginosa* in one study [30]. Finally, numerous studies noticed allergic reactions and prolongation of neutropenia due to myelosuppression from a prophylactic treatment with TMP-SMZ [21,31].

PROPHYLAXIS WITH FLUOROQUINOLONES

The introduction of the fluorinated quinolones offered a new possibility to prevent infections in neutropenic patients. They have good activity against *Pseudomonas aeruginosa*, against almost all other important clinically active gram-negative microorganisms, and against even some aerobic gram-positive bacteria, but almost no activity against anaerobes, leaving thereby the resident flora needed for colonization resistance: all this was the starting point for many investigations. As quinolones are well absorbed by the alimentary tract, their use should result in systemic prophylaxis as well [32]. Several studies have clearly shown that fluoroquinolones significantly reduce the occurrence of gram-negative bacterial infections [33]. Multiple trials comparing quinolones to placebo demonstrated beneficial effects for ciprofloxacin, norfloxacin, and ofloxacin. Several studies, comparing fluoroquinolone with TMP-SMZ plus colistin, showed that the efficiency of the quinolones is equivalent or superior to TMP-SMZ for the prophylaxis of gram-negative bacteremias. A drawback of prophylaxis with quinolones is the insufficient effectiveness for gram-positive bacterial infections [34,35]. All studies showed that quinolones are extremely well tolerated, without significant nausea, diarrhea, allergy, or other toxicity. Because of this, quinolone compliance is generally much better when compared to the compliance of TMP-SMZ or nonabsorbable antibiotics. When quinolones were compared to each other, ciprofloxacin showed to be superior to ofloxacin and pefloxacin in the prevention of gram-negative bacteremia, but there was no difference in the occurrence of gram-positive infections or infection-related mortality [36,37]. Altogether, the beneficial effect of fluoroquinolone prophylaxis on some parameters such as the number of gram-positive infections, fever, the need for systemic antibiotics, and infection-related mortality is uncertain [38].

An additional matter of concern is the selection of multiresistant organisms during prophylactic treatment with fluoroquinolones. It has been shown that prophylactic use of ciprofloxacin and norfloxacin leads to an increased number of resistant *Escherichia coli* strains [39,40]. Additionally, prophylaxis with levofloxacin seems to select resistant viridans group streptococci [41].

To reduce the number of breakthrough gram-positive bacteremias, the coadministration of an additional antibiotic has been investigated. The combination of a quinolone and rifampin resulted in a reduced number of gram-positive bacterial infections in one study [42] but negative results were also reported [43]. A study that compared the combination of pefloxacin and penicillin V versus pefloxacin alone demonstrated a decrease in the occurrence of febrile episodes and bacteremias due to streptococci in the penicillin group [44]. Finally, it has recently been shown that a regimen consisting of colistin and ciprofloxacin is more effective in preventing infections with gram-negative bacilli and *Staphylococcus aureus*, without the emergence of significant resistance when compared to a combination of neomycin and colistin [45]. Future studies will show whether the newer fluoroquinolones with enhanced activity against gram-positive organisms (e.g., levofloxacin, moxifloxacin, gatifloxacin) are more effective for prophylaxis during neutropenia than the drugs used in the past.

In summary, it can be said that the fluroquinolones seem to be superior to other available prophylactic regimens in the prevention of gram-negative bacteremias. However, there is some concern about the increased number of infections with gram-positive organisms, the emergence of resistant strains, and the failure of many studies to demonstrate a clear reduction of mortality rates. Consequently, the Infectious Disease Society of America (IDSA) has recommended that routine prophylaxis for bacterial infections in neutropenic patients with antibiotics should be avoided [46].

ANTIFUNGAL PROPHYLAXIS

As more and more patients are treated with high-dose chemotherapy or undergo bone marrow transplantation, leading to both severe and prolonged neutropenia, the incidence of fungal infections has markedly increased during the last decade. The predominant pathogens that cause fungal infections in cancer patients are species of *Candida* and *Aspergillus*, so most investigations on prophylactic treatment have been focused on these organisms. Other fungi, such as *Fusarium, Cryptococcus,* and *Trichosporon* species, are rare, and no particular prophylaxis has been established for these pathogens.

CANDIDA

Colonization of the alimentary tract and other body sites is probably the first step preceding systemic candidosis. Another origin of systemic *Candida* infections is contaminated central venous catheters. Strict hygienic measures are likely to help prevent invasive infections. Besides, several antifungal agents have been investigated for prophylaxis.

ORAL POLYENES

Nystatin and oral amphotericin B have been used to reduce the candidal colonization of the digestive tract. Unfortunately, only a small number of controlled clinical studies are available. Although some studies showed a reduced incidence of fungal infections due to *Candida*, many other trials did not show any benefits of nystatin prophylaxis [47]. Moreover, nystatin is poorly tolerated and has therefore never been recommended for regular prophylaxis. Orally administered amphotericin B has been used in several studies. As with nystatin, there is no clear evidence for a beneficial effect [48]. Because of its unpalatability and consequent problems with compliance, oral amphotericin B seems to be unsuitable for fungal prophylaxis.

AZOLES

Several azoles have been investigated and shown to be effective in preventing *Candida* infection in neutropenic patients. Some early studies using miconazole and ketoconazole reported that these agents could decrease the incidence of invasive candidiasis [49]. Because of severe side effects (especially of ketoconazole) and the introduction of better tolerated azoles, prophylactic therapy with miconazole and ketoconazole was discontinued [50].

The newer azoles, fluconazole and itraconazole, offer several advantages. Particularly fluconazole is extremely well absorbed, leading to reliable systemic prophylaxis with fewer side effects than the previously used agents. Studies that compared fluconazole to placebo reported a decreased colonization by fungi and consequently less invasive fungal infections in fluconazole recipients [51,52]. A recent meta-analysis of randomized-controlled clinical trials verified these findings but also showed that fungal infection–related mortality was only reduced in patients who had prolonged neutropenia or underwent hematopoietic stem cell transplantation [53]. When fluconazole was compared to nystatin or intravenous amphotericin B, it proved to have a better prophylactic efficacy and fewer toxic side effects [54,55].

However, the major drawback of fluconazole is the relatively narrow spectrum of activity that is limited to certain species of *Candida* and the lack of efficacy against *Aspergillus*. Additionally, there is an increased concern about infections with non–*Candida albicans* species (such as *C. krusei* and *C. glabrata*) among patients treated prophylactically with fluconazole [56,57].

Prophylaxis with itraconazole was difficult for a long time because of poor oral absorption in the presence of chemotherapy-induced mucositis [58]. However, the introduction of a new oral liquid formulation of itraconazole has been shown to improve the bioavailability. Several studies demonstrated that itraconazole prophylaxis has significantly reduced the occurrence of systemic fungal infections due to *Candida* species when compared to placebo [59]. Other trials revealed that itraconazole is superior to oral amphotericin B plus nystatin and equivalent to fluconazole to prevent systemic candidiasis [60,61]. The effect of itraconazole on candida infection–related mortality is controversial, but it is likely that a decrease in mortality can only be found in severely neutropenic patients [53].

ASPERGILLUS

In contrast to candidosis, aspergillosis is acquired from the exogenous environment. *Aspergillus* species usually found in cancer patients are *A. fumigatus* and *A. flavus*. In some patients, *Aspergillus* species may colonize the airways before causing an infection. As diagnosis of aspergillosis is difficult and mortality high, there is great interest in preventing *Aspergillus* infections. Several studies have shown that strict hygienic measures such as removal of plants from rooms and the use of high-efficiency particulate filtration are very effective [62,63].

ORAL POLYENES/FLUCONAZOLE

Both oral polyenes and fluconazole are ineffective in preventing invasive aspergillosis. Several studies revealed that even high doses of fluconazole are not able to lower the incidence of aspergillosis when compared to placebo [64,65].

ITRACONAZOLE

Several studies using itraconazole for aspergillus prophylaxis have reported encouraging results. One study, comparing itraconazole and fluconazole, showed that in the itraconazole group fewer patients developed aspergillosis. Additionally, patients with itraconazole needed significantly less IV amphotericin B than patients with fluconazole [66]. Other clinical trials supported these findings, although the reduced incidence of aspergillosis was not always statistically significant [67]. Thus more studies will be required to clarify the utility of itraconazole in preventing aspergillosis.

INTRAVENOUS AND INHALED AMPHOTERICIN B

Inhaled formulations of amphotericin B were investigated in several clinical trials, but the results are controversial. Bad taste and other side effects were leading to poor compliance, and as a result no clear reduction in the occurrence of invasive aspergillosis in patients treated with inhaled amphotericin B was observed [68,69]. Intravenous drug administration is not a favorable type of application for a prophylactic regimen. However, because of the failure of the prophylactic regimens mentioned above, intravenous amphotericin B was used for aspergillus prophylaxis. Low-dose amphotericin B did not show a beneficial effect when compared to placebo [70]. Unlike low doses, therapeutic doses of amphotericin B were able to reduce the incidence of aspergillosis in some studies, but nephrotoxicity and other side effects limited its utility [71,72]. Unfortunately, the better tolerated liposomal amphotericin B (AmBisome) did not prove to have a beneficial effect compared to placebo [73].

ANTIVIRAL PROPHYLAXIS

As viral infections are predominantly associated with defects in cellular immune function, they are less frequent in cancer patients than bacterial and fungal infections. However, there is an increased risk of viral infections for patients undergoing bone marrow transplantation and those with severe neutropenia because of high-dose chemotherapy. Particular to cancer patients is reactivation of viruses that belong to the group of human herpes viruses: herpes simplex virus (HSV), cytomegalovirus (CMV), and varicella zoster virus (VZV). Prophylactic efforts have focused on these pathogens. Other viruses are less common and particular prophylactic strategies for them are not available.

HSV

Viral infections in cancer patients are most likely caused by reactivation of latent HSV. It has been reported that without antiviral prophylaxis 60 to 80% of all patients undergoing bone marrow transplantation or high-dose chemotherapy experience HSV reactivation. Thus prevention of HSV disease is of particular interest in seropositive patients [74]. Several studies revealed that reactivation of HSV types 1 and 2 could be prevented by oral and intravenous acyclovir [75,76]. A recent study demonstrated that the oral administration of the new drug valacylovir has the same efficacy in preventing HSV infection as acyclovir. It was well tolerated and less expensive than acyclovir [77].

CMV

Approximately 40 to 100% of all adults are seropositive for CMV [78]. Patients undergoing bone marrow transplantation are at increased risk of developing CMV reactivation, which can lead to interstitial pneumonia, hepatitis, retinitis, and encephalitis. Thus the first step in preventing CMV disease is to avoid CMV-seropositive organs and blood products in CMV-seronegative recipients [79]. In CMV-seropositive patients, high-dose intravenous acyclovir was shown to reduce the incidence of CMV disease [80]. Even more effective than acyclovir in preventing CMV is intravenous ganciclovir. Ganciclovir can decrease the occurrence of CMV disease, but its effect on infection-related mortality is less clear [81]. Unfortunately, ganciclovir is very toxic and can lead to prolonged neutropenia. A new strategy called preemptive treatment has been evaluated for the prevention of CMV disease in transplant recipients. In this setting, ganciclovir was only given to patients who developed CMV viremia (detected by culture or antigen detection systems). Reactivation of CMV developed in significantly fewer patients, and overall survival was greater than in a placebo group [82]. A recent study compared foscarnet to ganciclovir for preemptive therapy of cytomegalovirus infection. Foscarnet showed similar efficacy and less hematotoxicity than ganciclovir and might therefore be the best choice for preemptive therapy [83].

VZV

Primary VZV infection occurs mostly in young children, leading to the clinical manifestation of chicken pox. In cancer patients and other immunocompromised hosts, latent VZV can reactivate, causing dermatomal or disseminated herpes zoster. The use of acyclovir as prophylaxis for VZV reactivation only delays the onset of herpes zoster and causes the occurrence of VZV resistance [84,85]. Primary infection of VZV-seronegative patients can be avoided by strict isolation from infectious persons. After exposure to infectious individuals, intravenous VZV immunoglobulin may help to prevent the occurrence and severity of disease manifestations [86].

PNEUMOCYSTIS CARINII PROPHYLAXIS

Pneumonia due to *Pneumocystis carinii* (PCP) is a common complication in patients undergoing bone marrow transplantation. It can also be found in cancer patients with prolonged neutropenia because of high-dose chemotherapy. In the 1970s several studies demonstrated the efficacy of TMP-SMZ for the prevention of PCP [20]. Multiple clinical trials have clearly shown that TMP-SMZ decreases incidence as well as mortality from PCP [87]. Today, TMP-SMZ is still the drug of choice for the prevention of *Pneumocysts* infection and is recommended by the IDSA for all patients at risk for PCP [46]. However, the use of TMP-SMZ is limited because of its side effects. Particularly allergic reactions and myelosuppression may be reasons to stop TMP-SMZ prophylaxis. Moreover, TMP-SMZ resistance in *P. carinii* has developed within the last few years [88]. When TMP-SMZ is not tolerated, the newer drug atovaquone may be helpful. Atovaquone is effective for PCP prophylaxis with less toxicity than TMP-SMZ [89]. Other available agents for patients intolerant of TMP-SMZ are aerosolized pentamidine and dapsone [87].

COLONY-STIMULATING FACTORS AND GRANULOCYTE TRANSFUSIONS

More than 30 years ago, the quantitative relationship between the number of circulating leukocytes and infections in cancer patients was recognized [2]. Thus the transfusion of granulocytes has long been considered as a logical approach to the treatment and prophylaxis of infections in neutropenic patients. However, the first clinical trials in the 1960s and 1970s reported inconsistent efficacy and serious side effects because of leukocyte incompatibility. Particularly the lack of availability of sufficient quantities of neutrophils and the development of new antibiotic and antifungal drugs led to a waning interest in the infusion of granulocytes [90]. Interest in this measure came back in the 1990s when the hematopoietic growth factors G-CSF and GM-CSF (granulocyte and granulocyte-macrophage colony-stimulating factor) became available. These new drugs allow for the mobilization of more neurophils in donors before leukapheresis, creating the possibility of larger quantities to transfuse. Several studies reported a reduced relative risk of infection and death from infection in transfused patients versus control. In particular, the transfusion of adequate doses of compatible leukocytes seems to be a crucial factor [91,92]. Unfortunately, other studies reported no clear benefit from prophylactic granulocyte transfusion [93]. More studies will be needed to clarify the usefulness and efficacy of granulocyte transfusion as a prophylactic measure.

A further strategy that has been evaluated during the last decade is the direct application of G-CSF and GM-CSF to neutropenic patients. The utility of these agents has provided the opportunity to shorten considerably the duration of neutropenia following chemotherapy. Several studies evaluated the beneficial effect of prophylactic administration of colony-stimulating factors. A recently presented meta-analysis of the available randomized controlled studies has confirmed the efficacy of prophylactic granuloctye colony-stimulating factors [94]. It was reported that they are effective in reducing the risk of febrile neutropenia and documented infection. However, the reduction in the risk of infection-related mortality was not statistically significant and will need further evaluation. Besides bone pain, there were no remarkable side effects reported. Colony-stimulating factors may therefore be an excellent tool to reduce the incidence of infections in neutropenic patients.

In summary, prophylaxis of bacterial, fungal, viral and protozan infections will continue to be a dynamic area of research. These infections have a high mortality rate in the immunocompromised cancer patient. In addition, once infection occurs, the antimicrobial treatment duration is prolonged, and future cancer-related treatment must be delayed or withheld. In the battle to cure cancer, prevention of infection will be as important as the intensive anticancer regimens developed.

REFERENCES

1. Bodey GP, Rosenbaum B. Effect of prophylactic measures on the microbial flora of patients in protected environment units. Medicine (Baltimore) 1974; 53:209–228.
2. Bodey GP, Buckley M, Sathe YS, Freireich EJ. Quantitative relationships between circulating leukocytes and infection in patients with acute leukemia. Ann Intern Med 1966; 64:328–340.
3. Viola MV. Acute leukemia and infection. JAMA 1967; 201:923–926.
4. Nauseef WM, Maki DG. A study of the value of simple protective isolation in patients with granulocytopenia. N Engl J Med 1981; 304:448–453.
5. Sherertz RJ, Belani A, Kramer BS, Elfenbein GJ, Weiner RS, Sullivan ML, Thomas RG, Samsa GP. Impact of air filtration on nosocomial Aspergillus infections. Unique risk of bone marrow transplant recipients. Am J Med 1987; 83:709–718.
6. Klastersky J. Science and pragmatism in the treatment and prevention of neutropenic infection. J Antimicrob Chemother 1998; 41(suppl D):13–24.
7. Mackowiak PA. The normal microbial flora. N Engl J Med 1982; 307:83–93.
8. Riddell MI. A review of the literature on preoperative prophylaxis of the bowel with antimicrobial agents. Am J Med Sci 1952; 223:301.
9. Yates JW, Holland JF. A controlled study of isolation and endogenous microbial suppression in acute myelocyte leukemia patients. Cancer 1973; 32:1490–1498.

10. Ribas-Mundo M, Granema A, Rozman C. Evaluation of a protective environment in the management of granulocytopenic patients. A cooperative study. Cancer 1981; 48:419–424.
11. Storring RA, Jameson B, McElwain TJ, Wiltshaw E. Oral non-absorbed antibiotics prevent infection in acute non-lymphoblastic leukaemia. Lancet 1977; 2:837–840.
12. Levine AS, Siegel SE, Schreiber AD, Hauser J, Preisler H, Goldstein IM, Seidler F, Simon R, Perry S, Bennett JE, Henderson ES. Protected environments and prophylactic antibiotics. A prospective controlled study of their utility in the therapy of acute leukemia. N Engl J Med 1973; 288:477–483.
13. Schimpff SC, Green WH, Young VM, Fortner CL, Cusack N, Block JB, Wiernik PH. Infection prevention in acute nonlymphocytic leukemia. Laminar air flow and reverse isolation with oral, nonabsorbable antibiotic prophylaxis. Ann Intern Med 1975; 82:351–358.
14. King K. Prophylactic non-absorbable antibiotics in leukaemic patients. J Hyg (London) 1980; 85:141–151.
15. Klastersky J, Debusscher L, Weerts D, Daneau D. Use of oral antibiotics in protected units environment: clinical effectiveness and role in the emergence of antibiotic-resistant strains. Pathol Biol (Paris) 1974; 22:5–12.
16. van der Waaij D, Berghuis-de Vries JM, Lekkerkerk-van der Wees JE. Colonization resistance of the digestive tract in conventional and antibiotic-treated mice. J Hyg 1971; 69:405–411.
17. Vollaard EJ, Clasener HA. Colonization resistance. Antimicrob Agents Chemother 1994; 38:409–414.
18. Jehn U, Ruckdeschel G, Sauer H, Clemm C, Wilmanns W. Comparative study of the value of selective decontamination of the digestive tract in acute leukemia patients. Klin Wochenschr 1981; 59:1093–1099.
19. Guiot HF, van den Broek PJ, van der Meer JW, van Furth R. Selective antimicrobial modulation of the intestinal flora of patients with acute nonlymphocytic leukemia: a double-blind, placebo-controlled study. J Infect Dis 1983; 147:615–623.
20. Hughes WT, Kuhn S, Chaudhary S, Feldman S, Verzosa M, Aur RJ, Pratt C, George SL. Successful chemoprophylaxis for Pneumocystis carinii pneumonitis. N Engl J Med 1977; 297:1419–1426.
21. Dekker AW, Rozenberg-Arska M, Sixma JJ, Verhoef J. Prevention of infection by trimethoprim-sulfamethoxazole plus amphotericin B in patients with acute nonlymphocytic leukemia. Ann Intern Med 1981; 95:555–559.
22. Gurwith MJ, Brunton JL, Lank BA, Harding GK, Ronald AR. A prospective controlled investigation of prophylactic trimethoprim/sulfamethoxazole in hospitalized granulocytopenic patients. Am J Med 1979; 66:248–256.
23. Starke ID, Donnelly P, Catovsky D, Darrell J, Johnson SA, Goldman JM, Galton DA. Cotrimoxazole alone for prevention of bacterial infection in patients with acute leukaemia. Lancet 1982; 1:5–6.
24. Kramer BS, Carr DJ, Rand KH, Pizzo PA, Johnson A, Robichaud KJ, Yucha JB. Prophylaxis of fever and infection in adult cancer patients. A placebo-

controlled trial of oral trimethoprim-sulfamethoxazole plus erythromycin. Cancer 1984; 53:329–335.

25. Henry SA, Armstrong D, Kempin S, Gee T, Arlin Z, Clarkson B. Oral trimethoprim/sulfamethoxazole in attempt to prevent infection after induction chemotherapy for acute leukemia. Am J Med 1984; 77:663–666.

26. Kauffman CA, Liepman MK, Bergman AG, Mioduszewski J. Trimethoprim-sulfamethoxazole prophylaxis in neutropenic patients: reduction of infections and effect on bacterial and fungal flora. Am J Med 1983; 74:599–607.

27. Gualtieri RJ, Donowitz GR, Kaiser DL, Hess CE, Sande MA. Double-blind randomized study of prophylactic trimethoprim/sulfamethoxazole in granulocytopenic patients with hematologic malignancies. Am J Med 1983; 74:934–940.

28. Wilson JM, Guiney DG. Failure of oral trimethoprim-sulfamethoxazole prophylaxis in acute leukemia. Isolation of resistant plasmids from strains of enterobacteriaceae causing bacteremia. N Engl J Med 1982; 306:16–20.

29. EORTC International Antimicrobial Therapy Project Group. Cotrimoxazole in the prevention of infection in neutropenic patients. J Infect Dis 1984; 150:372–379.

30. Verhoef J. Prevention of infections in the neutropenic patient. Clin Infect Dis 1993; 17(suppl 2):S359–S367.

31. Wade JC, de Jongh CA, Newman KA, Crowley J, Wiernik PH, Schimpff SC. Selective antimicrobial modulation as prophylaxis against infection during granulocytopenia: trimethoprim-sulfamethoxazole vs. nalidixic acid. J Infect Dis 1983; 147:624–634.

32. Crump B, Wise R, Dent J. Pharmacokinetics and tissue penetration of ciprofloxacin. Antimicrob Agents Chemother 1983; 24:784–786.

33. Cruciani M, Rampazzo R, Malena M, Lazzarini L, Todeschini G, Messori A, Concia E. Prophylaxis with fluoroquinolones for bacterial infections in neutropenic patients: a meta-analysis. Clin Infect Dis 1996; 23:795–805.

34. Dekker AW, Rozenberg-Arska M, Verhoef J. Infection prophylaxis in acute leukemia: a comparison of ciprofloxacin with trimethoprim-sulfamethoxazole and colistin. Ann Intern Med 1987; 106:7–11.

35. Donnelly JP, Maschmeyer G, Daenen S. Selective oral antimicrobial prophylaxis for the prevention of infection in acute leukaemia—ciprofloxacin versus cotrimoxazole plus colistin. Eur J Cancer 1992; 28A:873–878.

36. D'Antonio D, Piccolomini R, Iacone A, Fioritoni G, Parruti G, Betti S, Quaglietta AM, Accorsi P, Dell'Isola M, Favalli C. Comparison of ciprofloxacin, ofloxacin and pefloxacin for the prevention of the bacterial infection in neutropenic patients with haematological malignancies. J Antimicrob Chemother 1994; 33:837–844.

37. GIMEMA Infection Program. Prevention of bacterial infection in neutropenic patients with hematologic malignancies: a randomized, multicenter trial comparing norfloxacin with ciprofloxacin. Ann Intern Med 1991; 115:7–12.

38. Engels EA, Lau J, Barza M. Efficacy of quinolone prophylaxis in neutropenic cancer patients: a meta-analysis. J Clin Oncol 1998; 16:1179–1187.

39. Perea S, Hidalgo M, Arcediano A, Ramos MJ, Gomez C, Hornedo J, Lumbreras C, Folgueira D, Cortes-Funes H, Rodriguez-Noriega A. Incidence and clinical impact of fluoroquinolone-resistant Escherichia coli in the faecal flora of cancer patients treated with high dose chemotherapy and ciprofloxacin prophylaxis. J Antimicrob Chemother 1999; 44:117–120.
40. Carratala J, Fernandez-Sevilla A, Tubau F, Dominguez MA, Gudiol F. Emergence of fluoroquinolone-resistant Escherichia coli in fecal flora of cancer patients receiving norfloxacin prophylaxis. Antimicrob Agents Chemother 1996; 40:503–505.
41. Razonable RR, Litzow MR, Khaliq Y, Piper KE, Rouse MS, Patel R. Bacteremia due to viridans group streptococci with diminished susceptibility to levofloxacin among neutropenic patients receiving levofloxacin prophylaxis. Clin Infect Dis 2002; 34:1469–1474.
42. Munoz L, Martino R, Subira M, Brunet S, Sureda A, Sierra J. Intensified prophylaxis of febrile neutropenia with ofloxacin plus rifampin during severe short-duration neutropenia in patient with lymphoma. Leuk Lymphoma 1999; 34:585–589.
43. Gomez-Martin C, Sola C, Hornedo J, Perea S, Lumbreras C, Valenti V, Arcediano A, Rodriguez M, Salazar R, Cortes-Funes H, Hidalgo M. Rifampin does not improve the efficacy of quinolone antibacterial prophylaxis in neutropenic cancer patients: results of a randomized clinical trial. J Clin Oncol 2000; 18:2126–2134.
44. International Antimicrobial Therapy Cooperative Group of the European Organization for Research and Treatment of Cancer. Reduction of fever and streptococcal bacteremia in granulocytopenic patients with cancer. JAMA 1994; 272:1183–1189.
45. Prentice HG, Hann IM, Nazareth B, Paterson P, Bhamra A, Kibbler CC. Oral ciprofloxacin plus colistin. prophylaxis against bacterial infection in neutropenic patients. A strategy for the prevention of emergence of antimicrobial resistance. Br J Haematol 2001; 115:46–52.
46. Hughes WT, Armstrong D, Bodey GP, Bow EJ, Brown AE, Calandra T, Feld R, Pizzo PA, Rolston KV, Shenep JL, Young LS. 2002 guidelines for the use of antimicrobial agents in neutropenic patients with cancer. Clin Infect Dis 2002; 34:730–751.
47. DeGregorio MW, Lee WM, Ries CA. Candida infections in patients with acute leukemia: ineffectiveness of nystatin prophylaxis and relationship between oropharyngeal and systemic candidiasis. Cancer 1982; 50:2780–2784.
48. Menichetti F, Del Favero A, Martino P, Bucaneve G, Micozzi A, D'Antonio D, Ricci P, Carotenuto M, Liso V, Nosari AM, Barbui T, Fasola G, Mandelli F, Behre GF, Schwartz S, Lenz K, Ludwig WD, Wandt H, Schilling E, Heinemann V, Link H, Trittin A, Boenisch O, Treder W, Siegert W, Hiddemann W, Beyer J. Preventing fungal infection in neutropenic patients with acute leukemia: fluconazole compared with oral amphotericin B. The GIMEMA Infection Program. Ann Intern Med 1994; 120:913–918.
49. Meunier-Carpentier F, Cruciani M, Klastersky J. Oral prophylaxis with mico-

nazole or ketoconazole of invasive fungal disease in neutropenic cancer patients. Eur J Cancer Clin Oncol 1983; 19:43–48.

50. Working Party Report. Chemoprophylaxis for candidosis and aspergillosis in neutropenia and transplantation: a review and recommendations. J Antimicrob Chemother 1993; 32:5–21.

51. Laverdiere M, Rotstein C, Bow EJ, Roberts RS, Ioannou S, Carr D, Moghaddam N. Impact of fluconazole prophylaxis on fungal colonization and infection rates in neutropenic patients. The Canadian Fluconazole Study. J Antimicrob Chemother 2000; 46:1001–1008.

52. Slavin MA, Osborne B, Adams R, Levenstein MJ, Schoch HG, Feldman AR, Meyers JD, Bowden RA. Efficacy and safety of fluconazole prophylaxis for fungal infections after marrow transplantation—a prospective, randomized, double-blind study. J Infect Dis 1995; 171:1545–1552.

53. Bow EJ, Laverdiere M, Lussier N, Rotstein C, Cheang MS, Ioannou S. Antifungal prophylaxis for severely neutropenic chemotherapy recipients: a meta analysis of randomized–controlled clinical trials. Cancer 2002; 94:3230–3246.

54. Bodey GP, Anaissie EJ, Elting LS, Estey E, O'Brien S, Kantarjian H. Antifungal prophylaxis during remission induction therapy for acute leukemia fluconazole versus intravenous amphotericin B. Cancer 1994; 73:2099–2106.

55. Young GA, Bosly A, Gibbs DL, Durrant S. A double-blind comparison of fluconazole and nystatin in the prevention of candidiasis in patients with leukaemia. Antifungal Prophylaxis Study Group. Eur J Cancer 1999; 35:1208–1213.

56. Wingard JR, Merz WG, Rinaldi MG, Johnson TR, Karp JE, Saral R. Increase in Candida krusei infection among patients with bone marrow transplantation and neutropenia treated prophylactically with fluconazole. N Engl J Med 1991; 325:1274–1277.

57. Wingard JR, Merz WG, Rinaldi MG, Miller CB, Karp JE, Saral R. Association of Torulopsis glabrata infections with fluconazole prophylaxis in neutropenic bone marrow transplant patients. Antimicrob Agents Chemother 1993; 37:1847–1849.

58. Boogaerts MA, Verhoef GE, Zachee P, Demuynck H, Verbist L, De Beule K. Antifungal prophylaxis with itraconazole in prolonged neutropenia: correlation with plasma levels. Mycoses 1993; 32(suppl 1):103–108.

59. Nucci M, Biasoli I, Akiti T, Silveira F, Solza C, Barreiros G, Spector N, Derossi A, Pulcheri W. A double-blind, randomized, placebo-controlled trial of itraconazole capsules as antifungal prophylaxis for neutropenic patients. Clin Infect Dis 2000; 30:300–305.

60. Boogaerts M, Maertens J, van Hoof A, de Bock R, Fillet G, Peetermans M, Selleslag D, Vandercam B, Vandewoude K, Zachee P, de Beule K. Itraconazole versus amphotericin B plus nystatin in the prophylaxis of fungal infections in neutropenic cancer patients. J Antimicrob Chemother 2001; 48:97–103.

61. Huijgens PC, Simoons-Smit AM, van Loenen AC, Prooy E, van Tinteren H, Ossenkoppele GJ, Jonkhoff AR. Fluconazole versus itroconazole for the prevention of fungal infections in haemato-oncology. J Clin Pathol 1999; 52:376–380.

62. Uzun O, Anaissie EJ. Antifungal prophylaxis in patients with hematologic malignancies: a reappraisal. Blood 1995; 86:2063–2072.

63. Denning DW, Stevens DA. Antifungal and surgical treatment of invasive aspergillosis. Review of 2,121 published cases. Rev Infect Dis 1990; 12:1147–1201.

64. Lortholary O, Dupont B. Antifungal prophylaxis during neutropenia and immunodeficiency. Clin Microbiol Rev 1997; 10:477–504.

65. Philpott-Howard JN, Wade JJ, Mufti GJ, Brammer KW, Ehninger G. Randomized comparison of oral fluconazole versus oral polyenes for the prevention of fungal infection in patients at risk of neutropenia. Multicentre Study Group. J Antimicrob Chemother 1993; 31:973–984.

66. Morgenstern GR, Prentice AG, Prentice HG, Ropner JE, Schey SA, Warnock DW. A randomized controlled trial of itraconazole versus fluconazole for the prevention of fungal infections in patients with haematological malignancies. U.K. Multicentre Antifungal Prophylaxis Study Group. Br J Haematol 1999; 105:901–911.

67. Prentice AG, Donnelly P. Oral antifungals as prophylaxis in haematological malignancy. Blood Reviews 2001; 15:1–8.

68. Schwartz S, Behre G, Heinemann V, Wandt H, Schilling E, Arning M, Trittin A, Kern WV, Boenisch O, Bosse D, Lenz K, Ludwig WD, Hiddemann W, Siegert W, Beyer J. Aerosolized amphotericin B inhalations as prophylaxis of invasive aspergillus infections during prolonged neutropenia: results of a prospective randomized multicenter trial. Blood 1999; 93:3654–3661.

69. Behre GF, Schwartz S, Lenz K, Ludwig WD, Wandt H, Schilling E, Heinemann V, Link H, Trittin A, Boenisch O, et al. Aerosol amphotericin B inhalations for prevention of invasive pulmonary aspergillosis in neutropenic cancer patients. Ann Hematol 1995; 71:287–291.

70. Perfect JR, Klotman ME, Gilbert CC, Crawford DD, Rosner GL, Wright KA, Peters WP. Prophylactic intravenous amphotericin B in neutropenic autologous bone marrow transplant recipients. J Infect Dis 1992; 165:891–897.

71. Reents S, Goodwin SD, Singh V. Antifungal prophylaxis in immunocompromised hosts. Ann Pharmacother 1993; 27:53–60.

72. Richard C, Romon I, Baro J, Insunza A, Loyola I, Zurbano F, Tapia M, Iriondo A, Conde E, Zubizarreta A. Invasive pulmonary aspergillosis prior to BMT in acute leukemia patients does not predict a poor outcome. Bone Marrow Transplant 1993; 12:237–241.

73. Kelsey SM, Goldman JM, McCann S, Newland AC, Scarffe JH, Oppenheim BA, Mufti GJ. Liposomal amphotericin (AmBisome) in the prophylaxis of fungal infections in neutropenic patients: a randomised, double-blind, placebo-controlled study. Bone Marrow Transplant 1999; 23:163–168.

74. Reusser P. Current concepts and challenges in the prevention and treatment of viral infections in immunocompromised cancer patients. Support Care Cancer 1998; 6:39–45.

75. Prentice HG. Use of acyclovir for prophylaxis of herpes infections in severely immunocompromised patients. J Antimicrob Chemother 1983; 12(suppl B):153–159.

76. Epstein JB, Ransier A, Sherlock CH, Spinelli JJ, Reece D. Acyclovir prophylaxis of oral herpes virus during bone marrow transplantation. Eur J Cancer B Oral Oncol 1996; 32:158–162.

77. Dignani MC, Mykietiuk A, Michelet M, Intile D, Mammana L, Desmery P, Milone G, Pavlovsky S. Valacyclovir prophylaxis for the prevention of Herpes simplex virus reactivation in recipients of progenitor cells transplantation. Bone Marrow Transplant 2002; 29:263–267.

78. Wood MJ. Viral infections in neutropenia—current problems and chemotherapeutic control. J Antimicrob Chemother 1998; 41(suppl D):81–93.

79. Goodrich JM, Boeckh M, Bowden R. Strategies for the prevention of cytomegalovirus disease after marrow transplantation. Clin Inf Dis 1994; 19:287–298.

80. Meyers JD, Reed EC, Shepp DH, Thornquist M, Dandliker PS, Vicary CA, Flournoy N, Kirk LE, Kersey JH, Thomas ED, et al. Acyclovir for prevention of cytomegalovirus infection and disease after allogeneic marrow transplantation. N Engl J Med 1988; 318:70–75.

81. Winston DJ, Ho WG, Bartoni K, Du Mond C, Ebeling DF, Buhles WC, Champlin RE. Ganciclovir prophylaxis of cytomegalovirus infection and disease in allogeneic bone marrow transplant recipients. Results of a placebo-controlled, double-blind trial. Ann Intern Med 1993; 118:179–184.

82. Goodrich JM, Mori M, Gleaves CA, Du Mond C, Cays M, Ebeling DF, Buhles WC, DeArmond B, Meyers JD. Early treatment with ganciclovir to prevent cytomegalovirus disease after allogeneic bone marrow transplantation. N Engl J Med 1991; 325:1601–1607.

83. Reusser P, Einsele H, Lee J, Volin L, Rovira M, Engelhard D, Finke J, Cordonnier C, Link H, Ljungman P. Randomized multicenter trial of foscarnet versus ganciclovir for preemptive therapy of cytomegalovirus infection after allogeneic stem cell transplantation. Blood 2002; 99:1159–1164.

84. Han CS, Miller W, Haake R, Weisdorf D. Varicella zoster infection after bone marrow transplantation: incidence, risk factors and complications. Bone Marrow Transplant 1994; 13:277–283.

85. Jacobson MA, Berger TG, Fikrig S, Becherer P, Moohr JW, Stanat SC, Biron KK. Acyclovir-resistant varicella zoster virus infection after chronic oral acyclovir therapy in patients with the acquired immunodeficiency syndrome (AIDS). Ann Intern Med 1990; 112:187–191.

86. Straus SE, Ostrove JM, Inchauspe G, Felser JM, Freifeld A, Croen KD, Sawyer MH. NIH conference. Varicella-zoster virus infections. Biology, natural history, treatment, and prevention. Ann Intern Med 1988; 108:221–237.

87. Fishman JA. Prevention of infection due to pneumocystis carinii. Antimicrob Agents Chemother 1998; 42:1309–1314.

88. Armstrong W, Meshnick S, Kazanjian P. Pneumocystis carinii mutations associated with sulfa and sulfone prophylaxis failures in immunocompromised patients. Microbes Infect 2000; 2:61–67.

89. Colby C, McAfee S, Sackstein R, Finkelstein D, Fishman J, Spitzer T. A prospective randomized trial comparing the toxicity and safety of atovaquone

with trimethoprim/sulfamethoxazole as Pneumocystis carinii pneumonia prophylaxis following autologous peripheral blood stem cell transplantation. Bone
Marrow Transplant 1999; 24:897–902.

90. Strauss RG. Therapeutic granulocyte transfusions in 1993. Blood 1993; 81:1675–
1678.

91. Vamvakas EC, Pineda AA. Determinants of the efficacy of prophylactic
granulocyte transfusions: a meta-analysis. J Clin Apheresis 1997; 12:74–81.

92. Adkins DR, Goodnough LT, Shenoy S, Brown R, Moellering J, Khoury H, Vij
R, DiPersio J. Effect of leukocyte compatibility on neutrophil increment after
transfusion of granulocyte colony-stimulating factor-mobilized prophylactic
granulocyte transfusions and on clinical outcomes after stem cell transplantation. Blood 2000; 95:3605–3612.

93. Illerhaus G, Wirth K, Dwenger A, Waller CF, Garbe A, Brass V, Lang H, Lange
W, Treatment and prophylaxis of severe infections in neutropenic patients by
granulocyte transfusions. Ann Hematol 2002; 81:273–281.

94. Lyman GH, Kuderer NM, Djulbegovic B. Prophylactic granulocyte colony-
stimulating factor in patients receiving dose-intensive cancer chemotherapy: a
meta-analysis. Am J Med 2002; 112:406–411.

38

Immunization Against Infectious Diseases in Cancer Patients

Rama Ganguly
University of South Florida College of Medicine
Tampa, Florida, U.S.A.

John N. Greene
University of South Florida College of Medicine
and Moffitt Cancer Center and Research Institute
Tampa, Florida, U.S.A.

Prevention of infectious diseases in cancer patients is an important clinical problem, since the approach to cancer treatment of neoplastic diseases has been intensified significantly during recent decades. Cancer patients are frequently predisposed to infections because of their immunosuppression. The disease itself or/and its treatment precipitates this immunological decline: leukemia, lymphoma, generalized malignancy, or treatment with chemotherapy, radiation, or prolonged high-dose corticosteroids. There is a preponderance of infectious agents that can infect immunocompromised cancer patients for which no vaccine is available [1,2] (Table 1). In these situations, the use of antibiotics remains the main focus in clinical practice [3].

Inactivated vaccines and some live vaccines may be given to cancer patients under certain conditions following the recommended schedule in

TABLE 1   Nosocomial Infections in
Cancer Patients

Staphylococcus aureus, coagulase-negative
Streptococcus alpha hemolytic
Enterococcus sp.
Corynebacterium JK
Enterobacteracea
Pseudomonas aeruginosa
Stenotrophomonas maltophilia
Candida sp.
Aspergillus sp.
Fusarium sp.

---

normal healthy adults and children. Guidelines for vaccination against infectious diseases in normal health and altered immunocompetence are frequently updated by the Centers for Disease Control and Prevention (CDC) [4]. Cancer patients often recover from their immunosuppression with the passage of time after treatment-induced remission, but they may have significant losses of immunity against certain infectious diseases to which they were vaccinated prior to diagnosis [5,6]. The clinician should assess to what degree a cancer patient is immunocompromised and accordingly time the vaccination procedure to obtain optimal benefit. For example, pneumococcal infection in hematological malignancies could be quite severe [7], and the

TABLE 2   Immunization Recommendations Against Infectious Diseases in Cancer Patients

Vaccine	Recommendation	Comment
Pneumococcal	Yes	Lung cancer, acute and chronic lymphocytic leukemia, Hodgkin's disease, non-Hodgkin's lymphoma, and multiple myeloma, asplenia
Haemophilus influenzae Type b virus conjugate	Yes	Children with any cancer, asplenia
Influenza	Yes	Seasonal for any cancer
Varicella zoster virus	Yes	Consider if in remission and no longer immunosuppressive
Measles	No	Individual consideration and local epidemiology

health care provider should consider if the available polysaccharide and conjugate vaccines would render benefits. Health care practitioners should also pay attention to the local community incidence of infectious diseases, when immunization or additional preventive measures may be indicated in cancer patients. For example, measles virus, as it reemerges in certain communities and geographic locations, can be a threat to cancer patients, causing severe disease and death [7,8]. The available live virus vaccine has the propensity of causing severe complications in cancer patients undergoing treatment. However, it can be given to a patient who has an epidemiological threat of infection and has discontinued chemotherapy for at least 3 months [7,9]. Much less has been reported regarding infection and immunity to vaccines in adult patients with solid tumors compared to those with hematological malignancies. It is suggested that similar principles may be followed in vaccinating them as applies to patients with leukemia and lymphoma [7,10, 11] (Table 2).

INFECTION AND IMMUNITY STATUS IN CANCER PATIENTS

Both radiation and chemotherapy induce immunosuppression in patients with neoplastic diseases. This may be measured in terms of lymphopenia, primary antibody titer, T and B lymphocyte counts, proliferative response to mitogen, and delayed hypersensitivity–type reaction [11-15]. Chemotherapy differs from radiation in that it shows a "rebound" or "overshoot" phenomenon in the recovery phase, which has been determined by conventional immunological techniques, e.g., T and B cell counts, mitogen response, and antibody titers [10,11,15]. Cancer patients often recover their immune capabilities with time and cessation of treatment. Thus when treatment was discontinued 1 week both before and after vaccination, attenuated live VZV vaccine produced significant protection (80%) in children with leukemia [16]. Children with solid tumors also could benefit, following a similar protocol with this vaccine [17]. Human immunoglobulin preparations can be given to cancer patients for passive immunizations. Immunoglobulins against hepatitis A and B, rabies, measles, tetanus and vericella zoster can be safely administered if indicated [18].

Vaccination with live organisms is contraindicated in immunosuppressed cancer patients owing to severe complications [4,18]: BCG, oral polio vaccine (OPV), yellow fever vaccine, measles, mumps, and rubella (MMR) vaccine. Patients with cellular immunodeficiency should not be given VZV vaccine. Contacts of immunosuppressed patients should avoid receiving OPV, but can receive inactivated oral polio vaccine (IPV) as well as MMR and VZV vaccines. Of the latter two vaccines, live agents spread to contacts rarely. Inactivated vaccines, including pertussis (whooping cough), typhoid, cholera, influenza, and formaldehyde treated toxoids of tetanus and diphtheria can be safely administered to cancer patients and their contacts. Most adults in the United States are protected by vaccination against most preventable infectious diseases. However, recovery of immunological functions following treatment may take up to 2 years or more in adult patients [11]. International travel might require some immunization, but live vaccines are contraindicated in immunosuppressed patients, for example yellow fever vaccine. However, successful vaccination has been reported with yellow fever vaccine 5 years after bone marrow transplantation in three individuals [19]. Thus it has been suggested that immunization with yellow fever vaccine can be considered and the patient given a choice when one must visit an endemic area, along with an advance for mosquito avoidance and other preventive measures [7,18]. All inactivated vaccines, recombinant, polysaccharide, conjugates, and subunit are recommended for immunocompromised cancer patients in usual doses and schedules, although optimal responses are often not achieved [4]. In addition, pneumococcal, meningococcal, and Hib vaccines are recommended specifically for immunosuppressed patients with functional or anatomic asplenia [4,20]. Vaccination during chemotherapy or radiation therapy could produce little protection and therefore should be avoided. Thus according to the recommendations of the Advisory Committee on Vaccination Practices (CDC) patients receiving vaccines while immunosuppressed or in the 2 weeks before starting therapy should be considered unimmunized and should be revaccinated >3 months after therapy is discontinued [18]. Patients with leukemia in remission whose chemotherapy has ended at least 3 months ago can receive live virus vaccines.

HEMATOPOIETIC STEM CELL TRANSPLANTATION

Hematopoietic stem cell transplantation (HSCT) is becoming a preferred treatment for certain cancers, with infections the major obstacles for a successful outcome. Thus these patients need special consideration for vaccination. HSCT patients with allogenic grafts are more severely immune-impaired than autologous recipients, due to graft-vs.-host disease (GVHD) and/or immunosuppressive therapy. Transplant patients do not respond to vaccines well during the early posttransplant phase of immunosuppression. The antibody titers to vaccine-preventable diseases decline following both autologous and allogenic transplants during the next 1–4 years [4]. These include antibodies to tetanus, poliovirus, measles, mumps, diphtheria, rubella, and encapsulated bacteria. HSCT patients are at increased risk from cytomegalovirus (CMV), VZV, *Streptococcus pneumoniae*, and *H. influenzae*, particularly if GVHD is present. Effective immunity has been elicited in BMT patients when the vaccine was given as early as 3 to 6 months after transplant, particularly if chronic GVHD is absent [21,22]. When revaccinated repeat-

TABLE 3 Recommendations for Immunization in Stem Cell Transplant Patients Against Infectious Diseases

Vaccine	Allogenic SCT recipient	Autologous SCT recipient	Comments
Tetanus Toxoid + diphtheria toxoid	Yes	Yes	2 to 3 doses 12, 14, or 24 months after SCT
Polio (inactivated vaccine)	Yes	Yes	Same as above[a]
Measles	Yes	Yes	24 months after SCT if no GVHD
Rubella	Yes	Yes	24 months after SCT if no GVHD
Influenza (submit)	Yes	Yes	Seasonal 6 mo after SCT
Haemophylus influenzae b (Hib) (conjugate) vaccine	Yes	Yes	2 doses, 12,14, 24 mo or after SCT
Hepatitis B virus vaccine (subunit)	Regional	Regional	In countries of prevalence, 12,14, 24 mo following SCT
Pneumococcal vaccines (polysaccharide/ conjugate)	Yes	Yes	At 12 and 24 months if no GVHD
Varicella zoster virus (VZV) vaccine	Contraindicated	Contraindicated	Vaccinate susceptible family members and close contacts

[a] Oral polio vaccine contraindicated; GVHD—graft vs host disease; SCT—stem cell transplant.
Source: Modified from [7,37].

edly, stable immunity is generated against these infections [23,24]. Therefore routine revaccination after HSCT has been recommended in these patients regardless of the source of the transplanted stem cells. The health care providers and household and other close contacts of HSCT recipients should be vaccinated, if indicated, against influenza, measles, and varicella [4]. Autologous BMT patients are not prone to several vaccine-preventable infections immediately following transplant, unlike allogenic recipients, but they also lose protective immunity to poliovirus, measles, and tetanus during long-term follow-up [23,25]. See Table 3 for vaccine recommendations in patients following stem cell transplantation [7].

SPECIFIC VACCINES

Pneumococcal Vaccine

Patients with hematological malignancies and Hodgkin's disease with splenectomy are especially vulnerable to pneumococcal infections and may have severely impaired immune response to the polysaccharide vaccine if it is given after treatment. Immunization elicits a good response if it is given before therapy [26,27]. A similar situation exists in patients with carcinoma of the head and neck [28]. Lymphoma patients should receive pneumococcal vaccine soon after diagnosis and before chemotherapy or radiotherapy [7]. Allogenic BMT patients, who are prone to severe pneumococcal infection, should be vaccinated when GVHD is not present and at least 6 months have elapsed following transplant [21,29]. Autologous BMT patients may be immunized before harvesting stem cells and at least 3 months after transplantation. In Hodgkin's disease, the immune response is always better if vaccination is performed prior to therapy for splenectomy [27,30].

Haemophilus Influenzae Type b Vaccine

Leukemic children are at heightened risk for Hib infection. Conjugate Hib vaccine is indicated in children with cancer, preferably in the early phase of their cancer treatment. During intense chemotherapy, immunization produces suboptimal response and should be avoided [31,32]. Allogenic BMT patients are also vulnerable to Hib infection, and the vaccine produces good response if given after at least 3 months of transplantation and when GVHD is not present [22,29].

Influenza Vaccine

Influenza vaccine is recommended for immunocompromised patients. The severity of influenza infection varies with the type of cancer and the stage of treatment. Not much has been written about influenza vaccine responses in cancer patients subjected to modern chemotherapy regimens. During induction chemotherapy, patients with leukemia in particular develop more infectious complications than those with other hematological malignancies. Only a 40% response to the vaccine and substantial vaccine failure (24%) have been reported in adult patients with lymphoma and children with leukemia [33–35]. However, the vaccine may be beneficial in preventing complications, reducing the severity of the disease and death. Thus other strategies of prevention should be considered against nosocomial transmission of influenza, i.e., vaccination of household contacts and hospital caregivers along with selective antivirials such as rimantadine or oseltamivir. Allogenic BMT patients also suffer from severe influenza infection, particularly during the early posttransplant phase of immunosuppression. Immune responses improve substantially in both autologous and allogenic BMT recipients if vaccinated at least 6 months to 2 years after transplantation [36].

Tetanus Toxoid, Diphtheria Toxoid, and Inactivated Polio Virus Vaccine

Immunity to these vaccines declines in patients with leukemia and lymphoma as well as following BMT. Booster immunizations against these infections should be considered in all patients with cancer. Repeated doses of these vaccines should be used to induce stable protective immunity, including inactivated poliovirus vaccine. Vaccination is recommended beginning 12 months after BMT with inactivated, recombinant, subunit, polysaccharide, and Hib vaccines [37]. Immunization with tetanus toxoid, diphtheria toxoid, and inactivated poliovirus is recommended also after autologous BMT [7,23]. The CDC does not recommend varicella, meningococcal, or pneumococcal conjugate vaccines for BMT recipients owing to a lack of experience in their use in this setting [4].

Hepatitis B Vaccine

Severe infection with hepatitis B virus is rarely encountered in BMT patients in the USA but may be considered in countries with high HBV prevalence (Table 3).

LIVE VACCINES

Varicella Zoster Vaccine

Children with cancer have a high mortality rate if they develop primary VZV infection. Household exposure to VZV results in a more severe illness in secondary cases. Thus immunization with VZV vaccine is indicated in seronegative patients with cancer [38]. Vaccine administration should be adjusted to the cancer chemotherapy schedule. The existing live attenuated Oka stain vaccine is effective and safe in children with leukemia in remission with high seroconversion rate (98% after two doses), low side effects, and, in case of vaccine failure, attenuated infection [39,40]. Ayclovir can be used if breakthrough vaccine-acquired disease occurs. Varicella immunity lasts at least 5 years after immunization. Immunization of healthy seronegative family contacts may also be considered when the child with cancer is treated with intensive therapy since the vaccine virus is rarely transmitted. VZV infection can be severe during the immediate posttransplant phase of BMT, when vaccination is not effective. More data are needed regarding the use of this vaccine in preventing primary or reactivated VZV infection in the BMT recipients. Patients with immunosuppression and ongoing GVHD should not receive this vaccine. Autologous BMT patients when seronegative may receive this vaccine.

Measles Virus Vaccine

Measles virus infection results in a high mortality rate in cancer patients. The live attenuated vaccine is contraindicated during chemotherapy, during immunosuppression, and in the presence of GVHD. However, it can be given 3 months after the cancer therapy is terminated, if the epidemiological risk for measles increases. Family members without immunity to measles may consider measles immunization. Vaccine safety has been shown at 2 years following transplantation [41]. Among autologous BMT patients, risks of side effects from measles vaccination seem to be low. Measles immunization should be considered on an individual basis and depending upon the epidemiological indications.

Cytomegalovirus Vaccine

CMV is one of the most important pathogens after BMT, but unfortunately there is little experience with the live vaccine currently available in BMT recipients. Several different experimental vaccines, subcomponent and vector based, are being tested for clinical development.

Other Live Vaccines

Mumps, rubella, BCG, and yellow fever vaccines are not recommended during active cancer therapy, because those agents have the propensity for producing persistent and disseminated infections and complications in immunosuppression. Inactivated polio vaccine can be safely administered, but live poliovirus vaccine should be avoided, even in close contacts. Rubella, mumps, and yellow fever vaccines, however, may be considered in individual cases under certain conditions weighing risks and benefits, for example, for women of childbearing age and planning pregnancy, or when a traveler must visit an area where yellow fever virus infection is endemic. In BMT patients, the yellow fever vaccine has been given safely after 5 years of transplantation and rubella vaccine 2 years after BMT, when GVHD and immunosuppression were not present [19,41]. BCG vaccine has a potential for disseminated infection when T cell functions are depleted. It is therefore avoided in BMT patients and in cancer patients with deficient cellular immunity.

CONCLUSION

The major types of pathogens involved with immunological dysfunction observed predominantly with neoplastic diseases are shown in Table 4. Unfortunately, the only pathogens listed in Table 4 that can be prevented are the encapsulated organisms, *S. pneumonia* and *H. influenzae*. Vaccines are generally not useful during the active phase of cancer therapy. However,

TABLE 4 Immune Dysfunction in Neoplastic Diseases and Infectious Agents Involved

Immune defect	Risk factor	Pathogens
(a) Phagocytic dysfunction (granulocytopenia)	Acute leukemia, Stem cell transplantation Chemotherapy Aplastic anemia	Bacteria (Table 1) Fungi (*Candida* spp., *Aspergillus* spp., *Fusarum* spp.) Virus (HSV)
(b) Cellular immunodeficiency	Hodgkin's disease, non-Hodgkin lymphoma (ALL, CLL) Stem cell, transplantation Corticosteroid use	Bacteria (Table 1, and *Nocardia* spp., *Mycobacterium* spp.) Fungi (endemic mycosis, *Aspergillus* spp.) Virus (HSV, CMV, VZV, HHV-6) Protozoa (PCP) Parasites (*Strongyloides stercoralis*)
(c) Humoral immunodeficiency	Multiple myeloma Stem cell transplantation, CLL	Bacteria (*Streptococcus pneumoniae, Haemophilus influenzae*) Virus (VZV)

ALL = acute lymphocytic leukemia; CLL = chronic lymphocytic leukemia; HSV = herpes simplex virus; CMV = cytomegalovirus; VZV = varicella zoster virus, HHV-6 = human herpes virus 6.

prior to chemotherapy or shortly after remission, vaccines are useful for disease prevention when the immune system is able to mount a response.

REFERENCES

1. Brown AE. Infectious complications of neoplastic disease. In: Infections in Medicine. 1993; 12:64.
2. Carlisle PS, Gucalp R, Wiernik PH. Nosocomial infections in neutropenic patients. In: Infection Control and Hospital Epidemiology. 1993; 14:320–324.
3. Khardori N, Bodey GP. Infections in hematologic malignancies. Hematology 1991; 14:363–424.
4. Centers for Disease Control and Prevention. General recommendations on immunization: altered immunocompetence. Morbidity and Mortality Weekly Report (MMWR) 2002; 51:22–23.
5. Ljungman P, Duraj V, Magnius L. Response to immunization against polio after allogeneic marrow transplantion. Bone Marrow Transplant 1991; 7:89–93.
6. Ljungman P, Levensohn-Fuch I, Hammarstrom V. Long-term immunity to measles, mumps, and rubella after allogeneic bone marrow transplantation. Blood 1994; 84:657–664.
7. Ljungman P. Immunization in the immunocompromised host: patients with cancer. In: Plotkin SA, Orenstein WA, eds. Vaccines. 3rd ed. Philadelphia: W. B. Saunders, 1999:98–110.
8. Kaplan L, Daum R, Smaron M, et al. Severe measles in immunocompromised patients. JAMA 1992; 4:139–140.
9. Peter G, ed. Report of the Committee on Infectious Diseases. Red Book. 24th ed. Elk Grove Village, IL: American Academy of Pediatrics, 1997:344–357.
10. Fairlamb DJ. Immunization against infectious disease in adult oncology. Clinical Oncology 1992; 4:139–140.
11. Harris J, Sengar D, Stewart T, et al. The effect of immunosuppressive chemotherapy on immune function in patients with malignant disease. Cancer 1976; 37:1058–1069.
12. Hoppe RT, Fuks ZY, Stober S, et al. The long-term effects of radiation in T and B cell lymphocytes in the peripheral blood after regional irradiation. Cancer 1975; 40:2071–2078.
13. Kun LE, Johnson RE. Hematologic and immunologic status in Hodgkin's disease 5 years after radical radiotherapy. Cancer 1975; 36:1912–1916.
14. Stoner RD, Hale WM. Ionising radiations and the immune process. In: Leone CA, ed. New York: Gordon and Breach, 1961:183.
15. Mukerji B, Mukhopadhyay M. Radiation–drug interactions in the treatment of cancer. In: Sokol GH, Maickel RP, eds. New York: John Wiley, 1980:155–174.
16. Gershon AA, Steinberg S, Gelb L, Galasso G, Borkowsky W, LaRussa P, Ferrara A. A multicenter trial of live attenuated varicella vaccine in children with leukaemia in remission. Postgrad Med J 1985; 61(suppl 4):73–78.

17. Heath RB, Malpas JS. Experience with the live oka-strain varicella vaccine in children with solid tumors. Postgrad Med J 1985; 61(suppl):107–112.

18. Centers for Disease Control and Prevention. Recommendations of the Advisory Committee on Immunization Practices (ACIP): use of Vaccines and Immunoglobulins in Persons with Altered Immunocompetence. Morbidity and Mortality Weekly Report (MMWR) 1993; 42:1–18.

19. Rio B, Marjanovic Z, Levy V, et al. Vaccination for yellow fever after bone marrow transplatation. Bone Marrow Transplant 1996; 17(suppl):S95.

20. Center for Disease Control and Prevention. Update on Adult Immunization: Recommendations of the Immunizatin Practices Advisory Committee (ACIP). Morbidity and Mortality Weekly Report (MMWR) 1991; 40:1–94.

21. Parkkali T, Kayhty H, Ruutu T, Volin L, Eskola J, Ruutu P. A comparison of late and early vaccination with *Heaemophilus influenzae* type b conjugate and pneumococcal polysaccharide vaccines after allogeneic BMT. Bone Marrow Transplant 1996; 19:961–967.

22. Barra A, Cordonnier C, Preziosi MP, Intrator L, Hessel L, Fritzell B, Preud'homme JL. Immunogenicity of *Haemophillus influenzae* type b conjugate vaccine in allogeneic bone marrow recipients. J Infect Dis 1992; 166:1021–1028.

23. Engelhard D, Handsher R, Naparstek E, Hardan I, Strauss N, Aker M, Or R, Baciu H, Slavin S. Immune responses to polio vaccination in bone marrow transplant recipients. Bone Marrow Transplant 1991; 8:295–300.

24. Ljungman P, Wiklund-Hammarsten M, Duraj V, Hammarstrom L, Lonnqvist B, Paulin T, Ringden O, Pepe MS, Gahrton G. Responses to tetanus toxoid immunization after allogeneic bone marrow transplantation. J Infect Dis 1990; 162:496–500.

25. Pauksen K, Duraj V, Ljungman P, Sjolin J, Oberg G, Lonnerholm G, Fridell E, Smedmyr B, Simonsson B. Immunity to and immunization against measles, rubella and mumps in patients after autologous bone marrow transplantation. Bone Marrow Transplant 1992; 9:427–432.

26. Feldman S, Malone W, Wilbur R, Schiffman G. Pneumococcal vaccination in children with leukemia. Med Pediatr Oncol 1985; 13:69–72.

27. Levine AM, Overturf GD, Field RF, Holdorf D, Paganini-Hill A, Feinstein DI. Use and efficacy of pneumococcal vaccine with Hodgkin's disease. Blood 1979; 54:1171–1175.

28. Amman A, Schiffman G, Adiego J, et al. Immunization of immunosuppressed patients with pneumococcal polysaccharide vaccine. Rev Infect Dis 1981; 3: S160–S167.

29. Guinan EC, Molrine DC, Antin JH, Lee MC, Weinstein HJ, Sallan SE, Parsons SK, Wheeler C, Gross W, McGarigle C, et al. Polysaccharide conjugate vaccine response in bone marrow transplant recipients. Transplantation 1994; 57:677–684.

30. Donaldson SS, Vosti KL, Berberich FR, Cox RS, Kaplan HS, Schiffman G. Response to pneumococcal vaccine among children with Hodgkin's disease. Rev Infect Dis 1981; 3:S133–S143.

31. Ridgway D, Wolff L, Deforest A. Immunization response varies with intensity of acute lymphoblastic leukemia therapy. Am J Dis Child 1991; 145:887–891.

32. Shenep JL, Feldman S, Gigliotti F, Roberson PK, Marina N, Foreschle JE, Fullen GH, Lott L, Brodkey TO. Responses of immunocompromised children with solid tumors to a conjugate vaccine for *Haemophilus influenzae* type b. J Pediatr 1994; 125:581–584.

33. Kempe A, Hall CB, McDonald NE, Foye HR, Woodin KA, Cohen HJ, Lewis ED, Gullace M, Gala CL, Dulberg CS, et al. Influenza in children with cancer. J Pediatr 1989; 115:33–39.

34. Steinherz PG, Brown AE, Gross PA, Braun D, Ghavimi F, Wollner N, Rosen G, Armstrong D, Miller DR. Influenza immunization of children with neoplastic diseases. Cancer 1980 Feb 15; 45(4):750–756.

35. Lo W, Whimbey E, Elting L, Couch R, Cabanillas F, Bodey G. Antibody response to a two dose influenza vaccine regimen in adult lymphoma patients on chemotherapy. Eur J Clin Microbiol Infect Dis 1993; 12:778–782.

36. Englehard D, Nagaler A, Hardan I. Antibody response to a two dose regimen of influenza vaccine in allogeneic T-cell depleted and autologous BMT recipients. Bone Marrow Transplant 1993; 11:1–5.

37. Centers for Disease Control and Prevention. Guidelines for Preventing Opportunistic Infections Among Hematopoietic Stem Cell Recipients: Recommendation of CDC, the Infectious Disease Society of America, and the American Society of Blood and Marrow Transplantation. Morbidity and Mortality Weekly Report (MMWR) 200; 49(no. RR-10):1–128

38. American Academy of Pediatrics. In: Ickering LK, ed. Red Book: Report of the Committee on Infectious Diseases. 25th ed. Elk Gove Village, IL, 2000:60.

39. Gershon A, Steinberg S. Persistence of immunity to varicella in children with leukemia immunized with live attenuated varicella vaccine. N Eng J Med 1989; 320:892–897.

40. Brunell P, Geiser CF, Novelli V, Lipton S, Narkewicz S. Varicella-like illness caused by live varicella vaccine in children with acute lymphocytic leukemia. Pediatrics 1987; 79:922–927.

41. Ljungman P, Fridell E, Lonnqvist B, Bolme P, Bottiger M, Gahrton G, Linde A, Ringden O, Wahren B. Efficacy and safety of vaccination of marrow transplant recipients with a live attenuated measles, mumps, and rubella vaccine. J Infect Dis 1989; 159:610–615.

39

Role of the Microbiology Laboratory

Loveleen Kang and Ramon L. Sandin
University of South Florida College of Medicine
and Moffitt Cancer Center and Research Institute
Tampa, Florida, U.S.A.

ROLE OF THE MICROBIOLOGY LABORATORY

Currently available antineoplastic therapeutic approaches have markedly improved survival rates in cancer patients. However, infections are a major concern in the management of cancer patients. The clinical microbiology laboratory plays an important role in diagnosing such life-threatening infections. Several aspects of diagnostic laboratory medicine of specific importance to this category of immunocompromised individuals have been chosen for discussion. Issues such as the sources of clinical specimens, selected protocols and techniques (immunosuppressed patients, bone marrow, bone, transfusion reaction protocols), the relevance and interpretation of isolates, the role of new molecular diagnostic techniques, and fungal and viral susceptibility testing are reviewed.

CLINICAL SPECIMENS IN THE MICROBIOLOGY LABORATORY

Specimen Types

Invasive procedures such as tissue biopsies, bronchoscopically obtained biopsies, bronchoalveolar lavages (BAL), and bronchial washing and brushing, and fluids obtained by thoracentesis and paracentesis, offer the best chance of the recovery of a pathogen. Moreover, specimens obtained from sterile body sites are most useful in identifying the causative organisms and less likely to be contaminants. In debilitated cancer patients an ideal diagnostic sample for isolation of the pathogen may be difficult to obtain. Even the most commonly submitted sterile body site specimen, peripheral blood, may be hard to obtain from immunocompromised patients. For some individuals, sputum cultures for respiratory infection workups, and blood obtained from central lines for blood cultures, may be the only specimens available. In disseminated infections, especially by fungal agents, the recovery of a pathogen from skin or mucous membranes is helpful in making a diagnosis. However, it is very important to adhere to strict criteria to exclude the contaminating normal flora from being considered as the actual pathogen(s).

Blood Cultures

Cancer patients, especially patients with hematological malignancies, have altered microbial flora, owing to damage to anatomic barriers and to granulocytopenia and subsequent microbial invasion following intensive myelosuppressive therapy. All these factors increase the incidence of bacteremia and show a more morbid outcome in cancer patients. In view of the seriousness of bacteremic episodes, it is important to use the most efficient blood culture techniques, which offer a speedy and accurate isolation of the pathogens. The original traditional blood culture method, which used bottles containing enriched nutrient broth, and which entailed daily visual evaluation by the technologist, is labor-intensive and time-consuming.

Automation has accelerated the diagnosis of bacteremia significantly. Semiautomated blood culturing systems were introduced approximately three decades ago [1]. Prototypic systems, such as Bactec 460 (Becton-Dickinson, Cockeysville, MD), incorporated 14C-containing substrates in the blood culture media. When microorganisms use the ^{14}C-labeled substrate, $^{14}CO_2$ is produced, which was aspirated from the blood culture bottle head space by a needle and measured by a radioactive counter. Subsequent blood culture systems were nonradiometric, so CO_2 contents in the bottle head space were measured by an infrared analyzer. When the concentration of CO_2

reaches a predetermined threshold, the bottle is flagged as a potentially positive specimen. A Gram stain and subculture is performed subsequently to identify the pathogen. The advantage of this system is that it saves the technologist time, as the bottles with no growth do not have to be subcultured and can be discarded at the end of the predetermined incubation period (i.e., 5 or 7 days). However, the bottles still have to be inserted and removed from the instrument manually for testing.

The latest generation of automated blood culture instruments shows a completely noninvasive, continuous monitoring and a hands-off system. These instruments agitate and incubate the blood culture bottles. Noninvasive methods are used to measure microbial metabolism, thus decreasing the potential for cross-contamination of samples owing to the introduction of needles. The systems are "continuous monitoring" because the bottles are read every 10 minutes. There is no need to remove bottles from the instrument for a reading to occur. The bottles remain in the instrument until they are flagged as positive or discarded as negative after a predetermined time period. A prototype of this generation of instruments is the BacT/Alert microbial detection system from BioMerieux (Durham, NC). The BacT/Alert MDS system [2,3] uses a colorimetric photosensor and reflected light to monitor the presence of CO_2 dissolved in the culture medium. The CO_2 sensor inside the bottle is bonded to the bottom of the bottle and is separated from the broth by a membrane, which allows CO_2 to permeate through it. When CO_2 is produced by the growing microorganism(s), there is a color change from dark green to yellow. A scanner continuously monitors the photosensors for the color change, and once the color change is detected, the instrument alerts the technologist by the buzz of an alarm or the turning on of a light signal. The progress of the growth in the bottle can also be printed out as a curve of time versus reflectance units. Blood culture bottles specifically manufactured for cultures of bacterial isolation containing soybean casein digest broths even allow the growth of yeasts of the genera *Candida* and Cryptococcus readily [4]. Other continuous monitoring blood culture systems are also available. The BACTEC 9000 Fluorescent Series (BACTEC 9240, 9120, and 9050) from Becton-Dickinson (Lockeysville, MD) uses fluorescence as the detection mechanism. The BACTEC 9240 and 9050 also provide advanced algorithms for individual bottle types, for special circumstances such as low blood volume or pediatric specimens, or to detect slow-growing organisms such as Haemphilus and Neisseria. The ESP 128 or 384 uses the pressure of gases inside the bottle for detecting microbial growth.

Automated, continuous-monitoring mycobacterial testing systems are also now available. The BACTEC MGIT 960 system from Becton-Dickinson (Cockeysville, MD) has plastic tubes for added safety. MB/BacT from

BioMerieux (Durham, NC) is an automated system for continuous noninvasive monitoring of blood as well as nonblood specimens for mycobacterial detection.

Respiratory Samples

The number of potential pathogens that may cause respiratory disease and later disseminated disease in neutropenic cancer patients and that may be detected in clinical samples from the respiratory tract is quite large. For this reason, any respiratory tract specimen received in the laboratory should be evaluated with a comprehensive protocol that includes cultures, stains, antigen detection methods, and other tools for identifying the responsible pathogen(s).

The comprehensive approach used to identify the microbial agent(s) of pulmonary pathology in immunosuppressed patients at the University of South Florida's H. Lee Moffit Cancer Center is referred to as the immunosuppressed patient protocol (IPP) and includes

1. Routine bacterial culture with Gram stain
2. Fungus culture and smear (calcofluor white stain)
3. Culture and smear for acid-fast bacilli (AFB) (includes *Nocardia* spp. culture) (Kinyoun's stain)
4. *Nocardia* spp. smear (modified acid-fast stain)
5. *Legionella* spp. culture and smear (flourescent stain)
6. Respiratory viral panel for herpes simplex virus 1 and 2, cytomegalovirus (CMV), respiratory adenoviruses, respiratory syncitial virus (RSV), influenza A and B viruses, parainfluenza 1,2,3 viruses, varicella-zoster virus, enteroviruses and *chlamydia* spp.
7. Pneumocystis carinii detection by flourescent stain

Acceptable specimens include BAL, bronchial washings, bronchial brushings, tracheal aspirates, nasopharyngeal aspirates, and pulmonary biopsy tissues obtained bronchoscopically or via an open lung procedure. Sputa are accepted at our institution owing to the difficulty in obtaining invasive specimens from debilitated patients, but throat swabs are not accepted. The respiratory bacterial culture involves the inoculation of the specimen on three media plates: (1) blood agar, (2) chocolate agar, and (3) MaConkey's agar; and thioglycollate broth as enrichment medium. The inoculated media are incubated at 37°C for 2 days. If a tissue biopsy obtained by bronchoscopy or via thoracotomy is received, anaerobic plates are also inoculated and incubated accordingly. Cultures for fungi are inoculated on Sabouraud's dextrose agar plates with and without chloramphenicol, and blood-brain-heart infusion agar (BBHIA) plates with gentamycin and chloramphenicol, followed by incubation for 4 weeks at 30°C. For isolation of acid-fast bacilli, the treated specimen is inoculated into the BacT/Alert MB system (Bio Merieux) broth bottles and incubated at 35°C, with a 7H-10 solid medium also inoculated as backup and incubated at 36°C with CO_2 for up to 6 weeks. The solid and broth media for isolation for acid-fast bacilli also allow the growth of *Nocardia* spp. AFB smears are stained with the auramine fluorescent stain for screening, and all positives are confirmed with the Kinyoun acid-fast stain. *Nocardia* smears are stained with the modified acid-fast procedure using 2% H_2SO_4 as decolorizer. For isolation of *Legionella*, nonselective buffered charcoal yeast extract (BCYE) plates are the media of choice. These are incubated at 37°C for 7 days. *Legionella* smears are stained with the *Legionella*-Poly-ID test kit by Remel (Lenexa, TX), which utilizes fluorescent antibody-mediated detection.

The basic assay of the respiratory viral panel is the shell vial assay. Shell vials are 3-cm^3 vials with a round cover slip that fits on the bottom of the vial. A monolayer of tissue culture cells is present on the upper cover slip surface. For the respiratory viral panel at this institution we inoculate the shell vials containing human embryonic pulmonary fibroblast cell line MRC-5, R-mix (A549 + Mink Lung cells), and ELVIS (enzyme linked virus inducible system) containing baby hamster kidney cells. MRC-5 and R-mix are obtained from Diagnostic Hybrids (Athens, OH), while ELVIS is obtained from Bio Whittaker (Wakersville, MD). The clinical sample is inoculated into the shell vials followed by centrifugation and incubation at 37°C. After 24 hours or more of incubation, early or immediate-early viral protein antigens are synthesized in the tissue culture cells, which are detected by monoclonal antibodies labeled with fluorescein isothiocyanate (FITC), in either a one-step or a two-step procedure. For screening we use pools of antibodies directed at different viruses (Respiratory Viral Screen Direct Immunofluorescence Assay, Light Diagnostics, Chemicon International, Temecula, CA). Any positve signal is then evaluated with monoclonal antibodies to individual viruses to identify the specific viral agent. The shell vial assay is backed up by inoculation into traditional tube cultures containing MRC-5 and monkey kidney cell lines. These tube cultures are incubated at 37°C for 14 days and evaluated regularly for cytopathic effect.

Pneumocystis carinii cysts and trophozoites are detected in direct smears of respiratory specimens including sputum, bronchoalveolar lavage, and lung biopsy by a direct immunofluorescent antibody assay using a DFA kit (Light Diagnostics, Chemicon International, Temecula, CA) [5,6]. The kit uses anti-*Pneumocystis carinii* antibodies that detect all stages of the parasite life cycle: cyst wall, intracystic bodies, tachyzoites, and extracellular matrix protein. The antibodies are labeled with fluorescein isothiocyanate (FITC), which exhibits an apple-green fluorescence.

Bone Culture

Bone is received infrequently in our center's microbiology laboratory. Whenever bone is received, it is homogenized as well as possible in a tissue grinder. If homogenization of the bone is not possible, it is swabbed over the surface of various plates as described. The homogenized bone is divided into five parts for routine culture, acid-fast bacillus culture, fungal culture, smears, and future use in a $-70°C$ freezer. For routine culture the specimen is inoculated on a chocolate agar plate and an anaerobic blood agar plate; then it is placed in thioglycollate broth. The chocolate agar plate is incubated at $35°C$ in the presence of CO_2 hr. The anaerobic blood agar plate is incubated anaerobically in a non$-CO_2$ environment for 48 hours. For AFB culture, the homogenized tissue is inoculated or the bone is swabbed over the surface of a 7H11 plate and incubated at $35°C$ in the presence of CO_2 for 6 weeks. Isolation of fungal organisms is done after inoculation of the homogenized bone (or swabbing the bone) over the surface of a Sabouraud dextrose agar plate followed by incubation at $30°C$ for 4 weeks.

Bone Marrow/Stem Cell Cultures

Bone marrow/peripheral blood stem cell transplantation involves the intravenous administration of bone marrow/stem cells previously harvested from a related, unrelated, or autologous donor, to a recipient whose hematopoietic and immune systems have been ablated by chemotherapy or combined chemoradiotherapy. It is very important to maintain sterility of the bone marrow/stem cells from the time of harvesting from the donor until the time of transplantation to the recipient. H. Lee Moffitt Cancer Center has a relatively busy Blood and Marrow transplant unit, which performs approximately 160 bone marrow/stem cell transplants per year. Specimens received from the Bone Marrow unit include (1) Bone Marrow Fresh Harvest; (2) Bone Marrow Post Process (after the bone marrow is processed by the Bone Marrow laboratory, a sample is submitted to the microbiology laboratory), and (3) Bone Marrow thaw bags (as the numerous thawed bags of bone marrow are infused into the patient, bone marrow samples are submitted to the microbiology laboratory).

Bone Marrow Fresh Harvest is received in BacT/Alert pediatric blood culture bottles and a 1.5 mL Pediatric isolator tube. BacT/Alert blood culture bottles are processed as routine cultures. The bone marrow is withdrawn with a syringe from the 1.5 mL Pediatric isolator tube and inoculated on 7H11 plate and Sabouraud dextrose plate for isolation of mycobacteria and fungi, respectively. Smears are stained with Calcofluor and Kinyoun's stain to look for fungi and AFB. If no BacT/Alert blood culture bottles are submitted, the bone marrow from the pediatric isolator tube is also inoculated on a chocolate agar plate and thioglycollate broth.

Bone marrow post process samples and bone marrow thaw bag samples are submitted in BacT/Alert pediatric blood culture bottles for sterility testing. These specimens are set up for routine cultures only. The bone marrow specimens are withdrawn with a syringe and inoculated to a chocolate agar plate and thioglycollate broth followed by incubation at 35°C in the presence of CO_2 for 48 hours.

Transfusion Reactions (Whole Blood, RBC's, Platelets, etc)

When a patient experiences a transfusion reaction, the blood component(s) are returned to the blood bank where a transfusion reaction workup is initiated. Blood components will be submitted to the microbiology laboratory if bacterial contamination is suspected. The blood component is subjected to culture to look for the presence of aerobic and/or anaerobic pathogens.

A "sampling site coupler" is inserted into one of the access points of the blood component bag. The tip of the sampling coupler is cleaned with 70% alcohol followed by 2% tincture of iodine. The tip is allowed to dry. The aerobic (green top) and anaerobic (purple top) BacT/Alert blood culture bottles are obtained, and their tops are cleaned with 70% alcohol. Using a 20 mL syringe, approximately 21 mL of blood component is withdrawn from the bag through the sampling coupler tip, without touching it; 10 mL of blood component is placed in each blood culture bottle, and 1 mL is inoculated into a tube of thioglycollate broth. One drop of blood is smeared on a glass slide for the Gram stain.

If the volume of the blood component is less than 2 mL, the above procedure will not be feasible, in which case the component is inoculated onto a chocolate agar plate and two thioglycollate tubes. The chocolate agar plate and one thioglycollate tube are incubated at 37°C for 48 hours, and the second thioglycollate tube at room temperature for 5 days. If all cultures are negative, blood component bags are discarded, while bags are kept for one month if any of the cultures are positive [7].

Relevance and Interpretation of Isolates

The relevance of microbes isolated from specimens collected from immunosuppressed patients is often different from when such isolates are recovered from immunocompetent patients. Contaminating or saprophytic fungi, elements of normal flora present in stools or respiratory specimens, and several viral agents may be considered unremarkable when recovered from immunocompetent individuals but may be the true pathogens in cancer patients.

Saprophytic or free-living fungi are important pathogens in immuno-suppressed cancer patients [8–10]. Saprophytes are being isolated from cancer patients at the University of South Florida's H. Lee Moffitt Cancer Center in increasing numbers from respiratory samples and skin biopsy tissues. Histologic evaluation of tissue slides, if available, may confirm that such saprophytic fungi are the actual pathogens. Species in the genera *Aspergillus*, *Penicillium*, *Fusarium*, *Paecilomyces*, *Pseudallescheria*, and *Scedosporium* are among the most frequent isolates in our bone marrow transplant (BMT) population [11–13].

Several microorganisms that are normal flora in respiratory or stool samples from immunocompetent patients may be potential pathogens when recovered in large quantities from debilitated patients. For instance, when species of the genus *Candida* are found in abundant numbers in stool specimens alone or with other normal stool flora, they are routinely reported, in case treatment may be warranted in the presence of clinical correlation.

Dormant or latent agents capable of reactivation may cause significant morbidity and mortality in cancer patients. Such agents require identification when present in clinical samples from immunocompromised patients, but their involvement as the sole cause of an infection syndrome requires clinical correlation. Such a dilemma is epitomized by infections caused by the herpes family of viruses. Although CMV, one of the herpes viruses, may be shed asymptomatically in urine and saliva from immunocompetent hosts, its presence in peripheral blood from cancer patients may implicate it as a pathogen, especially in symptomatic patients. We are using the Digene Hybrid Capture CMV 1 version 2 signal amplification assay to detect the presence of viral DNA in peripheral blood samples from stem cell transplant patients. With any positive test result the patient is placed on ganciclovir preemptively until the test returns to negative [14]. This approach saves other patients with no positive test results from receiving prophylactic ganciclovir. Reactivation of latent or dormant agents, such as *Mycobacterium tuberculosis*, *Strongyloides stercoralis*, or deep or systemic fungal pathogens, usually correlates well with symptomatic disease in cancer patients.

Hence the interpretation of culture results of agents capable of causing reactivation syndromes requires clinical correlation between the pathology, infectious diseases, and the bone marrow service, to ascertain their true relevance in immunosuppressed patients.

Automated Identification and Susceptibility Testing Systems

The identification and susceptibility testing of microbes has been miniaturized and automated to a great extent. Final biochemical identification of most microbes follows the metabolic use of sugars and other substrates, and

enzymatic reaction profiles. The original method involved the use of tubes of agar or nutrient broths that contained specific biochemicals or sugar substrates and that were inoculated with a pure culture of the organism and incubated. Growth in these media was determined visually by turbidity in the medium or by the colors produced when reactions occurred between preformed enzymes and substrates in the presence of an indicator [15]. Large numbers of tubes are required for correct identification. Thus "miniaturized" systems became available more than a decade ago. The API strip (Bio-Merieux, Durham, NC) [16] is an example of such a miniaturized system, but such are still labor intensive and not used as the sole method of diagnosis in high-volume laboratories in cancer hospitals.

Miniaturized and automated systems such as the Vitek 2 Automicrobic system (Bio-Merieux, Durham, NC) [17] are available for microbial identification and susceptibility testing. Cards containing lyophilized reagents are commercially available (ID-GNB, AST-GNO4, ID-GPC, AST-GP55). The technologist prepares a suspension of an organism isolated in pure culture, and the system automatically inoculates a card with the suspension, incubates it, and determines growth by spectrophotometry. Absorbance patterns from each well yield a numerical profile that the instrument matches automatically to data stored in its memory banks. Final identification is then made by the instrument as to genus and species, with a percentage probability. The Vitek 2 ID YST card (Bio-Merieux Vitek, Hazelwood, MO) is now available for the identification of medically important yeast and yeastlike organisms. Unfortunately, very fastidious microorganisms still remain unlikely candidates for automated identification and testing.

Antifungal and Antiviral Susceptibility Testing

Antifungal susceptibility testing can predict outcome in several clinical situations, especially in immunocompromised patients. Susceptibility testing is most helpful in infections caused by non-*albicans* species of *Candida*. The susceptibility testing of azoles is increasingly important in the management of Candidiasis in critically ill patients. Despite the establishment of standardized methods and interpretive breakpoints for several antifungal agents used for yeast pharmacotherapy, antifungal susceptibility testing is not routinely performed in low-volume laboratories, owing to the difficulty in maintaining proficiency and the labor intensiveness of home-brewed assays. At the University of South Florida's H. Lee Moffitt Cancer Center we are evaluating Sensititre YeastOne (Trek Diagnostic Systems, Inc., Westlake, Ohio), a broth microdilution antifungal susceptibility testing method. This method identifies the susceptibility of *Candida* spp. to fluconazole, itraconazole, and 5-flucytosine. Susceptibility testing for filamentous fungi is still not widely available.

Studies are ongoing to evaluate the in-vivo correlation with the in-vitro data for molds.

Immunocompromised patients with viral infections can develop resistance to antiviral drugs. Two methods are used for the determination of antiviral resistance: phenotypic and genotypic. Phenotypic assays measure the direct effect of antiviral drugs on the replication of the total virus population in a clinical sample. Prototypic phenotypic assays like the plaque reduction assay require several weeks for subpassage of a viral strain to get adequate results and are labor intensive. Genotypic assays are designed to determine changes in the nucleotide sequence of a test strain of virus, known to cause drug resistance, and to compare with the wild-type reference strain of the virus. These changes may be single-point mutations (insertions, deletions, or substitutions) or multiple mutations. Commercial systems are being developed to identify the nucleotide sequence changes responsible for antiviral resistance.

Role of Molecular Techniques for Microbial Identification

The areas of clinical microbiology and clinical virology within the field of diagnostic pathology were the first to be strongly influenced by the use of DNA probes and amplification techniques. Prior to the development of amplification techniques, such as PCR, DNA probes were prepared either in-house or commercially and were used directly on clinical specimens for microbial detection. However, laboratory studies showed that if the number of target molecules in a clinical sample is low, the sensitivity of either in-house or commercially available nucleic acid probes may be unacceptably low [18]. The sensitivty of both in-house and commercially available probes increased remarkably when used after an amplification step. Amplification of intact microbes via culture has been used in microbiology laboratories for a long time. Unfortunately, culture amplification may still entail a lengthy period of time, such as several weeks, as in *Mycobacterium tuberculosis* (MTB), which may not be practical. However, if the amplified "entity" is a submicrobial clinical molecule such as DNA or RNA, then PCR and other non-PCR amplification techniques may produce rapid amplification of target. Selected clinical scenarios exist in infectious diseases, especially in immunocompromised patients, where the use of PCR and other amplification techniques is advantageous [19] (Table 1) [20].

A great number of microbiology and virology laboratories perform amplification techniques for various targets, and the FDA has approved various molecular amplification techniques for use in the diagnosis of infectious diseases. Several commercial companies have developed PCR and non-PCR amplification systems and are offering the technology in kit form. Such kits

TABLE 1   Clinical Scenarios in Infectious Diseases in Which the Use of PCR and Other Amplification Techniques may be Advantageous

Clinical scenario	Example(s)
Detection of slow-growing organisms	*Mycobacterium tuberculosis*, agents of deep mycoses
Detection of organisms that are highly infectious or dangerous to culture	HIV, *Coxiella burnetii*, *Coccidiodes immitis*
Detection of agents involved in encephalitis where a rapid and sensitive diagnosis may obviate obtaining a brain biopsy	Herpes simplex virus, enterovirus
Detection of microbes for which routine, commercially available culture methods are lacking in diagnostic laboratories	*Treponema pallidum*, 37°C phase of *Coccidioides immitis*, *Toxaplasa gondii*, *Pneumocystis carinii*
Detection in asymptomatic newborns where serology may be misleading	Congenital HIV infection
Detection of viruses in invasive specimens (CSF, peripheral blood, bone marrow aspirates, etc.) from patients undergoing bone marrow or solid organ transplantation where greater sensitivity is advantageous	Parvovirus, enterovirus, or CMV
Determination of the load of virus or other pathogen for prognostic purposes or for monitoring therapeutic drug effectiveness	HIV quantitation
Determination of the level of expression (i.e., transcription) of a pathogen's DNA by direct measurement of RNA	RT-PCR for CMV, HSV
Detection of antimicrobial resistance genes by amplification of sequences known to mediate such resistance	Isoniazid resistance in *M. tuberculosis*
Reclassification of previously uncultured organisms into the correct position in their genealogical tree	Sequencing of amplified 16s rRNA by RT-PCR or 16s rDNA targets by PCR
Determination of the safety or infectivity of blood products	Presence of HIV or HTLV I/II in blood products

Source: Adapted from R. L. Sandin. Molecular biology of Infectious Diseases, in Clinical Laboratory Medicine. 2d ed. Philadelphia, PA: Lippincott Williams and Wilkins, 2002, p. 187.

TABLE 2 Selective List of FDA-Approved Assays in Infectious Diseases Utilizing Molecular Amplification Techniques

---

Roche Molecular Systems
  (A) HIV-1
     Amplicor HIV-1 Monitor 1.0, 400 copies detection limit, microwell plate, format (MWP)
     Amplicor HIV-1 Monitor 1.0, ultrasensitive, 50 copies detection limit, MWP
     Amplicor HIV-1 Monitor 1.5, 50 copies/mL detection limit, with expanded subtype
       detection capability (Detect Group M subtypes A–G of virus, MWP)
  (B) *Mycobacterium*
     Amplicor *Mycobacterium tuberculosis*, MWP
  (C) *Chlamydia trachomatis*
     Amplicor *C. trachomatis*, MWP format
     COBAS automated system for *C. trachomatis*
Gen-Probe Transcription-Mediated Amplification Systems (TMAs)
  (A) *Mycobacterium*
     AMTDT-1 (Amplified *M. tuberculosis* Direct Test, version 1)
     AMTDT-2 (enhanced AMTDT or E-MTD)
  (B) *Chlamydia trachomatis/Neisseria gonorrhoeae*
     Amplified *C. trachomatis* Direct Test
     APTIMA Combo 2 assay for detection of rRNA of *C. trachomatis* and *N. gonorrhoeae*
  (C) HIV-1/HCV
     Multiplex amplification of HIV-1 and hepatitis C, for blood bank use only
Digene Diagnostics Hybrid Capture Systems
  (A) Human Cytomegalovirus
     CMV Hybrid Capture 1 (tube format), version 1-5,000 copies/mL of whole blood
      detection limit qualitative
     CMV Hybrid Capture 1 version 2-700 copies/mL of whole blood detection limit,
      qualitative
  (B) Human Papillomavirus
     HPV Hybrid Capture I (tube format)
     HPV Hybrid Capture II (MWP)
Abbott Corporation (Ligase Chain Reaction or LCx) Systems
  (A) *Chlamydia trachomatis*
     LCx *C. trachomatis*, male and female urine and genital swabs
  (B) *Neisseria gonorrhoeae*
     LCx *N. gonorrhoeae*, male and female urine and genital swabs
BioMerieux, Inc.
  (A) HIV-1
     Nuclisens HIV-1 QT, for quantitation of HIV-1, NASBA
     Visible Genetics, Inc.
  (A) HIV-1
     Trugene HIV-1 Genotyping kit and open gene DNA sequencing system

---

Abbreviations: FDA, Food and Drug Administration; HIV, human immunodeficiency virus; MWP, microwell plate.
Source: Adapted from R. L. Sandin. Molecular biology of Infectious Diseases, in Clinical Laboratory Medicine. 2d ed. Philadelphia, PA: Lippincott Williams and Wilkins, 2002, p. 188.

are in various stages of development: the R&D stage, undergoing clinical trials, approved for investigational use only, or fully approved by the FDA for use with clinical specimens. Table 2 [21] summarizes some of these kits. Diagnostic microbiology methods are presently being supplemented by these new molecular techniques, but in the future, it is likely that more molecular tests will become standard in large hospital microbiology laboratories that cater to the needs of cancer patient populations.

REFERENCES

1. Ryan MR, Murray PR. Historical evaluation of automated blood culture systems. Clinical Microbiology Newsletters 1993; 15:105–108.
2. Hardy DJ, Hulbert BB, Mignefeault PC. Time to detection of positive BacT/Alert blood cultures and lack of need for routine subculture of 5- to 7-day negative cultures. J Clin Microbiol 1992; 30:2743–2745.
3. Wilson ML, Weinstein MP, Reimer LG. Controlled comparison of the Bact/Alert and BACTEC 660/730 nonradiometric blood culture systems. J Clin Microbiol 1992; 30:323–329.
4. Ruge D, Valdes R, Sandin RL. Clinical Comparison of the Bact/Alert, Bactec 660 and the Isolator Blood Culture Systems for the Isolation of Fungi. Washington, D.C.: American Society for Microbiology, 1995:5.
5. Isenberg H. Clinical Microbiology Procedures Handbook. Washington, D.C.: American Society for Microbiology, 1992.
6. Light Diagnostics "*Pneumocystis Carinii* DFA" kit package insert, June 2001. Chemicon International, Temecula, CA. For questions or problems call Technical Services at 1-800-437-7500 for assistance.
7. American Association of Blood Banks Technical Manual. 13th ed. 1999:623–624.
8. Alvarez M, Ponga BL, Rayon C. Nosocomial outbreak caused by Scedosporium prolificans (inflatum): four fatal causes in leukemic patients. J Clin Microbiol 1995; 33:3290–3295.
9. Fakih MG, Barden GE, Oakes CA, Berenson CS. First reported case of Aspergillus granulosus infection in a cardiac transplant patient. J Clin Microbiol 1995; 33:471–473.
10. Leigheb G, Mossini A, Boggio P. Sporotrichosis-like lesions caused by a Paecilomyces genus fungus. Int J Dermatol 1994; 33:275–276.
11. Brown MA, Greene JN, Sandin RL. Clinical manifestations of filamentous fungi in neutropenic patients. Fifth Annual Meeting of SHEA (Soc. Hosp. Epidemiol. Amer.), April 2–4, 1995, San Diego, CA. Infect Control Hosp Epidemiol 1995; M54:42.
12. Brown M, Green JN, Sandin RL, Laszlo DS. Cutaneous manifestations of filamentous fungi. Clin Infect Dis 1995; 21:777.
13. Gompf S, Paredes A, Quilitz R, Greene JN, Hiemenz JW, Sandin RL.

Paecilomyces lilacinus osteomyelitis in a bone marrow transplant patient. Infect In Med 1999; 16:766–770.

14. Crowder L, Ruge D, Johnson J, Greene JN, Goldstein S, Field T, Sandin RL. Use of the Digene Hybrid Capture CMV Signal Amplification Assay ver. 2.0 (HC) in a Cancer Hospital Helps Modify Gasciclovir Use for Cytomegalo-virus from a Prophylactic to a Pre-emptive Approach [abstr C-138]. Abstract Book of the Annual Meeting of the American Society for Microbiol. P. 180. Session 126/C.

15. Hollis DG, Sottnek FD, Brown WJ, Weaver RE. Use of the rapid fermentation test in determining carbohydrate reactions of fastidious bacteria in clinical laboratories. J Clin Microbiol 1980; 12:620–623.

16. Otto LA, Pickett MJ. Rapid methods for identification of gram-negative non-fermentative bacilli. J Clin Microbiol 1976; 3:566–575.

17. Ryan C. Cost reductions and QC software on a microbiology identification and susceptibility system. American Clinical laboratory 1988; 14:295.

18. Enns RK. DNA probes: an overview and comparison with current methods. Lab Med 1988; 19:295.

19. Sandin RL, Rinaldi M. Special considerations for the clinical microbiology laboratory in the diagnosis of infections in the cancer patient. Infect Dis Clin NA 1996; 10:413.

20. Adapted from R.L. Sandin. Molecular biology of infectious diseases. In: Clinical Laboratory Medicine. 2d ed. Philadelphia, PA: Lippincott Williams and Wilkins, 2002:187.

21. Adapted from R.L. Sandin. Molecular biology of infectious diseases. In: Clinical Laboratory Medicine. 2d ed. Philadelphia, PA: Lippincott Williams and Wilkins, 2002:188.

Index

Acanthamoeba, 455, 463
Acinetobacter, 19, 51, 55, 117, 155, 166
Acute lymphoblastic leukemia (ALL),
   23–45
  bacterial infections, 26–28
  epidemiology, 24
  fungal infections, 30–32
  granulocyte transfusions, 35–36
  hematopoetic growth factors, 34–35
  history, 23–45
  immunity and infection, 24–26
  prophylaxis of infection, 32–43
  protozoal infections, 32
  viral infections, 28–30
Acute myelogenous leukemia (AML),
   47–64
  antimicrobial prophylaxis, 60
  bacterial infections, 50–56
  compared to acute lymphoblastic
   leukemia, 24
  empirical therapy, 57–59
  epidemiology, 47–50, 60

[Acute myelogenous leukemia (AML)]
  fungal infections, 51, 56
  high neutropenic risk, 48–49, 56
  immunity and infections, 49–50, 52
  pathogen-specific therapy, 59–60
  viral infections, 51–52
Adenovirus, 19–20
  hemorrhagic cystitis, 20, 157, 159
  latent/reactivation, 19–20
  neutropenia, 19
  pneumonia, 156
Aeromonas hydrophila, cutaneous
   infections, 346–347
AIDS, 471–474
Air filtration, high-efficency particulate
   air (HEPA), 19, 425
Alcaligenes, 19, 56, 117, 155
ALL (*See* Acute lymphoblastic
   leukemia)
Allogeneic stem cell transplant (*See*
   Hematopoietic stem cell
   transplantation [HSCT])

AML (*See* Acute myelogenous leukemia [AML])
Amphotericin B, 59, 432–434, 435–440, 483–485
  lipid formulations, 59, 432–434, 436–439
  stem cell transplant, 155
Anaerobic infection, acute myelogenous leukemia, 56
Antibiotic lock therapy (ALT), 389–390, 397
Antibiotics, history of prior exposure to, 18
Antigen presenting cells (APCs), 11
Antimicrobial
  effect on gastrointestinal flora, 18
  infection due to exposure, 18
  multi-drug resistant pathogens, emergence of, 18–19
  prophylaxis, 18
  treatment, 19
Ascaris lumbricoides, 460
Aspergillus, 19–20, 67, 78, 93, 277, 286, 419–422, 424, 427–431,438–441, 482–485, 516
  acute lymphoblastic leukemia, 30–31
  acute myelogenous leukemia, 57
  contact with, 19
  cutaneous manifestation, 353–354
  Hodgkin's disease, 146–147
  latent/reactivation, 20
  lung cancer, 194–195
  multiple myeloma, 118
  non-Hodgkin's lymphoma, 137
  stem cell transplant, 153, 154, 158–159
Autologous stem cell transplant (See Hematopoietic stem cell transplantation [HSCT])

Bacillus, 19, 28, 158
  acute myelogenous leukemia, 55
  cutaneous manifestation, 348

Bacteremia, 17, 20
  brain tumor patients, 172
BCG (Bacillus Calmette-Guérin), 334, 504
  infectious complications, 241–242
Biliary tract, 6
BK virus, 19–20
  hemorrhagic cystitis, 20, 157, 159
  latent/reactivation in neutropenia, 19–20
Bladder
  mucosal injury, 5
  obstruction, 5
  risk of bacterial contamination, 5
  urinary catheters, 5
Bladder conduit infections, 333
Blastocystis, 453, 462
Blastomycosis, 20, 67, 158
  cutaneous manifestation, 357–358
Blood culture, 510–512
BMT (*See* Bone marrow transplantation [BMT])
Bone culture, 514
Bone marrow culture (stem cell culture), 514–515
Bone marrow failure, 9
  aplastic anemia, 9
  myelodysplasia, 9
  neutropenia, 9
Bone marrow transplantation (BMT)
  acute myelogenous leukemia, 80
  chronic myelogenous leukemia, 93
Brain abscess, 286–287
  brain tumor patients, 172–173
Broad-spectrum antibiotics, 6, 57
  acute lymphoblastic leukemia, 57
  effect on bacterial flora, 6
  pathogen overgrowth, 6
Bronchiolitis obliterans, 297
Bronchiolitis obliterans with organizing pneumonia (BOOP), 297, 369
  stem cell transplant, 158
Bronchoscopy, 300–301

Cancidas (caspofungin), 59, 155,
    435–440
Candida, 67, 78, 93, 118, 137, 286,
    419–421, 424, 426–427, 429,
    435–438, 440–441, 482–484, 516
  acute lymphoblastic leukemia,
    30–31
  acute myelogenous leukemia, 57
  catheter-related infection, 393–394
  chronic disseminated, 420, 426, 437
  cutaneous manifestation, 276,
    352–353
  esophagitis, 436
  Hodgkin's disease, 146
  non-*albicans*, 18–20, 420–422
  pneumonia, 427
  stem cell transplant, 153, 154
Candida albicans, 420–422
  risk of candidemia, 18–19
Candida tropicalis, neutropenia, 19
Candidemia, 426, 436
  Candida tropicalis, 19
  neutropenia, 19
Candiduria, 427, 436
Capillaria philippinensis, 462
Capnocytophaga ochracea, 19, 153, 346
Caspofungin, 59, 155, 435–440
Catheter-related infections, 379
  bloodstream, 379
  exit site, 390
  port pocket, 390
  tunnel, 390, 396–397
Cell-mediated immunity, 10–11
  chronic lymphocytic leukemia, 75
  chronic myelogenous leukemia, 90
Cellulitis
  breast cancer, 205–209
  recurrent, 255–260
  sarcoma, 266–268
Central venous catheter (CVC), 7,
    20, 24, 66
  antibiotic-coated, 397–399
  risk of infection, 7
  stem cell transplant, 151, 157–158
Cestodes, 458–459

Chemoembolization
  infectious complications, 230,
    236
Chemotherapy
  complications, 4
  fever induced by, 9
  mucosa damage, 4
Chemotherapy-induced infections
    (*See* also Neutropenia)
  acute lymphoblastic leukemia, 23
  acute myelogenous leukemia, 47
  chronic lymphocytic leukemia, 75,
    77–78
Cholangitis, 6, 229, 315–316
Cholecystitis, 6
Cholangiocarcinoma, infectious
    complications of, 231
Chronic lymphocytic leukemia (CLL),
    73–86
  antibody response, 81
  bacterial infections, 74–81
  chemotherapy induced infections,
    77–78
  epidemiology, 73–74
  fungal infections, 74
  immunity and infection, 74–76
  immunization/vaccination, 81
  pathogenesis, 74–78
  prophylaxis of infections, 80
  viral infections, 76
Chronic myelogenous leukemia
    (CML), 87–98
  bacterial infections, 92
  bone marrow transplantation, 93
  epidemiology, 87–91
  fungal infections, 93
  immunity and infection, 89–92
  prophylaxis of infections, 92–94
  viral infections, 92
Chronic obstructive pulmonary
    disease (COPD) infections,
    188
Citrobacter, 19, 55, 117, 154
CLL (*See* Chronic lymphocytic
    leukemia)

Clostridia, 56
  cutaneous manifestation, 348–349
  neutropenia, 19
Clostridium difficile, 56, 154, 254, 255,
  319–322
Clostridium perfringens, 15, 49
Clostridium septicum, 4, 17, 27, 49, 325
  acute myelogenous leukemia patients
    at high risk, 49
  colon cancer, 219–220
  stem cell transplant, 153
CML (*See* Chronic myelogenous
  leukemia)
CMV (*See* Cytomegalovirus)
Coagulase-negative *Staphylococci*,
  17–18
Coccidioidomycosis, 67
  cutaneous manifestation, 358–359
  stem cell transplant, 158
Colitis, 254–255
Colonization, 15–18
Corticosteroids
  acute myelogenous leukemia, 49
  chronic lymphocytic leukemia, 76–77
  GVHD, 20
Corynebacteria, 18–19
Corynebacteria jeikeium, 28, 55
  cutaneous manifestation, 349
Cryptococcus, 20, 67, 131, 277, 286, 423,
  429, 440–441
  cutaneous manifestation, 276,
    356–357
  Hodgkin's disease, 146–147
Cryptosporidia, 453–454, 462–463
Curvularia, 423
CVC (*See* Central venous catheter)
Cyclospora, 453–454
Cystitis, pathophysiology of, 5
Cytomegalovirus (CMV), 19–20,
  92–93, 118, 277, 486, 500, 504
  acute lymphoblastic leukemia, 29
  cutaneous manifestation, 361
  gastroenteritis, 322–324
  latent/reactivation, 19
  neutropenia, 19

[Cytomegalovirus (CMV)]
  pneumonia, 294–295
  prophylaxis, 20
  non-Hodgkin's lymphoma, 137
  stem cell transplant, 153, 155–157,
    159

Decubitus ulcer, in brain tumor
  patients, 170–171
Demodex folliculorum, 460–461
Dientamoeba, 453
Diffuse alvealer hemorrhage (DAH),
  296–297
  stem cell transplant, 158
Digestive tract, 15–17

E. coli, 16, 19, 154, 231, 252, 478, 482
  acute lymphoblastic leukemia, 23
  acute myelogenous leukemia, 49–50,
    55
  gastrointestional tract, 16
  multiple myeloma, 115–116
  neutropenia, 19
Ectoparasites, 460
Empyema, lung cancer resection, 189
Endocarditis
  acute leukemia, 49
  Aspergillus, 309
  Candida, 309, 310
  native valve, 307–308
  prosthetic valve, 308
  Staphylococcus aureus, 308
  Staphylococcus, coagulase-negative,
    309
  Streptococci viridans, 308
  Streptococcus bovis, 308–309
Endogenous flora, neutropenia, 17,18
Endotracheal intubation, risk of
  infection, 6–7
Engraftment
  exogenous infection, 19
  infection prevention, 18–20
Entamoeba, 453, 462–463
Enterobacter, 19, 55, 117, 154
Enterobacteriaceae, 4, 19, 231, 252

Enterococci, 16, 19, 54, 117, 154
  vancomycin-resistant, 27, 54–55, 117
Enterocolitis, neutropenic, 4–5, 27, 49, 154, 324–327
Enterocytozoan, 454–455
Epstein-Barr virus (EBV), 472
  nasopharyngeal carcinoma, 177, 181
Escherichia (*See E. coli*)
Esophagitis, and radiation, 191, 222, 318

Febrile (*See* Fever)
Febrile neutropenia (*See* Neutropenia)
Fever
  acute myelogenous leukemia, 49
  bacteremia, 9
  chemotherapy-induced, 9
  infection, 9
Fistula, 370
  postsurgical, 243
Fluconazole, 18, 59, 431–434, 435–437, 483
  stem cell transplant, 154
Fludarabine, 75–80
  chronic lymphocytic leukemia, 78–80
  non-Hodgkin's lymphoma, 129, 131
Fluoroquinolones, prophylaxis, 18, 24, 33, 60, 481–482
Fungal infections, 15–20
  fluconazole, effect of, 18
  prophylactic agents, 18
Fungi
  air filtration, 19
  sinopulmonary infections, 19
Fusarium, 19, 20, 57, 155, 286, 421–423, 425, 428
  cutaneous manifestation, 354–355
Fusobacterium, 19, 153, 166, 179

Gangrene
  gynecological malignancy, 252
  Meleney's, 253
  synergistic bacterial, 253

Gastrointestinal (GI) tract
  adverse effects on endogenous flora, 15–18
  antimicrobial effects, 18
  coagulase-negative *Staphylococcus,* 18
  engraftment, 20
  Enterobacter, 16
  gram-negative bacteria, 16
  infections, 16–20
  neutropenia, 16
  nosocomial infections, 15, 18
  Pseudomonas aeruginosa, 16
  Viridans streptococci, 18
Genitourinary tract
  colonization, 17
  gram-negative bacteria, 17
  group B *Streptococci,* 17
  infections, 17
  Lactobacillus, 17
GI (*See* Gastrointestinal tract)
Giardia, 452, 454, 462–463
GNB (*See* Gram-negative bacteria [GNB])
Graft-versus-host disease (GVHD), 93, 107, 153, 155, 158, 425, 500, 502, 504–505
  changes in skin structure, 3
  diarrhea, 322
Gram-negative bacteria (GNB)
  acute lymphoblastic leukemia, 24
  acute myelogenous leukemia, 55–56
  epidemiology, 15–20
  hairy cell leukemia, 66
  hospitalization, 23
  multidrug-resistant (MDR), 19
  stem cell transplant, 152
Gram-positive bacteria
  acute lymphoblastic leukemia, 24
  acute myelogenous leukemia, 52–55
  hairy cell leukemia, 66
  infections, 7, 15–20
  stem cell transplant, 152
Gram stain, 511

Granulocyte colony stimulating factor
(GCSF), 434–435, 487–488
    acute lymphoblastic leukemia, 34–35
    non-Hodgkin's lymphoma, 135–136
Granulocyte monocyte colony
    stimulating factor (GM-CSF),
    434–435, 487–488
    acute lymphoblastic leukemia, 34–35
    non-Hodgkin's lymphoma, 136
Granulocyte transfusions
    acute lymphoblastic leukemia,
    35–36
    treatment and complications, 10
Granulocytes, in functional defect in
    hairy cell leukemia patients, 66
Granulocytopenia (*See* Neutropenia)
Granulomatous disease, hairy cell
    leukemia, 68
GVHD (*See* Graft-versus-host disease
    [GVHD])

HHV-6 pneumonia, 295
Hairy cell leukemia (HCL), 65–72
    bacterial infections, 66
    diagnostic problems in infection
    management, 68
    epidemiology, 65–66, 69
    fungal infections, 67
    immunity and infection, 65–66
    mycobacterial infections, 67
    prophylaxis of infection, 68
    viral infections, 67
HCL (*See* Hairy cell leukemia)
Hematopoietic stem cell
    transplantation (HSCT), 3, 19–20,
    151, 500–512
    chronic myelogenous leukemia,
    93–94
    graft-versus-host disease, 20
    multiple myeloma, 107, 113, 118
Hemophilus influenzae, 7, 165, 178, 284,
    498, 500, 502, 505
    Hodgkin's disease, 147
    multiple myeloma, 113
    stem cell transplant, 151

Hemorrhagic cystitis, 157, 333
    BK virus, 19,
    adenovirus, 157
HEPA (high-efficiency particulate air
    filtration), 19, 425
Hepatitis B virus, 501, 503
Hepatocellular carcinoma, 227–231
Herpes simplex virus (HSV), 4, 118,
    274, 276, 485–486
    acute lymphoblastic leukemia,
    28–29
    acyclovir-resistant, 156–157
    drug resistance, 4
    following HSCT, 4
    latent/reactivation, 4, 19–20
    mucocutaneous, 360
    neutropenia, 18–20
    non-Hodgkin's lymphoma, 132,
    135
    prophylaxis, 4
    stem cell transplant, 153, 155
Herpes zoster virus (HZV) (*See also*
    Varicella zoster virus [VZV])
    cutaneous manifestation, 276, 357
Histoplasmosis, 20, 67,
    cutaneous manifestation, 276, 357
    Hodgkin's disease, 147
    stem cell transplant, 158
HIV, 471–474
Hodgkin's disease, 145
Hospitalization, 23
    nosocomial infections, 6–7, 15–18
    patient's risk of infection while in
    ICU, 18
Host defenses, 1–12, 15
HSCT (*See* Hematopoietic stem cell
    transplantation [HSCT])
HSV (*See* Herpes simplex virus)
Human herpes virus-6 (HHV-6)
    acute lymphoblastic leukemia, 29
    stem cell transplant, 155, 157, 159
Human herpes virus-8 (HHV-8),
    472–473
    multiple myeloma, 104–105, 120
· Human papillomavirus (HPV), 472

Humoral immunity, 10–11
Hymenolepsis nana, 458–459
Hyperbaric oxygen, 370
Hypogammaglobulinemia
  chronic lymphocytic leukemia, 74
  multiple myeloma, 109

ICU (*See* Intensive care unit)
Immunization, 497–500
  chronic lymphocytic leukemia, 81
Immunocompromised host, 2
Immunodeficiency
  cell-mediated, 10–12, 66, 75, 505
  graft-versus-host disease, 20
  humoral, 10–11, 109–110, 505
Immunoglobulin, intravenous
  chronic lymphocytic leukemia, 81
  multiple myeloma, 119
Infections, 15–20
  basal cell carcinoma (BCC), 275
  complications, 6
  cutaneous malignancy, 271–278
  cutaneous T-cell lymphoma (CTCL),
    276, 277
  engraftment, 20
  ICU, patient risk, 6–7
  implants and tissue expanders,
    212–215
  malignant melanoma, 275–276
  squamous cell carcinoma (SCC),
    275
Influenza, 20, 498, 501–503
Intensive care unit (ICU)
  central venous catheter, 7
  endotracheal intubation, 6
  infectious complications, risk of, 6
  mechanical ventilation, 7
Intra-abdominal abscess, 254
Intravascular devices (*See* Central
    venous catheter)
Intravenous immunoglobulin (IVIG)
    (*See* Immunoglobulin,
    intravenous)
Intubation, 6–7
Isospora, 453–454

Itraconazole, 59, 431–434, 435–439,
    483–485
IVIG (*See* Immunoglobulin,
    intravenous)

Kaposi's sarcoma, 472–473
Klebsiella, 19, 50, 55, 115–116, 154, 166,
    231, 478
Kostmann's syndrome, 9

Lactobacillus, 55, 154, 255
  vaginal colonization, 17
Legionella, 78, 513
  hairy cell leukemia, 67
  lung cancer, 193–194
  pneumonia, 294
  stem cell transplant, 158
Leishmania, 458, 463
Leuconostoc, 19, 55, 154
Listeria monocytogenes, 27, 67, 78–80,
    286
Lung abscess, 295–296
Lung biopsy, 301
Lymphedema, 17, 207

MDS (*See* Myelodysplastic syndrome
    [MDS])
Macrophages, 11
Malassezia, 57, 422
  catheter-related infection, 394–395
  cutaneous manifestation, 359–360
Measles, 498, 501, 504
Mechanical ventilation
  in ICU, 7
  oropharyngial colonization, 16
  pneumonia, 7, 16
Meningitis, 284–286
  acute leukemia, 49
  aseptic, 285
  chemical, 285
  neurosurgical, 284–286
  postoperative, 284–286
Microbial flora, 15–20
Microsporidia, 453–455
Molds (*See* Fungi)

Monocytopenia, in hairy cell leukemia, 66
Moraxella catarrhalis, 178
MRSA (*See Staphylococcus aureus*, methicillin-resistant)
Mucormycosis (*See* Zygomycosis)
Mucosites, 4, 18, 24, 66, 179
　anaerobic, 316–318
　Candida, 317
　herpes simplex virus, 317
　stem cell transplant, 152, 153
Mucous membrane
　immunity, 76
　inhibitory agents, 3
　protective barrier, 3
　stem cell transplantation, 3
Multidrug resistance (MDR), and gram-negative bacterial infection, 18–20
Multiple myeloma (MM)
　B cell, 109–110
　cell-mediated, 110
　human herpes virus-8 (HHV-8), 104–105
　infection risk, 112
　immune defects, 109
　neutropenia, 111
Mycobacterium bovis, 241
Mycobacterium non-tuberculosis, 20, 67, 80, 92, 275, 286
　breast cancer, implants, 214
　catheter-related infection, 391, 395
　COPD, 188, 194
　cutaneous manifestation, 350–352
　hairy cell leukemia, 67
　Hodgkin's disease, 146
　lung cancer, 194
　non-Hodgkin's lymphoma, 138
　pneumonia, 292–293
　stem cell transplant, 158
Mycobacterium tuberculosis, 20, 516, 518
　cutaneous manifestation, 349–350
　hairy cell leukemia, 67
Mycoplasma, 67, 290

Myelodysplastic syndrome (MDS), 99–102
　bacterial infections, 100–101
　epidemiology, 99
　fungal infections, 100–101
　immunity and infection, 100
　infectious complications, 9, 100–101
　pancytopenia, 99
　viral infections, 101

Natural immune deficiency, 8
　aplastic anemia, 8
　hematological malignancies, 8
　inherited neutropenic states, 8
Necrotizing fasciitis, 254, 341
Neisseria gonorrhoeae, 5
Nematodes, 459–460
Neuroendocrine tumor
　infectious complications, 235–237
Neutropenia, 505
　acute lymphoblastic leukemia, 24
　acute myelogenous leukemia, 47–64
　bacteremia, 18
　causes of, 9
　chemotherapy induced, 9, 24, 47, 65, 75
　chronic lymphocytic leukemia, 65, 81
　cyclic, 9
　drug therapy, 9
　empiric therapy, 432–435
　endogenous flora, 17, 18
　engraftment, 19
　febrile, 9, 18
　functional deficiency, 9
　GI tract infections, 18
　hairy cell leukemia, 65, 66
　Hodgkin's, 146, 148
　idiosyncratic host reaction, 9
　increased risk for infection, 9
　Kostmann's syndrome, 9
　multiple myeloma, 111
　prophylaxis, 431–434
　resolution of, 20

[Neutropenia]
  toxicity grades, 130
  translocation of enteric flora, 65
  treatment of, 18–20
Neutrophil, 7–9
Nocardia, 20, 78, 80, 286, 513
  cutaneous manifestation, 352
  Hodgkin's disease, 146
  pneumonia, 293
  non-Hodgkin's lymphoma, 128,
    133–135
  stem cell transplant, 152, 154, 155
Non-Hodgkin's lymphoma, 127,
  471–473
  indolent, 129
  intermediate, 133
  high grade, 133
Nosocomial infections
  engraftment, 19
  GI flora, 18
  gram-positive bacteria, 7, 23
  intensive care unit, 18
  mechanical ventilator, 6–7
  Pseudomonas aeruginosa, 7
  risk, 15

Oropharynx, 15–16, 18
  Coagulase-negative *Staphylococcus*,
    18
  colonization by GNB, 15–16
  pneumonia, 16
  Viridans streptococci, 18
Osteomyelitis, 369
  basilar skull, 180
  mandibular, 179–180
  sternum, 339
  symphysis pubis, 338
  vertebral, 338
Osteonecrosis, 369–370
  mandible, 339
Osteoradionecrosis (*See* Osteonecrosis)

Paecilomyces, 20, 155
Pancytopenia, in myelodysplastic
  syndrome (MDS), 99

Parainfluenza, 20
Parasites, 451–463
Parotitis, 179
Parvovirus B 19, acute lymphoblastic
  leukemia, 29–30
Pathogens
  latent/reactivation, 19
  multidrug-resistant, 18–20
PCR (polymerase chain reaction), 302,
  518–520
Pediococcus, 19, 154
Perianal infections, prevention and
  treatment, 4–5
Peritonitis, 254, 314–315
Phagocytic cell defects in chronic
  lymphocytic leukemia, 75–76
Plasmodium, 456–457
Pneumocystis carinii, 167–168, 277, 294,
  487, 503, 504, 513
  acute lymphoblastic leukemia, 32
  brain tumor, 167–168
  chronic lymphocytic leukemia,
    78–81
  hairy cell leukemia, 67
  Hodgkin's disease, 146
  non-Hodgkin's lymphoma, 131, 135
  stem cell transplant, 158–159
Pneumonia, 6–7, 16, 20
  aspiration, 166–167, 181
  brain tumor patients, 164–165
  cellular immune defect, 292, 293
  CMV, 294–295
  community acquired, 113–114, 290
  HHV-6, 295
  humoral immune defect, 295
  idiopathic, 297
  Legionella, 295–296
  necrotizing, 189, 297
  neutropenia, 291–292
  nosocomial, 6–7, 115, 290
  viral, 294–295
  Pneumocystis carinii, 167–168, 294
  postobstructive, 189
  postoperative, 190
  stem cell transplant, 158–159

[*Pneumocystis carinii*]
  varicella, 295
  ventilator-associated neurosurgical
    patient, 165–166
Pneumonitis
  drug-induced, 296
  radiation, 190, 191, 297, 369
Prophylaxis, 18, 431–434, 478–479,
    480–488
  acute lymphoblastic leukemia, 32–34
  acute myelogenous leukemia, 60
  multiple myeloma, 118
Pseudallescheria (*See Scedosporium*)
Pseudomonas aeruginosa, 4, 78,
    115–116, 178, 231, 252, 275, 277,
    478, 481
  acute lymphoblastic leukemia, 27
  acute myelogenous leukemia, 49–51,
    55–56
  catheter-related infections, 386–395
  cutaneous infection, 346
  hairy cell leukemia, 66
  neutropenia, 6, 7, 16, 19
  stem cell transplant, 152, 154
Pyelonephritis, 239, 334
Pyomyositis, 341

Quinolones (*See* Fluoroquinolones)

Radiation-related infections, 367–370
Radiation therapy
  infectious complications of head and
    neck cancer, 182–183
  lung cancer, 190–191
  osteoradionecrosis, 182
Radiofrequency ablation, infectious
    complications of, 236
Renal abscess, 241
Respiratory syncytial virus (RSV), 20
  acute lymphoblastic leukemia, 30
  stem cell transplant, 156–157
Rhizopus (*See* Zygomycosis)
Rhodococcus equi, 28, 55, 67
Rituximab and non-Hodgkin's
  lymphoma, 131

Salmonella, 16, 78, 172, 239
Sarcoptes scabei, 461–462
Sarcocystis, 462
Scabies, 461
Scedosporium, 20, 67, 286, 421, 423,
    428
  acute lymphoblastic leukemia, 32
  stem cell transplant, 155
Septic arthritis, 339–340
  breast cancer, 210
  sternoclavicular, 340
Seroma, 265–266
Serratia, 19, 55, 117, 154, 166
Sinusitis, 178–179
Skin, 2–3
  central venous catheter, 17
  chemotherapy, 17
  hairy cell leukemia, cutaneous
    lesions, 68
  immunocompromised host, 2
  risk of infection, 2–3, 18
  source of infections, 18
Smoking, infections and, 178
Soft-tissue infection in multiple
    myeloma, 116–117
Splenectomy
  chronic lymphocytic leukemia, 76
  Hodgkin's disease, 147
Sporotrichosis, 67
Staphylococcus, 53, 66
Staphylococcus aureus, 17, 66, 117, 165,
    178–179, 237, 241, 255–259, 265,
    267, 276–277, 285, 482
  breast cellulitis, 207, 209
  catheter-related infection, 382–384,
    392–393
  methicillin-resistant, 19, 117,
    178–179, 237, 374
  stem cell transplant, 152
  surgical site infection, 373
Staphylococcus, coagulase-negative,
    52–53, 285
  catheter-related infections, 383–384
  stem cell transplant, 152
Staphylococcus haemolyticum, 19, 53

Stenotrophomonas maltophilia, 19, 28, 51, 55–56, 117
  catheter-related infections, 395
  cutaneous infection, 347
  stem cell transplant, 155
Stent infections, 332–333
Stomatococcus, 28, 55
Streptococci, 16–17 (*See also Streptococci viridans*)
Streptococci group A, cellulitis, 207, 209, 255–259
Streptococci group B
  lymphedema, 17
  vaginal colonization, 17
Streptococci viridans, 53–54, 179
  cutaneous manifestation, 348
  fluoroquinolone administration, 18
  stem cell transplant, 152
Streptococcus bovis
  colon cancer, 219–221
  stomach cancer, 222
Streptococcus pneumoniae, 54, 78, 165, 178, 284, 498–500, 502, 505
  Hodgkin's disease, 147–148
  lung cancer, 192–193
  multiple myeloma, 113–115, 117
  stem cell transplant, 151
Strongyloides stercoralis, 20, 67, 319, 459–460, 462–463, 516
Surgical site infection
  breast cancer, 202–204, 211–212, 375
  colorectal cancer, 376
  cystectomy, 243
  esophageal cancer, 375–376
  gynecological cancer, 376
  head and neck cancer, 181–182, 374–375
  lung cancer, 375–376
  sarcoma, 264–265
  sternal, 210, 211
Surgical wound infection (*See* Surgical site infection)
Susceptibility testing, 517

Taenia solium, 459
Taxanes
  complications/adverse reaction, 4
  T-cell receptor (TCR), 11
Toxocara canis, 460
Toxoplasmosis 20, 67, 277, 286, 455–456, 462–463
Transfusion reaction, 515
Trichinella, 462
Trichomonas, 455
Trichosporin, 57, 421–423, 428
  cutaneous manifestation, 355–356
Trimethoprim/sulfamethoxazole (TMP/SMZ)
  prophylaxis, 33, 60, 480–481, 487
  stem cell transplant, 152
Trypanosoma, 457
Typhlitis (*See* Enterocolitis, neutropenic)

Urinary tract infection (UTI), 5–6, 239, 331–334
  brain tumor patients, 168–170
  gynecological malignancy, 252
  multiple myeloma, 115
Urine
  cause of stagnation, 5
  glycoprotein, 5
  microorganism overgrowth, 5
  urine catheters, 5, 6
UTI (*See* Urinary tract infections)

Vaccination, 499–500
  chronic lymphocytic leukemia, 81
Vaccine
  BCG, 504
  cytomegalovirus, 504
  diphtheria, 503
  Haemophilus influenza type b, 502
  hepatitis B, 503
  influenza, 502–503
  measles, 504
  mumps, 504
  pneumococcal, 502
  polio, 503

[Vaccine]
  rubella, 504
  tetanus toxoid, 503
  Varicella zoster, 503–504
  yellow fever, 504
Vancomycin, 59
  drug resistance to, 19
Varicella zoster virus (VZV), 3, 19–20,
    118, 276, 486, 500–501
  acute lymphoblastic leukemia, 29
  cutaneous manifestation, 361–362
  Hodgkin's disease, 147–148
  immunoglobulin, intravenous, 3
  multiple myeloma, 118
  non-Hodgkin's lymphoma, 132, 135
  pneumonia, 294
  stem cell transplant, 153

Ventilator (*See* Mechanical
    ventilation)
Viral pneumonia, 294–295
Viridans streptococci (*See Streptococci
    viridans*)
Voriconazole, 59, 433–434, 435–439

Wound infections, necrotizing,
    252–253

Xanthogranulomatous pyelonephritis,
    239, 334

Zygomycosis, 20, 57, 286, 421,
    423–424
  cutaneous manifestation, 359
  stem cell transplant, 155, 158–159

Milton Keynes UK
Ingram Content Group UK Ltd.
UKHW020006071024
449327UK00031B/2673